PLASTIC SURGERY

Editor

JOSEPH G. McCARTHY, M.D.

Lawrence D. Bell Professor of Plastic Surgery and
Director of the Institute of Reconstructive Plastic Surgery
New York University Medical Center
New York, New York

Editors, Hand Surgery Volumes

JAMES W. MAY, JR., M.D.

Director of Plastic Surgery and Hand Surgery Service
Massachusetts General Hospital
Associate Clinical Professor of Surgery
Harvard Medical School
Boston, Massachusetts

J. WILLIAM LITTLER, M.D.

Past Professor of Clinical Surgery
College of Physicians and Surgeons
Columbia University, New York
Senior Attending Surgeon
The St. Luke's–Roosevelt Hospital Center
New York, New York

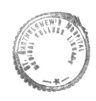

PLASTIC SURGERY

VOLUME 3
THE FACE
Part 2

W.B. SAUNDERS COMPANY

A Division of Harcourt Brace & Company

Philadelphia ▪ London ▪ Toronto
Montreal ▪ Sydney ▪ Tokyo

W.B. SAUNDERS COMPANY
A Division of
Harcourt Brace & Company

The Curtis Center
Independence Square West
Philadelphia, PA 19106

Library of Congress Cataloging-in-Publication Data

Plastic surgery.
   Contents: v. 1. General principles—v. 2–3.
The face—v. 4. Cleft lip & palate and craniofacial
anomalies—[etc.]
   1. Surgery, Plastic.   I. McCarthy, Joseph G., 1938–
[DNLM: 1. Surgery, Plastic. WO 600 P7122]

RD118.P536   1990   617'.95   87–9809

ISBN 0–7216–1514–7   (set)

25/7/94

Editor: W. B. Saunders Staff
Designer: W. B. Saunders Staff
Production Manager: Frank Polizzano
Manuscript Editor: David Harvey
Illustration Coordinator: Lisa Lambert
Indexer: Kathleen Garcia
Cover Designer: Ellen Bodner

Volume 1 0–7216–2542–8
Volume 2 0–7216–2543–6
Volume 3 0–7216–2544–4
Volume 4 0–7216–2545–2
Volume 5 0–7216–2546–0
Volume 6 0–7216–2547–9
Volume 7 0–7216–2548–7
Volume 8 0–7216–2549–5
8 Volume Set 0–7216–1514–7

Plastic Surgery

Last digit is the print number: 9   8   7   6   5   4   3

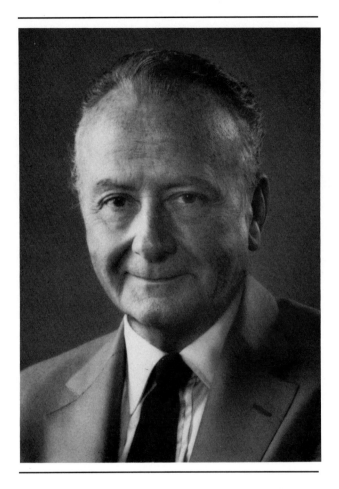

John Marquis Converse
(1909–1981)

This book is dedicated to John Marquis Converse. His enthusiasm for plastic surgery was unrivaled and his contributions to the field were legendary. Through his many writings he not only educated and inspired the plastic surgeon in the era after World War II, but also helped to define modern plastic surgery. This book is a testimony to his professional accomplishments.

Contributors

SHERRELL J. ASTON, M.D.
Associate Professor of Surgery (Plastic Surgery), New York University School of Medicine; Attending Surgeon, University Hospital and Manhattan Eye, Ear & Throat Hospital, New York, New York.

DANIEL C. BAKER, M.D.
Associate Professor of Surgery (Plastic Surgery), New York University School of Medicine; Attending Surgeon, University Hospital, Bellevue Hospital Center, Manhattan Eye, Ear & Throat Hospital, and Manhattan Veterans Administration Hospital, New York, New York.

ALFONSO BARRERA, M.D.
Attending Surgeon, Memorial City Medical Center Hospital and West Houston Medical Center Hospital, Houston, Texas.

FRITZ E. BARTON, JR., M.D.
Professor and Chairman, Division of Plastic Surgery, Department of Surgery, The University of Texas Health Science Center at Dallas; Chief, Plastic Surgery Service, Children's Medical Center; Assistant Chief, Plastic and Reconstructive Surgery Service, Baylor University Medical Center; Attending Surgeon, Parkland Memorial Hospital, Dallas Veterans Administration Hospital, Presbyterian Medical Center, and Gaston Episcopal Hospital, Dallas, Texas.

BURT BRENT, M.D.
Clinical Associate Professor of Plastic Surgery, Stanford University School of Medicine; Clinical Faculty, Stanford University Hospital; Staff Surgeon, El Camino Hospital, Palo Alto, California.

H. STEVE BYRD, M.D.
Associate Professor of Plastic and Reconstructive Surgery, The University of Texas Health Science Center at Dallas; Attending Surgeon, Children's

Medical Center, Baylor University Medical Center, Presbyterian Hospital, and St. Paul Hospital, Dallas, Texas.

THOMAS D. CRONIN, M.D.
Clinical Professor of Plastic Surgery, Baylor College of Medicine; Attending Surgeon, St. Joseph Hospital, Houston, Texas.

JOEL J. FELDMAN, M.D.
Associate in Plastic Surgery, Harvard Medical School; Consultant Plastic Surgeon, Shriners Burns Institute and Massachusetts General Hospital, Boston, Massachusetts; Attending Surgeon, Mount Auburn Hospital, Cambridge, Massachusetts.

JOSEPH G. McCARTHY, M.D.
Lawrence D. Bell Professor of Plastic Surgery, New York University School of Medicine; Director, Institute of Reconstructive Plastic Surgery, New York University Medical Center; Attending Surgeon, University Hospital, Bellevue Hospital, Manhattan Eye, Ear and Throat Hospital, and Veterans Administration Hospital, New York, New York.

KITARO OHMORI, M.D.
Associate Professor of Plastic Surgery, Juntendo University School of Medicine; Director, Department of Plastic and Reconstructive Surgery, Tokyo Metropolitan Police Hospital, Tokyo, Japan.

THOMAS D. REES, M.D.
Clinical Professor of Surgery (Plastic Surgery), New York University School of Medicine; Chairman, Department of Plastic Surgery, Manhattan Eye, Ear & Throat Hospital, New York, New York.

JACK H. SHEEN, M.D.
Associate Clinical Professor of Plastic and Reconstructive Surgery, University of California, Los

Angeles, School of Medicine; Attending Surgeon, UCLA Medical Center, Los Angeles, California.

CHARLES H. M. THORNE, M.D.
Assistant Professor of Surgery (Plastic Surgery), New York University School of Medicine; Attending Surgeon, Manhattan Eye, Ear & Throat Hospital, University Hospital, Bellevue Hospital, and Manhattan Veterans Administration Hospital, New York, New York.

DONALD WOOD-SMITH, M.D., F.R.C.S.E.
Professor of Surgery (Plastic Surgery), New York University School of Medicine; Chairman, Department of Plastic Surgery, New York Eye & Ear Infirmary; Attending Surgeon (Plastic Surgery), Bellevue Medical Center; Attending Surgeon, New York University Hospital, New York Veterans Administration Hospital, and Manhattan Eye, Ear & Throat Hospital, New York, New York.

BARRY M. ZIDE, D.M.D., M.D.
Assistant Professor of Surgery (Plastic Surgery), New York University Medical Center; Attending Surgeon, Bellevue Hospital Center, Manhattan Veterans Administration Hospital, and Manhattan Eye, Ear & Throat Hospital, New York, New York.

Preface

Where does a book begin? Initially, I think of a warm September afternoon in a hotel in Madrid when I first organized an outline of the chapters while waiting for an international surgery meeting to begin. However, a scientific book is only an extension of earlier publications. This text is descended from *Reconstructive Plastic Surgery*, edited in 1964 by my predecessor John Marquis Converse, and reedited in 1977. I had been Assistant Editor of the latter. Many of the ideas and principles, if not the exact words, that were integral to the teaching and writing of Dr. Converse live on in the present volumes. *Reconstructive Plastic Surgery* in turn was derived from his earlier collaboration with V. H. Kazanjian, *The Surgical Treament of Facial Injuries*, published in 1949, 1959, and 1974.

Earlier textbooks by Nélaton and Ombrédanne (1904), Davis (1919), Gillies (1920), and Fomon (1939) had played a germinal role in the development of modern plastic surgery. However, even these books represented only a continuum of publications extending back over the centuries to Tagliacozzi and Sushruta. Indeed, there are also the many surgeons who never published but who by their teachings contributed greatly to the body of knowledge that is represented in the present publication. Their concepts, too, have found their way into the plastic surgery literature for the edification of another generation of students.

My own career has been greatly influenced by my teachers, and their spirit has remained an integral part of my personal and professional life. This heritage of the plastic surgeon–teacher represents the spirit of this book.

The title defines the subject—*Plastic Surgery*. Adjectives such as *reconstructive* or *esthetic* are misleading and redundant and represent artificial divisions of this surgical specialty. The parents of the infant undergoing cleft lip repair are more interested in the *esthetic* aspects of the procedure, which traditionally has been regarded as *reconstructive*. The contemporary face lift, long perceived as an *esthetic* operation, represents a surgical reconstruction of the multiple layers of the soft tissues of the face. Plastic surgery, a term first popularized by Zeis in 1838, is preferred.

With the deliberate exception of parts of Chapters 1 and 35, originally written by Dr. Converse and revised through subsequent editions of various books, few paragraphs in these volumes remain unchanged from the 1977 edition. Many of the authors, however, have used material from the previous editions. Line drawings prepared for these editions by Daisy Stillwell have been reproduced again where appropriate. With the death of Ms. Stillwell, I was fortunate to recruit yet another outstanding medical artist, Craig Luce, to draw hundreds of new illustrations to reflect the continuing developments in this specialty.

The purpose of this book is to define the specialty of plastic surgery. To accomplish this goal, contributions have been sought from the acknowledged leaders of this discipline in all of its ramifications. The clinical applications of plastic surgery, practiced over the whole of the human anatomy, range from skin grafting to the management of uncommon craniofacial clefts, to replantation of the lower extremity. Its practice varies from uncomplicated procedures to sophisticated multistage reconstructions that ally the plastic surgeon with other specialists. The chapters that follow vary in the same way from the short and direct to the lengthy and complex. More than any other, this type of surgery strives for the restoration or improvement of form as well as the restoration of function. The teaching of plastic surgery thus lends itself to illustration. The contributors to this book have been encouraged to use drawings and photographs liberally as an enhancement of the principles and techniques described in the text. Special attention has been given to the sizing and placement of more than 5000 illustrations submitted in accordance with this plan. The contributors and publisher have also made every effort to acknowledge and cite the work of other authors. In a text of this magnitude any omission, while understandable, is regrettable.

In Volume 1 will be found discussions of the essential principles basic to all plastic surgery: wound healing, circulation of the skin, microneurovascular repairs, skin expansion, and grafting of tendons, nerves, and bone, as well as their associated methods of repair. This is the largest of the volumes and testifies to the broadening scope of the field. Much of what is now fundamental to the training of a plastic surgeon was only imagined a generation ago.

After the discussion of general principles in Volume 1, the organization of the text is by anatomic regions. Volumes 2 and 3 are devoted to the face; here, as throughout the book, each chapter draws upon the expertise of acknowledged master surgeons particularly experienced in the subjects on which they have written.

Clefts of the lip and palate as well as severe craniofacial anomalies make up Volume 4. In addition to plastic surgery, these chapters incorporate contributions from the allied fields of embryology, craniofacial growth and development, orthodontics, prosthodontics, speech pathology, and neurosurgery.

Volume 5 covers tumors of the skin and head and neck and Volume 6 the trunk, lower extremity, and genitourinary system. Of particular note, the text details recent advances in reconstruction that involve newly developed flaps of ingenious design and considerable sophistication.

The application of plastic surgical principles and techniques of the upper extremity are discussed in Volumes 7 and 8 under the editorship of Drs. James W. May, Jr., and J. William Littler. The latter, one of the most esteemed and influential hand surgeons of the modern era, edited the upper extremity section in 1964 and 1977. He has been joined in this edition by Dr. May, who is qualified in both hand surgery and microsurgical reconstruction. Both, who are my personal friends, brought their usual enthusiasm, experience, and equanimity to bear on this project. Because surgery of the upper extremity is practiced so extensively, ample space has been afforded for the comprehensive description of the reconstructive procedures specifically designed for the restoration of injured parts. Much of the current progress in plastic surgery of the upper extremity has been made possible by the gradual perfection of microvascular techniques, and these newer developments have been incorporated into the text.

Continuing change, the hallmark of all medical and surgical practice, dictates the need for a reference book such as this and makes its accomplishment a challenging task for everyone involved. With the writing of these words the lengthy process of revising, updating, and improving is ended. The book is committed to the press with the promise that it is both complete and current, in the belief that readers will find it an invaluable resource, and with the hope that it makes a contribution to the body of plastic surgery knowledge and to the education of tomorrow's plastic surgeon.

JOSEPH G. McCARTHY, M.D.

Acknowledgments

The authors or contributors, all with heavy clinical responsibilities and demands, have contributed greatly and are responsible for this text. In addition to outlining their personal views, they have conducted exhaustive literature searches and have organized their illustrative material. They represent the heart and soul of the book.

I wish also to acknowledge my fellow faculty members at the Institute of Reconstructive Plastic Surgery, since their work and concepts, as well as their encouragement, have been so important in the development of this text: Sherrell J. Aston, Donald L. Ballantyne, Robert W. Beasley, Phillip R. Casson, David T.W. Chiu, Peter J. Coccaro, Stephen R. Colen, Court B. Cutting, Barry H. Grayson, V. Michael Hogan, Glenn W. Jelks, Frances C. Macgregor, Thomas D. Rees, Blair O. Rogers, William W. Shaw, John W. Siebert, Charles H. M. Thorne, Augustus J. Valauri, Donald Wood-Smith, and Barry M. Zide. Dr. Frank Cole Spencer, George David Stewart Professor of Surgery and Chairman of the Department of Surgery at the New York University Medical Center, has always championed the goals of the Institute and has especially encouraged development in the newer areas of craniofacial surgery and microsurgery.

I should also pay tribute to Ms. Karen Singer, who did so much of the bibliographic study, and Wayne Pearson and Harry Weissfisch, who provided photographic support. I must also acknowledge my associates at the Institute, Robert E. Bochat, Linda Gerson, Donna O'Brien, Caren Crane, Marilyn Deaton, Margy Maroutsis, Marjorie Huggins, and others for acts of kindness and support during the years of preparation of this book.

Mr. Albert Meier, Senior Editor at Saunders, had a major share in the organization and editing of this book. A friend and colleague since 1974 when we began the Second Edition, I have benefited immensely from his advice and counsel. He has also shown an unusual sense of understanding throughout this project. Special thanks are also due to David Harvey, Frank Polizzano, and Richard Zorab of the W. B. Saunders Company for their support.

I am also grateful to the residents and fellows at the Institute of Reconstructive Plastic Surgery, whose boundless enthusiasm is ever encouraging and who have given generously of their time to proofread manuscripts and galleys: Christopher Attinger, Constance Barone, Richard Bartlett, P. Craig Hobar, William Hoffman, Armen Kasabian, Gregory LaTrenta, George Peck, Rosa Razaboni, Gregory Ruff, John Siebert, R. Kendrick Slate, Henry Spinelli, Michael Stevens, Charles Thorne, and Douglas Wagner.

Special thanks are also due to my colleagues and friends at the National Foundation for Facial Reconstruction, whose support and encouragement have provided a unique environment at the Institute that is conducive to writing and research.

Finally, I want to thank my family, Karlan, Cara, and Stephen, for their love and understanding during the demanding years of this project, especially those times spent at a desk when I may have appeared distracted or lost in thought. They remain my main support and life focus.

I also want to thank my friends, especially Charles and Heather Garbaccio, who had the ability to offer those special moments of lightheartedness, good cheer, and camaraderie.

JGM

Contents

PLASTIC SURGERY

35

Joseph G. McCarthy
Donald Wood-Smith

Rhinoplasty

Rhinoplasty, one of the most commonly performed procedures in plastic surgery, in many ways symbolizes the art and practice of this discipline: attention to the psychosocial status of the patient, modification of form, and improvement in nasorespiratory function. It is the surgical procedure that the trainee struggles to learn and the practitioner continues to modify throughout his career.

Occupying the most prominent position on the face, the nose has been the source of well-known sayings ("plain as a nose in a man's face") and has drawn the attention of writers through the ages:

A great nose indicates a great man—
Genial, courteous, intellectual
Virile, courageous

CYRANO DE BERGERAC

Different nasal appearances have elicited various social connotations: large nose—sinister personality, small nose—weak personality, red or erythematous nose—alcoholism or substance abuse, and deviated nose—criminal or psychopathic behavior.

The surgeon undertaking a rhinoplasty must take into consideration the psychologic motivation of the patient and the associated social attitudes, especially in planning a change in nasal form. He must also be prepared to repair deformities in any part of the nose: skin, lining, septum, airway, turbinates, and so forth. There is no place for the "cosmetic nasal surgeon"; the surgeon must be experienced in all aspects of nasal surgery.

HISTORY

The history of plastic surgery has paralleled the development of rhinoplastic techniques (see Chap. 1). However, as late as the twentieth century little faith in the success of purely corrective procedures was expressed by Nélaton and Ombrédanne in their classic textbook *La Rhinoplastie* published in 1904: "The surgeon could not pretend to correct a slight malformation. If a nose be slightly deviated or humped, or show a slight saddle deformity—these are unfortunate defects . . . but we do not believe that the correction of such defects can be achieved by surgery." However, a review of the literature of the last decade of the nineteenth century and the early part of the twentieth century indicates that nasal corrective procedures were being performed but mostly through external incisions.

In the United States, corrective nasal surgery was pioneered by a small number of surgeons, among whom Roe, Goodale, and Mosher are outstanding. Roe appears to have been the first to employ an intranasal approach as early as 1887. Extracts from some of Roe's papers reveal his understanding of both the functional and psychologic aspects of corrective rhinoplasty (Converse, 1970; Rogers, 1986):

> *If the deformity of the nose is found to be associated with a local disturbance inside the nose, obstructing the passages, we should invariably remove or correct this local condition, whether it be deviation or thickening of the septum, enlargement of the turbinates, a polyp or other growths, or even adenoids and large tonsils. To preserve perfect nasal respiration is of the utmost necessity, not only to the health and comfort of the patient, but to the satisfactory correction of the nasal deformity.*
>
> *While symmetrical relations of the different portions of the nose to one another are of the greatest importance, the symmetrical relation as to the size and shape of the nose to the general contour of the face must also be carefully considered, in order to approach the ideal from an artistic point of view.*
>
> *We are able to relieve patients of a condition which would remain a lifelong mark of disfigurement, constantly observed, forming a never ceasing source of embarrassment and mental distress to themselves, amounting, in many cases, to a positive torture, as well as often causing them to be objects of greater or less aversion to others.*

Roe was the first surgeon to use an intranasal approach, but it was Joseph (1931) who popularized corrective nasal surgery through internally placed incisions. His influence was predominant during the first third of this century (Natvig, 1982) and surgeons from around the world traveled to his clinic in Berlin to learn his technique. His teachings were collected in a widely read textbook published in 1931. The Joseph technique was introduced in the United States by Aufricht and Safian. The literature concerned with corrective nasal plastic surgery is abundant.

A comprehensive bibliography was compiled by McDowell, Valone, and Brown (1952). In recent years the emphasis has been placed on modifying rhinoplastic techniques with refinements in incisions, instrumentation, and cartilage grafts (Sheen, 1978; Sheen and Sheen, 1987; Rees, 1980).

Before rhinoplastic procedures are undertaken, an understanding of the anatomy, esthetics, ethnic variations, and physiology of the nose is a prime requisite.

ANATOMY

The nose is shaped as a pyramid. The nasal pyramid is an osteocartilaginous structure, covered with soft tissues that include skin, subcutaneous tissue, muscle, and epithelium.

The surface anatomy of the nose is shown in Figure 35–1 and this is the terminology that will be used in the text. The osteocartilaginous framework of the nose is illustrated in Figure 35–2. The nose can be divided into three components (Sheen, 1978): the *bony vault* (frontal processes of maxilla and nasal bones), the *upper cartilaginous vault* (upper lateral cartilages), and the *lower cartilaginous vault* (medial and lateral crura, alae, alar lobules, nostril vestibules and sills, columella, and membranous septum).

The nasal pyramid has two openings at its base, the *external nares* (Fig. 35–3). These inlets for the nasal airway admit air into the nasal vestibules, delimited posteriorly by the *internal nares,* frequently referred to as the nasal valves (Mink, 1920). It is these valvelike structures that control the air flow into the nasal fossae proper, paired cavities separated in the midline by the nasal septum. The convergence and divergence of the nasal valves open and close the internal nares, thus controlling the air flow into the nasopharyngotracheal airway. The nasal fossae drain the accessory sinuses and the lacrimal apparatus. A small portion of the nasal mucous near the cribriform plate is specifically olfactory in function.

Covering Soft Tissues of Nose. At the tip, the skin of the nose is tightly bound to the alar cartilages; in contrast, the skin and musculature are loosely attached and mobile over the lateral cartilages and nasal bones. The skin is rich in sebaceous glands over the caudal portion of the nose. The arteries and veins of the nose are situated in the soft tissues; the plane of dissection in nasal operations should therefore be close to the os-

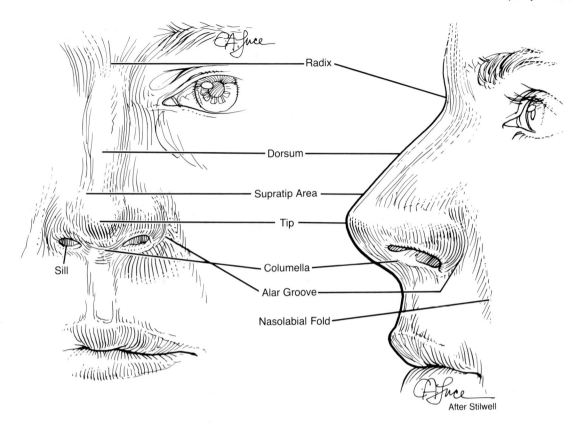

Figure 35–1. Surface anatomy of the nose.

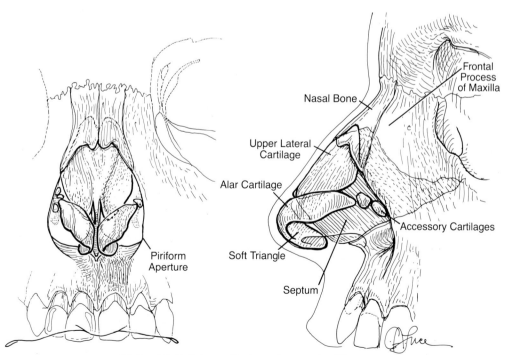

Figure 35–2. Osteocartilaginous framework of the nose.

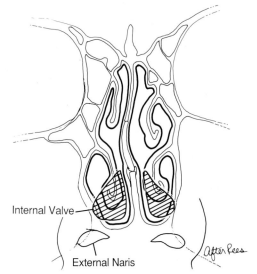

Figure 35–3. The external and internal nares. Note the relationship of the nasal vestibule (crosshatched) to the entire nasal cavity and especially to the inferior turbinate.

teocartilaginous framework to avoid injury to the vessels and unnecessary bleeding.

Essential External Landmarks of Nose. The *dorsum* or *bridge* of the nose is formed in part by the bony nose and in part by the cartilaginous nose (see Fig. 35–1). It is essential that a uniform terminology be employed to designate the various portions of the nose.

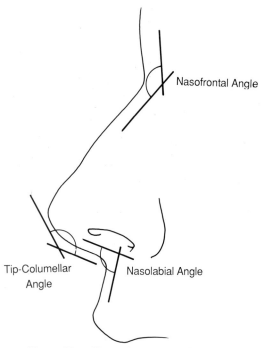

Figure 35–4. The surface angles of the nose.

The *nasofrontal angle* (Fig. 35–4) is the area where the nose joins the forehead, the *radix* or *root* of the nose (the radix nasi).

Above (cephalad to) the tip of the nose is the *supratip* area. This area usually overlies the septal angle of the quadrangular cartilage of the septum. The *septal angle* is a convenient term for the angle formed by the caudal and dorsal borders of the septal cartilage (Converse, 1955).

The *tip* of the nose is formed by the junction of the two alae of the nose. Confusion has resulted from the use of the term "lobule." The noun "lobule" originates from the Greek *lobos,* which became in late Latin *lobus,* a term that designated a hanging structure such as the lobe of the ear. The nose consists of fixed and mobile structures. If one wishes to use the term "lobule," it is acceptable as a descriptive term for the lower mobile part of the nose: tip, alae, columella, and membranous septum.

The base or caudal portion of the nasal pyramid is formed by the nostrils and the *columella.* The nostrils can also be designated as the external nares, in contradistinction to the internal nares.

The nostrils or nares are the point of entry of air into the nose. The columella joins the tip of the nose to the upper lip and separates the two external nares. The *sills* are the slightly protuberant floors of the nostrils. The junction of the base of the columella with the upper lip defines the *nasolabial angle.* Sheen (1978) emphasized the *columellar-lobular junction* as an important landmark in grafting techniques of the nasal tip. The *tip-columellar angle* is formed by the intersection of the surface plane of the columella with that of the tip (see Fig. 35–4).

Other essential landmarks of the external nose include the *alar groove,* which is at the junction of the ala with the cheek and which in its midportion meets the *nasolabial fold.* The alar groove extends over the cephalic border of the alar cartilage, where it forms a shallow furrow.

Bony Structures of Nose. The anatomy of the nose varies from individual to individual within the same ethnic group and according to the individual's ethnic background.

The bony portion of the nose (see Fig. 35–2) is formed by the paired nasal bones; these are joined in the midline and are supported posteriorly by the nasal spine of the frontal bone and laterally by the frontal process of the maxilla. The osseous lateral walls of the nose are formed by the nasal bones and frontal processes of the maxilla (bony vault).

The nasal bones are quadrangular, thick, and narrow above and thin and wide below (Fig. 35–5 and see Fig. 35–2); their anterior surface is concave from above downward in the upper portion, convex from side to side. The thicker and stronger cephalic portion of the nasal bones is further reinforced by the nasal spine of the frontal bone, which lends additional support to this part of the bony bridge. The caudal borders of the nasal bones show a concave curve, the lateral portion of each bone extending downward along the edge of the piriform aperture (Fig. 35–5*B*). The frontal process of the maxilla is a plate of bone, thick below and thinner above, which projects upward and medially from the body of the maxilla, forming the edge of the piriform aperture (Fig. 35–5*C*), the lower boundary of the lateral nasal wall. The posterior border of the frontal process of the maxilla forms the lacrimal groove with the neighboring lacrimal bone (Fig. 35–5*C*).

The frontal process of the maxilla forms the anterior lacrimal crest. The medial canthal tendon inserts upon the anterior and posterior lacrimal crests, and some fibers reach the suture line between the nasal bone and the frontal bone.

Cartilaginous Structures of Nose

Lateral (Upper Lateral) Cartilages. During embryologic development, the nasal cartilages are formed from a portion of the chondrocranium, the cartilaginous nasal capsule, which is a paired structure. This explains embryologic abnormalities such as duplication of the septum or duplication of the entire nose as seen in midline cleft syndromes.

The lateral cartilages are paired structures, roughly triangular in shape, attached to the nasal bones and frontal processes of the maxilla above and to the septal cartilage in the midline (Fig. 35–6). The attachment of the lateral cartilages to these structures and to the septum is described later in the text. The lower third of the lateral cartilages diverges

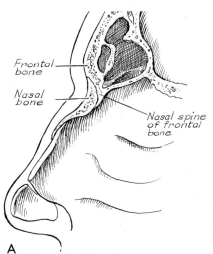
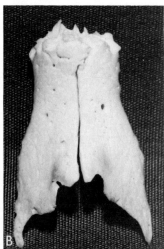
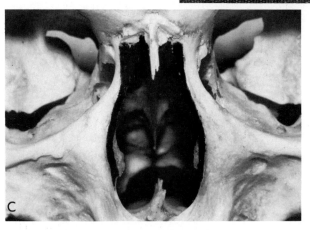

Figure 35–5. The bony framework of the nose. *A,* Sagittal section illustrating the thicker cephalic portion of the nasal bones reinforced by the nasal spine of the frontal bone. *B,* The nasal bones. *C,* The piriform aperture.

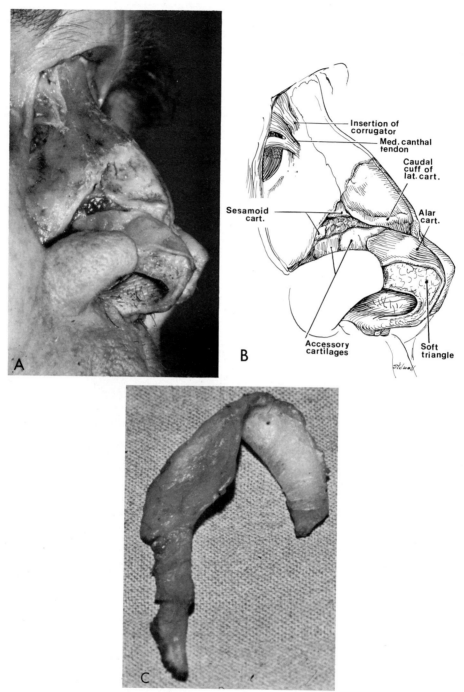

Figure 35–6. Dissection of the nose to demonstrate cartilage relationships. *A,* The nasal bone, frontal process of the maxilla, upper lateral and alar cartilage, and accessory cartilages are shown in the dissection and outlined in *B. C,* The right alar cartilage with the accessory cartilages. (From Firmin, F., and Le Pesteur, J.: Reflexions sur l'auvert cartilagineux nasal. Ann. Chir. Plast., 22:1, 1977.)

from the septum, becomes mobile, and constitutes the internal valves of the nose.

The lower portion of each lateral cartilage is thicker and turns on itself, forming a cuff (Fig. 35–6). This characteristic was noted by Testut and Jacob (1929) and other anatomists, who also described small sesamoid cartilages that are present between the lateral cartilage and the alar cartilage that overlaps the lateral cartilage. The small sesamoid cartilages appear to act as roller bearings, facilitating the movement of the alar cartilage over the lateral cartilage (Firmin and Le Pesteur, 1977).

The lateral margin of the lateral cartilage is joined to the edge of the piriform aperture except in its lower portion, where the area of the junction varies.

The cartilages of the nose are subjected to movements by the nasal musculature (Fig. 35–7) that play an important role in nasal physiology (Zide, 1985). The closure of the nasal valves is affected by compression of the cephalic portion of the lateral crura of the alar cartilages that overlap the lateral cartilages (Van Dishoek, 1937). The preservation of the mobility of the caudal portion of the nose is essential for the function of these muscles. Their function is inhibited in facial paralysis; the cartilages of the nose are immobile owing to paralysis of the musculature, and an inadequate nasal airway is noted on the paralyzed side (Fig. 35–8).

The alar cartilages are connected to the lateral cartilages by loose connective tissue that facilitates their cephalic displacement over the lateral cartilages.

The cartilaginous external nose is situated caudad and anterior to the piriform aperture. The piriform aperture, the base of the nasal pyramid, is a pear-shaped skeletal opening to the nasal fossae. It is bounded above by the lower borders of the nasal bones and laterally by the frontal processes of the maxilla, the thin, sharp margins of which extend downward, where they curve medially to join each other at the anterior nasal spine.

Nasal Septum and Septal Cartilage. The nasal septum is a midline structure that divides the nasal cavity into two lateral chambers. The septal framework is composed of bony and cartilaginous constituents: the four bony components of the osseous septum (the perpendicular plate of the ethmoid, the vomer, the nasal crest of the maxilla, the nasal crest of the palatine bone), and the septal cartilage. The septal cartilage has a posterior extension into the ethmoid plate (Fig. 35–9).

The septal cartilage is a quadrangular lamina that forms the major portion of the framework of the caudal portion of the septum; it protrudes in front of the piriform aperture. The septal angle is located immediately cephalad to the alar cartilages in an area referred to as the supratip area. This finding can be demonstrated by digital pressure on the nasal tip applied in a caudal direction. Blanching of the overlying skin is observed at the septal angle.

The lower portion of the septal cartilage is firmly bound to the vomer and the premaxillary wings, the perichondrium of the cartilage being continuous with the periosteum of the vomer. The caudal part of the septal cartilage is more mobile and flexible. The perichondrium of the septal cartilage extends outward to join the periosteum of the wider groove in the premaxillary wings and the flat surface of the nasal spine, thus simulating a joint capsule within which lateral movements of the septal cartilage are possible. The plasticity of this portion of the septum increases the flexibility of the septal cartilage. The caudal margin of the septal cartilage is separated from the columella (and medial crura) by the juxtaposition of two mucocutaneous flaps that form the *membranous septum*.

The mobility of the lower portion of the septal cartilage and of the membranous septum permits side to side movement and, together with the resilient lateral and alar cartilages, accounts for the shock-absorbing role of these structures in preventing nasal fractures as well as more severe craniofacial injuries.

The cephalic portion of the dorsal border of the septal cartilage, intimately connected with the cephalic portion of the lateral cartilages, extends under the nasal bones, where it is received in a shallow bony groove. The posterior border is connected to the perpendicular plate of the ethmoid; the posterior extension of the septal cartilage separates a portion of the ethmoid plate from the vomer (see Fig. 35–9).

The cephalic portion of the septal cartilage is usually thicker, constituting at its junction with the ethmoid plate a strong, fixed, *central pillar* supporting the nasal bones. The preservation of the central pillar is of considerable importance in rhinoplasty when all the struc-

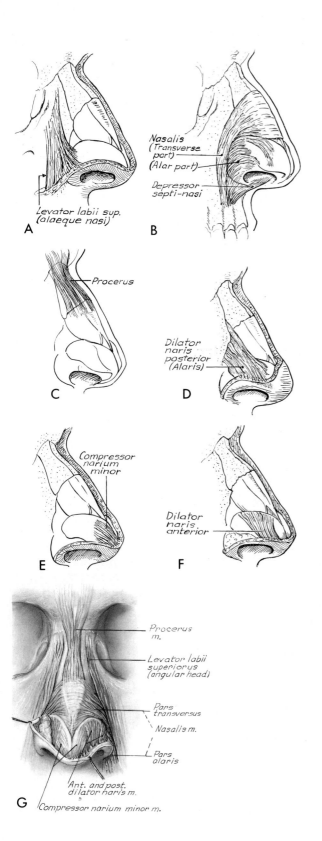

Figure 35–7. The muscles of the nose.

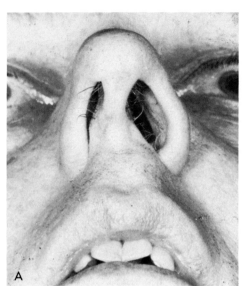 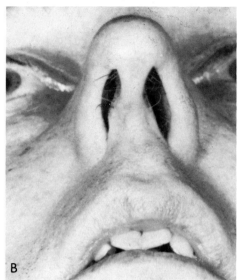

Figure 35–8. Loss of function of the ala in facial paralysis. *A*, The nose during inspiration. On the unaffected left side, the naris opens; on the paralyzed right side, the ala is immobile. *B*, The paralyzed right ala also remains collapsed during expiration.

tures of the nose have been mobilized and only the central pillar remains to support the dorsum.

The relationship of the upper lateral cartilages to the nasal bones is established during the embryologic development of these structures. The overlapping of the nasal bones over the cephalic portion of the lateral cartilages may extend for 8 to 10 mm (see Fig. 35–2; Fig. 35–10). The fusion of the perichondrium and the periosteum through dense connective tissue results in an intimate

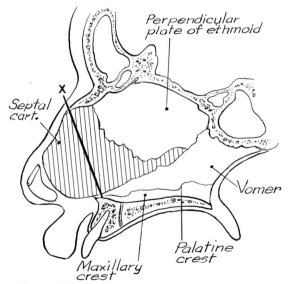

Figure 35–9. The nasal septum. The line *X* indicates the line of demarcation between the fixed and the flexible portion of the nasal septum.

relationship between the cartilage and bone. The overlapping area is oval in shape. The maximal length of the oval is at the junction of the nasal bones; as the frontal process is reached, the overlap is only a few millimeters. This intimate relationship is of clinical significance in fractures and in rhinoplastic procedures; it explains why the lateral cartilage is displaced medially with the bony lateral wall following lateral osteotomy.

The dorsal border of the cartilaginous nasal septum undergoes alteration in width and configuration in the area of the nasal bones and bifurcates into a Y, forming a supraseptal groove between the limbs of the Y (Fig. 35–10). The groove is readily seen and palpated in some individuals, but it is usually indistinguishable on the surface, being masked by the perichondrium, connective tissue, the aponeurosis of the nasalis muscle, and subcutaneous tissue. The supraseptal groove is wide near the junction with the nasal bones and tapers toward the septal angle.

The nasal hump, often a prominent portion of the dorsum, is formed by the nasal bones, the widened portion of the septal cartilage, and the lateral cartilages. The dorsal hump is fusiform, narrow above, wide near the junction of the lateral cartilages and nasal bones, and narrow above the septal angle. The nasal hump varies in its osseous and cartilaginous composition.

The lateral and septal cartilages are intimately connected near the nasal bones. In the series of sections obtained from cadaver

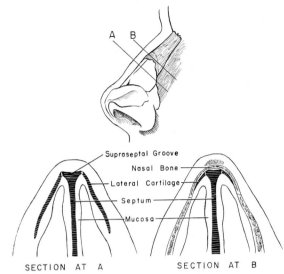

Figure 35–10. Serial sections of the external nose through a frontal plane. The upper drawing illustrates the levels *A* and *B* at which cross sections have been made. The sectional view *A* demonstrates the relationship of the lateral and septal cartilages. The sectional view *B* shows the relationship of the lateral and septal cartilages with the nasal bones.

dissections (Converse, 1955), there was a gross appearance of cartilaginous continuity. Histologic examination, however, showed a separation between the ends. There was intervening dense connective tissue; continuity of the perichondrium was seen in every specimen. In the specimens studied by Straatsma and Straatsma (1951) and Natvig and associates (1971), continuity of the septal and lateral cartilages was seen on histologic examination. However, Natvig (1975) reexamined a series of specimens and confirmed the findings of Converse (1955).

The septal and lateral cartilages are separated by a narrow cleft that becomes wider toward the septal angle. Fibroareolar tissue in this area permits inward and outward movement of the lateral cartilages. The mobile caudal portion of the lateral cartilages, activated by the nasal musculature, regulates the flow of air that penetrates into the nasal fossae and constitutes the internal nares (the nasal valves). In the course of a corrective rhinoplasty, the integrity of the nasal valve must be preserved.

Alar (Lower Lateral) Cartilages. The alar cartilages are paired structures that form the cartilaginous framework of the tip of the nose (see Fig. 35–2; Fig. 35–11). Each cartilage consists of two portions, a medial crus and a lateral crus, which are joined at the most prominent point of the tip of the nose, the dome of the alar cartilage. The medial crura curve downward to form the skeletal framework of the columella. As they extend downward, they diverge at their lower ends (the foot plates of the medial crura), the maximal divergence being reached at the widened base of the columella. Each medial crus is intimately adherent to the skin of the columella.

In dissected specimens, when viewed from their caudal aspect (the "worm's eye view"), the lateral crura and the domes show a distinct downward curve of their caudal portions (Fig. 35–11). The caudal margin is lower than the dome and the more cephalic portion of the lateral crus.

The size, shape, and orientation of the alar cartilages, particularly the lateral crura, vary. The medial crura assume various curves and shapes (Natvig and associates, 1971). In an anatomic study of cadavers, Zelnick and Gingrass (1979) observed five variations in the configurations of the lateral crura:

1. Entirely smooth and convex.
2. Convex anteriorly, concave posteriorly.
3. Concave anteriorly, convex posteriorly.
4. Concave anteriorly and posteriorly but convex centrally.
5. Entirely concave (rare).

The height and width of the lateral crura were variable. Average height was 11 mm and average width 22 mm. There were also sexual and ethnic variations. The configuration of the medial crura was variable but there was a suggestion of three patterns.

The lateral portion of the lateral crus, which occupies little more than the medial half of the ala, is joined to the edge of the

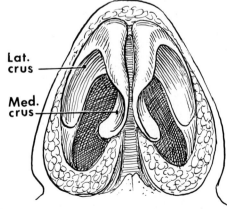

Figure 35–11. The alar cartilages. Note the downward curve of the caudal portions and the flare of the medial crura.

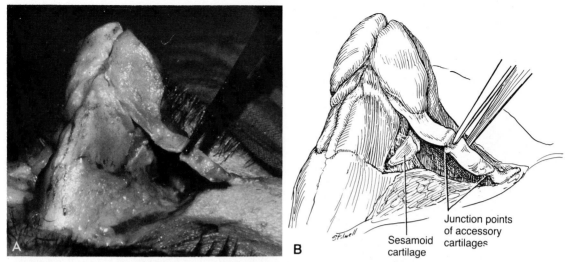

Figure 35–12. The accessory cartilages. *A,* Dissection of the nasal framework (viewed from above), demonstrating the accessory cartilages that join the lateral crus to the edge of the piriform aperture. *B,* Drawing illustrating the accessory cartilages (three in number in this specimen) joined to each other and to the alar cartilages by the continuity of the perichondrium. (Courtesy of Firmin and Le Pesteur, 1977)

piriform aperture by accessory and sesamoid cartilages.

Accessory Cartilages of Nose. The term "sesamoid" may be applied to the minuscule cartilages between the lateral and alar cartilages and also the small cartilages in the superolateral portion of the ala. The term "accessory" cartilages is suggested to designate the larger cartilages that join the lateral crus to the edge of the piriform aperture through the continuity of the perichondrium of these structures. Described by Testut and Jacob (1929), their presence has been·confirmed by Firmin and Le Pesteur (1977).

Although variable in size and shape, the accessory cartilages establish a bridge be-

tween the alar cartilage and the edge of the piriform aperture (Figs. 35–12, 35–13). Thus, the alar cartilage and its accessory cartilages form a cartilaginous three-quarter ring at the base of the nasal pyramid (Fig. 35–14).

Nostril Border. The border of the nostril is supported by dense collagenous tissue arranged in resilient longitudinal bundles. The lateral crus is closer to the caudal margin of the external naris border in its medial third but extends away from the margin in its lateral portion.

Soft Triangle. The dome, point of union of the lateral and medial crura, is separated from the margin of the nostril by a triangular-shaped area known as the soft triangle

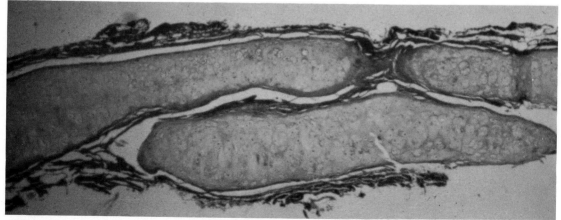

Figure 35–13. Photomicrograph of a histologic section showing the continuity of the perichondrium joining the accessory cartilages. (Courtesy of Firmin and Le Pesteur, 1977)

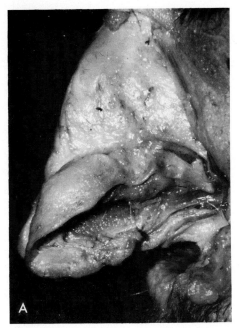
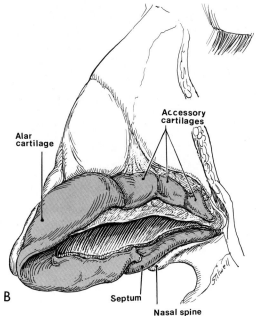

Figure 35–14. The narial ring formed by the alar and accessory cartilages. *A,* Dissection of the cartilages showing the alar cartilage (medial crus, dome, lateral crus, and accessory cartilages). *B,* Drawing illustrating the various structures shown in *A.* The alar cartilage and its accessory cartilages form a 3/4 circle narial ring. (Courtesy of Firmin and Le Pesteur, 1977.)

(Fig. 35–15) (Converse, 1955). The soft triangle consists of two juxtaposed layers of skin, the covering skin of the nose and the vestibular skin, separated by loose areolar tissue. An incision through the soft triangle should be avoided, as subsequent healing may result in a disfiguring notch. The marginal or rim incision for exposure of the alar cartilage should follow the caudal margin of the cartilage and *not* the margin of the nostril.

Weak Triangle. The lateral crura of the alar cartilages diverge in the supratip area, leaving a triangular-shaped area between them into which the septal angle is fitted. In this area, in many noses, the dorsum is supported only by the septal angle (Fig. 35–16*A*). As described earlier in the text, the alar cartilages, which overlap the lateral cartilages, are connected by aponeurotic-like tissue, which also maintains the attachment of the alar cartilages to the septal angle and acts as a suspensory ligament of the tip of the nose (Fig. 35–16*B*).

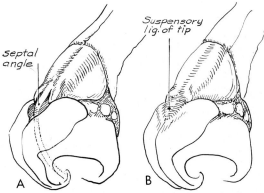

Figure 35–15. The soft triangle of the nose, consisting of two juxtaposed layers of skin separating the dome of the alar cartilage from the nostril border. The soft triangle is represented by the shaded area. Skin incisions should be avoided in this area.

Figure 35–16. The weak triangle and the suspensory ligament of the nose. *A,* The soft tissues have been removed to show that the septal angle supports the area of the dorsum between and above the diverging lateral crura (the weak triangle). This area is subject to many anatomic variations. *B,* The aponeurosis joining the structures (the suspensory ligament of the nasal tip).

Columella. The columella extends from the tip of the nose to the lip, joining the lip at the upper portion of the philtrum and separating the external nares. The posterior portion of the columella is wider than the anterior portion owing to the divergence of the medial crura of the alar cartilages, the lower ends of which embrace the caudal margin of the septal cartilage (see Figs. 35–1, 35–11). The lower portion of the columella is also wider because of the divergence of the lower portions of the medial crura; the contour of the columella depends largely on the shape and degree of divergence of these cartilaginous structures.

The columella is penetrated by the paired depressor septi nasi muscles, which arise from the incisive fossae of the maxilla (see Fig. 35–7). The muscle inserts into the caudal portion of the septum and a few fibers extend into the cephalic portion of the ala of the nose. Its principal function is to tense the membranous septum. In some patients it is overactive, depressing the tip when the patient smiles or even speaks. In these patients, the muscle can be excised in toto. The insertions of the muscle cause the mucoperichondrium of the caudal portion of the septum to be more adherent and thus more difficult to detach when the septal cartilage is being surgically exposed.

The medial crura curve down from the domes, thus assuming a vertical position. Before the crura reach their vertical and sagittal position in the lower portion of the columella, they form a facet at the turning point, a flat surface that breaks the continuity between the tip and the columella. This area is the tip-columella angle (see Fig. 35–4; Fig. 35–17), flanked on each side by the soft triangles. Below the angle, the remainder of the columella shows a gentle curve with a caudal convexity.

Vestibule. The vestibule, the antechamber of the nasal fossa (Fig. 35–18), forms the caudal portion of the floor of the nose and extends under the dome of the alar cartilages. The vestibule is separated from the nasal fossa proper by the caudal border of the lateral cartilage. From a physiologic standpoint, this is the most important anatomic structure of the nose. It is easily visible when one retracts the ala; the lower border of the lateral cartilage protrudes. This area was termed the "limen nasi" (the threshold of the nose) by Zukerhandl (1892); Mink (1920) referred to it as the nasal valve. The fold formed

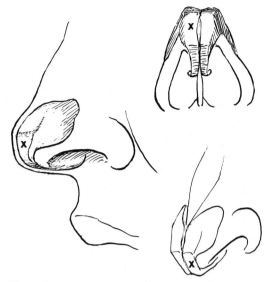

Figure 35–17. The tip-columellar angle. Between the tip and the base of the columella there is a break in the continuity of the cephalic curve of the columella.

by the protruding caudal border of the lateral cartilage is prolonged downward and medially along the crest of the piriform aperture to form the posterior vestibular fold (Fig. 35–19). The crest with its overlying posterior vestibular fold delimits the vestibule cephalad along the floor of the nose and separates the vestibule from the nasal fossa proper.

The vestibule is delimited caudad by a medial extension of the alar border, the anterior narial fold. Thus, along the floor of the nose, the vestibule is delimited by the anterior narial fold caudad and by the posterior vestibular fold cephalad. The relationship of

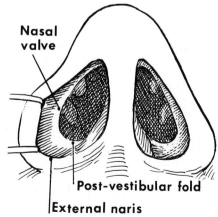

Figure 35–18. The nasal vestibule. The internal naris (the nasal valve), formed by the lower border of the lateral cartilage and prolonged along the floor of the nose as the posterior vestibular fold, constitutes the cephalic limit of the nasal vestibule.

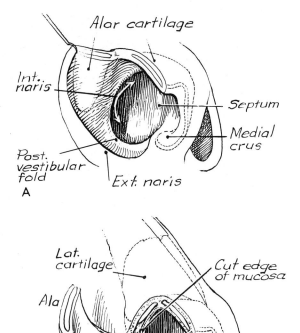

Figure 35–19. The internal and external nares. *A,* The internal naris (the nasal valve) is formed by the caudal border of the lateral cartilage. *B,* Dissection showing that the posterior vestibular fold extends along the border of the piriform aperture, across the floor of the vestibule to the columella.

the nasal vestibule to the entire nasal cavity is illustrated in Figure 35–3.

The lining of the vestibule differs from that of the nasal fossa proper. The squamous epithelial lining of the vestibule contains numerous hairs (the vibrissae) and sebaceous glands. The nasal valve controls the flow of air into the nasal fossa; thus, the vestibule serves as an air-conditioning apparatus, warming, filtering, and moistening the inspired air.

The caudal border of the lateral cartilage is the portal of entry into the nasal fossa, which is lined by mucous membrane. The "respiratory" portion of the nasal fossa is lined by a delicate, pseudostratified, ciliated, columnar epithelium. Because of the important physiologic function of the nasal mucous membrane, its integrity must be preserved.

Over the nasal septum, the nasal mucous membrane is intimately connected to the underlying perichondrium and periosteum.

In the most cephalic portion of the nasal fossa, the mucous membrane has an olfactory function. Over the cephalic portion of the septum and the superior turbinate, the epithelium is no longer ciliated and is yellowish in color; it consists of supporting cells and olfactory cells that connect with the olfactory nerves.

Turbinates. There are three pairs of turbinates: the superior, middle, and inferior (see Fig. 35–3). The superior is ethmoidal in origin and located beneath the cribriform plate. Partially covered by olfactory epithelium and more yellow in color, it has few mucous glands or cavernous sinuses. It is not involved in nasal respiration.

The middle turbinate, ethmoidal in origin, overlies the maxillary ostium. While it secretes mucus, it has little effect on nasal respiration.

Because of its size and rich supply of cavernous sinuses, the inferior turbinate plays a major role in regulating the nasal airway (see under Physiology).

ESTHETICS

When one looks at the nose, one does not observe it in isolation. Intuitively it is related in the observer's eyes to the forehead, the brow or supraorbital rims, the medial canthi (the "naso-orbital valley" of Converse), the eyes or orbits, the maxilla or "platform" of the nose, the lips, and the chin. The stature or height of the patient must also be considered. For example, the small, highly sculpted nose on a taller person is as incongruous as the large nose on a person of small stature.

The topography of the face is characterized by a series of interconnecting lines and curves often defined by the underlying craniofacial skeleton (Fig. 35–20). As emphasized by Sheen (1978), the nose should flow naturally into these lines and curves. There is a natural, uninterrupted curve from the brow to the lateral aspect of the nose (Fig. 35–20). It is defined by the supraorbital rim, the frontal process of the maxilla, and the medial canthi. Disruption of this curve is especially apparent in the patient with a saddle nose deformity (Fig. 35–21) or post-traumatic telecanthus (Fig. 35–22). These relationships must be preserved with rhinoplasty techniques. Other

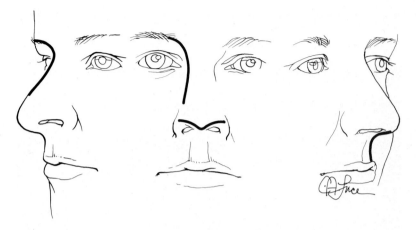

Figure 35–20. Topographic curves. There is a natural, uninterrupted curve from the medial brow to the lateral aspect of the nose (after Sheen). Others include the nasofrontal junction, the lobular-alar rim, and the nasolabial junction.

curves define the lobular-alar rim (Fig. 35–20, *center*) and nasolabial junction (Fig. 35–20, *right*).

On a frontal view the nasal configuration also shows a series of curves. The nose is narrow at its root, then becomes broader, showing a gentle convexity in the region of the hump to narrow again immediately above the tip of the nose. The dorsum of the nose should be adequate in width and height to prevent a hyperteloric appearance between the eyes (see Fig. 35–22); the lower the dorsum, the wider apart the eyes appear. The tip of the nose should be differentiated from the remainder of the nose and be well defined. The base of the nose is in the shape of a

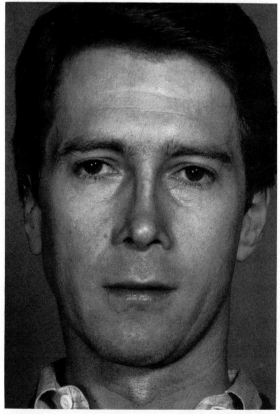

Figure 35–21. Postsurgical nasal deformity illustrating interruption of the curve from the medial brow to the lateral aspect of the nose and the curve of the lobular-alar rim ("pinched tip" deformity).

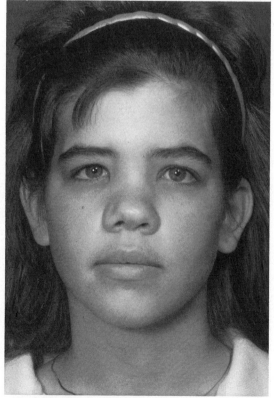

Figure 35–22. Post-traumatic telecanthus with interruption of the curve from the medial brow to the lateral aspect of the nose.

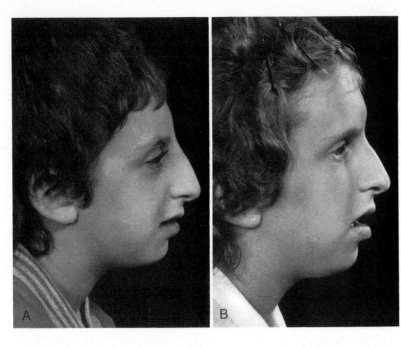

Figure 35–23. The role of the supraorbital ridge (brow) in determining nasal profile. *A,* A 12 year old girl before frontal bone advancement and cranial vault enlargement for the treatment of papilledema. *B,* Postoperative view. A rhinoplasty was not performed. The increased brow projection reduces the relative projection of the nose.

rounded triangle, and the nares are tear shaped.

The anterior projection of the supraorbital rim is also variable among individuals. With recession of this structure, a normal-sized nose appears large (Fig. 35–23).

In similar fashion, the nose relates to the maxilla or perinasal region. *The underlying bony skeleton defines soft tissue contours.* A small nose is often a component of nasomax-

illary hypoplasia, and surgical correction entails advancement of the entire nasomaxillary complex (Fig. 35–24). A normal-sized nose appears large if the maxilla is hypoplastic. A corrective (reduction) rhinoplasty would yield only a flattened appearance to the face, whereas augmentation or advancement of the hypoplastic maxilla would restore facial relationships.

Vertical maxillary excess or the long face

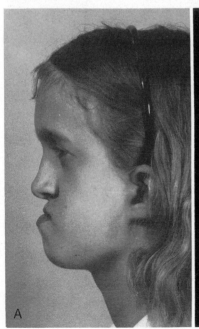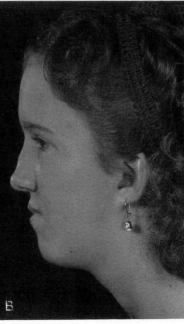

Figure 35–24. Nasomaxillary hypoplasia. *A,* Preoperative view. Note the generalized hypoplasia of the midface skeleton with a normal-sized nose. *B.* Appearance after a Le Fort II advancement osteotomy *without* a rhinoplasty. Note the improved midface contours, lip relationships, and nasolabial angle. There was associated nasal tip elevation with the midface advancement.

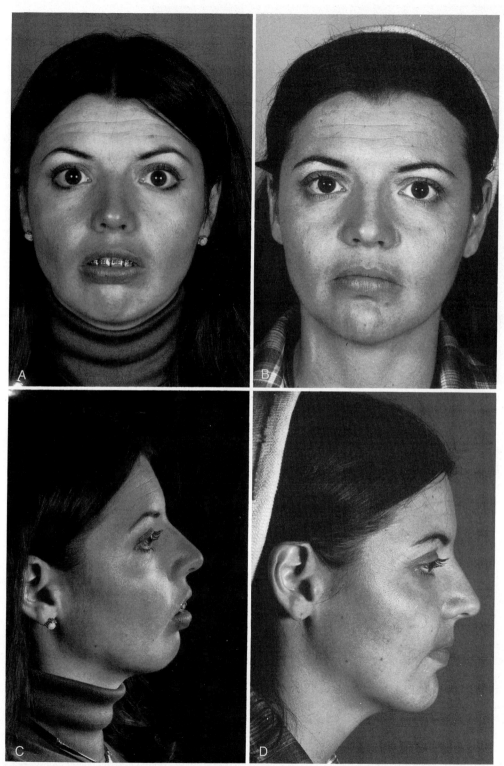

Figure 35–25. Long face syndrome (vertical maxillary excess). *A,* Preoperative frontal view. Note the incisor show, poor lip posture, and microgenia. *C,* Preoperative profile. Note that the nose looks enlarged. *B, D,* After vertical impaction of the maxilla (Le Fort I) and genioplasty. Even though nasal surgery was *not* performed, there are improved facial relationships. A rhinoplasty alone would have ignored the true pathology.

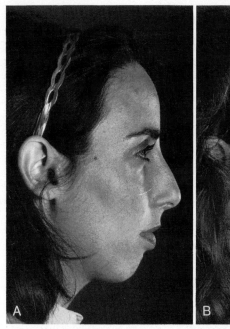
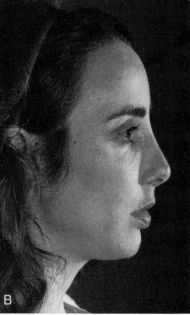

Figure 35–26. Rhinoplasty combined with genioplasty. *A,* Preoperative appearance with moderate microgenia. *B,* After rhinoplasty and genioplasty (horizontal osteotomy of the anteroinferior border of the mandible). Note the improvement in the facial profile and the labiomental angle.

syndrome is associated with incisor show at rest, gingival exposure on smiling, and an obtuse nasolabial angle. Primary surgical attention should be directed toward correcting the underlying skeletal pathology before considering rhinoplasty surgery (Fig. 35–25). Maxillary advancement surgery also affects nasal, especially tip, position (see Fig. 35–24).

The chin is, like the nose, a prominent facial projection. It is not uncommon to see a patient with a large dorsal hump and microgenia. Chin surgery should be considered with the rhinoplasty, and the horizontal osteotomy (or genioplasty) is the preferred technique in moderate to severe microgenia (Fig. 35–26).

The tip is the most subtle component of the nose and in many ways is responsible for its elegance and definition. The tip can also be the bane of the surgeon since it integrates the dorsum, columella, domes, and nostrils.

Sheen (1978) described four essential landmarks of the refined tip (Fig. 35–27):

1. Lateral projection of the left dome.
2. Lateral projection of the right dome.
3. Point of tip differentiation from the dorsum.
4. Columellar-lobular junction.

These points form two triangles with a common base, the *intercrural distance.* In the ideal, three light reflexes should be apparent on the nasal tip—the two domes and the

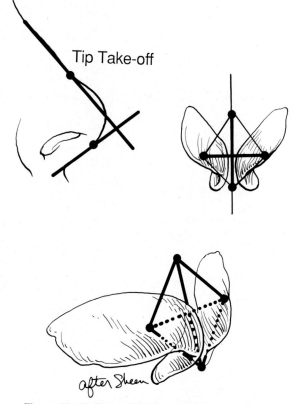

Figure 35–27. Sheen (1978) defined four essential landmarks of the refined nasal tip: projections of the right and left nasal domes, the point of tip (take-off) differentiation from the dorsum, and the columellar-lobular junction. The line between the domes is designated the intercrural distance.

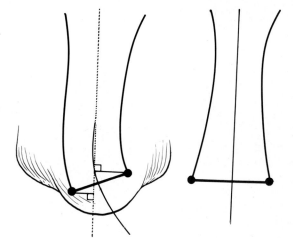

Figure 35–28. In the asymmetric tip the distortion of the intercrural distance is readily apparent (see Fig. 35–27) (after Sheen).

central arch that joins them. On oblique view, the intercrural distance must be sufficient to project the far dome beyond the near one. Deviations of the tip are associated with distortion of these relationships (Fig. 35–28). The columella should be 2 to 3 mm lower than and parallel to the alar rims.

ETHNIC VARIATIONS

Migrations of populations and military conquests have resulted in an admixture of ethnic groups and the interaction of genetic factors. Thus, there are innumerable variations of nasal structural characteristics. Wen (1921) studied the ontogeny and phylogeny of nasal cartilages in primates and in man. He noted structural differences in the nasal cartilages of black and white individuals.

From a clinical standpoint, among the people of the Western world, it is difficult to stereotype a patient's nose according to ethnic origin. Usually Caucasians (the Caucasoids) have noses that vary from the short nose of the Irish, the thin straight nose of the Scandinavians, and the longer nose of the French to the more aquiline nose of the Italians. The population of the Middle East (Armenoids) tends to have a convex dorsum, but again there are exceptions. The sabras of Israel, for example, are quite different in appearance from Middle European or Russian Jews. There is one characteristic, however, frequently seen in Armenoids: the dislocation of the alar cartilages from the septal angle. When digital pressure is exerted over the tip of the nose, the tip is easily depressed from the septal angle, which then protrudes con-

Figure 35–29. Differences in nasal anatomy among the major racial groups. *Left,* In the Caucasian there is an elongated leptorrhine-type nostril with a narrow piriform aperture. *Center,* In the Oriental there is an obliquely directed or mesorrhine nostril. *Right,* In the Negroid there are horizontally oriented and flattened (platyrrhine) nostrils with the widest piriform aperture. Note also the differences in nasal bone size and shape. (After Rees, 1980.)

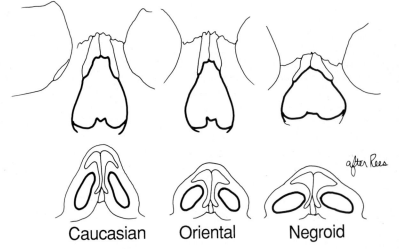

after Rees

Caucasian   Oriental   Negroid

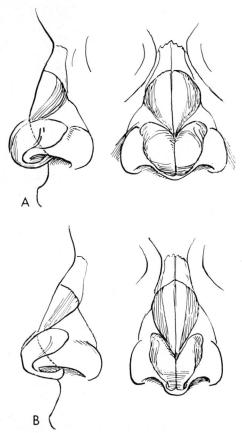

Figure 35–30. Anatomic relationships of the nasal cartilages in the Caucasian and in the Negroid nose. *A,* In the Negroid nose, the septal angle is rounded and contributes no support to the tip cartilages. *B,* The cartilages in the Caucasoid nose. (After Wen, I. C.: Ontogeny and phylogeny of the nasal cartilages. Contributions to Embryology, Carnegie Institution, Washington, *414*:109, 1921.)

spicuously under the skin in the supratip area.

The nasal bones tend to be large in Western Europeans but they progressively decrease in size in Eastern Europeans, Orientals, and the black race (Fig. 35–29). There are also distinct nostril features. Vertical (leptorrhine) nostrils are observed in whites, oblique (mesorrhine) in Orientals, and horizontal (platyrrhine) in blacks. There are also significant differences in the cartilages (Fig. 35–30).

The black nose has a flat, depressed, and broad radix with a straight or slightly depressed dorsum. The tip is thick and bulbous but the alar cartilages are paradoxically small and thin (Fig. 35–31). The nostrils are thick and flaring.

The Oriental nose has a flat or concave dorsum (Fig. 35–32). In contrast to the black nose the radix and dorsum are narrower; the tip is more defined and the alae, while flaring, are narrower.

Of the three major races, the variation in nasal form is greatest within the white race. Rogers (1974) defined the following types:

1. *Nordic*: convex profile, narrow radix, sharp tip, and narrow nostrils and alae.

2. *East Baltic*: less narrow than the Nordic nose, less dorsal convexity, thicker alar cartilages, and broader tip.

3. *Alpine* (Central and Eastern Europe): a more concave and foreshortened nose, and medium-sized tip.

4. *Dinaric* (Balkan): large and long nose with drooping tip.

5. *Armenoid* (Middle East): large, convex noses with great height and length and wide tip. The large alar cartilages curve posteriorly and expose the inner aspect of the columella on profile view.

6. *Mediterranean* (Italy, Spain): straight or convex dorsum with thin radix and tip.

PHYSIOLOGY

In addition to being an important esthetic landmark and the end organ of olfaction, the nose is the principal respiratory airway, the anatomy and physiology of which are often disturbed. A knowledge of respiratory rhinology is essential and should be acquired by those who intend to perform corrective nasal surgery.

The vestibules filter the air through their lining, which contains mucus-secreting glands and vibrissae, entrapping foreign bodies and conditioning the temperature of the air current before its passage through the nasal valve. The air currents are further moistened by the secretions of the pseudostratified, ciliated, columnar epithelium of the nasal cavity (fossa). The air currents are influenced by a number of factors, including the structure and function of the cartilages of the external nose, the shape and directions of the nasal septum, the size of the nasal turbinates, and the thickness of the nasal mucosa. Suppurative, allergic, and vasomotor diseases affecting the sinuses and nasal cavities cause swelling of the turbinates and

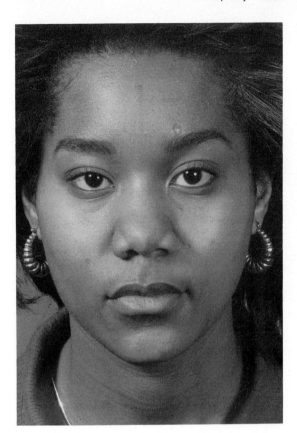

Figure 35–31. Example of a black nose.

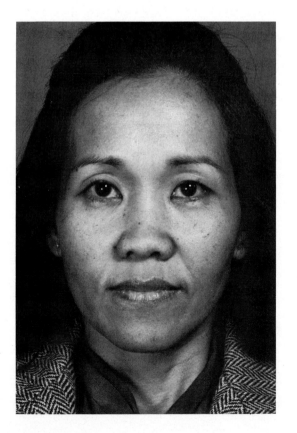

Figure 35–32. Example of an Oriental nose.

nasal mucosa and restrict the dimensions of the nasal airway.

The most important function of the nose is to supply an adequate flow of properly conditioned air to the lungs. To achieve this the nose has other functions: olfaction, filtration, heating and humidification of inspired air, the ability to clean itself, and phonation. Its direct communication with the paranasal sinuses results in an effect on the resonance of the voice. The average length of the nasal air passage in an adult is 10 cm. Within this distance, air of high or low moisture content, which is hot or cold, is converted to air approximately 31° to 37°C in temperature with a 75 per cent relative humidity. Approximately 70 kilocalories of energy are required to perform the functions of humidification and heating. Exposure of inspired air to the nasal mucosa is enhanced by the anatomic arrangement of the turbinates and their relation to the nasal septum. The average width of the airway or column of air in the nose is 1 mm as it passes over, under, or beside the turbinates and septum. The air flow from the external naris passes to the internal nasal valve, where the airway narrows, increasing the velocity of flow while narrowing the column of air. From this point the flow continues along the middle meatus, between the inferior turbinate and septum, and along the upper border of the middle turbinate. It bends in a 60 to 130 degree parabolic curve, and a smaller amount passes through the inferior meatus and along the floor (Fig. 35–33). On expiration the same airway is utilized but in the reverse direction.

Air flow may be either *laminar* or *turbulent* (Rees, 1980). In laminar flow the speed and direction tend to be uniform (see Fig. 35–33). By contrast, in turbulent flow there are irregular currents that vary according to time and direction, with resultant decrease in air flow efficiency and increase in resistance. Scarring of the internal valve or septal deviations increase the amount of turbulent air flow.

Larger particles of foreign material (15 microns and above) become trapped by the vibrissae or by the mucus blanket that coats the entire nasal mucosa. This is secreted by the goblet cells, present in all the nasal mucosa except the olfactory epithelium of the cephalic portion of the nasal cavity. In this region the glands of Bowman secrete a serous fluid, whose function is to dissolve air-borne substances into a liquid for interpretation by the bipolar olfactory cells.

Lysozyme is an enzyme contained in nasal mucus and thought to be bactericidal. The nasal mucosal vascular apparatus responds to irritants, and submucosal vascular spaces (lakes) are responsible for engorgement or enlargement and shrinkage of the turbinates. The turbinates appear to be in a constant state of flux, one side being engorged while the contralateral side carries most of the air flow with cyclic alternations. Approximately 1 liter of water is added to inspired air daily. One-third or more is recovered during nasal expiration. Thus, in cold, dry, high altitude climates, the nose drips from secretion of more moisture than can be contained in its small volume.

The *nasal cycle* is characterized by unilateral nasal obstruction at any given moment—an alternating congestion and decongestion of the turbinates on each side. The normal individual is subjectively unaware of this phenomenon.

The ciliary action of the pseudostratified, ciliated, columnar epithelium is continuous toward the nasopharynx. The cilia weaken and die from drying or become inactivated by strong drugs. Sinus air interchanges with nasal air pressure every two hours.

The physiology of nasal air flow appears to be highly complex, and the objective findings by various methods of measurement currently available are not adequate to explain many aspects of nasal ventilation. There undoubtedly are subjective factors involved in patients in whom objective findings of a sat-

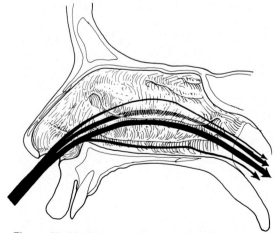

Figure 35–33. The main air current follows a parabolic curve through the middle meatus over the inferior turbinate. A lesser amount passes through the inferior meatus along the nasal floor, and a smaller volume over the middle turbinate.

isfactory airway contrast with the complaint of nasal obstruction; other patients with apparent mechanical obstruction of the nose on physical examination do not seem to be aware of it. It appears that some patients can utilize their defective structures, while others with fairly satisfactory nasal structures do not know how to use them.

Anatomic Factors Influencing Nasal Ventilation

Nostrils and Vestibule. The nasal tip and nostrils play a major role in nasal air flow and resistance. Excessively narrow nostrils (usually iatrogenic) impair air flow, as do dislocated and recessed tips (Fig. 35–34*B*). In the long nose with an acute nasolabial angle the air flow is directed past the anterior naris and vestibule to a point high in the nasal cavity. A noticeable improvement in nasal breathing is observed when the tip is elevated by finger pressure from the examining physician. In the patient with a retroussé tip and obtuse nasolabial angle (or saddle deformity), the air flow is directed inferiorly along the floor of the nose (Fig. 35–34*C*) (Rees, 1980).

The alar cartilages are subjected to movements by the nasal musculature (see Fig. 35–7) and play an important role in nasal physiology. Malfunction of the external musculature and of the alar cartilages is seen in certain postrhinoplasty patients who show an indrawing and collapse of the alae during respiration. Patients with this type of mal-

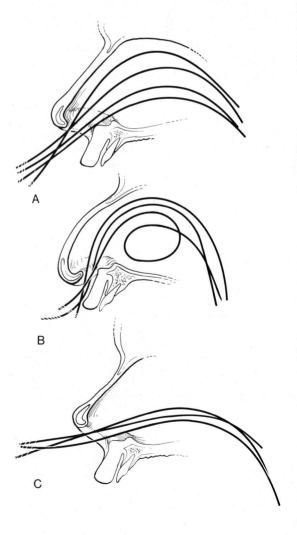

Figure 35–34. Inspiratory air current. *A,* Normal nose with parabolic curves. *B,* Dislocated nasal tip and acute nasolabial angle with misdirection of the air currents toward the nasal dorsum and development of eddies and symptoms of nasal obstruction. *C,* Increased nasolabial angle with direct passage of the air current along the nasal floor into the pharynx. There is incomplete humidification. (After Rees, 1980.)

function usually have elongated external nares with slitlike openings.

Internal Valve. The internal valve or ostium internum is narrowed on deep inspiration (Fig. 35–35) because of the increase in negative pressure in the upper respiratory tract. With the change in contour of the internal valve, airway resistance is increased and air flow patterns are modified. On expiration, airway pressure becomes positive and the area of the internal valve is widened.

With disruption of the internal valve and loss of the structural integrity of the lower cartilaginous vault, inspiratory effort (negative intranasal pressure) is characterized by "alar collapse" or severe narrowing of the nostrils. This condition is most commonly seen in patients in whom there was an excessive resection of alar cartilages during rhinoplasty.

A septal deviation, synechium, or scarring at the internal valve area can interfere with the function of the valve and cause nasal obstruction. Because of these problems some surgeons have advocated a submucous approach to separating the septum from the upper lateral cartilages. However, the attachment of these structures is routinely incised in full-thickness fashion in the corrective rhinoplasty without causing symptoms of nasal obstruction.

Septum. Septal pathology can be varied and can consist of soft tissue hypertrophy and adhesions as well as cartilaginous thickening and angulation. The septum is subject to trauma as the result of a faulty position of the fetus in the uterus and birth trauma.

Septal deviations resulting from early childhood trauma show a developmental increase with growth and often cause deviation of the external nose. Septal fractures also occur as a result of injuries after nasal growth has been completed and are a common accompaniment of nasal bone fractures.

A deviated septum is also found as a congenital malformation, sometimes showing a hereditary tendency; the lateral dislocation of the caudal portion of the septum is an example. Deviation of the septum is also a usual deformity in congenital malformations such as cleft lip and palate.

Most of the population have some degree of septal deviation that must be carefully examined before a nasal operation. However, it must be emphasized that deviation of the septum is the rule rather than the exception, and many patients with severe septal deviation are often free of symptomatology of nasal obstruction.

If the surgeon is confronted preoperatively with a deviated septum in a patient without symptoms of nasal obstruction, he must realize that the patient could become symptomatic following nasal bone infracture. A high

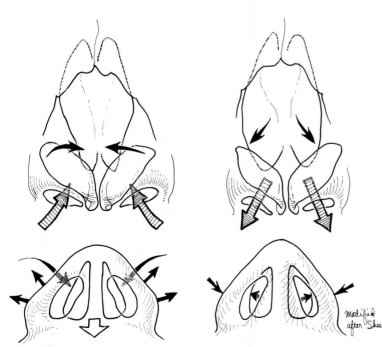

Figure 35–35. The internal valve. *Left,* On deep inspiration the internal valve is narrowed but the nostrils flare. *Right,* On expiration the upper lateral cartilages move away from the septum and the internal valve is enlarged. The nostrils relax to their normal position. (After Sheen, 1978.)

septal deviation could also interfere mechanically with the infracture of the nasal bones and mar the esthetic result of the rhinoplasty.

Turbinates. The middle and inferior turbinates play an important role in nasal respiration. Covered by a thick and highly vascular mucous membrane, the inferior turbinate is especially rich in cavernous sinuses. Because of its erectile properties it can change size and shape and thereby function as an airway valve and maintain proper airway resistance. It is a sensitive organ and the vasomotor supply is from both divisions of the autonomic nervous system. Sympathetic stimulation results in vasoconstriction and reduction in volume (increase in airway) and the opposite is true with parasympathetic stimulation (Rees, 1980). Chronic enlargement progressively leads to hypertrophy and polypoid degeneration as well as symptoms of nasal obstruction.

CORRECTIVE SURGERY

General Considerations

Examination and Diagnosis. The shape and size of the nose are evaluated by direct inspection: the convexity or concavity of the dorsum, the width or projection of the tip, the deviation of the nose, the shape and position of the columella, and the thickness and quality of the skin. The thickness of the skin is of considerable importance. Skin thickened by hypertrophic sebaceous glands is rigid and drapes inadequately over the remodeled caudal framework of the nose. The alar cartilages are readily identified in the long nose with thin skin, but their outline is more difficult to identify when the skin is thick. When a tip operation is done in a nose with thick skin, one usually encounters thin, nearly atrophic alar cartilages, whereas in the nose with thin skin the cartilages are usually well developed. Tip-plasty is a less successful procedure in the former. The relationship of the nose to the forehead, midface, and chin is also assessed.

Palpation along the dorsum is helpful in detecting a curvature of the dorsal border of the septum and the position of the septal angle. Digital pressure over the tip will show the location of the septal angle and the relationship of the alar cartilages to the septal angle. This test is particularly important. If the alar cartilages are dislocated caudally

from the septal angle and the membranous septum is unduly elongated, resection of the caudal portion of the septum is contraindicated because the deformity would be accentuated.

Careful intranasal examination of the septum, nasal floor, and turbinates with a speculum under adequate lighting and, if necessary, after application of a topical vasoconstrictor, such as 1 per cent Neo-Synephrine, usually shows any abnormality. The simplest test for nasal obstruction is to occlude one nostril at a time and listen and evaluate the passage of air while the patient breathes through the opposite nasal passage. Malfunction of the internal valve can be confirmed by elimination of the obstruction through dilation of the nasal vestibule with a speculum.

Planning the Operation. The patient who requests an esthetic improvement may not have a functional problem. The surgeon should question the patient concerning the functional impairment, if one is present, resulting from the deformity. He should also note the individual's psychologic reaction to what may seem to be a relatively minor defect as well as to a deformity of greater magnitude. The patient's motivation to cooperate with the surgeon in achieving a satisfactory result should be evaluated.

Critical listening to the patient is of particular importance in esthetic surgery. Beware of patients with unrealistic expectations and particularly of those who cannot be specific as to what they think is wrong. These patients are dangerous because they may never be satisfied. By carefully listening, the surgeon may detect a deep-seated psychologic disturbance that precludes the operation (see Chap. 3). The surgeon may undertake an operation that may not satisfy the patient: *a satisfactory result is what the patient perceives as a satisfactory result.*

Photography is useful in determining the indications for an operation. Professional photographs (see Chap. 1) taken with standardized position, lighting, and exposure permit the patient to see himself as he really is. The photographs should include the full face, both profiles, both obliques, a smiling view (which will show the caudal displacement of the tip), and a basal or "worm's eye" view that highlights the alar rims and any asymmetries.

The photograph is useful because it permits the patient first to react to his own image, second to point out to the surgeon what he thinks is wrong, and third to give the surgeon an opportunity to describe what corrective measures should and could achieve a satisfactory result. In this way an understanding is reached between the patient and the surgeon before the operation, thus avoiding a postoperative misunderstanding.

Certain modifications made on a profile matte-finished photograph are useful to show the patient how his appearance can be improved. Dorsal "humps" can be shaded with a No. 2 lead pencil and suggested augmentation of the chin can be done with a China white ink pen (Fig. 35–36). The patient thus has a preoperative concept of how he will look after the operation. Recent advances in computer imaging also permit this. *The surgeon, however, must be able to achieve what he has proposed.*

Misunderstandings between the patient and surgeon, some resulting in legal action, usually stem from a lack of communication. Careful explanation of the possibilities and impossibilities is essential. There is a tendency to shape the nose according to preconceived standards of beauty applicable to all patients. As stated earlier in the text, this often leads to a stereotyped nose that is obviously a "surgical" nose. A "natural"-looking nose, even though less "perfect," is preferable.

In planning a nasal plastic correction, it is essential to consider the entire face and even the patient's stature. In a broad face, it would be an error to overshorten the nose. When the patient's upper lip is shortened by the impingement of the nose and septum upon this structure, shortening of the nose provides not only a suitable nasal contour but also a more satisfactory length of the upper lip. The position and shape of the chin should also be considered, since an underdeveloped chin increases the relative prominence of the nose. In the patient shown in Figure 35–37, adequate nasal length was maintained for a harmonious face-nose relationship, while chin augmentation was indicated because of a deficiency of the mental symphysis (see Chap. 29).

Increase in the projection and augmentation of the chin by a variety of methods, which include an inorganic chin implant or genioplasty (horizontal advancement osteotomy) (see Chap. 29), may be necessary in order to obtain facial balance. Diminution of the forward projection of the chin is required in mandibular prognathism.

The success of the operation depends as much on the esthetic judgment of the surgeon as on his technical skill. Aufricht (1961) pointed out that a change in the shape of the nose is a serious undertaking equivalent to changing the entire face.

Aside from considerations involving the patient's facial type, the particular anatomy of the nose in which corrective surgery is being contemplated should be taken into account. The long, thin nose with fine, textured

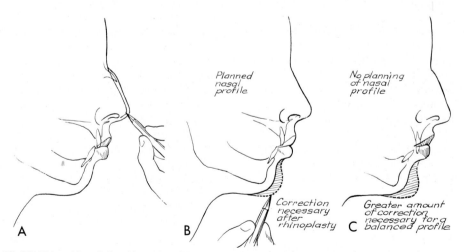

Figure 35–36. Nose-chin relationships; planning of a balanced profile. Such planning may be done on photographic prints prepared without a glossy finish. *A,* Proposed change in the nasal profile. Note the prominence of the nose in relation to the underdeveloped chin. *B,* The nasal profile has been modified, and the outline of the chin is also traced to provide a guide for the chin augmentation. *C,* The nasal profile has not been changed, but the overall appearance is improved. A greater amount of chin augmentation is necessary to achieve an acceptable facial profile.

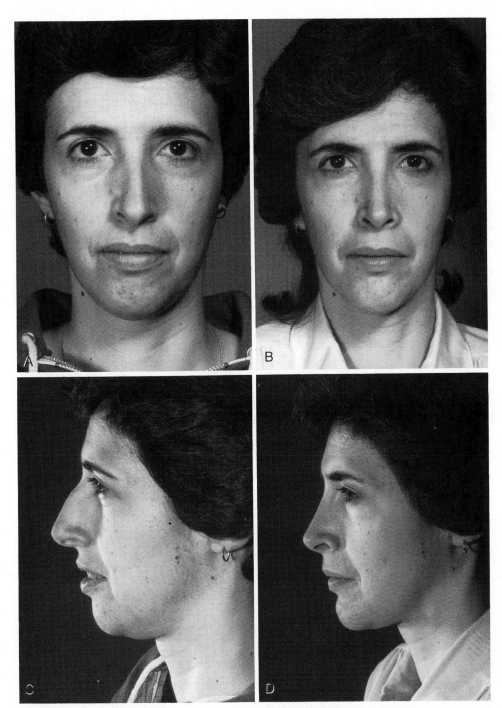

Figure 35–37. The importance of the chin in facial profile. Combined rhinoplasty and insertion of a chin implant. *A, C,* Preoperative views. Note the dorsal hump and projecting tip of the nose. There is microgenia but the occlusal status is acceptable. *B, D,* Appearance after rhinoplasty and insertion of a chin implant. There has been an associated reduction in the submental soft tissue excess.

skin is ideal for surgery. The broad nose with thick skin is always an unfavorable candidate. It seems paradoxical that the long nose with thin skin frequently has overdeveloped cartilages, so that any change in their contour can be embarrassingly evident through the thin skin. On the other hand, the patient with thick skin, which hides the reductive incisions through the cartilage, frequently has thin cartilages, making changes in contour difficult and at times impossible.

Anesthesia

Local anesthesia is commonly employed for corrective nasal plastic surgery.

The importance of correct preoperative medication must be emphasized. An adequately sedated patient experiences minimal bleeding during the operation, whereas an anxiety-ridden patient may bleed profusely. No direct relationship exists between the quantity of the medication administered and the resultant sedation because of the variable susceptibility of different individuals. Patients with a history of heavy alcohol or sleeping pill ingestion require larger doses of medication. A patient of small stature is susceptible to respiratory depression from only small doses.

A subliminal type of anesthesia can be achieved by the careful selection and dosage of sedative drugs. The patient is sleeping through most of the procedure and is mostly unaware that he is undergoing an operation. An example of a preoperative medication protocol is the following:

1. A hypnotic the night before operation, Seconal (secobarbital), 100 mg per os, or Dalmane (flurazepam), 30 mg per os.

2. Preoperative medication: two hours before surgery, Valium (diazepam), 10 to 15 mg per os; one hour before surgery, Pantopon (hydrochlorides of opium alkaloids), 10 to 15 mg intramuscularly, and Thorazine (chlorpromazine), 10 to 15 mg intramuscularly. An intravenous infusion is started before the operation and is used to administer incremental amounts of Valium (2.5 mg at a time) to maintain sedation as needed. Valium is preferred as a preoperative and intraoperative sedative because it is amnestic. Intravenous narcotics (morphine sulfate) can also be used as a supplementary drug.

Dosage of all agents should be adjusted to meet the needs of the individual patient.

Individuals of small stature should receive reduced amounts of all agents. The introduction of the oximeter has permitted careful intraoperative monitoring of blood oxygen saturation.

Hypotensive general anesthesia administered via an endotracheal tube provides a relatively bloodless field. This more complex technique is not advisable in the average corrective rhinoplasty. A considerable diminution in the amount of bleeding during a conventional anesthesia with intratracheal intubation (when required) can be obtained by local infiltration of lidocaine (Xylocaine)-epinephrine (Adrenalin) solution before induction.

Careful reassurance on the part of the surgeon is necessary at all times for the apprehensive patient; gaining the patient's confidence is an indispensable condition for satisfactory anesthesia.

Topical and Infiltration Anesthesia. Both topical and infiltration anesthesia are required in rhinoplasty surgery. The sensory innervation of the nose is illustrated in Figures 35–38 and 35–39. It is derived from two main sources: the anterior ethmoidal nerve and the sphenopalatine ganglion.

Topical anesthesia precedes infiltration anesthesia. Before draping, a 4 per cent cocaine solution is sprayed into each nasal fossa, providing superficial topical analgesia and vasoconstriction. After the patient has been prepared and draped, cotton pledgets are dipped in a solution of 5 per cent cocaine and introduced into the nasal cavity. The cotton should be squeezed to eliminate excess cocaine and thus avoid dripping of the drug into the nasopharynx.

One pledget is introduced through the nasal passage, under the dorsum to the root of the nose, where the anterior ethmoidal nerve enters the nasal cavity (Fig. 35–40). The other pledget is placed into the middle meatus situated beneath the middle turbinate and backward over the sphenopalatine ganglion. It is essential, however, to avoid any discomfort that will arouse the sedated patient. Unless the middle meatus is readily accessible, the cotton is placed between the septum and the middle turbinate.

Topical application is followed by *infiltration anesthesia* with local anesthetic solution. A solution of 1 per cent lidocaine (or procaine) mixed with a fresh solution of 1:1000 epinephrine at a concentration of 1:50,000 is employed.

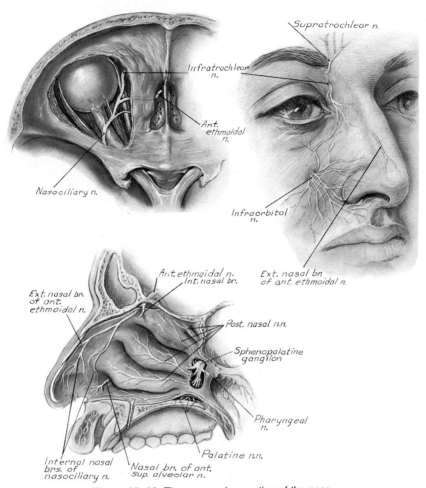

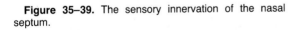

Figure 35–38. The sensory innervation of the nose.

Figure 35–39. The sensory innervation of the nasal septum.

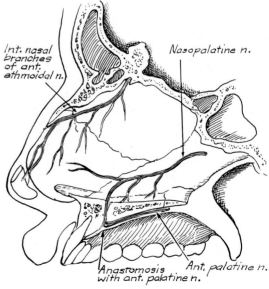

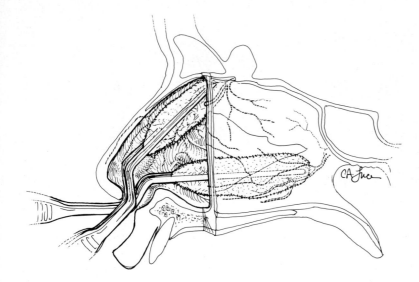

Figure 35–40. Topical nasal anesthesia. A cotton pledget, dampened in cocaine solution, is individually placed under the dorsum and in the middle meatus beneath the middle turbinate.

With a small volume of solution the entire nose may be injected, blocking the branches from the supra- and infratrochlear nerves and from the infraorbital, nasopalatine, and external nasal nerves. The anesthetic solution may also be injected in stages. Adverse reactions such as tachycardia, palpitations, headache, nervousness, restlessness, and anxiety are avoided.

The internal naris (the nasal valve) is exposed by retracting the ala. The solution is injected through a fine gauge needle into the tissues immediately above the caudal border of the lateral cartilage and directed toward the radix of the nose (Fig. 35–41). The plane of infiltration should follow the outer surface of the cartilage and bone. Another injection is made at the junction of the lateral cartilage and septum (Fig. 35–41C). A third injection is made in the region of the septal angle (Fig. 35–41D). Additional solution is injected between the layers of the membranous septum to block the nasopalatine nerve (Fig. 35–41E). The left ala is retracted, and an injection similar to the one on the right side is made. Additional injections on the left side are unnecessary.

Block anesthesia is also feasible by injection

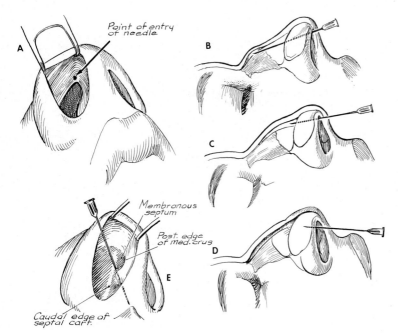

Figure 35–41. Corrective rhinoplasty under local anesthesia. *A,* Point of insertion of the needle. *B,* The needle is introduced between the alar and the lateral cartilages and passes over the lateral cartilage, the solution being injected at the root of the nose. *C,* As the needle is withdrawn, an injection is made at the junction of the lateral cartilage with the septum. *D,* The injection is continued on toward the septal angle. *E,* With a shorter needle the anesthetic solution is infiltrated within the two layers of the membranous septum at its base.

around the base of the nasal pyramid; however, in this technique the hemostatic benefits of the local infiltration of epinephrine are lost.

Adequate sedation, a suitable concentration of epinephrine, and careful dissection are factors that contribute toward the control of bleeding during the operation.

In children and in the occasional patient who reacts unfavorably to local anesthesia, general anesthesia administered by endotracheal intubation may be indicated.

Basic Technique

Some Preliminary Landmarks. The patient is placed on the operating table inclined at a 30 degree angle, only the head tilted downward (Fig. 35–42). After topical anesthesia and before infiltration anesthesia, it is essential to locate various landmarks before the first incision is made.

Good illumination is essential. A fiberoptic headlight provides the best illumination of the intranasal structures (Fig. 35–43). A fiberoptic angulated retractor enables the surgeon to see accurately any irregularity of the structures along the dorsum (Fig. 35–44).

Palpation along the dorsum indicates the position of the septal angle. The relationship of the septal angle to the alar cartilages determines the advisability of resecting a portion of the caudal part of the septal cartilage. If the tip is dislocated downward from the septal angle, it is no longer supported by

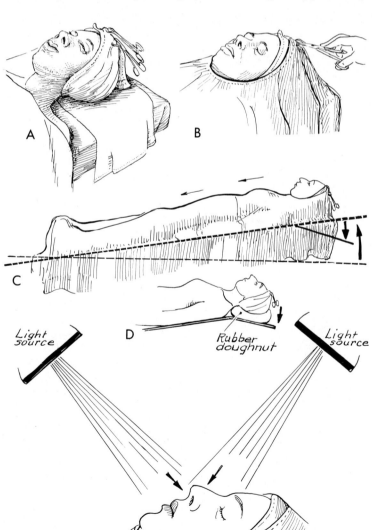

Figure 35–42. Position of the patient on the operating table, draping, and lighting. *A, B,* Draping the patient. *C,* Inclination of the table 30 degrees. *D,* The head is tilted back and rested on a rubber pad. *E,* Position of the operating lights.

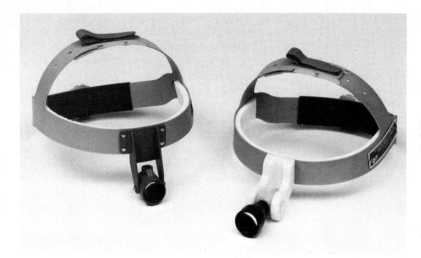

Figure 35–43. Two types of fiberoptic headlights that provide excellent visibility for intranasal surgery. (Designs for Vision, Inc.)

this structure. An attempt to shorten the nose by resecting cartilage from the caudal portion of the septum would only increase the downward dislocation of the tip. The septum must not be shortened; on the contrary, it may be necessary to reattach the alar cartilages to the septal angle by the invagination procedure (see Fig. 35–120).

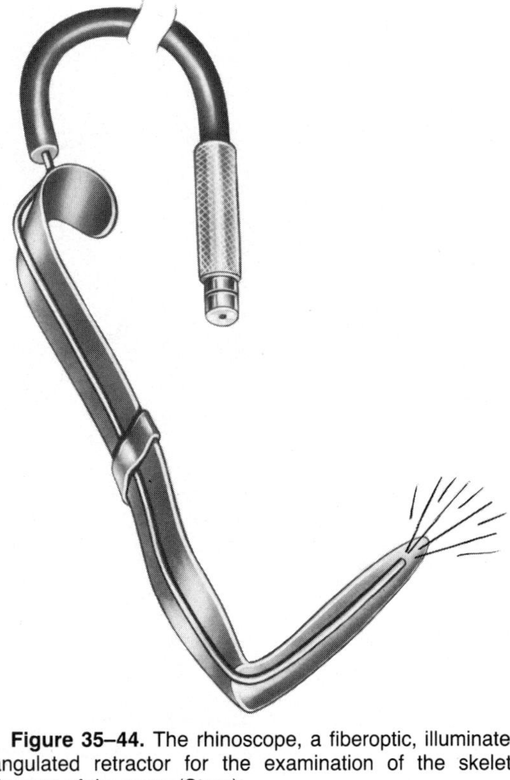

The degree of protrusion of the septal angle should also be considered in relation to the proposed profile line. In the humped nose, the septal angle may be situated high in relation to the alar cartilages. The position of the septal angle may be determined by inspection and palpation, and slight downward pressure on the tip of the nose will cause it to protrude.

Surface landmarks may be indicated on the skin of the nose. Upward traction of the skin of the supratip area causes blanching of the skin at the domes of the alar cartilages, thus locating the position of these structures (Fig. 35–45). A line can be drawn at the cephalic margin of each alar cartilage. An ink line divides the lateral crus into a cephalic and a caudal portion; the cephalic portion includes

Figure 35–44. The rhinoscope, a fiberoptic, illuminated, angulated retractor for the examination of the skeletal dorsum of the nose (Storz).

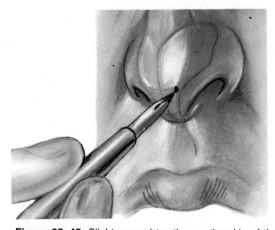

Figure 35–45. Slight upward traction on the skin of the supratip area causes blanching of the skin at the domes of the alar cartilages. The position of the dome can thus be located and marked with ink.

the undesirable convexity of the tip and is of variable width. Such ink landmarks are an aid during the operation.

The size and shape of the columella, its degree of protrusion in relation to the base of the alae, and the angle at which it meets the lip are noted. Abnormalities or deviations of the septum or turbinates should also be noted after careful examination by means of a headlight.

The various deformities demand different approaches and procedures. An order of procedure is helpful, however, not only in teaching but also in the operative treatment of the most common nasal deformity.

Evolution of Techniques. Before describing in detail the author's approach to the corrective rhinoplasty, it is helpful to review the evolution of the techniques.

The Joseph technique, introduced in the United States by Aufricht and Safian, has been employed as a routine procedure for rhinoplasty, minor modifications being devised by individual surgeons. The usual order of procedure is to make bilateral intercartilaginous incisions, skeletonize the nose, resect the dorsal osteocartilaginous hump with a saw, perform lateral osteotomies with a saw, perform a medial osteotomy and outfracture (Aufricht), and lastly carry out a Joseph- or Safian-type tip operation.

The operation is successful in the hands of experienced surgeons. Those less experienced often obtain good results in the correction of the large hump nose. Because too much hump was often resected by less experienced surgeons, it was frequently observed that many patients showed a concave dorsum and "operated" look. It also became evident that teaching the beginner the art of modifying the profile of the nose with a saw was a difficult undertaking.

Fomon (1960), Cottle (1960), and Aufricht (1961) performed routine septal resection procedures as part of the rhinoplasty to compensate for the narrowing of the nose. Fomon (1960) advocated complete resection of the septal framework, a technique that did not survive. Cottle (1960) used a "hemitransfixion" incision, an incision along the caudal border of the septum, as a routine approach to the septum and as a first procedure in the rhinoplasty. He was one of the first to advocate a "submucous" approach to spare the nasal valves.

Routine extensive septal operations are performed less often than previously. The septum is a source of the best transplant material in case the patient requires a secondary rhinoplasty; thus, limited amounts of cartilage are removed if the patient requires a cartilage graft in the course of the primary operation or has nasal airway obstruction (see the later section on septal surgery). Most patients have some degree of septal deviation, yet do not have symptoms of nasal obstruction.

Two principal modifications of the Joseph technique have evolved over the years: (1) the corrective surgery is begun at the caudal or cartilaginous portion of the nose and the remainder of the nasal skeletal framework is adapted according to the degree of projection of the tip; or (2) the bony dorsum is lowered as a first step and the cartilaginous portion is aligned to conform to the bony profile (Sheen, 1978).

In the Joseph technique, after resection of the osteocartilaginous hump, the tip is approached from the undersurface of the alar cartilage (from below). Sheen (1976) advocated realigning the entire cartilaginous dorsum through a subcutaneous approach (from above), retracting the soft tissues to obtain adequate exposure of the cartilaginous vault and approaching the nasal tip cartilages through rim incisions. These various techniques are individually discussed later in the text.

RHINOPLASTY: AN ORDER OF PROCEDURE

The operation follows an order of procedure composed of six stages. The advantage of this orderly approach is the complete control maintained by the surgeon in a step by step modification of the profile.

Stage 1: Uncovering the Nasal Framework

The ala is retracted and the vibrissae are cut with scissors (Fig. 35–46). The ala retractor straddles the most projecting and most caudal point of the dome, previously indicated by an ink mark. The caudal border of the lateral cartilage comes into view (Fig. 35–47). The intercartilaginous incision is made between the alar and lateral cartilages. When the ala is retracted, a line of mucous membrane is protracted with the alar cartilage. It is along this red line at the junction with the vestibular lining that the intercartilaginous

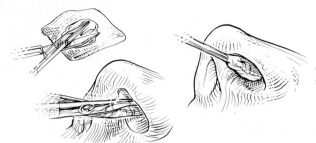

Figure 35–46. Cutting the vibrissae. The nasal vestibule is cleaned with a swab soaked in saline. The vibrissae are cut with scissors previously inserted in a lubricant for adherence of the hairs.

incision is made (Fig. 35–48A). The length of the incision, which should always extend to the midline, varies with the size of the hump to be removed and also depends on the amount of alar cartilage to be freed during the tip surgery.

It is a rule to avoid resecting vestibular lining, but in the case of the long nose with large vestibules, a small amount of vestibular lining is removed. In this situation the intercartilaginous incision is made a few millimeters caudad to the usual site between the lateral and alar cartilages. The excess vestibular lining is then removed when the caudal portion of the lateral cartilage is trimmed.

A double-blade Joseph knife (Fig. 35–49) is used to dissect the soft tissues from the lateral cartilage, extending the dissection to the midline (see Fig. 35–48B) and slightly over the midline. The plane of dissection should be as close as possible to the cartilage, thus preventing injury to the overlying musculature of the nose.

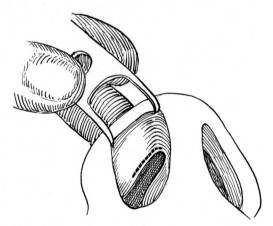

Figure 35–47. After retraction of the ala and eversion of the alar cartilage, the caudal border of the lateral cartilage (the nasal valve) comes into view. The incision is indicated by the line of junction between the red mucosa and the white vestibular skin. The incision can be extended laterally for increased exposure of the nasal dorsum.

An incision is then made in the periosteum near the caudal border of the nasal bones with the tip of the Joseph knife (see Fig. 35–48C). The handle of the knife should be maintained along a plane parallel with that of the dorsum of the nose to avoid buttonholing the skin with the tip of the instrument (Fig. 35–50).

A periosteal elevator is placed through the incision, and the periosteum is elevated to and over the midline (Figs. 35–51, 35–52). Similar procedures are repeated on the left side. Subperiosteal elevation over the nasal bones is routine, with less bleeding occurring than above the periosteal level. The elevated periosteum also serves to prevent adhesions of the overlying soft tissue to the modified nasal framework.

Transfixion Incision. The next procedure is known as the transfixion incision, a technique in which the soft tissues overlying the dorsum are separated from the septum (see Variations in Transfixion Incision, p. 1842). The procedure is facilitated if the surgeon moves to the head of the table and executes the maneuver from this position. A curved button knife (Fig. 35–53) is introduced through the intercartilaginous incision at the right internal naris into the subperiosteal pocket over the nasal bones (Fig. 35–54A). An incision is made with the button knife along the dorsal border of the septum (Fig. 35–54B) until the tip of the knife reaches the intercartilaginous incision at the internal naris of the opposite side (Fig. 35–54C). The tip of the button knife, which may be palpated with the operator's left index finger as it reaches the incision at the left internal naris, protrudes into the left vestibule, and the incision is continued to the septal angle (Fig. 35–55A). Prior to the incision along the caudal border of the septum, the membranous septum is tensed by a forward pull on the base of the columella by the assistant, employing hooks, and the tip of the nose is

Figure 35–48. The uncovering of the nasal framework. *A,* The intercartilaginous incision is of variable length, depending on the size of the hump to be resected, but always extends medially to the dorsal border of the septum. *B,* Sharp dissection over the lateral cartilage. *C,* The tip of the knife palpates the lower border of the nasal bone and incises the periosteum. A similar procedure is carried out on the contralateral side.

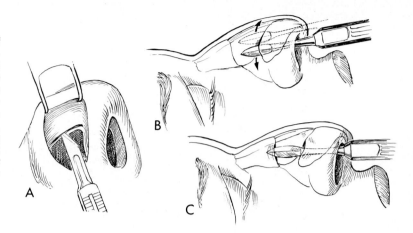

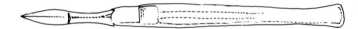

Figure 35–49. Modified Joseph knife.

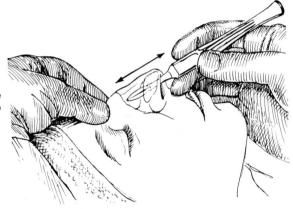

Figure 35–50. Position of the Joseph knife. The handle of the knife should be parallel to the dorsum of the nose to avoid perforation of the skin by the point of the knife.

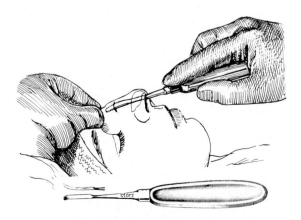

Figure 35–51. The periosteal elevator has been inserted through the incision in the periosteum to elevate the periosteum from the nasal bone. The periosteum is also raised on the contralateral side.

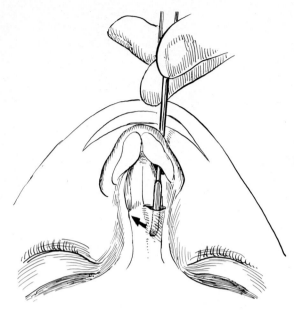

Figure 35–52. The periosteal elevator raising the periosteum over the bony dorsum.

Figure 35–53. Curved button knife used for the transfixion procedure.

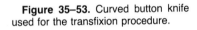

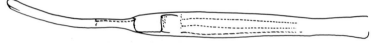

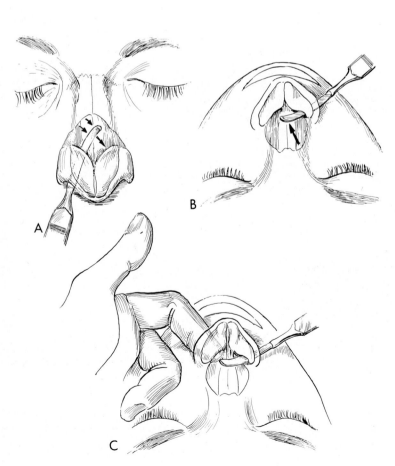

Figure 35–54. The transfixion incision. *A,* Position of the button knife, which has been placed in the subperiosteal pocket over the nasal bones and which separates the soft tissue structures from the dorsal border of the septal cartilage. *B,* Position of the button knife as it approaches the septal angle. *C,* The index finger of the left hand palpates inside the vestibule and feels for the tip of the knife projecting through the intercartilaginous incision.

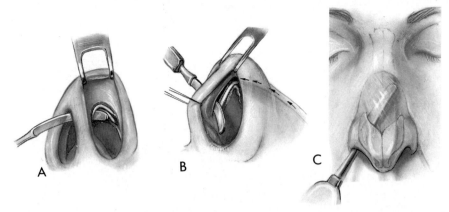

Figure 35–55. Completion of the transfixion procedure. *A,* The button knife is extruded through the intercartilaginous incision on the contralateral side. *B,* The incision is extended around the septal angle and downward along the caudal border of the septum. Note the upward retraction of the tip, and the forward traction on the columella by two hooks. *C,* The periosteal elevator verifies that the skeletal structures have been separated from the covering soft tissues.

retracted with a double-pronged retractor (Fig. 35–56); the button knife is then rotated approximately 90 degrees, cutting along the caudal margin of the septal cartilage toward the anterior nasal spine (see Fig. 35–55*B*).

A pair of scissors extends the transfixion incision toward the nasal spine if surgery on the nasal spine, the base of the septal cartilage or the depressor muscle is required. The periosteal elevator verifies that the exposure of the nasal framework is completed (Fig. 35–55*C*).

In the average rhinoplasty, it is preferable to elevate the soft tissues over an area only wide enough to permit resection of the nasal dorsal hump, leaving intact the soft tissue on the lateral aspect of the nose (Fig. 35–57). In large noses and in older patients, the raising of soft tissues over a wide area allows for a more complete redistribution of the skin over the reduced skeletal framework. An incision through the periosteum over the lateral aspect of the lateral wall on each side also assists in the redraping of the soft tissues in the large nose after modification of the underlying structural framework.

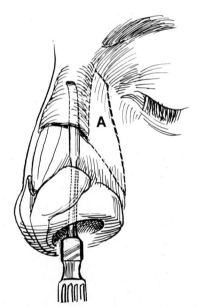

Figure 35–57. The outlined area delimits the area of undisturbed periosteum between the dorsal portion of the nose and the line of the lateral osteotomy, as indicated by the letter *A.* The periosteum over the dorsal portion of the nose is raised over an area only sufficient to permit resection of the dorsal hump. The larger the hump, the wider will be the area of subperiosteal elevation.

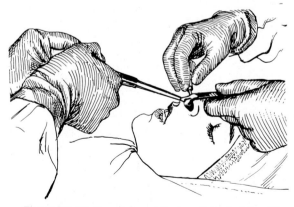

Figure 35–56. Completion of the transfixion incision. The operator retracts the tip upward; the assistant exerts forward traction upon the columella and the membranous septum.

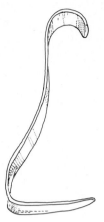

Figure 35–58. Angulated retractor used for examination of the dorsum and detachment of the lateral cartilages.

Stage 2: Lowering the Cartilaginous Septal Profile; Shortening the Septum; Correcting the Nasal Tip

An angulated Aufricht retractor (Fig. 35–58) elevates the soft tissues over the dorsum of the nose. The major portion of each lateral cartilage is separated from the septum with a No. 11 blade after the lateral cartilages are retracted with forceps (Fig. 35–59*A*). As illustrated in Figure 35–59*B*, the mucoperichondrium has been raised, after the anesthetic solution has been infiltrated between the mucoperichondrium and the cartilage. However, many surgeons consider this technique unnecessary in the large hump nose (see Submucous Approach, p. 1843).

Although separation of the lateral cartilages from the septum is necessary and inevitable during surgery on the nose with a large dorsal hump, this procedure should not be regarded as routine. When the hump is relatively small, it is possible to shave the cartilaginous dorsum without detaching the lateral cartilages from the septum.

An angulated retractor exposes the septal angle and the dorsal border of the septal cartilage and provides exposure of the structures. Under direct vision with angulated scissors (Fig. 35–60), the dorsal border of the septum is trimmed, starting at the septal angle, so that the nasal tip stands free without support from the septum (Fig. 35–61).

The medial portions of the lateral cartilages are not trimmed at this stage; they will be adjusted to the dorsal border of the septum during the fifth stage. Thus, they are trimmed only once.

At this point in the operation, the relationship between the nasal tip and the dorsum

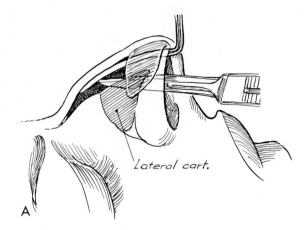

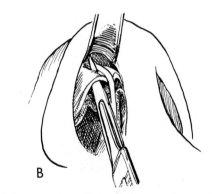

Figure 35–59. *A*, Severing the attachment of the lateral cartilage to the septum. *B*, The most cephalic portion of each lateral cartilage is not severed from the septum and remains attached to the nasal bone.

usually changes. For example, in the nose with a short columella, the tip, which has been tethered by this structure, assumes a more cephalad and projected position. The

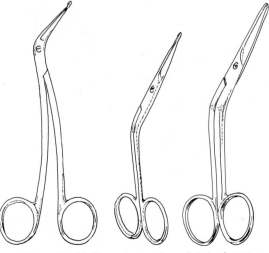

Figure 35–60. Three types of angulated scissors.

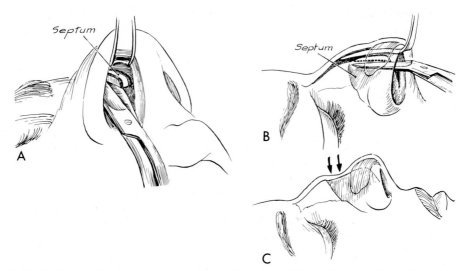

Figure 35–61. *A,* The angulated scissors lower the cartilaginous profile. *B,* The resection of the septal cartilage is along an oblique line. *C,* The dorsal hump is thus accentuated.

amount of shortening of the septum may then be less than originally planned. The change of position of the nasal tip is particularly noticeable in noses in which the tip, before the operation, was dislocated downward from the septal angle and in noses in which the position of the tip is influenced by overactive depressor septi muscles, an overdeveloped nasal spine, or septal cartilage protruding and invading the upper lip. Release of the tip from these contractile factors lengthens the columella and modifies the position of this important structure of the nose; often, little or no cartilage resection is required from the caudal edge of the septal cartilage.

When indicated, a segment of cartilage is removed from the caudal border of the septal cartilage. The columella is retracted by the assistant, exposing the caudal margin of the septum and the septal angle (Fig. 35–62). The cartilage is steadied by grasping it with tooth forceps, and a suitable amount is excised (Fig. 35–63). It is preferable to remove the cartilage with a knife from below (nasal spine) upward, following a curve that parallels the curve of the columella.

Prudence is required in shortening the septum. Overshortening is a frequent mistake that results in a flat nasal base owing to the disruption of the columella-ala triangle.

Excess septal cartilage over the nasal spine is removed, when indicated, thus correcting an excessively narrow nasolabial angle usually caused by a protrusion of the caudal

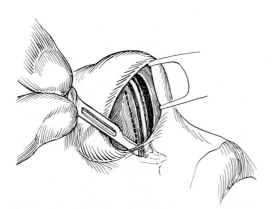

Figure 35–62. The retractor exposes the caudal edge of the septal cartilage; the segment to be resected is outlined.

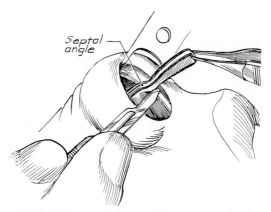

Figure 35–63. Shortening the septum. A segment of the caudal portion of the septum is resected.

margin of the septal cartilage into the lip. If the nasal spine is unduly protrusive and the upper lip is short, the nasal spine is trimmed or resected.

The change in the dorsal profile is evaluated by applying finger pressure over the septum; the protruding lateral cartilages are pressed down and out of the way.

At this point in the operation, the dorsal (bony) hump is accentuated and the tip appears protrusive (Fig. 35–64). The tip has also assumed a slightly more cephalic position.

Even when the tip of the nose appears adequate in shape and size preoperatively, surgery is required if the contour of the nasal dorsum is modified. The lateral crura of the alar cartilages are still shaped to fit the former convex dorsum. If they are not corrected, they will not fit the newly contoured dorsum, and a "polly-tip" deformity could result.

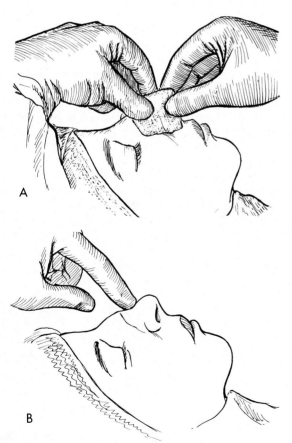

Figure 35–64. *A,* Gauze is placed over the nose, and blood is gently squeezed from the undermined spaces. *B,* At this point in the operation, the dorsal (bony) hump is accentuated.

Two main objectives of a corrective tip operation are (1) to resect excess cartilage and thus reduce the size of the nasal tip and permit its reshaping, and (2) to weaken the cartilage between the lateral and medial crura in order that the lateral crus may "lie down" and assume a position in harmony with the new profile line of the nose.

Tip Operation: A Technique. An injection of local anesthetic solution at the base of each ala ensures completion of the block anesthesia of the tip of the nose. Previous injections have blocked branches from the external nasal and nasopalatine nerves. A small amount of the anesthetic solution is also injected under the vestibular skin ("hydrodissection") to facilitate elevation of the bipedicle flap.

After retraction of the ala, an incision is made through the vestibular lining but not through the cartilage (Fig. 35–65A). The incision extends from the dome and runs laterally in a position parallel to the alar rims. The length of the incision and its position depend on the amount of cartilage to be resected cephalad. The extent of the cartilage to be resected varies and should not be standardized. The incision should be parallel to the caudal border of the lateral crus and is usually located at a distance not exceeding 3 or 4 mm from this border. Dissection in a caudad direction can confirm the position of the caudal margin. Preservation of the continuity of the cartilage along the caudal margin of the alar cartilage prevents a displacement of the lateral edges of the sectioned cartilage, which protrude as two small "horns" under the skin of the tip of the nose postoperatively. In the broad tip, it may be necessary to transgress the caudal border of the alar cartilage, removing a sizable piece of cartilage in order to reduce the width of the nasal tip. A suture should be placed to approximate the medial and lateral portions of the cartilage and prevent irregularities of contour of the caudal edge of the tip cartilages.

Angulated scissors (Fig. 35–66) elevate the bipedicle vestibular flap from the undersurface of the cartilage (Fig. 35–65B). An incision through the cartilage is then made (Fig. 35–65C), and the overlying cutaneous coverage of the cartilage is raised.

The transcartilaginous incision has divided the cartilage into cephalic and caudal segments; the cartilage situated cephalad to the cartilage-splitting incision is resected (Fig.

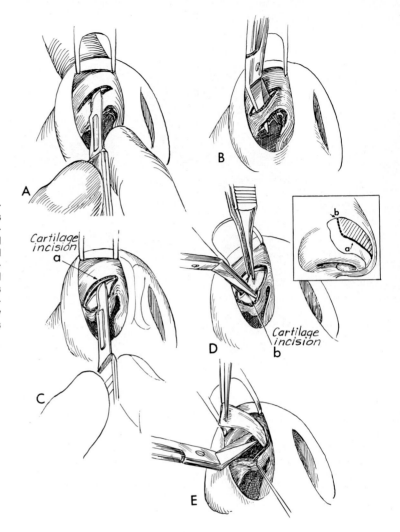

Figure 35–65. The nasal tip operation: a technique. *A,* An incision is made through the vestibular lining parallel to the caudal border of the lateral crus. *B,* The vestibular lining is raised from the cartilage. *C,* The transcartilaginous incision is made. *D,* The lateral portion of the lateral crus is divided, as indicated in the inset. The line of section is parallel to the proposed new profile of the nose. *E,* The cartilage is removed.

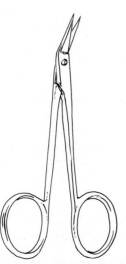

Figure 35–66. Small angulated scissors for tip surgery.

35–65*D,E*). In order to facilitate the procedure, the assistant holds the alar retractor in one hand, everting the ala with the middle finger, and a hook retracting the bipedicle flap of vestibular lining in the other hand. The operator's two hands are therefore free, and with the aid of forceps and small angulated scissors may proceed with the resection of the desired amount of alar cartilage (Fig. 35–67). The cartilage is sectioned at a suitable point and extruded. The sagittal cut through the lateral crus should be parallel to the caudal portion of the dorsum of the septum. The lateral portion of the lateral crus of the alar cartilage usually is not resected in the average case in order to avoid postoperative constriction of the nares. The extent of the cartilage resection is determined by the extent of the convexity of the tip. Excessive

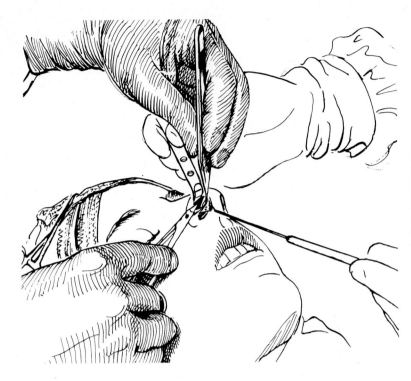

Figure 35–67. Position of the operator's and the assistant's hands during the tip operation. The assistant is retracting the ala and the vestibular skin flap by means of a hook and retractor. The operator's hands are holding the cartilaginous segment to be excised with forceps, and the small angulated scissors are used to complete the resection.

removal of cartilage results in a "pinched-tip" deformity, which may not become apparent until two or three years after the operation. Small, blunt-tipped (Stevens) scissors free the skin over the supratip area. If the tip is slightly bifid, small, angulated scissors (see Fig. 35–66) are placed in a retrograde fashion between the domes, severing the fibroareolar tissue between them, thus making it possible to approximate the domes (Fig. 35–68). If the domes are adequately approximated, this area is not disturbed.

The amount of cartilage to be resected should be carefully predetermined. However,

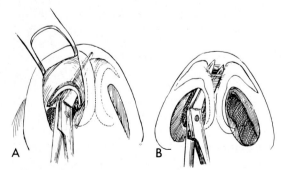

Figure 35–68. *A,* The small angulated scissors are placed between the medial crura and the domes. *B,* Dividing the fibroareolar tissue between the domes. This is an effective way to approximate the domes if there is mild bifidity of the tip.

the contour may not be entirely satisfactory; additional cartilage resection may be required. The cartilage at the dome may be reshaped by *partial-thickness* cuts. A short rim incision is made and the dome is exposed. A number of incisions made in the cartilage thus accentuate the angle of the dome.

In deformities of lesser degree, narrowing of the tip is obtained by resecting a measured strip of cartilage parallel to the superomedial border of the lateral crus of the alar cartilage (Fig. 35–69).

Three precautions should be observed in performing surgical modifications of the shape of the alar cartilage:

1. Avoid raw areas resulting from removal of vestibular lining; the healing of such defects by secondary intention results in scar formation and distorting contracture.

2. Avoid excessive removal of cartilage to avoid a "pinched" appearance. In the region of the dome, excessive removal may leave a gap between the pieces of cartilage, resulting in an unsightly groove in the skin of the tip of the nose.

3. Avoid sharp angles and protuberances due to overlapping cartilaginous fragments or improperly shaped cartilaginous grafts which may produce external irregular prominences. This is especially true in the patient with thin nasal skin.

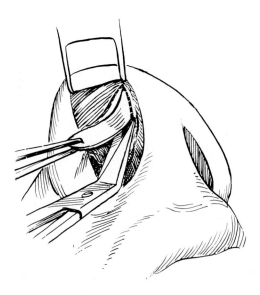

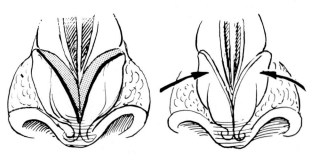

Figure 35–69. Minimal resection from the superomedial portion of each lateral crus when only a slight change of shape of the nasal tip is indicated.

Stage 3: Resecting the Bony Hump

Removal of the bony hump precedes the final correction of the profile (resection of the dorsal border of each lateral cartilage and the final trimming of the septum). A double-guarded osteotome of adequate width (usually 14 mm) is placed at the caudal border of the undisturbed area of the cartilaginous dorsum, the area where the cephalic portions of the lateral cartilages and septum are continuous with the bony dorsum. The lateral cartilages are reflected laterally to allow the placing of the osteotome. The amount of bone to be removed is determined by the projection of the tip.

Osteotome Technique. The osteotome is held in the right hand while the operator's left hand raises the skin of the dorsum to protect it from injury. The osteotome is advanced by carefully applied blows of the mallet administered by the assistant. Before completing the separation of the hump, a narrower osteotome (12 mm) is used to section the upper portion (Fig. 35–70). The hump, once freed, is removed by hump removal forceps (Fig. 35–71). Any irregular bony edges are smoothed with a sharp rasp.

Rasp Technique. The rasp bevels the lateral edges of the sectioned lateral walls, thus reproducing the rounded shape of the bony dorsum (Fig. 35–72). A dull-edged curette or

Figure 35–70. Resection of the bony hump with an osteotome. *A,* The shaded area represents the amount of bone to be resected along the bony dorsum. *B,* The osteotome is placed at the protruding end of the nasal hump. Note that the skin is raised in order to avoid injury during the procedure. *C,* One type of osteotome for hump resection.

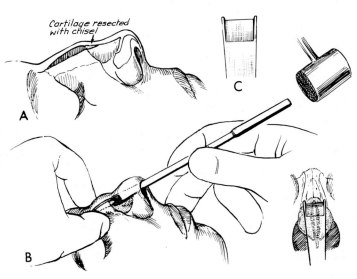

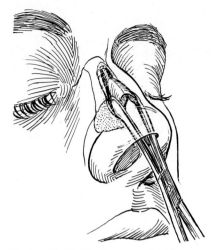

Figure 35–71. The hump removal forceps.

suction removes the debris that results from rasping.

For the removal of all but large bony humps, the rasp is often the most efficient instrument (see Sheen's Technique, p. 1841). A sharp rasp gradually reduces the bone and maintains the rounded dorsal border and the lateral convex curvatures of the bony dorsum.

At this point in the operation, the bony dorsum and the major portion of the septal border have been lowered; the lateral cartilages and a portion of the septum still protrude (Fig. 35–73).

Stage 4: Lateral (and Medial) Osteotomies of Lateral Walls of Nose

Lateral Osteotomy: Start Low, Finish High. The dorsal hump has been removed.

The lateral walls, therefore, must be approximated to avoid a "flat top" nasal vault. Inspection of the skeletal dorsum using an angulated retractor will show the remaining protruding dorsal septal border and the medial borders of the lateral cartilages. These structures will not be adjusted to the new profile line until after the lateral osteotomies have been completed.

Considerable changes in the concept of the osteotomy have arisen since the technique first advocated by Joseph, in which an angulated saw was used to section the base of the lateral wall of the nose (the frontal process). Undue emphasis has been placed on the need for a low osteotomy in the upper portion of the osteotomy line. The lacrimal sac was reported to be injured in a high proportion of osteotomies (Flowers and Anderson, 1968). As emphasized by Sheen (1976), the lateral osteotomy should be *high* rather than *low* in the region of the root of the nose in the average corrective rhinoplasty (Fig. 35–74). The reasons for this position include the following:

1. Attempting to narrow the root of the nose in most patients may be a mistake, because such a procedure may cause an illusion of an increased distance between the eyes.

2. If the line of osteotomy extends upward above the area of junction of eyelid and nasal skin and if this "frontier" is not transgressed, periorbital ecchymosis can be minimized or even prevented.

There are two techniques of lateral osteotomy, *extranasal* and *intranasal*.

When the *extranasal* or subcutaneous os-

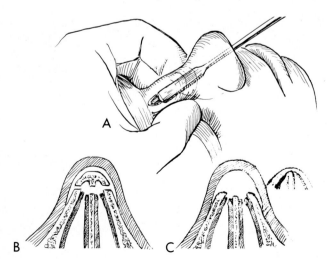

Figure 35–72. *A,* Rasping the bony edges after the resection of the hump. *B,* Frontal section showing the portion of the bony dorsum that has been resected. *C,* The bony edges are beveled with the rasp, so that when they are approximated following the lateral osteotomy, they will reproduce the rounded shape of the bony dorsum.

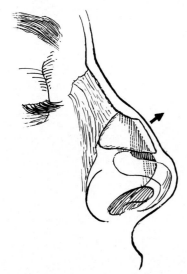

Figure 35–73. At this point in the operation, the nasal tip operation has been performed and a major portion of the dorsal border of the septum has been lowered. The bone has also been resected. The lateral cartilages and a portion of the dorsal border of the septum protrude. These structures will be trimmed *after* the lateral osteotomies.

teotomy technique is employed, the ala is retracted outward, and a longer needle is introduced into the vestibule lateral to the border of the piriform aperture; this is passed upward, following the contour of the bone. At the root of the nose, the needle remains above the eyelid-nose skin junction in order to minimize ecchymoses of the eyelids; the lidocaine-epinephrine solution blocks the branches from the intratrochlear and infraorbital nerves. A previously made injection immediately caudad to the inferior turbinate has blocked the nasal branches of the anterosuperior alveolar nerve.

When the *intranasal* or submucous osteotomy technique is employed, the edge of the piriform aperture is located by palpation with

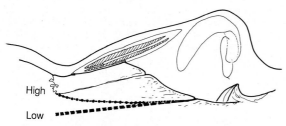

Figure 35–74. Low to high lateral osteotomy (Sheen, 1978). The osteotomy within the frontal process of the maxilla is begun at the piriform aperture *(low)* and extended *high* at the root of the nose. A low to low osteotomy is also illustrated.

an instrument and the needle is passed from the piriform aperture near the floor of the nose along the *medial* aspect of the frontal process, hugging the bone; thus, the needle is under the mucoperiosteum. The needle is inserted *low* and progresses to the root of the nose, where the tip of the needle is *high*, i.e., above the eyelid-nose skin junction.

Osteotome Technique: Extranasal Lateral Osteotomy. With practice, a satisfactory osteotomy is performed with a 3 mm wide osteotome or chisel (Fig. 35–75). The osteotome is placed in the vestibule at the edge of the piriform aperture; it pierces the lining of the vestibule and is tapped gently upward through loose subcutaneous tissue along the base of the lateral wall (Fig. 35–76). It is not necessary to elevate the periosteum along the base of the lateral wall. The osteotomy is started low at the piriform aperture and ends high near the junction of the frontal process and the nasal bone. After bilateral osteotomy, manual pressure fractures the bones medially, first on one side, then on the other.

Osteotome Technique: Intranasal Lateral Osteotomy. Another technique is the intranasal or submucous technique of lateral

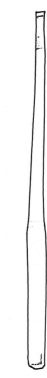

Figure 35–75. The 3 mm wide osteotome for the lateral osteotomy.

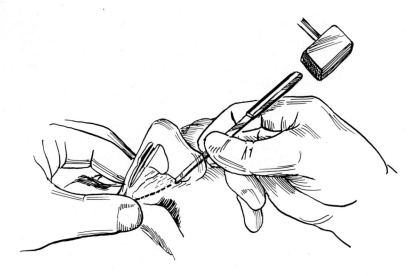

Figure 35–76. Extranasal lateral osteotomy with the 3 mm osteotome.

osteotomy (Hilger, 1968). The blunt end of the Joseph knife is used to locate the border of the piriform aperture at its base; an incision is made through the mucoperiosteum at the edge of the piriform aperture (Fig. 35–77A). The mucoperiosteum is raised from the *medial* aspect of the lateral wall of the nose by means of the Joseph periosteal elevator (Fig. 35–77B). The guarded osteotome (Fig. 35–78) is then introduced through a submucous tunnel. The osteotomy is performed from inside out instead of from outside in, as in the technique described above (Fig. 35–77C,D). The intranasal submucous osteotomy appears to cause a lesser degree of periorbital ecchymosis than the extranasal osteotomy.

Infracture. Digital pressure exerted alternately over one lateral wall, then over the contralateral wall, achieves the infracture. The cephalic portion of the lateral wall is not fractured. The *transverse* fracture at the junction of the infractured lateral wall and the undisturbed nasal bridge may occasionally result in a step; a rasp or osteotome will

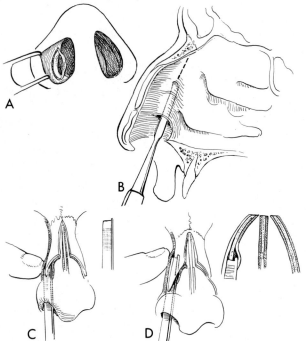

Figure 35–77. The intranasal lateral osteotomy. *A,* An incision made at the edge of the piriform aperture. *B,* Submucoperiosteal elevation along the base of the frontal process of the maxilla. *C,* A guarded osteotome (see Fig. 35–78) is introduced. *D,* The guarded osteotome progresses along the lateral wall, being tapped upward by a mallet. Note the finger palpating the edge of the osteotome at the base of the lateral wall of the nose.

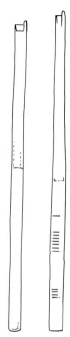

Figure 35–78. Guarded osteotomes for the intranasal lateral osteotomy. They are also used for outfracturing the lateral walls (medial osteotomy).

uniform line of osteotomy; by weakening the bone by a series of cuts with the osteotome, the lateral walls can be pressed inward.

Medial Osteotomy: Outfracturing Procedure. This procedure was advocated by Aufricht (1943) to fracture the remaining cephalic attachment of the lateral nasal wall after the lateral osteotomy and to loosen the lateral wall in order to facilitate the infracture.

An osteotome (Fig. 35–78) is placed in the space between the cut edge of the nasal bone and the septum to outfracture the lateral wall. A line of section upward through the remaining bone is established by the use of a mallet and osteotome (Fig. 35–79A). A characteristic dull sound is heard when the osteotome penetrates the frontal bone at the root of the nose. This "sign of the sound" indicates that the instrument is now solidly fixed in the bone. The osteotome is levered outward from the frontal bone, and the remaining attachment of the nasal bone and the frontal process is outfractured (Fig. 35–79B).

The purpose of outfracturing is threefold: (1) to disconnect the remaining upper attachment of the lateral nasal wall (the "transverse osteotomy"); (2) to ensure adequate loosening at the line of osteotomy; and (3) to establish sufficient space for the insertion of a rongeur to remove the remaining bony web.

The dorsal hump is usually situated consid-

readily plane down the protruding cephalic bone. It is not essential in the younger patient that the lateral wall be sectioned along a

Figure 35–79. Medial osteotomy. Outfracturing. *A,* The guarded osteotome is hammered into the solid bone at the root of the nose. *B,* The osteotome is rotated outward, outfracturing the lateral wall of the nose. Outfracturing is rarely indicated in the average corrective rhinoplasty; the technique is used for traumatic deformities and exceptionally wide noses.

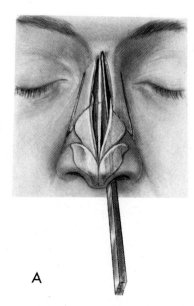

A

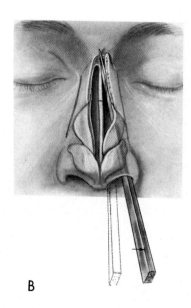

B

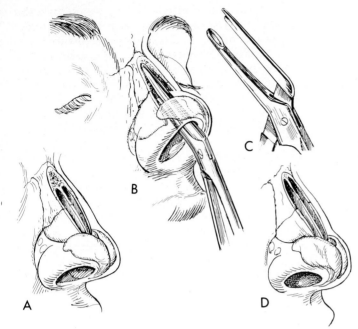

Figure 35–80. Removal of a bony wedge at the root of the wide nose. *A,* The bony wedge remaining on each side of the septum after resection of the hump. The bony wedge is formed by thick bone at the root of the nose, the superimposition of the nasal spine of the frontal bone, and the thick portion of the nasal bone. *B,* Rongeur in position removing the wedge of bone. *C,* Design of the rongeur. The upper blade is guarded to avoid including soft tissue into the cutting portion of the rongeur. *D,* The nasal dorsum after removal of the bony wedge on each side. This procedure facilitates the infracture and avoids an excessive width at the upper portion of the bony dorsum.

erably below the level of the nasofrontal angle. After removal of the hump, a gap exists in the continuity of the dorsum in the area from which the hump has been excised, and direct examination with a retractor shows the cut surfaces of the lateral bony walls and lateral cartilages separated in their midline by the cut surface of the septum. Above this area of the hump excision, however, the nasal dorsum shows an undisturbed vault where the bones remain in continuity. Infracture of the lateral walls at this stage would result in narrowing of the nose below the level of the undisturbed bony vault. It will be recalled that the root of the nose is formed of thick bones; the upper portions of the nasal bones are short and thick and are further reinforced by the thick nasal spine of the frontal bone.

Removal of a wedge of bone from this area on each side of the septum is required only when the area of the root of the nose is wide. The bony wedge can be removed after completion of the resection of the bony hump (Fig. 35–80). If the rongeur cannot be introduced for lack of space, the procedure is performed after the outfracture of the lateral walls. Removal of the wedge of bone provides sufficient space for medial displacement of the upper portion of the lateral walls of the nose. Thus, the nose is adequately narrowed in its upper portion, an important feature

when a large, wide nose is being reduced in size.

The lateral walls can now be infractured and displaced medially, joining each other in the midline (Fig. 35–81).

Following infracture, the lateral osteotomy line should be palpated to determine whether any stepping is present. This complication may result when the osteotomy has been placed at too high a level in the lower portion of the osteotomy rather than at the base of

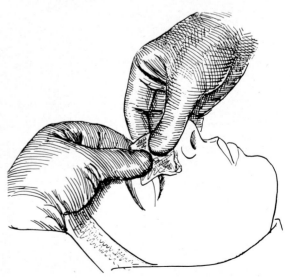

Figure 35–81. Infracture of the lateral walls.

the frontal process where it arises from the body of the maxilla. If the osteotomy is too high, a ridge lateral to the osteotomy line may result in a steplike protuberance at the base of the lateral wall. If such a complication occurs, the crest remaining at the base of the lateral wall should be fractured inwardly; a simple technique involves use of a narrow, tapered (2 mm) osteotome placed through the vestibule or skin at the upper end of the nasolabial fold.

Stage 5: Trimming Dorsal Border of Septal Cartilage, Medial and Caudal Borders of Lateral Cartilages

After the lateral osteotomies and the infracture, the bony nose has settled to a lower level. It is therefore preferable to make the final adjustment of the profile line and to trim the medial borders of the lateral cartilages and the septum at this stage of the operation. These procedures are performed under direct inspection, using an angle retractor with illumination (see Fig. 35–44) and angulated scissors.

The medial border of the right lateral cartilage is trimmed and adjusted to the new profile line with the angulated scissors (Fig. 35–82). This procedure provides a good view of the septum. The dorsal septal border is also trimmed appropriately. Finally, the left lateral cartilage is also adjusted.

The "Final Look." The esthetic result of a corrective nasal operation often depends on careful last-minute inspection and palpation. The "final look" at the dorsal skeletal structures under good illumination is most important; loose pieces of bone or cartilage and irregularities of contour of the cut edges of the bones and cartilage are removed. The dorsum of the nose is carefully palpated for irregularities. Additional correction may include rasping or the use of the osteotome in the upper portion of the dorsum; rasping the dorsal edge of the bone; and additional trimming of cartilage along the dorsal border of the septal cartilage, particularly in the region of the septal angle. "If the nose looks good on the inside, it will look good on the outside" (Diamond).

It must be emphasized that a deviation or excessive thickness of the dorsal portion of the septum is the usual cause of postoperative widening of the nose after osteotomy. Measures should be taken at this stage to correct such deviations; the techniques for this purpose are described later in this chapter. When an angle retractor is used with good illumination to elevate the soft tissues, an excellent opportunity is afforded to examine the shape, size, and position of the septum. An excessively thick dorsal portion of the septum may prevent approximation of the lateral walls in the midline and require thinning (Fig. 35–83).

Forestalling the Supratip Protrusion. A slight protrusion in the supratip region may spoil an otherwise satisfactory profile. This complication has two principal causes:

1. Inadequate reduction of the projection of the septal angle, which protrudes under the skin in the supratip area. The septal angle should be checked under direct vision. A gentle downward pressure at the columella-tip junction will cause it to blanch the skin if the angle is not sufficiently reduced.

2. Excessive reduction of the dorsum of the nose in patients with thick skin and large sebaceous glands. The unyielding skin does not adapt to the underlying framework and maintains a round protuberance at the tip and supratip area.

Final Procedures. The nose is compressed

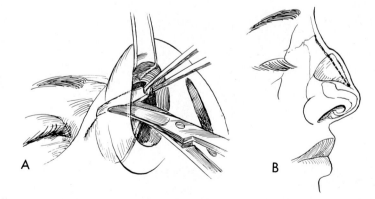

Figure 35–82. The final trimming of the dorsum. The medial edge of each lateral cartilage is trimmed with angulated scissors to the level of the dorsum of the septum, which itself has also been trimmed. The final profile of the nose is achieved.

A

B

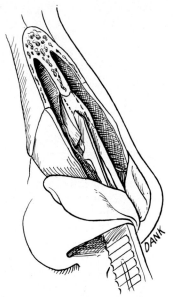

Figure 35–83. A thick septum as a cause for inadequate narrowing of the nose following osteotomy and infracturing of the lateral nasal walls. A frequent site of a wide dorsal edge of the septum is at the junction of the septal cartilage and the ethmoid plate (the tubercle of the septum). Thinning of the septal cartilage is obtained by paring with a knife.

upon completion of the operation; blood is squeezed from the undermined spaces by gentle finger pressure with gauze compresses. The transcartilaginous incision through the lateral crus of the alar cartilage is often sutured with plain catgut (Fig. 35–84). The intercartilaginous incision usually is not sutured. A single transfixion suture through the caudal septum and the columella approximates these structures.

Trimming Caudal Ends of Each Lateral Cartilage. After the suturing is completed, the last surgical procedure of the corrective

rhinoplasty is performed, if indicated. Respect for the integrity of the nasal valve has been emphasized earlier in the text. The purpose of such trimming is to adjust the lateral cartilages to the new nasal length. The lateral cartilage protrudes into the vestibule in a long nose that has been shortened. Resection of an excessive amount of the caudal portion of the lateral cartilage with attached mucoperichondrium is a frequent cause of disturbance of nasal physiology. Resection of lateral cartilage, if indicated, should be done with extreme caution. Overresection of the lateral cartilage also causes postoperative retraction of the ala. The cartilage may be trimmed prudently (Fig. 35–85). The ala should not be retracted excessively since this exaggerates the amount of overhang of the caudal border of the lateral cartilage.

Stage 6: Splinting the Nose

Intranasal packing may be dispensed with in the routine corrective nasalplastic operation. A dorsal strip of adhesive tape secures the lateral crura and obliterates any dead space between the septal angle and the soft tissues and cartilages. The application of the skin against the septum, as illustrated in Figure 35–86, is an important measure to prevent the dead space between the dorsal skin of the nose and the dorsal border of the septal cartilage. Additional strips are placed over the dorsum.

The postoperative nasal splint immobilizes the tissues and maintains them against the framework, thus preventing hematoma formation. Aquaplast, employed in the splinting technique, is softened in hot water (Fig. 35–87) and molded evenly over the nasal pyramid. It is hardened in situ.

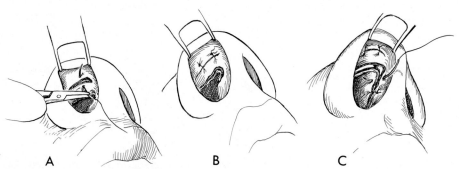

A   B   C

Figure 35–84. Suturing the transcartilaginous incision *(A, B)* and the transfixion incision *(C)*. The latter is usually full thickness.

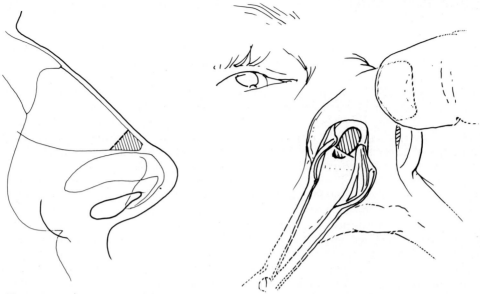

Figure 35–85. Resection of the caudal border of the upper lateral cartilage must be prudent to prevent foreshortening of the nose.

Figure 35–86. Stage 6: splinting the nose. *A,* One or more pieces of tape are strapped across the dorsal border of the septum in the supratip area. This important measure prevents a void between the dorsal skin and the septum. *B,* A strip of paper tape is placed sling-fashion around the tip of the nose to maintain contact between the columella and the septum. *C,* Pinching the tape to take up any slack. *D,* Completion of adhesive strapping of the nose.

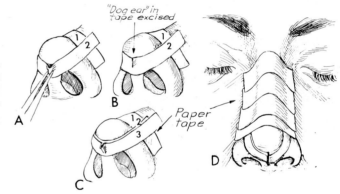

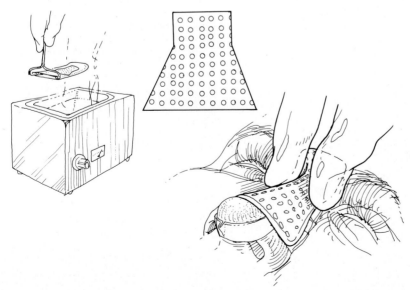

Figure 35–87. Application of the nasal splint. The splint is inserted into a hot water bath. When it is lucent and pliable, the plastic is removed, allowed to cool, and shaped to the nose.

Adjunctive Techniques

Modification of Alar Base. Careful consideration should be given to surgical modification of the alar bases. The facial features should be considered in their entirety, and frequently the wide, thick alae may "fit" the broad or rounded face. The alar base position is best evaluated from the "worm's eye" or basilar view. The risk of a slight asymmetry or noticeable scar should be weighed against the minor improvements resulting from this additional procedure.

After the nose has been remodeled, the tip of the nose may have been recessed in order to align it with the new profile line. The diminution in the projection of the tip causes a flaring of the alae (Fig. 35–88A). Bilateral resection of the alar base is required to eliminate the flare (Fig. 35–88B,C). This procedure may also be required when the alar base is excessively wide and thick.

Weir (1892) described an operation for the correction of flaring nostrils in black patients, consisting of excision of a portion of the base in the area of attachment of the nostril to the cheek. Joseph (1931) and Aufricht (1943) reduced the area of excision to the base of the nostril and the floor of the vestibule.

Slight, laterally directed pressure is exerted on the ala; a crease is then apparent in the anterior narial fold and the floor of the vestibule. The crease is outlined in ink. By exerting inward pressure on the ala, an evaluation can be made of the amount of excess tissue. The fold between the external naris and the upper lip is outlined (Fig. 35–88B). A second line is drawn over the skin of the ala, based upon the amount of tissue to be removed (Fig. 35–88B). This line rejoins the posterior extremity of the vestibular line, thus outlining a trapezoid area. Grasping the trapezoid area with a forceps and using a sawing movement with a No. 11 blade, inci-

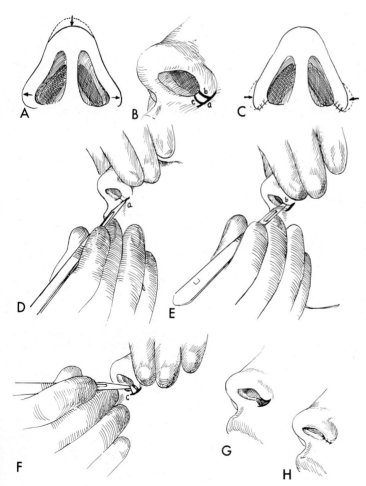

Figure 35–88. Resection of the alar base. *A,* When the tip of the nose is recessed in a corrective rhinoplasty, a flaring of the alae often occurs. This condition may also exist as a primary deformity. *B,* Outline of the area to be excised varies according to the individual case. *C,* Result obtained after the excision of an alar base segment and suture; note the shortening and medial displacement of the alar base. *D,* A pointed scalpel incises through the external narial fold. *E,* The scalpel sections through the lateral aspect of the segment to be excised. *F,* Excision being completed. *G, H,* The defect produced and the edges of the defect sutured.

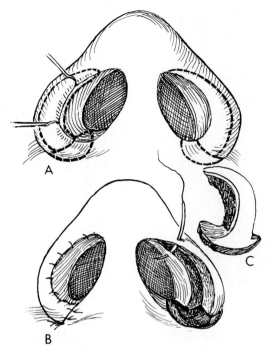

Figure 35–89. *A,* Outline of the alar margin excisions to thin a bulky rim. *B,* The edges of the excised area have been approximated and sutured. *C,* The excised tissue. (After Millard.)

sions are made following the outline of the segment to be resected (Fig. 35–88*D* to *F*). The segment is removed (Fig. 35–88*G*), and the edges of the wound are approximated and sutured (Fig. 35–88*H*). Special care is taken

to avoid resecting tissue from the floor of the vestibule.

Sculpturing Alar Margin. It is rarely necessary to excise tissue from the alar margin in Occidentals. Resection of the alar base is the only procedure occasionally required.

Removal of irregularities along the alar margin is a useful procedure in secondary rhinoplasty and in the correction of the nasal deformity of cleft lip and palate (see Chap. 56).

Millard (1967b) advocated the use of alar margin excisions to reduce a bulky rim (Fig. 35–89), a modification of a procedure previously advocated by Fomon (1960). It is also a useful technique to elevate a drooping ala and reform its natural curve when the alar margin is situated more caudal than the columella.

Modification of Columella-Ala Triangle and Nasolabial Angle. In a harmoniously shaped nose, the columella protrudes downward beyond a horizontal line drawn through the base of each ala; the columella is placed so as to form an open triangle with the alae (Fig. 35–90*A,B*). When the septal cartilage protrudes excessively into the upper lip, the columella-labia angle is obtuse (Fig. 35–90*C*). The resection of a suitably shaped piece of cartilage from the caudal end of the septal cartilage generally corrects this deformity (Fig. 35–90*D*). Usually, the septal cartilage is seen to protrude beyond the nasal spine,

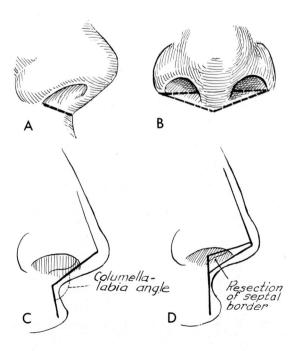

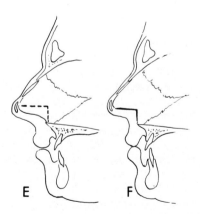

Figure 35–90. *A, B,* Columella-ala triangle. *C* to *F,* Columella-labia angle. This angle may be modified by resection of the lower portion of the caudal border of the septal cartilage.

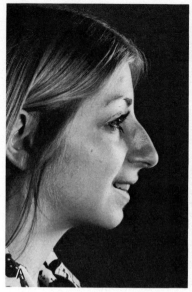 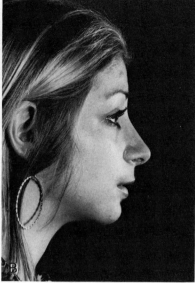

Figure 35–91. The protrusive nasal spine. *A,* Note the protrusion of the nasal spine under the upper lip and the obtuse columella-labia angle. *B,* After resection of the nasal spine.

and resection of cartilage is required to correct the deformity. A suture placed through the base of the columella and through the septal cartilage "snugs" the columella base upward against the septum.

The nasal spine may also be protrusive and must be resected. The protrusive nasal spine not only causes an increased projection of the columella base (Fig. 35–91) and shortens the upper lip but also contributes to the formation of a transverse crease in the upper lip when the patient smiles.

Cartilage Grafting of Nasal Tip. Cartilage grafting of the nasal tip in the primary rhinoplasty was emphasized by Sheen (1975a), Ortiz-Monasterio (1975), and Peck (1983). The usual indication is the tip with inadequate projection. Donor sources include the septum and concha.

Sheen's technique (1975a) consists of a meticulously shaped septal cartilage graft placed at the tip-columella angle with a cephalic tilt of 35 degrees (Fig. 35–92). An incision is made on the lateral aspect of the columella along the anterior border of the medial crus. The incision is placed above the lower border of the facet formed by the tip-columella junction (Fig. 35–93A). A subcutaneous pocket is then formed in front of the cartilages and upward to the domes, extending into the alar rim and hugging the caudal aspect of the downward turning curve of the medial crura (Fig. 35–93A). The cartilage graft is carefully shaped for the individual problem (Fig. 35–93B). It is usually flat along its upper border

and notched along its inferior border for better fixation, as the notch prevents rotation of the graft (Fig. 35–93C). Fixation of the graft is assisted by 4-0 chrome catgut guide sutures passed through the skin and through the graft. The incision is closed with 5-0 plain catgut sutures. Further fixation is provided by the taping of the nose. A patient in whom a large nose with a round tip was treated by

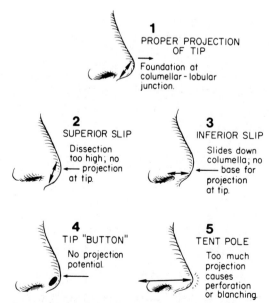

Figure 35–92. Correct position of the cartilage graft at the tip-columella junction. (From Sheen, 1975a.)

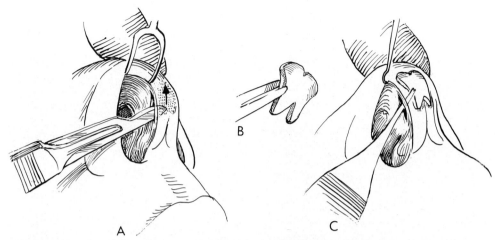

Figure 35–93. Placing the cartilage graft. *A,* Incision along the anterior edge of the medial crus and preparation of the subcutaneous pocket. *B,* Sculptured cartilage graft. *C,* The cartilage graft is imbedded. (After Sheen, 1975a).

this type of septal cartilage graft is shown in Figure 35–94.

Peck (1983) prefers to place the cartilage graft directly on the domes of the alar cartilages. He maintains that such placement gives more tip projection and less displacement of the graft.

The technique may not be indicated in patients with very thin skin, in whom the graft may cause blanching of the skin and may be very obvious.

Deepening of Obtuse Nasofrontal Angle. When the nasofrontal angle is obtuse, the condition may be corrected by the following technique. A flat osteotome is placed along the line of section for the removal of the hump, and the osteotome is tapped upward to the upper portion of the root of the nose in a line that is a continuation of the corrected dorsal profile (Fig. 35–95*A*). The fragment of bone is removed (Fig. 35–95*B*) after the attachment of bone is fractured by levering the bone with the osteotome along the line of section. One should not hesitate to use a fine-tapered, narrow osteotome introduced through the skin at the uppermost level of the line of section to deepen the angle if necessary. Irregularities are smoothed with a curved rasp after the wedge of bone is removed (Figs. 35–95*C,* 35–96).

Variations in Techniques

There is probably no area of plastic surgery that requires more judgment and careful planning than the corrective rhinoplasty. Each patient requires an individualized approach based on the morphology of the nose, the facial configuration, the overall body stature, and the ethnic/racial background. The stilted, formalized rhinoplastic result should be avoided; the nose must fit the face and the person. Thus, the surgeon must be conversant with the many variations in rhinoplastic technique.

While an order of procedure provides a precise and orderly approach to corrective rhinoplasty, variations in the types of deformities may require different techniques.

Single Hump Operation. In this procedure, the saw is used to cut the bony hump and the button knife is then passed under the hump, sweeping caudally to resect a portion of each lateral cartilage and the dorsal border of the septum. In this way the osteocartilaginous profile is modified in a single step. The technique is particularly applicable in a large nose with a prominent dorsal hump. This technique has the disadvantage of leaving the operator with a fait accompli: the hump is removed, the change of the profile is definitive, and the surgeon is committed.

Double Hump Operation. In this procedure, the tip is first adjusted to the septal angle and caudal border of the septum. The tip operation is performed, the lateral cartilages are separated from the septum, and the dorsal border of the septum is lowered to establish the cartilaginous profile as far cephalad as the caudal border of the nasal bones. The lateral cartilages are then adjusted to the dorsal border of the cartilaginous septum. The projection of the bony hump is now in-

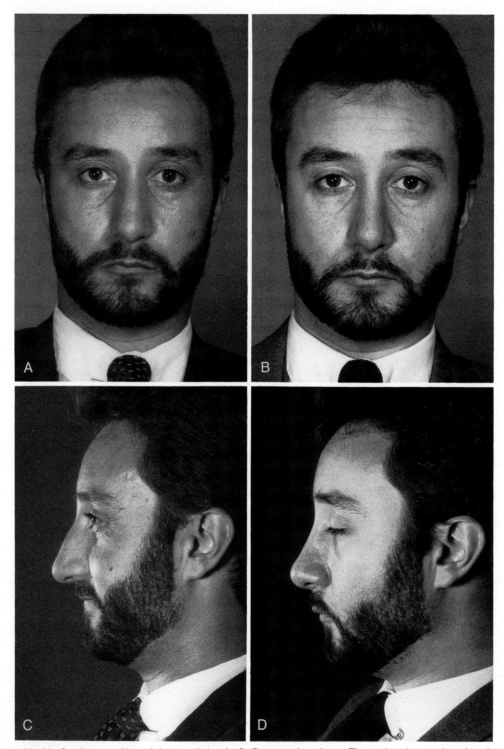

Figure 35–94. Cartilage grafting of the nasal tip. *A, C,* Preoperative views. The patient has a drooping tip without adequate projection. *B, D,* Postoperative appearance after corrective rhinoplasty and cartilage grafting of the tip (see Fig. 35–93).

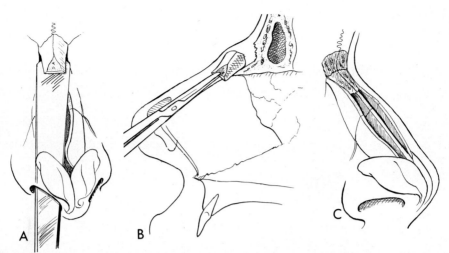

Figure 35–95. Deepening the nasofrontal angle. *A,* A wide osteotome, with rounded angles to avoid injury to the soft tissues, is placed along the line of resection of the dorsal hump and is tapped upward with a mallet. *B,* After the osteotome is levered upward, the attachment to the frontal bone is fractured (or if this is inadequate, the upper attachment to the frontal bone can be severed by sectioning with a narrow osteotome placed through the skin). The wedge of bone is removed. *C,* Deepened nasofrontal angle obtained by this procedure.

creased in relation to the modified cartilaginous profile. An osteotome or a rasp placed at the lower border of the nasal bones removes the hump. The cartilaginous nose is

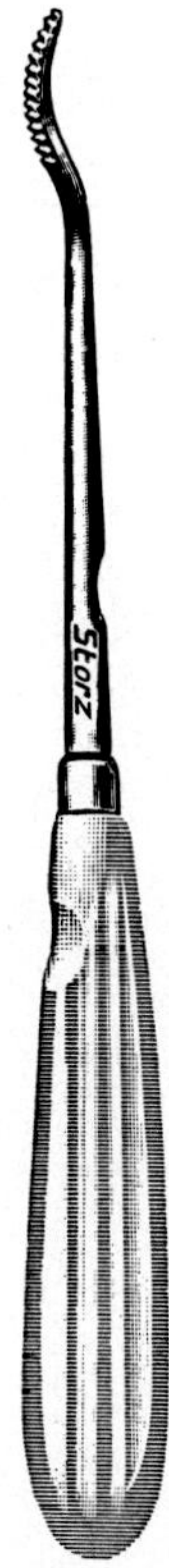

Figure 35–96. Curved rasp used to deepen the nasofrontal angle.

thus remodeled and the bony nose adjusted to the cartilaginous nose.

A disadvantage is a partial commitment on the part of the surgeon: he must be confident that the bony hump resection will "fit" the new profile of the cartilaginous nose. Another disadvantage of this technique is a slight irregularity that may appear at the junction of the bony and cartilaginous dorsum of the septum, usually caused by projecting cephalic portions of the lateral cartilages. Care must be taken to verify the position of these structures under direct vision at the end of the operation.

Sheen's Technique of Corrective Rhinoplasty. Although Sheen (1978) stated that he does not necessarily follow a routine order of procedure in correcting the average nasal hump deformity, he normally uses as an initial landmark the reduction of the bony hump. The bony nasal dorsum is reduced and contoured by a rasp (Fig. 35–97). When a suitable level of reduction has been achieved, the cartilaginous nose is reduced in harmony with the bony nose under direct vision with headlight illumination and adequate retraction. A No. 11 blade with its tip broken off is used for this purpose. The cartilaginous dorsum is progressively shaved until it is aligned in continuity with the bony dorsum. Sheen stated that, if the dorsal hump does not exceed 4 to 5 mm, it is possible to remove the cartilage in a submucous fashion without interrupting the continuity of the mucoperi-

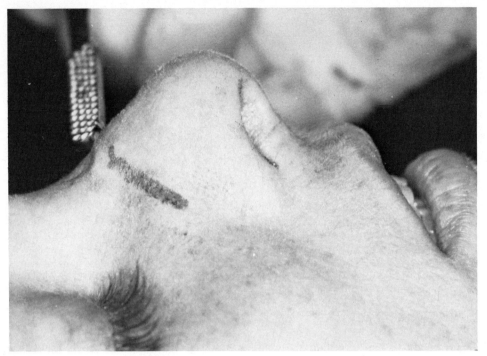

Figure 35–97. Use of the rasp to determine the degree of lowering of the nasal profile. The bony profile has been lowered to the desired level. The remainder of the nasal dorsum is then reduced to conform to the profile level established at the cephalic portion of the dorsum. (Courtesy of Dr. J. Sheen.)

chondrium. In the resection of larger humps, the cartilages and mucoperichondrium are removed together, thus avoiding excess nasal lining being left. The alar cartilages are also approached in a cartilage-splitting fashion for the tip operation. Rim incisions can also expose the cartilages (see Fig. 35–105). The cartilage is removed without resecting the vestibular lining. A series of partial-thickness incisions accentuate the angle of the domes when required. The lateral osteotomies are done with a chisel, *starting low and ending high* (see Fig. 35–74), and the lateral walls are infractured.

Variations in Transfixion Incision. The complete transfixion incision (Fig. 35–98A) is contraindicated when the nose does not require a change in the position of the tip and when only a minor dorsal hump removal or straightening of the nose is indicated. When additional exposure is required, the transfixion incision is extended in an inferior direc-

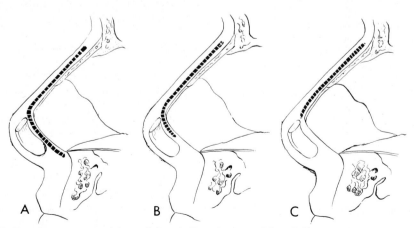

Figure 35–98. Complete versus partial transfixion. A, Complete transfixion. B, Transfixion interrupted below the septal angle. C, Transfixion interrupted at the septal angle.

tion around the septal angle for a short distance, sufficient to allow shortening of the septal cartilage in the region of the septal angle (Fig. 35–98*B*). Adequate exposure is thus obtained for modification of the dorsal septal profile line. The transfixion should be interrupted in the types of noses that do not require shortening; in such instances, the transfixion incision extends no further than the septal angle (Fig. 35–98*C*). Kaye (1983) believes that the complete transfixion incision is a significant cause of loss of tip projection in rhinoplasty.

Submucous Approach. The septal angle serving as a landmark, the mucoperichondrium is raised bilaterally from the septal cartilage (Fig. 35–99*A,B*), after subperichondrial injection of a solution of lidocaine-epinephrine. The mucoperichondrium is raised over an area sufficient to allow the required resection of the dorsal septal cartilage for modification of the profile (Fig. 35–99*B*). As the junction with the lateral cartilage is reached, the mucoperichondrial elevation is continued laterally along the undersurface of the cartilage. Thus, the continuity of the mucous membrane is not interrupted between the septum and the lateral cartilage.

The lateral cartilage attachment to the septum is divided without sectioning the underlying mucous membrane (Fig. 35–99*C*). The mucoperichondrium and mucoperiosteum are raised with a Joseph elevator from

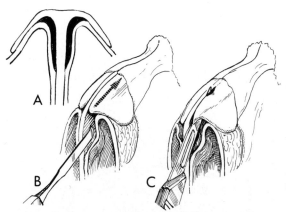

Figure 35–99. Submucous approach for resection of the skeletal structures to modify the nasal profile. *A,* Frontal section through the septum and lateral cartilages; the black areas illustrate the raised areas of mucoperichondrium from the septum and the lateral cartilages. *B,* Raising the mucoperichondrium along the septum and the undersurface of the medial portion of the lateral cartilages. *C,* Severing the attachment of the lateral cartilage to the septum. (After Robin).

the undersurface of each lateral cartilage and nasal bone. The mucous membrane thus being reflected downward away from the skeletal structures that are to be resected, the integrity of the highly specialized mucous membrane of the nose is preserved, as advocated by Anderson and Rubin (1958), Cottle (1960), Anderson (1966), and Robin (1969). This technique reduces the danger of stenosis from contracture at the critical nasal valve. At the end of the operation, a mattress suture of chromic catgut is placed through and through, approximating the mucous membrane flaps to the septal cartilage a few millimeters below the dorsal border of the septal cartilage.

The submucous approach is designed to safeguard the integrity and preserve the physiologic mechanism of the nasal valve. The technique is contraindicated in very large noses because of the excess of mucous membrane that remains after the reduction of the nose. The submucous approach also provides an excellent exposure of the septal framework when correction of a septal deviation is required during the rhinoplasty.

Recession of Nasal Dorsum. In long, thin noses that require surgical reduction in size, the dorsum of the nose may be delicately shaped. Surgeons have attempted to preserve this well-shaped, rounded structure.

Kazanjian, in a few patients, reduced a long nose with a well-shaped dorsum by recessing the dorsum after resecting a segment of septum and a segment from each lateral wall. This procedure was similar to that of Cottle, who advocated a "pushdown" of the dorsum in order to preserve the mucous membrane, which is resected with the hump to avoid interfering with nasal physiology. The entire nasal pyramid was mobilized, and the dorsum was then pushed down. The dorsal border of the septum must be trimmed to permit this maneuver. Skoog (1974) also popularized a technique in which the dorsal hump was replaced as a graft in order to preserve the delicate features of the nasal dorsum (Fig. 35–100). These techniques require considerable skill to achieve the type of result expected by the patient.

Variations in Technique of Tip Exposure. The *hockeystick incision*, popularized by Brown and McDowell (1951), is similar to the incision described earlier in the text (see Fig. 35–65) which divides the lateral crus of the alar cartilage into cephalic and caudal segments. The hockeystick incision owes its

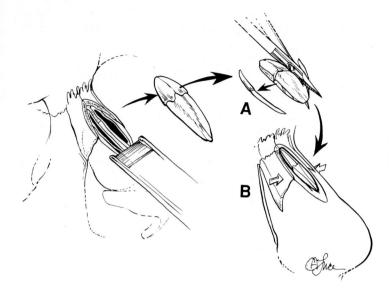

Figure 35–100. Skoog technique of replacing the dorsal hump after appropriate trimming *(A)* and lateral wall infracture *(B)*.

name to its shape, characterized by the curve of its medial portion, which extends caudad into the dome in order to preserve a bipedicle flap of vestibular skin.

The *retrograde technique* involves separating the overlying soft tissues and the vestibular lining from the cartilage through the intercartilaginous incision that was employed for the exposure of the nasal framework (Fig. 35–101). Excision of the required amount of cartilage from the cephalic portion of the lateral crus and from the region of the dome is done in a retrograde manner. The retrograde technique is convenient when only a small amount of lateral crus needs to be resected to achieve an adequate tip correction.

The *eversion technique* employs an incision with a caudal extension from the medial pole of the intercartilaginous incision. It permits eversion of the lateral crus and trimming of the excess cartilage under direct vision (Fig. 35–102). The eversion technique provides better exposure than the retrograde technique.

Joseph Tip Operation. The technique of nasal tip surgery developed by Joseph, with some modification, was widely employed. Guided by preliminary landmarks traced on the skin of the tip of the nose, the lateral crus is divided by a *transcartilaginous* incision into upper and lower segments (Fig. 35–103*A*). An incision is made a few millimeters cephalad to the caudal margin of the alar cartilage in the area of the dome. Scissors

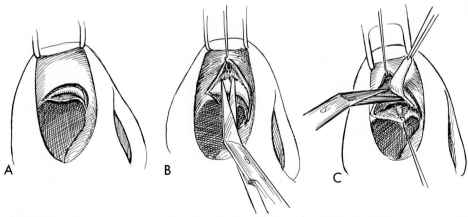

Figure 35–101. The retrograde technique. *A,* Intercartilaginous incision for exposure of the nasal framework. *B,* With angulated scissors, the vestibular skin has been raised; the soft tissues are elevated from the cartilage. *C,* The cartilage is resected from the cephalic portion of the lateral crus.

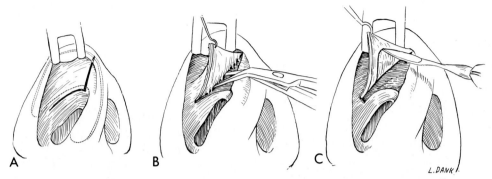

Figure 35–102. The eversion technique. *A,* From the medial end of the intercartilaginous incision, an additional posteroanterior incision is made. *B,* Subperichondrial separation of cartilage from the soft tissues. *C,* The cartilage is everted into an upside-down position, and necessary incisions preparatory to cartilage removal are being made.

free the soft tissue over the cartilage by subperichondrial elevation (Fig. 35–103*A*). At a chosen point in the region of the dome, an anteroposterior incision is made through the vestibular skin and cartilage, and a second oblique incision is made lateral to the first, delimiting a triangular or trapezoid piece of cartilage with its apex toward the margin of the nostrils (Fig. 35–103*B*). The segment of cartilage with its vestibular lining is removed. The continuity of the caudal border of the cartilage should not be interrupted; a narrow strip of cartilage is preserved and not included in the triangular or trapezoid resection. The cephalic segment of the lateral crus is also excised (Fig. 35–103*C,D*). The cut surfaces of the cartilage at the dome are approximated and after a similar procedure is carried out on the contralateral side, the tip is examined for shape. The technique is dangerous and mainly of historical interest.

Safian Tip Operation. The technique employed by Safian (1934) consisted of a posteroanterior incision medial to the dome (Fig. 35–104*A*) and a second incision separating the cartilage from the overlying soft tissues along the caudal margin of the alar cartilage (Fig. 35–104*A,B*). The cartilage is extruded, and excess cartilage from the caudal, cephalic, or medial portions of the lateral crus and dome is excised according to the clinical indications (Fig. 35–104*C* to *E*). An objection to the Safian operation is that it may sacrifice a major portion of the dome of the alar cartilage with a resulting tip deformity. The technique is of historic interest.

Rim Incisions; Delivery Techniques or Open Rhinoplasty. A wider exposure of the alar cartilage may be obtained by extending the marginal incision along the caudal border of the medial crus (Fig. 35–105). The so-called rim or marginal incision should be made

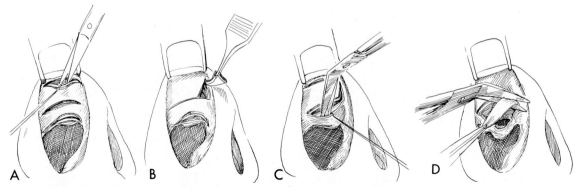

Figure 35–103. The Joseph tip operation (modified). *A,* The lateral crus of the alar cartilage, the dome, and a portion of the medial crus are freed from the overlying tissue. The alar cartilage has been divided into two segments by a transcartilaginous incision through the vestibular lining and cartilage. *B,* A triangular piece of cartilage and vestibular lining is resected from the dome. A quadrangular-shaped segment of cartilage is resected in a broad nasal tip. A narrow strip of caudal margin of the alar cartilage is preserved. *C,* The vestibular lining is raised from the upper segment of the lateral crus. *D,* The cephalic cartilaginous segment is resected.

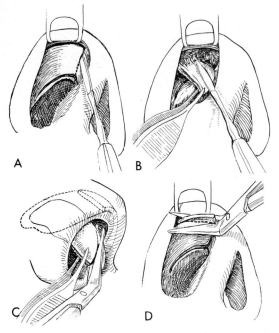

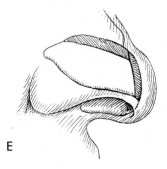

Figure 35–104. The Safian tip operation. *A,* The intercartilaginous incision has been made; the lateral crus is incised along its caudal margin, and an anteroposterior incision is made medial to the dome. *B,* Subperichondrial separation of cartilage from the soft tissues. *C,* Trimming the medial border of the cartilage. *D,* Trimming the caudal border of the cartilage. *E,* The original version of the Safian operation trimmed only the caudal and medial portions of the lateral crus of the alar cartilage. A modification of the Safian procedure, as illustrated, can be employed, which involves excision of the cephalic portion of the lateral crus instead of the caudal portion.

along the rim of the alar cartilage (Fig. 35–105*A,B*) and not along the rim of the nostril. It will be recalled that the caudal margin of the alar cartilage lies considerably cephalad to the caudal margin of the nostril (see Fig. 35–15). An incision through the soft triangle, which is formed only of soft tissues, may result in disfiguring nostril rim notching.

A subperichondrial exposure of the lateral and medial crura can be obtained by elevation of the soft tissues from the cartilage by means of scissors. The cephalic border of the lateral crus is freed from the caudal border of the lateral cartilage by the intercartilaginous incision. A hook is placed under the dome, and the skeletonized cartilage is extruded, the dome being readily accessible (Fig. 35–105*C*). The required cartilage excisions, incisions, and remodeling can be done under direct vision. By exerting gentle lateral traction with a skin hook, both domes come into view. Thus, the entire cartilaginous framework of the tip may be clearly examined and modified. This incision provides the optimal exposure

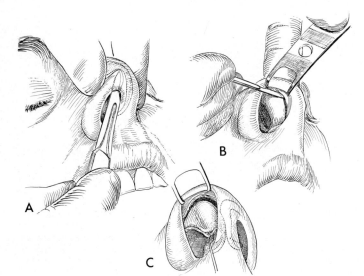

Figure 35–105. Delivery technique. Complete exposure of the tip cartilages by rim incisions. *A,* The tip of the knife is placed in the recess of the vestibule caudal to the dome; the tip is pinched to facilitate the procedure. *B,* The knife incises downward along the caudal margin of the medial crus. *C,* After a rim incision along the caudal border of the lateral crus, the cartilage is separated from the overlying tissues and delivered. One or both domes can be brought into view by lateral traction with a hook (delivery technique).

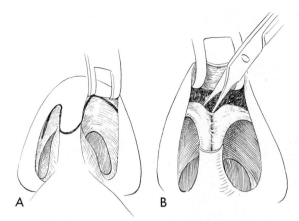

Figure 35–106. The Rethi incision. *A,* Rim incisions along the caudal borders of the lateral crura, domes, and medial crura are joined by a horizontal incision across the columella. *B,* Exposure obtained.

of the nasal tip cartilages and can be combined with an external incision (see below), the so-called *delivery technique* or *open rhinoplasty* (Gruber, 1988).

External Incisions. Rethi (1934) described a procedure consisting of bilateral rim incisions extending along the margin of each lateral crus and downward along the caudal border of each medial crus. A transverse incision through the skin of the columella joins the two marginal incisions at the junction of the upper third with the lower two-thirds of the columella (Fig. 35–106). The soft tissues of the tip of the nose are raised from the cartilage, giving a wide exposure of both domes. Gillies (1920) described an incision similar to Rethi's, the transverse incision extending through the base of the columella in order to make a less noticeable scar. The skin of the columella is raised from the medial crura, exposing the caudal borders of both medial crura and the domes. With this approach the surgeon has full exposure of the tip cartilages (the *delivery technique* or *open rhinoplasty.*)

DeKleine (1955) advocated an approach to the tip through a midcolumellar vertical incision.

Problem Noses

Some noses present unique problems for which specialized techniques are required.

Obtuse Nasofrontal Angle. It is not uncommon to encounter the patient with an obtuse nasofrontal angle. Often the planes of the forehead and nasal dorsum are one. As previously discussed (see Fig. 35–95), the nasofrontal angle must be recreated with appropriate osteotomies and bone resection.

Straight Nasal Dorsum. The esthetics of the nose demand graceful curves; straight lines are unnatural and are mentioned only as something to be avoided (Fig. 35–107). If the surgeon fails to exercise conservative judgment, a saddle deformity will result.

Short Nasal Bones. Sheen (1978) emphasized the pitfalls of a "standardized" technique in the patient with *short nasal bones.* In such a patient the support of the middle nasal vault is precarious, and infracture of the nasal bones combined with reduction of the nasal dorsum can result in collapse of the walls of the middle vault against the septum (Fig. 35–108).

As a preliminary, the surgeon should make the diagnosis of short nasal bones. On frontal inspection the surgeon can detect a narrowness of the central third of the nose with concavities on both sides of the nasal contour. Palpation in this region shows only minimal bony support. A lateral view radiograph confirms the above clinical findings.

Osteotomies and infracture of the nasal bones are to be avoided in patients with short nasal bones, otherwise the walls of the middle nasal vault will collapse. Sheen (1978) recommended reconstruction of the roof of the upper aspect of the cartilaginous vault with a graft of septal cartilage. The Skoog (1974) method of reinserting the resected dorsal hump (modified) is a possible alternative technique (see Fig. 35–100).

Tip Problems

Projecting Tip. An excessively projecting tip, the "Pinocchio nose," requires shortening and recession. First of all, a correct diagnosis must be made. Is the tip projecting or is the dorsum recessed? In the patient shown in Figure 35–109, the dorsal profile was elevated with a septal cartilage graft, and minimal tip surgery was performed.

Lipsett (1959) described a technique for skeletonizing the lateral crus, the dome, and the upper portion of the medial crus. An anteroposterior incision is made through the skin and medial crus. The lateral crus is then advanced medially, and the dome and upper portion of the columellar skin and cartilage are advanced downward. Multiple incisions through the cartilage lateral to the recessed dome form a new dome, and the excess tissue (cartilage and skin) is resected from the col-

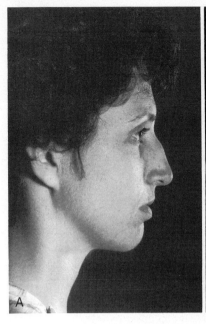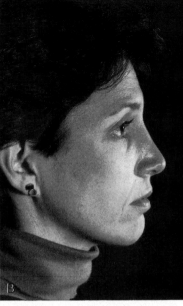

Figure 35–107. *A*, Preoperative appearance with drooping tip. *B*, Appearance after rhinoplasty: the slight irregularity along the dorsum avoids the long, straight appearance of the nose.

umella. The incision is sutured. Because the technique results in the formation of a new dome on each side, it is not devoid of complications, such as irregularity in shape and position of the reconstructed domes, and thus has lost popularity.

The author prefers a technique in which the domes are approached via bilateral rim incisions (see Fig. 35–105). The medial crura and the foot plates are delivered into the surgical field (Fig. 35–110) and an appropriate amount of cartilage is resected from the caudal aspect of each medial crus. With extensive mobilization of the lateral and medial crura there will be a noticeable recession of the nasal tip (Fig. 35–111).

Sheen (1976) described an alternative technique of lateral rotation as follows. After the usual tip operation and the resection of the cephalic segment of the lateral crus, the re-

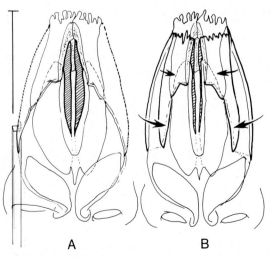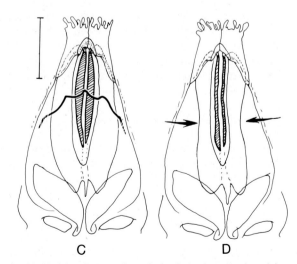

A   B   C   D

Figure 35–108. *A, B,* Nasal bones of normal length (at least one-half of the distance from the radix to the septal angle). After resection of the hump, lateral osteotomy, and infracture, the support of the lateral nasal walls is maintained. *C, D,* Short nasal bones. In contrast, after resection of the hump, lateral osteotomy, and infracture, there can be collapse of the lateral nasal walls against the septum with obvious surface concavities on both sides of the nose. (After Sheen, 1978.)

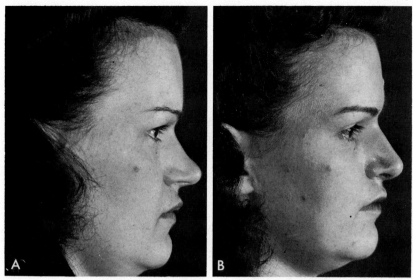

Figure 35–109. Correction of a projecting tip by increasing the dorsum of the nose. *A,* The tip projects because of the lack of projection of the dorsum. *B,* Result obtained by means of a septal cartilage transplant over the dorsum (see the technique illustrated in Figure 35–146). (Patient of J. M. Converse.)

maining caudal and lateral portion is everted and freed (Fig. 35–112*A*); the most lateral portion is amputated (Fig. 35–112*B*). The size of the resected segment depends on the amount of recession required. This procedure is the reverse of the technique described above. The recession is obtained by a lateral rotation, and what was dome becomes lateral

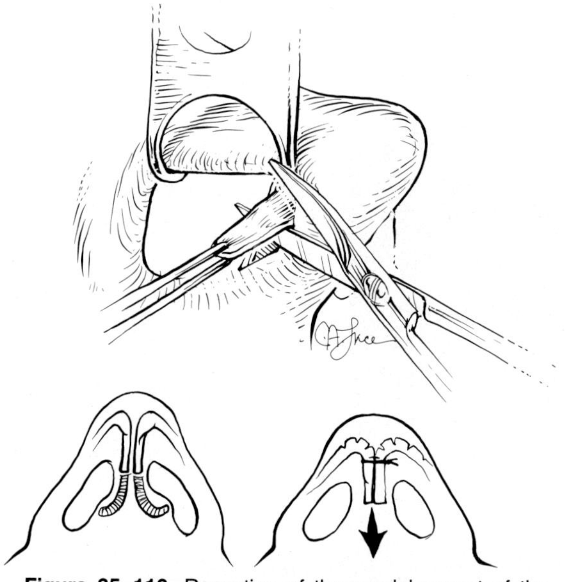

Figure 35–110. Resection of the caudal aspect of the medial crura to recess the projecting nasal tip. The arrow designates the direction of recession of the nasal tip. A suture coapts the medial crura.

crus, and what was medial crus becomes dome. To facilitate the formation of the new dome when the cartilage is thick, an incision partially extending through the cartilage medial to the dome eliminates any resistance (Fig. 35–112*C,D*). The correction may be combined with a medial crus resection as described above.

Excessively Pointed Tip. A sharp, narrow-tipped nose is due to the anatomic configuration of the domes. The dome ordinarily forms a gently curved arch at the point where the lateral and medial crura meet; a pointed tip results if the crura meet at a sharp angle. The technique suggested by Aufricht (1943) may be used to correct this type of deformity (Fig. 35–113). The alar cartilages are exposed by the Joseph technique; the cartilages are divided at the highest point of the dome without incising the vestibular lining. A suitable segment of cartilage can then be resected; if necessary, a number of strips of cartilage are resected until a suitable curvature is obtained.

The lateral rotation technique (see Fig. 35–112) graft can also be used to correct the pointed tip, and if the tip is not also projecting too much, a camouflaging conchal cartilage can be laid over the cartilaginous irregularities.

Inadequate Projection of Tip. The caudal portion of the tip of the nose should project slightly above the profile line of the dorsum.

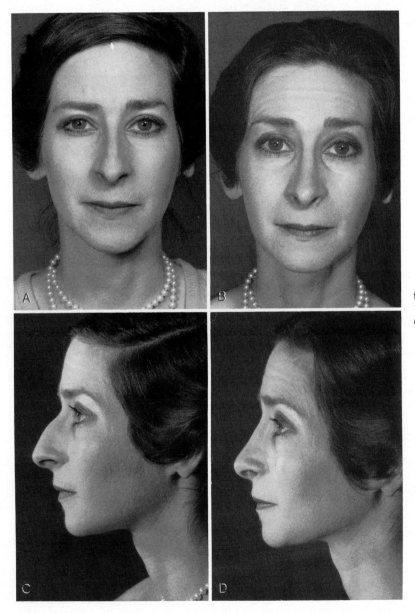

Figure 35–111. Correction of the projecting tip (see Fig. 35–110). *A, C,* Preoperative views. *B, D,* Postoperative views.

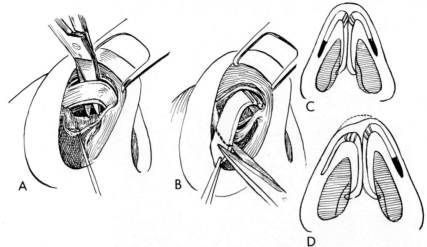

Figure 35–112. Correction of the projecting tip by the lateral rotation technique. *A,* After resection of the cephalic portion of the lateral crus, the cartilage is freed of its attachments. *B,* A segment is resected from the lateral end of the lateral crus. *C.* The cartilage is rotated laterally. Partial-thickness incisions through the cartilage medial to the domes facilitate the formation of the new domes. *D,* The right lateral rotation has been completed; the left rotation has not, and the dome is still in the original position. (After Sheen, 1978.)

Various procedures have been attempted to increase the projection of the tip.

Often the tip is tethered by the columella. After the transfixion procedure, and in some cases after resection of the depressor septi nasi muscle (see Fig. 35–122), or in most cases after release of the columella from the nasal spine, the nasal tip becomes tilted into a more cephalic and projected position.

Cartilage grafting, the graft being obtained from the septal or conchal cartilage, has been employed. The nasal tip grafting techniques of Sheen (1975a), Ortiz-Monasterio (1975), and Peck (1983) have been previously described under Adjunctive Techniques (p. 1838).

Increasing the projection of the tip is also discussed later in this chapter in the section on bone grafting and in the chapter on secondary rhinoplasty (Chap. 36).

Daniel (1987) has also described a technique of increasing tip projection without a cartilage graft. Through an open rhinoplasty *(delivery technique)*, the tip is refined either by a horizontal mattress suture through each domal segment or by suturing together cartilage flaps removed from the lateral crura.

Broad or Bulbous Tip. The wide or broad tip, the square-shaped tip, and the bulbous tip may require extensive excision of cartilage.

The alar cartilages of the broad tip have a wider curve, and the domes are often separated from each other in the midline. The contour of the square-shaped tip is determined by the wide, flat surface of the cartilaginous domes.

Bulbous tips are often characterized by thick soft tissues and relatively thin alar cartilages. The *delivery technique* (see Fig. 35–105) is employed to expose the tip cartilages. The domes are then contoured and approximated with nonabsorbable sutures under direct vision (Fig. 35–114). This maneuver gives more definition and projection to the nasal tip.

Sheen (1978) also obtained satisfactory results by the lateral rotation technique (Figs. 35–115, 35–116).

Bifid Tip. Approximation of the medial crura and the domes usually corrects the bifid

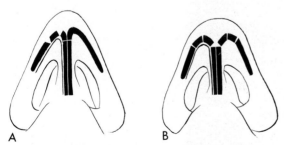

Figure 35–113. Correction of the exessively pointed tip. *A,* Remodeling of the shape of the tip of the nose by excision of cartilage from the dome of the right alar cartilage. *B,* Both sides completed. The cartilage segments remain attached to the vestibular lining. (After Aufricht, 1943.)

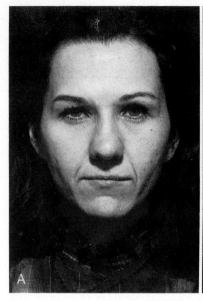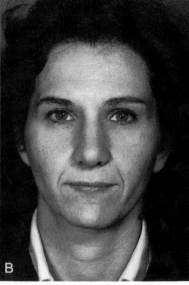

Figure 35–114. Correction of the broad, bulbous tip by the delivery technique (open rhinoplasty) and remodeling and suturing of the tip cartilages. *A*, Preoperative view. *B*, Postoperative view.

Figure 35–115. Technique of correction of the broad tip by the lateral rotation technique. *A*, Exposure of the caudal portion of the alar cartilage after resection of the cephalic segment. The cartilage is dissected from its bed (delivery technique). A segment is resected from the lateral portion of the lateral crus. *B*. The right lateral crus is placed back into its bed and recessed. Partial-thickness incisions at the area of the dome are usually required to aid the lateral rotation, which is maintained by taping. (After Sheen, 1978.)

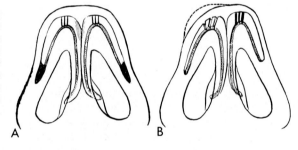

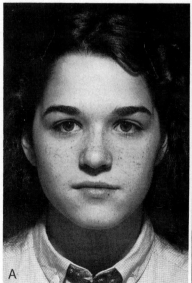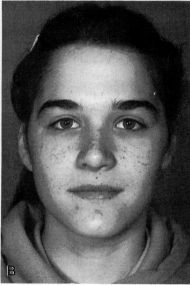

Figure 35–116. Correction of a round, bulbous tip by the technique illustrated in Figure 35–115. *A*, Preoperative view. *B*, Postoperative view.

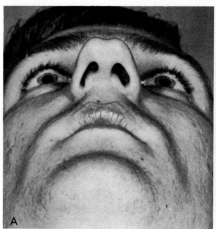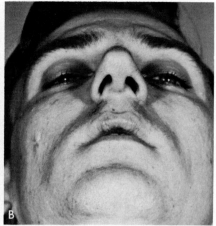

Figure 35–117. The bifid tip. *A,* Example of a bifid tip, characterized by a gap between the medial crura and the domes. *B,* Result obtained by bilateral rim incisions, resection of the intervening fibroareolar tissue, and approximation of the domes under direct vision (delivery technique). (Patient of Dr. J.M. Converse.)

tip deformity (Fig. 35–117). The various steps required for this procedure include exposure of the alar cartilages through rim incisions, removal of tissue between the medial crura, suitable scoring of the alar cartilages, excision of cartilage from the dome, and suturing of the domes under direct vision.

Deviated Nasal Tip. The tip of the nose can be severely deviated. The pressure of the laterally twisted septal angle may separate the alar cartilages from one another, resulting in bifidity of the tip and asymmetry. Distortion of the columella by a deviated septal cartilage may displace one medial crus laterally and separate the crura, widening and distorting the columella with lateral protrusion of the lower end of one of the medial crura (Fig. 35–118*A,C*).

Correction of an asymptomatic septal deflection is not indicated in the average corrective rhinoplasty. In the deviated nose, however, straightening of the cartilaginous septum is an essential procedure (Fig. 35–118*B,D*).

"Plunging" Tip. The long nose with the "plunging" tip is a condition that becomes more accentuated with aging. The anatomic basis of this deformity can vary.

In one type, the septum is long, invading the lip, and the ligamentous attachments of the alar cartilages to the septal angle are adequate. The deformity is essentially caused by the long nasal septum and lateral walls of an excessively long nose. These patients often have poorly developed alar cartilages and long, slitlike external nares.

The second type of long nose with a "plunging" tip shows, on digital distraction, a lack of continuity between the tip of the nose and the septal angle; the nasal tip is dislocated downward from its aponeurotic attachments to the septal angle, which protrudes in the supratip area. This is also an anatomic characteristic of the Armenoid nose (see the digital palpation test, Fig. 35–134). The treatment of each of the two varieties of "plunging" tip varies.

In the long nose of the first type, in which the nasal tip cartilages have an intimate connection with the septal angle, disruption of this relationship must be avoided. The following procedure has proved effective and given satisfactory results. Instead of the usual transfixion incision that follows the dorsal border of the septal cartilage and curves around the septal angle, the transfixion incision transects the septum cephalad to the septal angle (Parkes and Brennan, 1970). The *transeptal* transfixion incision is directed obliquely downward and forward to the mobile portion of the septal cartilage, anterior to the vomer groove, where the septal cartilage is mobile over the nasal spine (Fig. 35–119*A*). The caudal segment, being loosely connected in this area, may be retracted cephalad, overriding the fixed cephalic portion of the septum. In this manner the amount of required resection of the septum can be evaluated and the excess removed from the fixed portion of the septum (Fig. 35–119*B*). The caudal portions of the lateral cartilages usually must be detached from the septum and

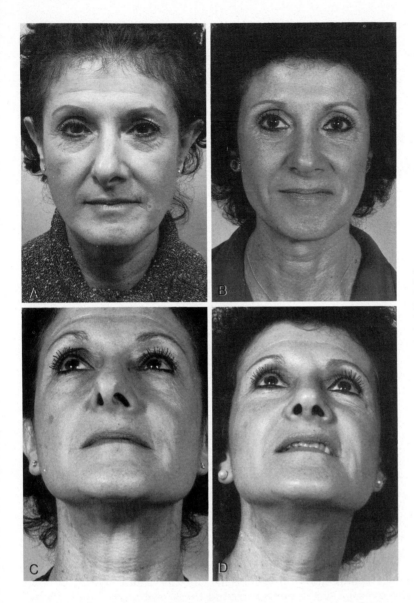

Figure 35–118. The deviated tip. *A, C,* Preoperative views showing deviation of the tip, columella, and medial crura. *B, D,* After rhinoplasty, septoplasty and straightening of the angle and caudal border of the septum. An eyelidplasty was also performed.

the necessary procedures carried out to shorten the cartilaginous nasal walls by excising a segment from each lateral crus. The transfixion incision is sutured with two through and through mattress catgut sutures (Fig. 35–119C). Trimming of the dorsal border of the septal cartilage is required to align the dorsal borders of the two cartilaginous segments in order to achieve a satisfactory profile line.

In the type of "plunging" tip in which the deformity is caused by a dislocation downward of the alar cartilages from the septal angle, it would be a mistake to further shorten the septum. Instead it is essential to obtain fixation of the tip to the septal angle.

To maintain the tip, the *invagination procedure* (Fig. 35–120) is employed. It consists of removing the mucous membrane from the caudal end of the septal cartilage, particularly at the septal angle, and placing the septal cartilage between the medial crura, achieving an overlap of the crura over the septal cartilage. The medial crura are maintained in this position by sutures (Fig. 35–121).

In the older patient, the tip of the nose tends to droop, and shortening of the nose may be indicated. The operative procedures described above can be performed but are not efficacious in this type of nasal "ptosis" with excess skin. Consequently, resection of skin

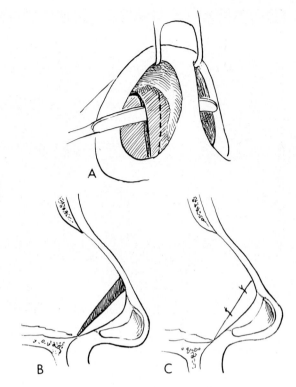

Figure 35–119. The *transeptal* transfixion incision. *A,* Transfixion posterior to the caudal border of the septal cartilage. *B,* Outline of the resected septum. *C,* The septal incision is sutured. (After Parkes and Brennan, 1970.)

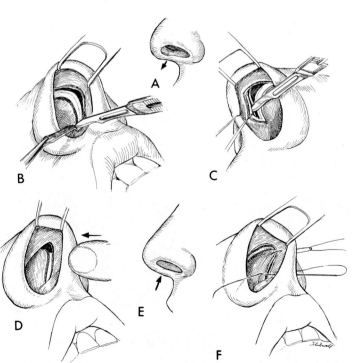

Figure 35–120. The invagination procedure. *A,* The tip of the nose tends to droop downward off the septal angle. *B,* The septal angle is denuded of mucous membrane. *C,* A pocket is made between the medial crura. *D,* The septal angle is invaginated between the medial crura. *E,* Suspension of the tip to the septal angle. *F,* Transfixion sutures approximate the structures. The upper transfixion suture invaginates the septal angle between the medial crura.

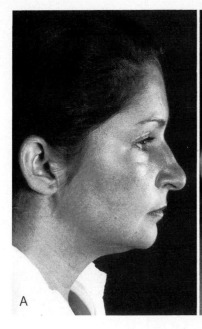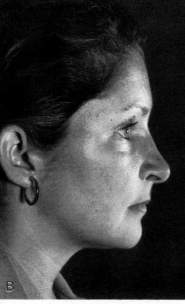

A   B

Figure 35–121. Plunging tip corrected by a rhinoplasty including the invagination technique (see Fig. 35–120). *A,* Preoperative view. *B,* Postoperative view.

may be necessary at the root of the nose. In extreme cases, a transverse incision across the root of the nose, with bilateral vertical extensions of each side over the frontal process of the maxilla, enables the surgeon to remove the excess skin without leaving conspicuous scars because of the nature of the loose skin in the older patient. The scars, however, can be objectionable.

"Smiling" Tip; Mobile Tip. In patients with mobile tips, the paired depressor septi nasi muscles are hyperactive. The tip undergoes a caudal displacement when the patient smiles. Treatment consists of resection of the paired depressor septi nasi muscles and their attachments to the incisive fossae. Furukawa (1974) demonstrated by electromyographic studies that the tip of the nose is pulled toward the columella-labia angle and also in a caudal direction by the depressor nasi muscle when the patient smiles.

The approach to the muscle is through the transfixion incision (Fig. 35–122), the muscle being resected from its position behind the columella, between the medial crura. Despite the resection of the depressor septi nasi muscles, none of the patients has complained of nasal airway impairment (Fig. 35–123). If the septal cartilage invades the lip, resection of cartilage at the caudal border is also necessary.

Nostril Problems

Malpositioned Lateral Crura. Malposition of the lateral crura is defined by Sheen (1978) as any displacement from their anatomic alignment with the nostril rims. Pertinent physical findings include a parenthesis-like appearance around the nasal tip, notches in the alar rim, broadening and flattening of the nasal tip, and a square nasal-alar base.

Through bilateral rim incisions (Fig. 35–124), the lateral crura can be skeletonized, delivered into the surgical field and then repositioned along the nostril rim so that the lateral crus extends into the alar lobule.

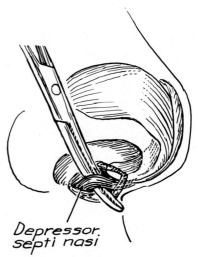

Depressor. septi nasi

Figure 35–122. Exposure for the resection of the depressor septi nasi muscle.

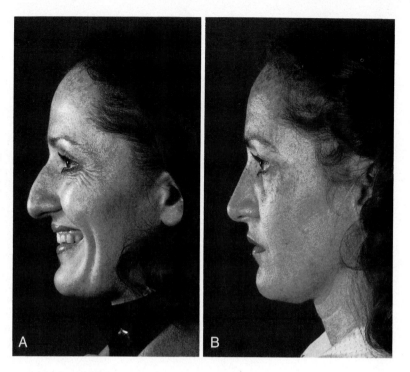

Figure 35–123. The "smiling" tip corrected by rhinoplasty and resection of the depressor muscles (see Fig. 35–122). *A,* Preoperative view on smiling. Note that the tip is also dislocated. *B,* Postoperative view.

Nostril Flare. Extreme flaring of the nostrils requires a combination of alar base resection and repositioning (see p. 1836). Millard (1980) described a technique, entitled the "alar cinch," in which the alar bases are transposed to a more medial position.

Thick Alar Rim. An extremely thick alar rim can be resculpted according to the techniques described on page 1837.

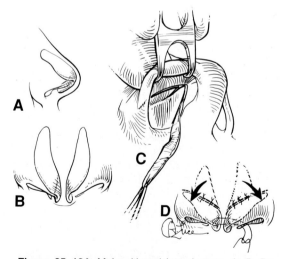

Figure 35–124. Malpositioned lateral crura. *A, B,* Preoperative appearance. Note that the lateral crura are not aligned with the nostril rims. *C, D,* Surgical correction consists of delivery of the lateral crura and repositioning them along the rim with sutures (Sheen, 1978).

Columellar Problems

Hanging Columella. The hanging columella can be associated with two types of pathologic anatomy: (1) the medial crura have an excessive curvature and length, the convexity of the cartilages being caudad; and (2) the membranous septum is excessively stretched, and the distance between the medial crura and the caudal border of the septal cartilages is increased.

In unusually severe cases, the medial crura must be approached via rim incisions and a delivery technique, and reduced in length by resection of a portion of their caudal end (Fig. 35–125).

Resection of an overdeveloped membranous septum may be achieved by excising the excess; an alternative is to sweep the transfixion incision caudally to the septal cartilage, excising a segment of septal cartilage along with the excess membranous septum.

Retracted Columella. The columella is an esthetic landmark of the nose, a column that divides the nares and supports the tip of the nose. Any noticeable discrepancy of the columella becomes conspicuous. The columella may be retracted and the columella-labia angle acute. This deformity may be caused by a deficiency of the caudal portion of the septal cartilage or underdevelopment of the premaxillary wings and nasal spine, as in Binder's syndrome (see Chap. 29). The colu-

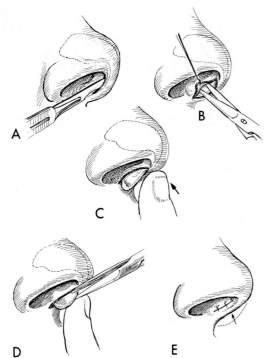

Figure 35–125. Correction of the hanging columella by excision of excess medial crus. *A,* Incision along the caudal margin of the medial crus. *B,* Freeing the medial crus from the overlying skin. *C,* The columella is retruded to an adequate position of correction; excess medial crus becomes evident. *D,* Trimming the medial crus. *E,* The incision along the caudal border of the medial crus is sutured. This procedure can be combined with resection of the caudal portion of the septal cartilage and/or nasal spine.

mella itself may be severely scarred as a result of injury that has also affected the membranous septum, the nasal spine, and the anterior floor of the nose. Many retracted columellas result from overshortening of the septum during a corrective rhinoplasty.

Careful examination is required in order to determine whether the columella is truly retracted, or whether the retraction is relative because the lateral walls of the nose are excessively long and the alae protrude caudally in relation to the columella. In such cases, the lateral walls, in addition to the entire nose, must be shortened. This type of deformity is usually associated with the long nose with the "plunging tip" (see p. 1853).

Various methods have been employed to correct the retracted columella. The most commonly used technique is the placement of a septal cartilage graft, through an incision in the columella, along the caudal border of the medial crus. After the columellar skin is undermined down to the nasal spine, the lower end of the transplant rests on, or is caudal to, the nasal spine, thus increasing the projection of the columella and improving the contour of the columella-labia angle (Fig. 35–126). A mattress suture placed through the medial crura prevents the transplanted cartilage from being displaced backward between the medial crura.

To correct retrusion of the base of the columella (acute columella-labia angle), Aufricht (1961) employed a transverse incision through the floor of the vestibule of the nose, undermining the soft tissue over the nasal spine, and transplanted septal cartilage in this area (Fig. 35–127). Resected alar and lateral cartilage may also be used for the transplant.

The retraction of the columella may be such that the insertion of a septal cartilage graft causes blanching of the skin, making it obvious that the soft tissues must be released. The "sleeve" procedure has been successful in obtaining release of the retracted soft tissues (Converse, 1964). The procedure involves the use of bilateral vertical and horizontal incisions through the mucoperichondrium on each side of the septum, the mucoperichondrium being raised from the septal cartilage as far as the caudal margin of the septal cartilage (Fig. 35–128). The columella may then be protracted, the mucoperichondrial flaps and the membranous septum following the advancement of the columella. The exposed areas of septal cartilage that result from the advancement of the mucoperichondrial flaps usually heal rapidly by secondary epithelization. In order to avoid exposure of the septal cartilage at the same position on both sides, the incisions through the mucoperichondrium and mucoperiosteum should be placed at different positions, one in front of the other.

The intraoral approach to the nasal spine uses a vestibular incision made on the buccal aspect of the vestibule; the nasal spine is exposed under direct vision. The graft is placed into the base of the columella and over the nasal spine.

Nasal septal cartilage is usually the preferred material for restoring columellar contour. Other procedures have been described to release the retracted columella: flaps of vestibular lining and alar cartilage (Fig. 35–129) were used by Millard (1974), and a composite graft of the concha of the auricle

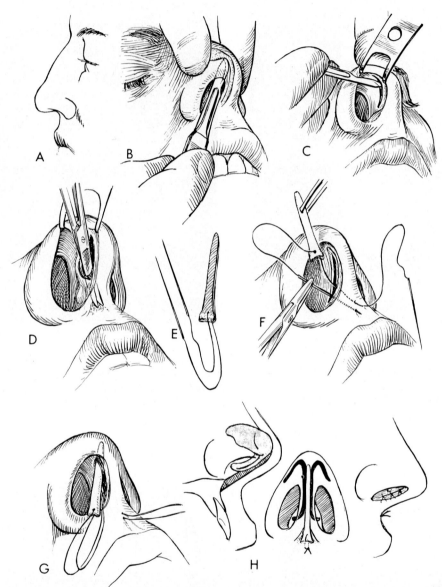

Figure 35–126. Increasing the projection of the retracted columella by a septal cartilage graft introduced through an anterior columellar approach. *A,* Typical appearance of a patient with retracted columella and overhanging tip and alae. *B,* The tip is pinched, and the knife is placed in the recess of the vestibule along the caudal border of the dome; the incision is extended downward along the caudal border of the medial crus. *C,* An incision along the medial crus is being completed. *D,* Scissors dissect between the medial crura anterior to the nasal spine. *E,* The septal cartilage graft with traction sutures. *F,* The septal cartilage graft is introduced caudal to the medial crura, guided by the traction sutures. *G,* The septal cartilage graft is introduced. *H,* Position of the cartilage graft *(left).* The cartilage graft is maintained anterior to the nasal spine *(center);* the traction sutures may be brought through the skin and tied over a piece of cotton to maintain the position of the graft. The columella incision is sutured *(right).*

Illustration continued on following page

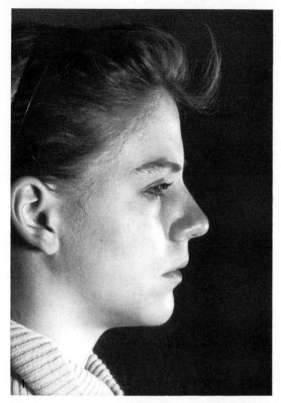
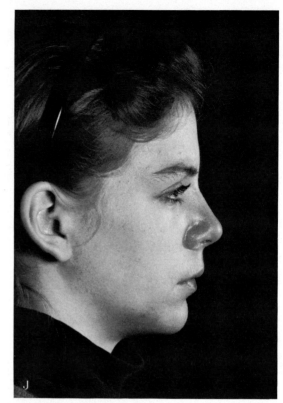

Figure 35–126 *Continued I,* Preoperative view. *J,* Postoperative view.

was advocated by Dingman and Walter (1969) to correct the retracted columella.

Correction of Wide Columellar Base. This condition often results from lateral traction on one medial crus by the deviated caudal end of the septal cartilage. One medial crus becomes separated from the other, leaving a wide gap between the cartilaginous structures. Attempts to narrow the base of the columella by means of mattress sutures through the skin result in failure. The follow-

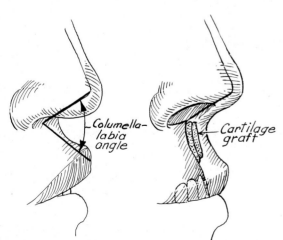

Figure 35–127. Opening the columella-labia angle by means of septal cartilage grafts. The cartilage grafts are introduced through an incision in the floor of the vestibule. (After Aufricht.)

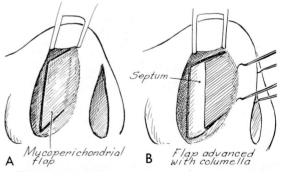

Figure 35–128. The sleeve procedure for the correction of columellar retraction (Converse, 1964). *A,* Incisions are made through the mucoperichondrium and mucoperiosteum to release a flap, permitting the increase in projection of the columella as shown in *B. B,* The flap has been advanced, with the columella leaving an area of exposed cartilage that reepithelizes spontaneously. A similar flap is designed on the contralateral side of the septum. The precaution should be taken, however, to place the areas of denuded septum one in front of the other in order to avoid the possibility of a septal perforation. This procedure is effective only if it is done in conjunction with a septal columella cartilage transplant, as shown in Figure 35–126.

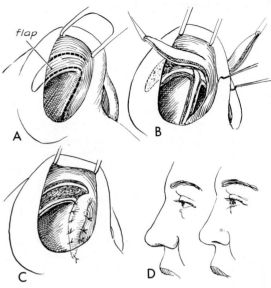

Figure 35–129. Increase in the projection of the columella by a flap of alar cartilage and vestibular lining. *A,* The flap of the cephalic portion of the alar cartilage with vestibular lining is outlined, as well as the incision in the membranous septum. *B,* The alar flap is raised. *C,* The flap has been transposed. *D,* The procedure not only increases the projection of the columella but also shortens the nose, correcting the overhanging nasal tip and alae. (After Millard.)

ing technique has been used with success. An incision is made along the caudal margin of the medial crus on each side (Fig. 35–130*A*), the overlying skin of each medial crus is separated from the cartilage (Fig. 35–130*B*), and the areolar tissue between the crura is resected (Fig. 35–130*C*). When the medial crura diverge excessively from each other, a transverse incision is made in the medial crus at the point of divergence in order to break the spring of the cartilage (Fig. 35–130*D*). A mattress suture approximates the medial crura (Fig. 35–130*D,E*) and the skin incisions are closed (Fig. 35–130*F*).

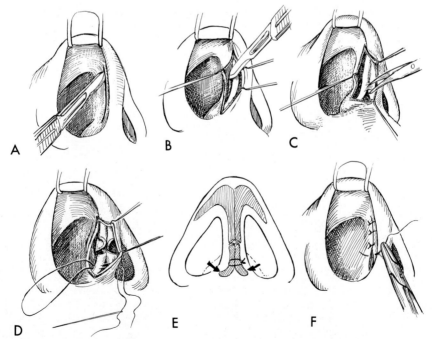

Figure 35–130. Narrowing the wide columella. *A,* An incision is made along the caudal margin of the medial crus. *B,* The skin is elevated from the lateral surface of the medial crus. *C,* The medial crura are separated in the midline. *D,* An incision is made through each medial crus at its point of divergence. *E,* Approximation of the medial crura by a buried mattress suture of chromic catgut. *F,* The cutaneous incision is sutured with 5-0 plain catgut.

THE DEVIATED NOSE

The deviated or twisted nose is most often of traumatic or congenital origin. The nasal dorsum should lie in the midsagittal plane of the face (Fig. 35–131A). In *partial* deviations, only a portion of the nose is involved. When the nasal dorsum is curved to one side (Fig. 35–131B), when two portions of the dorsum are twisted in opposite directions, as in an S-shaped deformity (Fig. 35–131C), or when the entire nose veers to one side, the condition is referred to as a *total* deviation (Fig. 35–131D). In most deviated noses the tip remains in the midline but in the last type (Fig. 35–131D), the tip of the nose is also deviated.

Nasal deviations may be classified into three broad categories: congenital, those acquired in childhood, and those acquired in adulthood.

Congenital Deviations (Prenatal). Some nasal deviations are caused by intrauterine injury and do not correct spontaneously. A genetic component is suggested when the parents or grandparents also show a similar deformity; a familial tendency has been especially noted in cases of dislocation of the caudal portion of the septal cartilage.

Deviations Acquired in Childhood (Postnatal). Deviation of the nose occurs not infrequently in the newborn after the trauma of delivery. Kirschner (1955) observed severe compression of the nose in every normal delivery. In posterior presentation, a greater amount of injury results because of more extensive rotation of the head. Most of these deviations tend to return to the midline spontaneously at the end of three months.

Injury occurring in the infant or young child as a result of a fall from the crib or while learning to walk is generally overlooked. Studies have been made of the frequency of accidents in early childhood (Kravits and associates, 1969). Deviation of the nose is also a common finding in the battered child syndrome.

Injuries suffered in early childhood cause deviation by fracture, hypertrophic callus, and dislocation of the bones at a time when the sutures are not yet closed. Deviation may also result from the disproportionate growth caused by trauma. The deviation becomes more accentuated as the nose grows and becomes progressively more conspicuous in the adolescent. Developmental changes in the child result in greater anatomic disturbances than those that occur in the adult.

Deviations Acquired in Adult Life. These deformities are produced by injury in adolescence or in adult life after or near the completion of nasal growth. The tip of the nose usually is in the midline, despite severe deflection of the dorsum.

Deviations of Bony Portion of Nose. These deviations usually show a unilateral dorsal hump, often thin ridged and prolonged downward by a cartilaginous portion, which is formed by the septal and upper lateral cartilages. The deformities are varied and include such conditions as simple deviations of the bony ridge; deviation with a dorsal hump due to hypertrophic callus or overriding fragments; widening; flattening; saddle deformity; or a combination of these deformities. The essential anatomic feature in such conditions is the disproportionate width of the

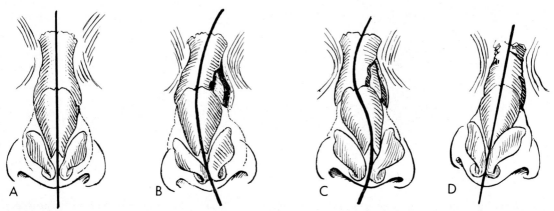

Figure 35–131. The straight nose and three principal types of nasal deviations. *A,* In the straight nose, the dorsum is aligned with the midsagittal plane of the face, which passes through nasion above and subnasale below. *B,* The C-shaped deviation. *C,* The S-shaped deviation. *D,* The generalized *(total)* deviation to one side. In the generalized deviation the tip is often deviated also.

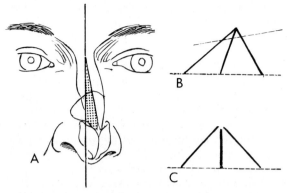

Figure 35–132. Disproportion between the lateral walls of the nose in nasal deviation. *A,* The shaded area represents the amount of bone and lateral cartilage excision required to equalize the lateral walls. *B,* Resection of the hump in a beveled manner equalizes the lateral walls. *C,* After septoplasty and correction of the disproportion between the lateral walls, the dorsum of the nose is realigned with the midsagittal plane of the face.

lateral walls of the nose, the side of the deviation being narrower (Fig. 35–132). Deflection of the septum is a common occurrence because of the close association of the nasal bones with the lateral and septal cartilages.

Deviations of Cartilaginous Portion of Nose. In addition to intranasal inspection, digital palpation of the dorsum of the deviated nose from the nasal bones to the tip provides information concerning the shape and position of the dorsal border of the septal cartilage; finger pressure just above the tip of the nose discloses the position of the septal angle. The dorsal border of the septal cartilage may be C shaped, have an S-shaped curvature, or show a generalized deviation to one side. The position and shape of the septal

angle and the caudal portion of the septum can be determined by placing the tip of the thumb in one vestibule and the tip of the forefinger in the other. When the nasal tip is gently elevated, the cephalic borders of the alar cartilages can also be seen protruding beneath the skin. The size, shape, and position of the alar cartilages can thus be determined.

The position and shape of the septum are confirmed by intranasal examination. Hypertrophy of the turbinates on the side opposite the deviation is noted in patients with severe deviation of the septum; the hypertrophy is a compensatory phenomenon to fill the void caused by the deviated septum. Spurs are also a frequent finding near the vomer–septal cartilage junction.

Because of long-standing deflection, the lateral cartilages may be asymmetric, the cartilage on the side opposite the septal deviation being wider (Fig. 35–133). The nasal tip feels soft to the touch and can be depressed by digital pressure when the septal angle is situated lateral to its midline position. A depression is noted just above the tip of the nose. The septal angle may protrude beneath one alar cartilage, splaying apart the alar cartilages and broadening the tip (see Fig. 35–133), which usually is also asymmetric in shape. The caudal septal border, protruding in the narial opening, causes widening and distortion of the columella. The medial crus is separated from its counterpart, its lower portion forming a protrusion.

When the septum has been crushed or fractured, it loses its supportive function. In such cases the tip of the nose may be pressed backward against the face without encoun-

Figure 35–133. A severe lateral deviation of the septum; note the disproportionate size and shape of the upper lateral and alar cartilages resulting from a deviation of the developmental type. The septal angle, no longer in the midline, elevates the dome of the left alar cartilage.

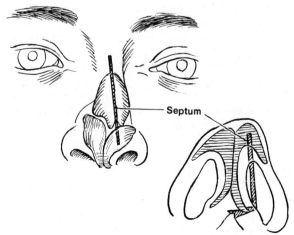

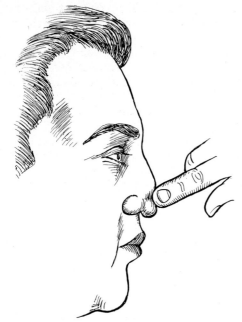

Figure 35–134. Digital palpation test. The septum has lost its supportive function. Palpation demonstrates that the tip of the nose can be depressed by digital pressure.

tering the septal angle; the septum no longer supports the tip of the nose (Fig. 35–134).

Variations also occur in the angulation or curvature of the septal cartilage in the sagittal and vertical planes. The anterocaudal portion of the cartilage may be dislocated to one side of the vomer, and the cephalic portion of the cartilage deviated toward the opposite side. The angulation may be so severe that the caudal portion of the septal cartilage lies transversely across one vestibule, with the free border of the cartilage protruding into the opposite vestibule, thus obstructing the airway.

More severe angulations occur along a line extending from the junction of the nasal bones with the perpendicular plate. The posterior part of the septum is often seen to be fairly straight in severe deflection of the caudal portion of the septum. The reverse condition also occurs; a septum with severe posterior deflection may be relatively straight in its anterior (caudal) portion.

Deviations of the septum may be complicated by a considerable increase in the thickness of the septum and by vomer-cartilage spurs. Thickening is caused by overlapping of fractured cartilaginous fragments and by fibrous tissue thickening after hematoma of the septum. The curvature or angulation of

the septal cartilage, dislocation from the vomer groove, or a change in shape may result in a decrease of the anteroposterior or vertical dimensions of the septum. The contraction after the healing of lacerated or destroyed mucous membrane can also cause a change in the position of the remaining portions of the septal cartilage after submucous resection. Characteristic deformities (retraction of the columella and depression or flatness of the cartilaginous dorsum cephalad to the alar cartilages) accompany these changes.

The Septum and the Deviated Nose. *The correction of septal deflection remains the key to the straightening of the deviated nose, but camouflage techniques may also be required.* Deviations that occur in the cartilaginous portion of the nose can be explained by a brief review of some anatomic characteristics of the nasal septum. The component parts of the septal framework are illustrated in Figure 35–135. The septal cartilage has two areas of fixation. The first is on the undersurface of the nasal bones, where the septal cartilage has an intimate relationship with the lateral cartilages and a shallow bony groove. The second area is the vomer groove; this area of fixation extends backward by means of a posterior extension of the septal cartilage into the perpendicular plate of the ethmoid.

The ethmoid plate plays a relatively unimportant role in supporting the bony vault.

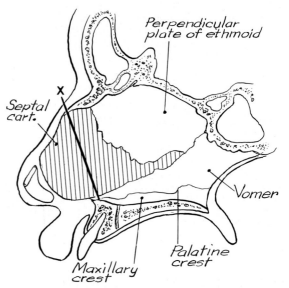

Figure 35–135. The component parts of the septal framework. Posterior to line *X* the septum is rigid.

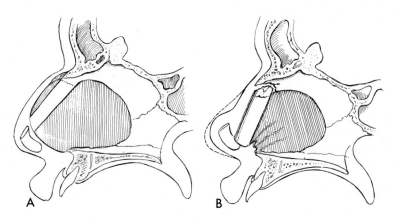

Figure 35–136. Collapse of the septum. *A,* Remaining portion of the septum after excision of the dorsal hump and resection of the caudal end of the septal cartilage *(shaded).* The remaining septal framework is supported by the perpendicular plate of the ethmoid. *B,* Fracture of the ethmoid plate, resulting in a downward displacement of the remaining septal framework. This may occur after osteotomy of the lateral nasal walls.

The area where the septal cartilage joins the perpendicular plate bone is usually thick, a resistant pillar that supports the portion of the vault formed by the lower part of the nasal bones and the lateral cartilages. This portion of the septal cartilage, the central pillar supporting the dorsal vault, must be preserved, if possible, in order to prevent the collapse of the dorsum. It is the remaining pillar of support after the other nasal structures have been loosened from the adjacent attachments by the osteotomies in the corrective rhinoplasty.

Collapse of the septal skeletal framework may occur after an extensive submucous resection performed in conjunction with a corrective rhinoplasty. After the osteotomy of the lateral walls of the nose, the remaining portion of the septum remains as a cantilever at the mercy of a fracture of the perpendicular plate of the ethmoid, and may collapse into the nasal cavity. When this unfortunate complication occurs, it is necessary to suspend the remaining dorsal portion of the septum and suture it to the lateral cartilages (Figs. 35–136, 35–137).

Septal Surgery in Rhinoplasty. Extensive submucous resection is rarely performed in the routine corrective rhinoplasty. Conservative measures include the following:

1. Resection of only a bony spur or an obviously obstructive portion of the septum.

2. Replacing the septum into the vomer groove by incising the base of the septal cartilage.

3. Shaving areas of thickened septal cartilage.

4. Straightening a curved dorsal border of the septum by conservative means.

5. Straightening the dislocated caudal portion of the septum.

6. If additional septal surgery (submucous resection) is required, a judicious approach is to limit the area of septal excision rather than risk a nasal collapse or cause a floppy septum.

Submucous Resection and Other Techniques to Straighten the Septum. It must be emphasized that septal deviations occur in most of the population and yet are not associated with symptoms of nasal obstruction. Consequently the surgical attempt to place the septum in a perfect vertical plane in the midline is not based on normal anatomic findings. *The surgical goals remain: (1) to obtain nasal airways that permit symptom-free air flow, (2) to accomplish this with as conservative a septal operation as possible, and (3) to obtain a nasal profile that appears nondeviated.*

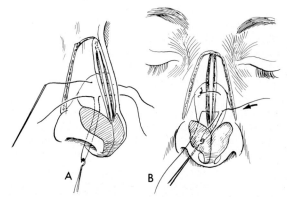

Figure 35–137. Technique of fixation after fracture of the septum and collapse of the nose. *A,* The septal cartilage is sutured to the lateral cartilages by transfixion sutures placed through the skin. After the sutures are exposed intranasally, each suture is drawn out by means of a hook, as shown in the drawing. *B,* The sutures are tied intranasally. An alternative technique is to obtain fixation to the lateral cartilages by means of externally placed mattress sutures tied over bolsters or soft lead plates.

The classic submucous resection of the nasal septum is usually a partial resection of the septal framework. The most important single operative step is to inject local anesthetic solution through a needle with a large bore and a short beveled point between the mucoperichondrium and the cartilage, thus separating the structures ("hydrodissection") and facilitating the operation. Extensive resection of the septal framework is unnecessary and endangers the stability of the nose. The operation should be performed only in cases in which there are specific indications; in many cases, more limited resection gives more satisfactory clinical results. A particular objection to the wide resection of the framework is the resulting flaccid septum (the "flapping flaps"). The replacement of resected septal cartilage fragments between the mucoperichondrial flaps has been advocated to avoid this complication, but this procedure is hazardous, since complications such as twisting of the transplanted cartilage may interfere with the airway. As previously emphasized, the tendency in recent years has been away from radical submucous resection of the septum and toward more conservative septoplasties.

After the mucoperichondrium is raised on one side, a wide exposure of the septal framework is obtained by retraction of the mucoperichondrial flap. A conservative submucous resection of the septal framework is made, removing only the most obstructive portion. The important technical point in the deviated nose is to straighten the septum while preserving its dorsal and caudal portions. The perpendicular plate of the ethmoid may be straightened by fracturing it with Bruening forceps. The vomer may be detached from the floor of the nose by means of an osteotome and replaced into the midline.

As stated earlier in the text, the turbinates, the inferior and particularly the middle, may be hypertrophied, reducing the void in the nasal cavity produced by the deviated septum. They may require outfracture, trimming, or electrocoagulation in order to complete the restoration of the airway after the septum has been straightened.

Principle of the Mucoperichondrial Splint. Through the transfixion or a separate incision, the mucoperichondrium is elevated on one side of the septal cartilage in order to obtain exposure. The mucoperichondrial elevation is limited on the contralateral side of the septum, sufficient to permit excision of *only the angulated portion of the septum.* When possible, the mucoperichondrium is left completely undisturbed; this maneuver ensures the continued nourishment of the septal cartilage, but, more important, the undisturbed mucoperichondrium acts as a splint, preventing overlapping of cartilage fragments after incision.

If the caudal portion of the septum is in the midline, straightening of the remaining dorsal and caudal portions of the septal cartilage may be done by means of incisions extending through the cartilage but not through the mucoperichondrium on the contralateral side (Fig. 35–138).

The septal framework is exposed by raising the mucoperichondrium and the mucoperios-

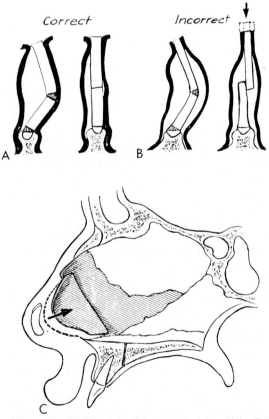

Figure 35–138. Principle of the mucoperichondrial splint. *A,* In an angulated deformity of the septum, a wedge is removed at the angulation; the septal cartilage is thus straightened. The mucoperichondrium left attached on one side prevents overlapping of the fragments, as in *B. C,* The same principle applies in preventing the anteroposterior overlapping following an incision through the septal cartilage. The intact mucoperichondrium on one side prevents overlap and shortening of the septal cartilage.

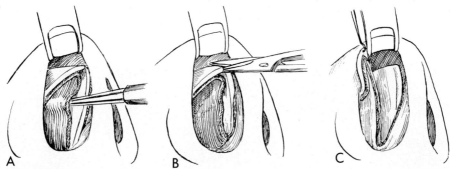

Figure 35–139. Complete exposure of the septal cartilage. *A,* The mucoperichondrium is raised from the septal cartilage. *B,* The lateral cartilage is detached from the dorsal border of the septum without incising through the mucoperichondrium. *C,* Exposure obtained on the concave side.

teum on the side *opposite* (concave) the direction of the deviation. The entire framework may be exposed on one side (Fig. 35–139) and the upper lateral cartilage is detached, as the latter usually must be trimmed to allow the return of the structures to the midline.

When the septal framework is angulated or curved, selective incisions through the cartilage and strip excisions will straighten it (Fig. 35–140). The incisions may extend to the dorsal border of the septal cartilage only if the lateral cartilages have not been separated from the septum and the cartilaginous vault is intact. In most rhinoplastic operations, at this stage the cartilages have already been separated from the septum. Such incisions should be avoided in order not to disrupt the continuity of the dorsal border of the septum.

When both sides of the septal cartilage must be exposed, mattress sutures of chromic catgut are employed to prevent overlapping of cartilage fragments, and fixation is maintained by an internal splint (see Fig. 35–144).

Swinging Door Operation. The swinging door operation permits straightening of the septal framework with minimal resection of the latter (Fig. 35–141). This type of operation should be reserved for septal deflections in which the caudal half of the septal cartilage or the entire nasal pyramid is angulated to one side (Fig. 35–142). The septal deflection is also characterized by a dislocation of the septal cartilage to one side of the vomer groove, with the caudal portion of the septal cartilage protruding into the vestibule. The vomer and the anterior nasal spine may be in the midline, the cartilage being dislocated from the vomer groove, or the vomer may be a component of the deviation (Fig. 35–143A).

In the *the swinging door procedure*, it may be possible to preserve the entire septal cartilage by straightening it and replacing it in the midline. After the usual exposure of the nasal framework and the transfixion incision that frees the septal cartilage along its dorsal and caudal borders, the lateral cartilage attachments to the septum are severed. The mucoperichondrium and mucoperiosteum are raised from only one side of the septum (see Fig. 35–139A). One should choose the side opposite to the deviation. The mucoperiosteum is raised from the vomer, and the mucoperiosteal elevation is extended to include the floor of the nose.

The point of angulation of the septal cartilage in the sagittal plane is cut through or resected in order to straighten the cartilage. The incisions are made through cartilage and do not extend through the mucoperichondrium on the opposite side (see Fig. 35–138).

The fibrous tissue between the dislocated septal cartilage and the vomer (Fig. 35–143A, B) is incised. The septal cartilage is retracted, an incision is made into the vomer groove, and fibrous tissue that fills the vomer groove is resected. The cartilage is separated from its vomer attachments and replaced in the groove (see Fig. 35–141B, C; Fig. 35–143C,D).

The flap of septal cartilage with mucoperichondrium attached, which has been freed by incisions separating the lateral cartilages from the septum and the septal cartilage from the vomer, is swung into the midline like a door swinging on its hinges (see Fig. 35–141B).

If the vomer is also deviated, it must be detached from the floor of the nose by means of an osteotome and replaced in the midline (Fig. 35–143C,D). If the septal cartilage

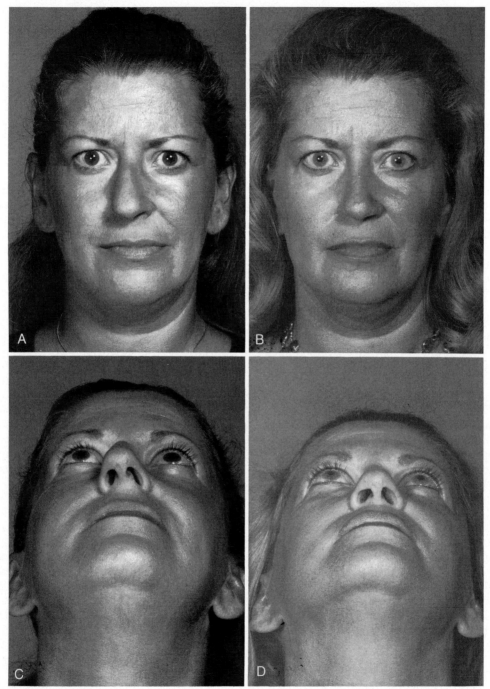

Figure 35–140. Developmental nasal deviation with C-shaped deformity of the dorsum. Note the protrusion of the septal angle under the right alar cartilage. *A, C,* Preoperative views. *B, D,* After septoplasty and corrective rhinoplasty.

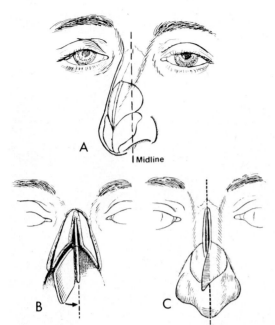

Figure 35–141. The swinging door procedure. *A,* The entire nose is deflected to one side. *B,* A strip of septal cartilage has been resected at the point of angulation, and the caudal portion of the cartilage is moved into the midline; fixation is established in the vomer groove (see Fig. 35–143*D*). The mucoperichondrium on one side of the septal cartilage remains attached. *C,* Restoration of symmetry between the two lateral cartilages after replacement of the structures in the midline; a portion of the dorsal border of the overlapping lateral cartilage must be excised.

shows a curvature in the frontal plane, a wedge excision is required to replace the septal angle into the midline (Fig. 35–143*C, D*). The structures should remain in the midline after the corrective surgery, without any tendency to fall back into their previously deviated position. It is essential to provide fixation of the septal cartilage: a hole is drilled through the nasal spine or the premaxillary wings (or both) by means of a small, round drill point activated by an air turbine. The caudal portion is maintained in fixation with a nonabsorbable suture or stainless steel wire (Fig. 35–143*D*).

Reshaping of the deformed columella may require section or resection of a portion of the lower end of one or both medial crura (see Fig. 35–130).

Other Techniques. Fry and Robertson (1967), applying the observations made by Gibson and Davis (1958), showed that when the mucoperichondrium is raised from both sides of the septal cartilage and the cartilage is scored on one side, the cartilage bends to the opposite side. The author of this chapter

attempted to apply this experimental finding to the clinical problem of straightening the septum but did not find it as reliable as the methods described above. Actual sectioning of the cartilage is necessary in angulated deviations and curvatures. An alternative technique, mentioned earlier in the text, is that of "morselization." An instrument with jaws having protruding asperities either on one jaw only or on both jaws is employed to produce multiple incisions through the cartilage. It is alleged that the septal cartilage loses its resilience. In general it is more prudent for the surgeon to ensure that the septum is straightened under direct vision at the operative procedure.

Internal Splint. When a number of incisions through the septal cartilage are required, mattress sutures of absorbable material may assist in the fixation of the fragments, in addition to the mucoperichondrial splint.

Nasal gauze packing helps to support the straightened septum. Sheets of Silastic rubber, Teflon, polyethylene, or other substances such as x-ray film may be cut to size, placed on each side of the septum, and joined by a *loosely* tied mattress suture. This type of internal splinting was described by Johnson (1964). The splints may be left in position for several weeks and are well tolerated.

Jost, Vergnon, and Hadjean (1973), by placing the holes through which the suture is passed in a decussated manner (Fig. 35–144*A,B*), were able to splint the major portion of the septum. This technique was used by the authors after incising the septum in a serpentine manner to prevent recurrent septal deviation (Fig. 35–144*C*).

Dislocated Caudal Border of Septal Cartilage

Anterior Columellar Approach. Dislocation of the caudal end of the septal cartilage from its position in the vomer groove causes it to protrude to one side of the columella. The protrusion obstructs the airway in some cases and nearly always distorts the appearance of the columella (Fig. 35–145; see also Fig. 35–140).

The swinging door procedure can be employed to replace the cartilage in the midline without resecting the cartilage (see Fig. 35–141).

The caudal portion of the septal cartilage may be so distorted in some cases that any plan to straighten the septal framework by conservative surgery must be abandoned. The

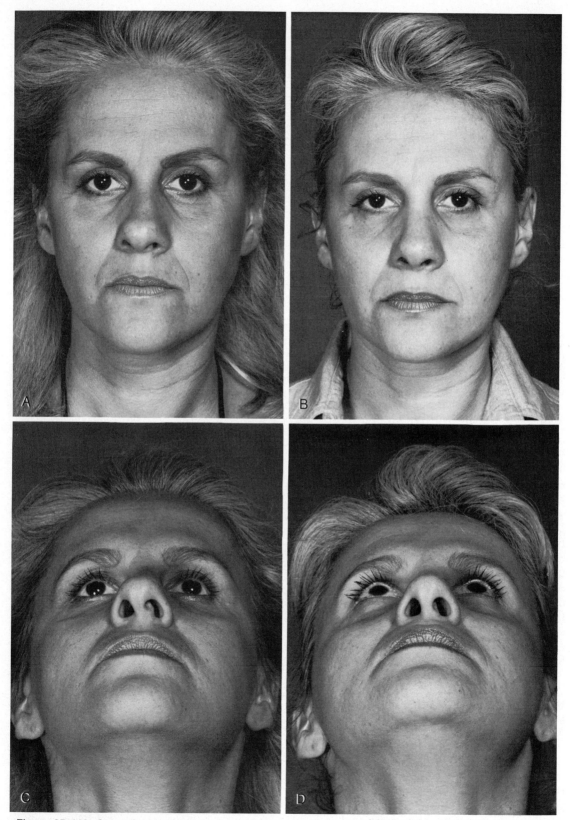

Figure 35–142. Generalized deviation of the nose corrected by the technique illustrated in Figure 35–141. *A, C,* Deviated nose of traumatic origin. The tip is deflected because of severe angulation of the septum to the right side. *B, D,* Postoperative appearance.

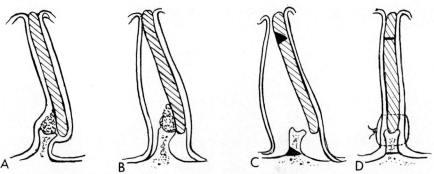

Figure 35–143. Straightening the caudal portion of the septal cartilage. *A,* Frontal section through the caudal portion of the septal cartilage dislocated out of the vomer groove. Fibrous tissue fills the vomer groove. *B,* The septal mucoperichondrium and mucoperiosteum over the vomer on the right side of the septum are raised. The mucoperiosteum is also elevated over the left side of the vomer. The mucoperichondrium over the left side of the septal cartilage remains intact. *C,* A wedge of cartilage is resected near the dorsal portion of the septal cartilage to allow straightening. The pad of fibrous tissue in the vomer groove is removed. *D,* The cartilage is straightened, replaced in the vomer groove, and anchored in position by a suture placed through a drill hole in the premaxillary wings or the nasal spine.

caudal portion of the septal cartilage is resected; resection of the vomer spurs often is also required in order to ensure an adequate nasal airway. Retraction of the columella is prevented by embedding a strip of septal cartilage into the columella through an inci-

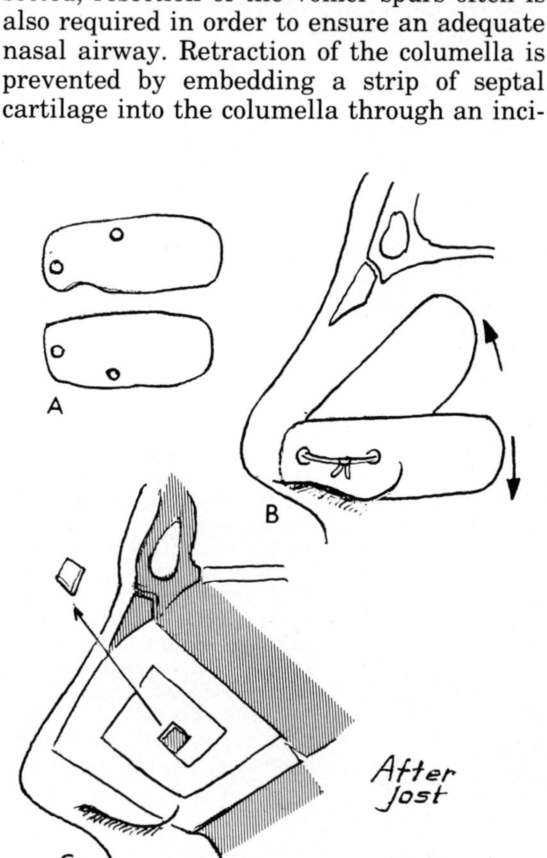

Figure 35–144. The internal splint. *A, B,* By placing the holes in each plate in a decussated manner, it is possible to splint the major portion of the septum when the suture is tightened. *C,* Spiral septal incision, which is varied according to the type of deviation, combined with removal of a small piece of septal cartilage. (After Jost.)

sion along the caudal border of the medial crus (see Fig. 35–126).

Total Resection and Transplantation of Septal Cartilage Over Dorsum of Nose (Camouflage Procedure). There are two types of nasal deviations in which a conservative type of septal straightening cannot be done.

The first is the deviated nose in which the septal cartilage is severely twisted in the frontal plane as well as in the sagittal plane; the dorsal border of the septal cartilage shows an accentuated, S-shaped curvature in both the sagittal and frontal planes (see Fig. 35–140). The septal cartilage must be resected because (1) it cannot be straightened by conservative septoplasty techniques and (2) there is the need to recover strips of septal cartilage for transplants placed into the columella (see Fig. 35–126) and over the nasal dorsum (see Fig. 35–146) (McKinney and Shively, 1979; Rees, 1986).

A second type of deviation in which the septum must be completely resected is the flat and deviated nose often seen after repeated trauma. In this type of deformity, the septum has lost its supportive function. Septal resection is necessary because the septum is so thick that it obstructs the airway ("boxer's septum"). Complete resection of the septum does not result in any change in the shape of the nose, because the septum has already lost its role as a supporting structure. This type of nose may require reconstruction by means of cartilage (septal, costal) or bone grafts to restore the contour of the dorsum.

Technique. The dorsal hump is resected.

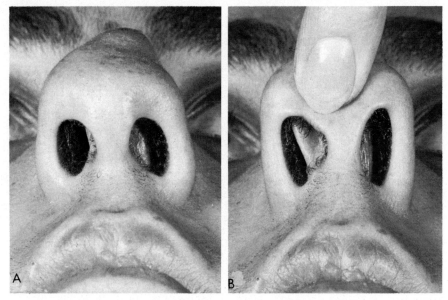

Figure 35–145. Dislocation of the caudal end of the septal cartilage. *A,* The caudal end of the septal cartilage protrudes into the left vestibule. *B,* Pressure over the tip accentuates the twisted shape of the cartilage; the cartilage now protrudes into the *right* vestibule. Note the bifidity of the tip caused by deviation of the septal angle.

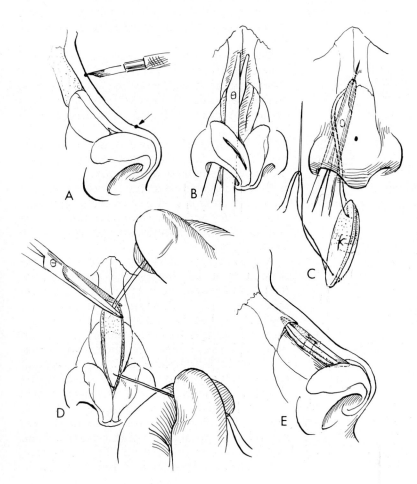

Figure 35–146. Technique of transplantation of septal cartilage to the dorsum of the nose. *A,* Two ink dots on the skin indicate the upper and lower limits of the transplant. *B,* Scissors undermining the area over the dorsum to be occupied by the transplant. *C,* The transplant (layered) is held by guide sutures of catgut; the upper guide suture is introduced into position by means of a straight needle, which pierces the skin through the upper ink dot. *D,* The guide suture is removed, and the plain catgut is left buried under the skin. *E,* The graft in position.

It is usually a small pseudohump resulting from the loss of contour of the cartilaginous dorsum of the nose. The lateral cartilages are not separated from the septum; thus, the continuity between the lateral cartilages and the septum is preserved.

It is possible to secure a sufficiently long, straight piece of cartilage (or cartilage plus ethmoid plate) for a suitable transplant, even in the most deviated septal cartilage. Additional cartilage may be harvested from the conchal portion of the auricular helix. A single piece of cartilage or a number of superimposed pieces may be required.

The cartilage graft is introduced through one of the incisions previously made to correct the tip and is placed over the lateral cartilages. The dorsal septal cartilage transplant may be placed with precision by the technique illustrated in Figure 35–146.

Two ink dots are made over the dorsum at points between which the cartilage is to be placed. The dots indicate the upper and lower limits of the transplant (Fig. 35–146*A*). This area is undermined with scissors (Fig. 35–146*B*). Sutures of plain catgut are passed with a straight cutting needle, which is placed through each extremity of the cartilage transplant (Fig. 35–146*C*). The needle carrying the cephalic traction suture is placed into the subcutaneous pocket and out through the skin (Fig. 35–146*C*); the needle with the caudal traction sutures is also placed into the pocket and through the skin. The sutures are cut before adhesive paper tape is placed over the dorsum to stabilize the graft (Fig. 35–146*D, E*).

Corrective Surgery for Deviated Nose That Requires Modification of Profile Line. When the profile must be modified in the course of straightening the deviated nose, the order of procedure is similar to that followed in a typical rhinoplastic operation. The septum must be straightened to avoid recurrence of the deviation by pressure of the septum against the lateral nasal wall. It is essential, however, to employ a conservative technique in order to preserve the support afforded by the septum and avoid nasal collapse.

Technique of Submucous Resection of Septum: Radical Operation. Although the radical resection of the septal framework is rarely used except in a severely damaged nose and septum, the procedure is occasionally indicated.

The technique of submucous resection of the septal framework was established in the early part of the century by Freer (1902) and Killian (1904). A wide resection of the skeletal constituents of the septum, involving the major portions of the septal cartilage, perpendicular plate of the ethmoid, and vomer, was advocated.

Care should be taken to expose the septal framework along a plane situated between the cartilage and mucoperichondrium. This procedure is assisted by ballooning out the mucoperichondrium and mucoperiosteum from the framework by a preliminary injection of anesthetic solution made with a large-bore needle with a short bevel. The plane of dissection is thus prepared, bleeding is eliminated, and the operation is rendered considerably easier by the resulting exposure (Fig. 35–147*A* to *C*).

Before making the incision for the submucous resection of the septal framework, the surgeon should plan to leave a strip of cartilage (1 cm or more in width) along the dorsal and caudal borders of the septum. If the caudal portion of the septum is deviated and requires straightening, the septum can be approached through the transfixion incision of the rhinoplastic procedure. Near the transfixion incision, the mucoperichondrium is intimately attached to the cartilage through the fibers of the depressor septi nasi muscle and often must be sharply dissected with the knife. It is essential at all times that the blue-white color of the septal cartilage be seen, a finding that indicates that the operator is in the correct plane of dissection. Failure to follow this plane of dissection results in tearing of the mucoperichondrium, with the danger of septal perforation if the tear occurs on both sides. Moreover, contraction of the healing mucoperichondrium can cause a depression of the nasal dorsum.

When the caudal portion of the septum is not deviated, an L-shaped incision is made behind the posterior vestibular fold (Fig. 35–147*D*) in order to avoid the formation of a cicatricial band on the floor of the vestibule. A horizontal incision that extends along the base of the septum near the floor of the nose provides dependent drainage, avoids a septal hematoma, and obviates the need for intranasal packing to prevent a collection of blood between the flaps. In severe traumatic septal deflection, the incision for the exposure of the septal framework is made on the concave side

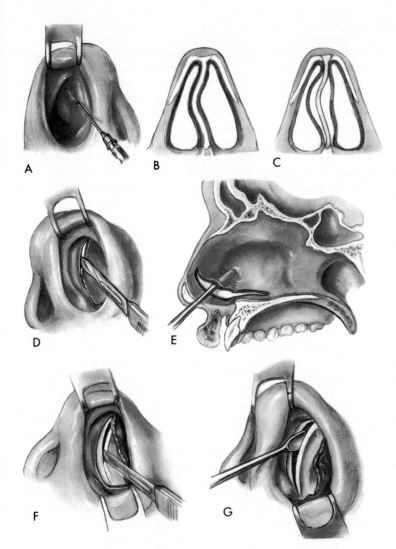

Figure 35–147. Radical submucous resection of the nasal septum. *A,* Submucoperichondrial infiltration of anesthetic solution. *B,* Frontal section, showing the deviation of the septal framework. *C,* The mucoperichondrium and mucoperiosteum have been raised from the septal framework on each side. *D,* Beginning of the L-shaped incision of the type used when the caudal portion of the septum does not need correction. The incision is started approximately 10 to 15 mm posterior to the caudal border and extends through the mucoperichondrium to the cartilage. *E,* The incision has been made down to the floor of the nose and it extends along the floor. Mucoperichondrial elevation is begun. *F,* After the flap of mucoperiosteum on the left side is raised, the incision is made through the septal cartilage a few millimeters posterior to the mucosal incision. The incision extends through the cartilages but not through the mucoperichondrium on the opposite side. *G,* Raising the mucoperichondrium on the opposite side.

of the septal deflection, the mucoperichondrium on the concave side being technically easier to raise (Fig. 35–147*E*).

After one side of the septal cartilage is exposed, an incision is made through the cartilage, a few millimeters posterior to the mucous membrane incision (Fig. 35–147*F*); the mucoperichondrium and mucoperiosteum are raised from the opposite side of the septal cartilage (Figs. 35–147*G*, 35–148*A*). A medium-length nasal speculum exposes the cartilage between its blades, retracting the septal flaps. An incision through the septal cartilage is made, parallel to the dorsal border of the septum, by means of angulated septal scissors (Figs. 35–148*B*, 35–149). The septal cartilage is then separated from the perpendicular plate of the ethmoid by cutting through the cartilage with an angulated knife

(Fig. 35–148*C*), and the remainder of the cartilage is resected from the vomer (Fig. 35–148*D*). Additional septal framework is resected as required (Fig. 35–150). A patient is illustrated in Figure 35–151.

Treatment of Enlarged Turbinates. It has been a traditional view that subtotal resection of the turbinates interferes with the essential functions of nasal humidification, warming, and filtering of inspired air. It was also felt that such surgery resulted in rhinitis sicca. More recently, however, other surgeons (Fry, 1973; Courtiss, Goldwyn, and O'Brien, 1978), after failing to document a single case of rhinitis sicca in the literature after subtotal resection of the inferior turbinates, have recommended this procedure for hypertrophic turbinates that impede nasal air flow.

While steroid injections, electrocautery,

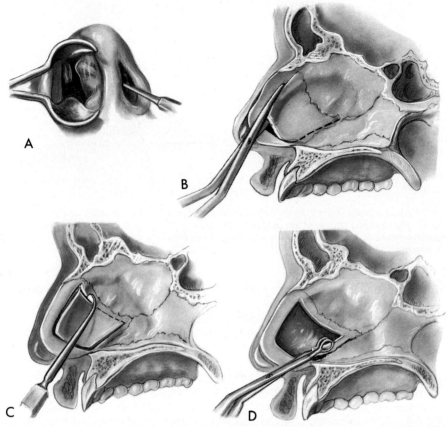

Figure 35–148. Radical submucous resection of the nasal septum. *A,* Elevation of the mucoperichondrium on the right side of the septum. *B,* Resection of the deviated septal framework with scissors; an adequate amount of cartilage is left along the dorsum for septal support. *C,* An angulated knife is employed to sever the cartilage from the perpendicular plate of the ethmoid. Cartilage, which has also been separated from the vomer, can then be removed intact and employed as a transplant when necessary. *D,* Resection of the remaining cartilage in the vomer groove. A portion of the vomer will also be resected when necessary to remove the obstructing portion of bone and spurs.

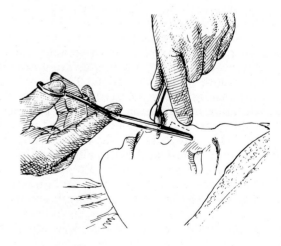

Figure 35–149. Position of the scissors held parallel to the nasal dorsum while the incision shown in Figure 35–148*B* is made.

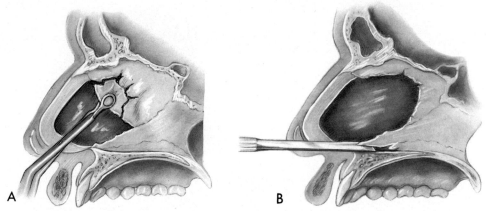

Figure 35–150. Radical submucous resection of the septum (continued). *A,* The deviated portion of the septal cartilage has been removed. The deviated portion of the perpendicular plate of the ethmoid is being resected. *B,* A portion of the vomer is resected by means of an osteotome. As a rule, only those portions of the septal framework that appear to cause obstruction are removed (see text).

and crushing and outfracture techniques have been recommended, the improvement in nasal airway symptoms is short-lived. Since the patient is prepared for nasal surgery, partial resection of the offending turbinate is the procedure of choice.

Technique. After the cocaine packs are removed, the inferior pole of the inferior turbinate is injected with anesthetic solution (Fig. 35–152*A,B*). It is important to balloon the hypertrophic mucosa sufficiently.

Through the nasal speculum a knife is introduced into the nasal cavity and the mucosa is incised down to bone over the antero-inferior edge of the turbinate. The mucoperi-osteum is elevated off the medial and lateral surfaces of the conchal bone. Angulated scissors are then introduced in a plane parallel to the plane of the turbinate, and an appropriate amount of hypertrophic mucosa and/or bone is resected (Fig. 35–152*C*).

Complications Following Corrective Surgery for Nasal Deviations. In addition to the complications that occur after corrective surgery for the nose, the major complication after surgery for the deviated nose is recurrence of the deviation. The most frequent cause of the recurrence is inadequate straightening of the nasal septum. The inexorable pressure exerted by a deviated septum prevents infracture of the nasal bone or presses a lateral wall out of alignment.

A dismaying complication after a corrective rhinoplasty is a postoperative deviation in a nose that was straight preoperatively. This complication can be explained as follows: the dorsal border of the septum was straight;

beneath the dorsal septal border, however, the septum was curved along a sagittal plane; when the dorsal border was resected, the curved portion of the septum became the new dorsal border, hence the postoperative deviation. Careful preoperative examination of the septum will suggest precautionary measures to avert such a complication. When the complication occurs, the remedy is a secondary operation to straighten the septum and realign the nasal structures.

A major complication is collapse of the remaining dorsal portion of the septal framework, which, after resection of the caudal portion of the septum, remains in position as a cantilever. Fracture of the cantilever at the perpendicular plate of the ethmoid (see Fig. 35–136) causes a collapse of the remaining septal framework, a loss of contour of the nasal dorsum, and a resultant saddle nose deformity. This complication is avoided by straightening the septum through conservative measures, thus preserving adequate septal support.

ESTHETIC RHINOPLASTY IN NON-CAUCASIANS

Choices of corrective nasalplastic procedures in black and Oriental patients often involve the techniques described in the previous pages in addition to the transplantation of bone or cartilage.

The population of the United States contains representatives of nearly every ethnic

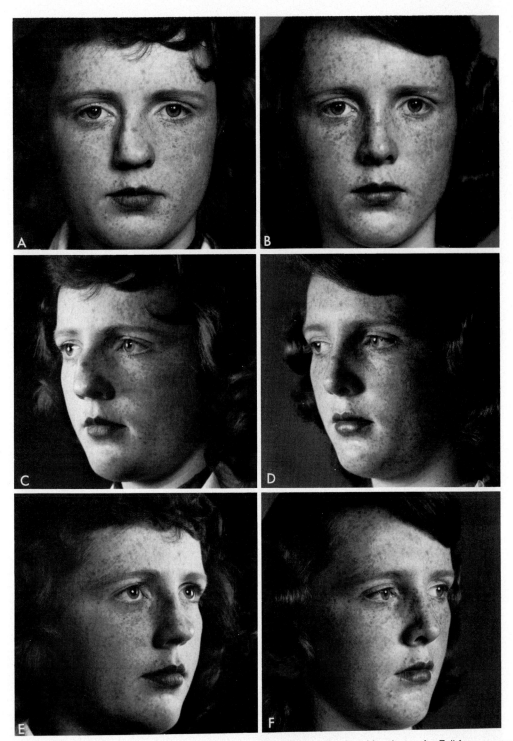

Figure 35–151. Straightening the deviated nose and concomitant corrective rhinoplasty. *A,.* Full-face appearance shows the C-shaped deviation, widening, and bifidity of the tip. *B,* Postoperative result. *C,* Preoperative three-quarter anterior view showing the osteocartilaginous dorsal bump. *D,* Postoperative three-quarter view. *E,* Preoperative three-quarter anterior view showing the bifidity of the tip. *F,* Postoperative view.

Illustration continued on following page

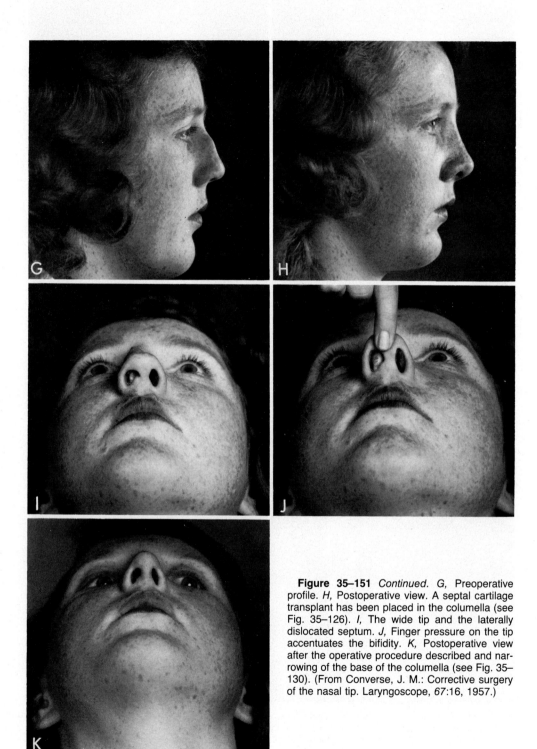

Figure 35–151 *Continued. G,* Preoperative profile. *H,* Postoperative view. A septal cartilage transplant has been placed in the columella (see Fig. 35–126). *I,* The wide tip and the laterally dislocated septum. *J,* Finger pressure on the tip accentuates the bifidity. *K,* Postoperative view after the operative procedure described and narrowing of the base of the columella (see Fig. 35–130). (From Converse, J. M.: Corrective surgery of the nasal tip. Laryngoscope, *67:*16, 1957.)

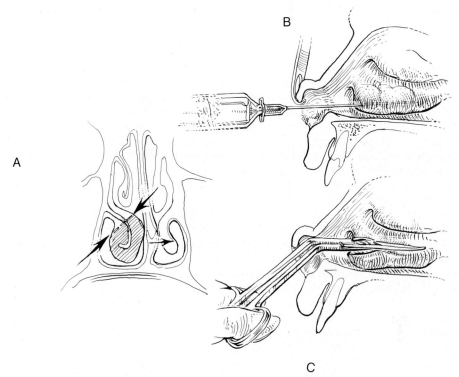

Figure 35–152. Technique of partial turbinectomy. *A, B,* Injection of the turbinate with anesthetic solution. The arrows note the level of mucosa-bone resection. The smaller arrow designates the direction of the septal deviation. *C,* Resection is accomplished with angulated scissors introduced through a nasal speculum.

group of the world's population. In their desire for assimilation, a considerable number of individuals from these diverse ethnic/racial groups request the removal of distinctive ethnic traits, notably correction of the nose.

The growing desire to acquire a more Occidental appearance has manifested itself in the Far East by patients' requesting the Oriental eye operation and an increase in the projection of the dorsum of the nose (see Chap. 44).

Anatomic Characteristics. The noses of the Oriental and the black have some features in common: the flat nasal dorsum, the short columella, the slanted external nares, and the flared nostrils (see Figs. 35–29, 35–31, 35–32). The nostril borders usually are delicately formed in the Oriental; in the black, however, they are generally thick. These characteristics can vary as a result of the admixtures of ethnic groups.

The basic skeletal variations between the nose of the Occidental and that of the patient of African origin were studied by Wen (1921) (see Fig. 35–30). He noted that, whereas the septal angle in the Caucasian is usually well defined, the dorsal border of the septum has

a downward curve with an ill-defined septal angle in the black patient (see Fig. 35–30). Wen also described a distinct difference in the structure of the alar cartilages between the two ethnic groups. In the black patient, the alar cartilages are often smaller and more frail, despite the external appearance of the wide-flaring nares. Matory and Falces (1986) recommended the use of the *nasal index* (nasal width to length multiplied by 100) in establishing racial differences in the nose on frontal view. The base of the triangle tends to be wide in non-Caucasian patients and ideally should be within the vertical lines dropped from the medial canthi.

Corrective Rhinoplasty in Orientals. The increase in the projection of the dorsum of the nose is a common procedure, following the Oriental eye operation in frequency. Uchida (1958) described various techniques for this purpose. Boo-Chai (1964) inserted a Silastic implant over the dorsum to increase the projection. Although no longitudinal studies have been reported, the Silastic implant appears to be more successful in the Oriental nose than in the Occidental nose, especially when it is used to correct a post-traumatic deformity in the latter. Boo-Chai also advocated alar base wedge excisions. Furukawa (1974) elaborated upon the various techniques for rhinoplasty in the Oriental nose (see Chap. 44).

Corrective Rhinoplasty in Blacks. Rees (1969), Falces, Wesser, and Gorney (1970), Rees and Wood-Smith (1972), and Matory and Falces (1986) described techniques for corrective rhinoplasty in black patients.

The techniques include increasing the projection of the dorsum of the nose by means of an iliac bone graft, lengthening the columella, and increasing the projection of the tip by weakening the alar cartilage in the region of the domes via partial- or full-thickness incisions. The medial crura and domes are maintained by a mattress suture. These procedures are combined with interalar narrowing, alar sill advancement (Matory and Falces, 1986), wedge excisions at the base of the alae (see Fig. 35–88), and also excision along the alar borders in selected cases (see Fig. 35–89). Although the possibility of keloid formation in the black patient must be considered, it has not been reported in the papers published on this subject.

POSTOPERATIVE CARE

The patient is placed in the Fowler position after returning to bed, the head being elevated in order to minimize postoperative bleeding. Pain is controlled by medication. A soft diet is prescribed during the first two postoperative days.

No intranasal treatment is required. Healing occurs faster and the incidence of postoperative bleeding is diminished if the patient is undisturbed. Postoperative edema, ecchymoses around the eyes, and occasionally subconjunctival hemorrhage are minimal when the high osteotomy technique is employed. Swelling and ecchymoses, which may peak 48 hours after the operation, begin to subside on the third day. Orbital ecchymosis, if present, gradually changes from a dark bluish color to a yellowish tinge at the end of the first week. Subconjunctival hemorrhage, which disappears more gradually and may extend for a period of two to three weeks, is a rare occurrence after the average rhinoplastic operation.

Ice compresses over the eyes, although soothing for the patient, do not appear to diminish the periorbital ecchymosis or hasten its disappearance.

The nasal splint and tapes are removed after a period varying from five to seven days. The patient is advised against blowing his nose to avoid provoking hemorrhage or subcutaneous emphysema by the passage of air through the lines of osteotomy.

After removal of the splint, the patient is instructed to apply cold cream or paraffin ointment (Vaseline) to the nasal vestibule to soften blood clots or crusts.

The undermined skin of the tip of the nose is denervated temporarily. Sebaceous glands, which are abundant in this area, are passive and filled with secretion. During the postoperative period, twice daily gentle washing with a strongly alkaline soap or a mildly detergent cream assists in the evacuation of the accumulated sebaceous secretion and facilitates the progressive contraction of the skin.

The patient is also informed that the nose may appear somewhat overcorrected and swollen but that the appearance will gradually improve (Fig. 35–153).

Edema may persist over a period of months, especially in the supratip area or the root of the nose. The time period is extended in direct proportion to the amount of reduction in size of the nose and the age of the patient. Contraction of the soft tissues over the modified

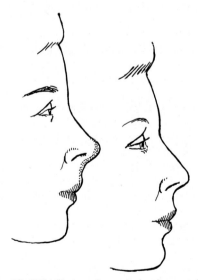

Figure 35–153. Change in contour after resolution of postoperative swelling. *Left,* Immediate postoperative appearance. *Right,* Appearance after subsidence of the postoperative swelling. (After Aufricht.)

skeletal framework occurs more slowly in the older patient and may require six months to a year.

Slight irregularities may appear after the edema subsides, causing considerable anxiety to the patient. These may occur along the dorsum of the nose at the point of junction of the lateral walls; although the condition usually is not visible, the patient can feel the irregularities on palpation.

COMPLICATIONS

Hemorrhage. This is usually the result of the detachment of a clot overlying an area denuded of mucous membrane. Avoidance of denuded areas minimizes the danger of bleeding after surgery. Postoperative hemorrhage is more frequent if a septal procedure has been performed. It usually is not severe and is easily controlled by removing clots, achieving hemostasis by the application of epinephrine or Oxycel gauze, and providing intranasal packing when required. Care should be exercised to avoid displacing the bony lateral walls of the nose by pressure from the packing. Occasionally, severe epistaxis may occur, requiring posterior nasal packing as well as packing of the anterior nasal fossae. This is fortunately a rare occurrence.

Infection. If hematoma is avoided and if small fragments of spicules of bone or cartilage are carefully removed before the completion of surgery, infection is rare. The usual site for an abscess, a rare occurrence, is in the upper portion of the line of osteotomy. Incision, drainage, and antibiotic treatment usually resolve this complication.

Mucous Cysts. Protrusions can be observed along the lines of dorsal resection or lines of osteotomy and represent herniation of nasal mucosa. Treatment usually involves excision.

Irregularity in Shape. Most complications are due to faulty planning or technique. These potential problems have been described earlier in this chapter, and secondary surgery is discussed in Chapter 36.

Progressive postoperative *widening of the bony dorsum* is usually caused by an undiagnosed high deviation of the septum. The following anatomic factors may impede the medial displacement of the lateral walls of the nose: excessive width of the dorsal border of the septum caused by the increase in skeletal width; hypertrophy of the mucous membrane; interposition of mucous membrane between the medially mobilized lateral nasal walls; and deviation of the dorsal portion of the septum. Such complications can be avoided by careful inspection and correction before the operation is completed.

Minor *curvature or deviation of the cartilaginous nasal dorsum* by undetected curvatures of the septal framework can spoil an otherwise satisfactory result. Careful examination of the septum prevents such a complication.

Irregularities in the area of the *dome* and *the lateral crus* are common complications. In order to avoid an irregularity along the caudal border, the transgression of the border by surgical incision is avoided in the routine corrective rhinoplasty. If the caudal border is transgressed, the border of the cartilage should be realigned by carefully placing a catgut suture, otherwise a "pinched" tip will result. Failure to realign the cartilage may result in a protrusion of the portion of the cartilage lateral to the incision. Other irregularities, such as disproportion in the shape of the domes, may occur and require secondary surgery to achieve symmetry (see Chap. 36).

Drooping of Tip. The tip of the nose appears to droop in the early postoperative period because swelling of the base of the columella and upper lip produces a temporary elevation of the tip. Subsidence of the swelling allows the tip to resume its position, and the patient interprets this event as a downward drooping of the tip (see Fig. 35–153). The tip of the nose will droop after a rhinoplasty if the cartilaginous lateral walls (alar cartilages) have been shortened inadequately in relation to the shortened septum. The elasticity of the cartilages pushes the tip downward, the nasal tip gradually resuming its preoperative position. Ironically, overshortening of the septum may be a cause of postoperative drooping of the tip. When the tip is downwardly dislocated from the septal angle before surgery, shortening the septum increases the loss of contact between the structures and is a basic technical mistake to be avoided.

Supratip Protrusion. A not uncommon postoperative complication is the supratip protrusion, which spoils an otherwise satisfactory profile. Various factors are responsible for this complication, the treatment of which is discussed in Chapter 36.

Saddle Deformity. Earlier in the text, the

need to avoid excessive resection of the dorsal hump was emphasized. In the nose with thick skin, it is particularly necessary to be prudent in the amount of resection along the dorsum in order to avoid the supratip protrusion.

A depressed area of the cartilaginous dorsum occurs if the septum has been removed in excess, particularly if the septal mucoperichondrial flaps have been badly torn, since the cicatricial contraction of the healing flap increases the tendency to depression along the dorsum.

Vestibular Atresia. It has been estimated that most postrhinoplasty patients show some evidence of synechia formation at the apex of the vestibule (Sheen, 1978). The resulting reduction in the perimeter of the vestibule can result in varying degrees of airway obstruction and the need for corrective surgery. This finding can usually be attributed to excessive resection of the caudal edge of the upper lateral cartilage.

Septal-Turbinate Synechiae. An adhesion or synechia forms as a result of the healing of the raw areas after a combined septoplasty and turbinectomy. Nasal obstruction is the consequence of this type of nasal airway closure.

Treatment consists of cutting through the adhesion and interposing nasal packing or a sheet of Silastic, which must be left in position for a minimum of seven days to allow for reepithelization of the raw areas.

Perforation of Septum. Iatrogenic septal perforation may result from an incorrectly performed operation to straighten the deviated septum. If the septal mucoperichondrial flap is lacerated on both sides and the intervening septal cartilage has been removed, a perforation of varying size results.

Loss of nasal mucous membrane, associated with a large septal perforation, results in serious impairment of nasal physiology, because the ciliated, columnar epithelium is indispensable for nasal function. Small perforations may produce a whistling sound and are more symptomatic than larger ones.

Large perforations, with a loss of a major portion of the septum, are intractable. Surprisingly, some patients tolerate large perforations relatively well, while the small perforation and the whistling sound may annoy the patient. All patients with septal perforations have crusts that must be removed, and the area of the perforation must be cleansed. Loss of olfaction and nasal obstruction with atrophic rhinitis may result when mucosal changes involve the entire nasal cavity. The daily use of emollients such as paraffin oil, sprayed to soften the crusts, and nasal irrigations with saline solution are necessary to rid the patient of the foul-smelling crusts.

When the septal framework has been entirely removed, it is difficult to separate the septal flaps. In smaller perforations, fortunately, the septal framework is usually present. Use of a rotation flap (Fig. 35–154A,B) is feasible in small and moderate-sized anterior perforations. Grafts of oral mucosa, adequately thinned (Fig. 35–154C to E), provide a covering for the raw surface of the flap. An anterior transposition flap (Fig. 35–154F,G) may also be used.

In larger perforations, the only successful technique in the author's experience has been the labial mucosal flap, raised from the labial aspect of the buccal sulcus, based at the level of the frenulum, and introduced into the nasal cavity (Fig. 35–154H to N).

Small perforations may be closed by using two hinge flaps of mucoperichondrium, one on each side. On one side the flap is hinged on a superior pedicle; on the other side the flap is hinged on an inferior pedicle (Fig. 35–155). Nasal packing maintains the raw surfaces of the flaps in apposition until healed.

The subject of septal perforations was discussed in detail by Meyer (1972), who closed large perforations by the following technique. The cartilage is buried at the distal end of a flap of mucous membrane in the labial gingival sulcus. The flap is so designed that mucous membrane at the distal end of the flap is folded under the cartilage; thus, the cartilage is enveloped by two layers of mucous membrane. After three weeks the flap is introduced into the nasal cavity, and the three-layered distal end of the flap is sutured into the septal perforation.

DEPRESSED NASAL DORSUM: TECHNIQUES OF BONE AND CARTILAGE GRAFTING

Depression of the dorsum of the nose (Fig. 35–156) may occur in the bony or the cartilaginous portion; when both are affected, the term *saddle nose* is often used to designate the deformity. Associated conditions can also interfere with respiratory function: e.g., thickening of the septal cartilage and collapse of the lateral and alar cartilages.

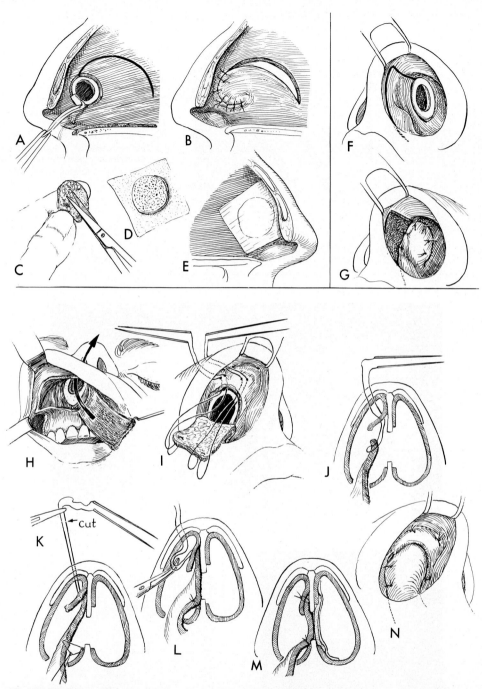

Figure 35–154. Techniques for the closure of septal perforations. *A,* Outline of a posterior rotation flap of mucoperichondrium. *B,* The flap is sutured in position. *C,* A mucosal graft is removed from the oral mucosa. The raw surface of the graft is trimmed, thus reducing the thickness of the graft. *D,* A mucosal graft placed on paper tape. *E,* The graft carried on the paper tape is applied to the raw surface of the rotation flap illustrated in *A* and *B* and maintained by nasal packing. *F, G,* Transposition flap for the closure of small perforations. *F,* A flap is outlined anteriorly from the membranous septum. *G,* The flap is transposed. *H* to *N,* In larger perforations a flap of mucosa from the upper lip is indicated. *I,* The mucosal flap from the upper lip is introduced into the nasal cavity; two catgut mattress sutures are placed through the distal end of the flap and are brought out through the raised mucoperichondrium and the cartilaginous nasal wall. *J,* Frontal section illustrating the maneuver in *I. K,* The sutures are cut and the needles removed. *L,* The sutures are reintroduced into the nasal cavity. *M,* The sutures are tied, providing fixation of the flap. A graft of mucosa *(C, D, E)* is applied to the raw surface of the flap on the contralateral side of the septum. *N,* The flap is sutured.

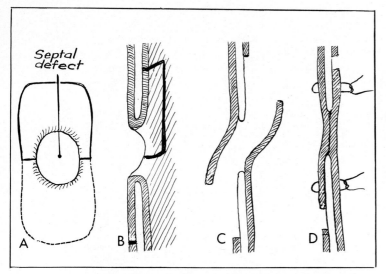

Figure 35–155. Technique for closure of small perforations. *A,* Healed perforation with cicatricial edges. *B,* Outline of a hinge flap. *C,* Frontal section of bilateral, hinged, turnover flaps of mucoperichondrium. *D,* The flaps are sutured to each other with mattress sutures.

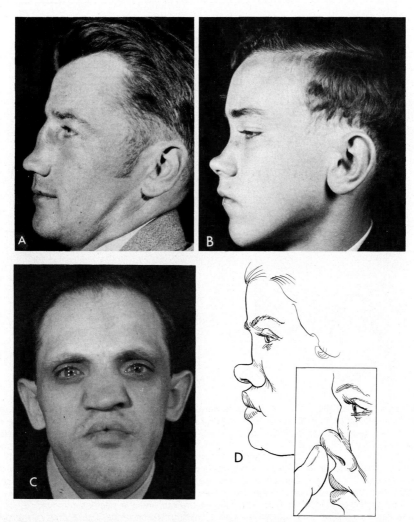

Figure 35–156. The depressed nasal dorsum. *A,* Traumatic depression of the cartilaginous portion of the nose. Note the drooping tip and retraction of the columella. *B,* Typical saddle nose deformity involving both the bony and cartilaginous portions. *C,* Flat nose resulting from widening of the bony dorsum and loss of septal support of the cartilaginous portion of the nose. *D,* When the cartilaginous framework is destroyed, the tip offers no resistance to digital pressure *(inset).*

Congenital saddle nose is unusual, most deformities of this type being traumatic in origin. Saddle nose was a typical deformity resulting from syphilis before the latter was largely eradicated by chemotherapy. Saddle deformities caused by syphilis, leishmaniasis, and leprosy are characterized by a loss of nasal lining as well as of the nasal framework. In these deformities it is often necessary to restore the nasal lining before restoring the nasal framework.

Depression of the cartilaginous portion of the nose is often seen after excessive resection of the septal cartilage as part of a corrective rhinoplasty. If the mucoperichondrial flaps have been lacerated, there is additional loss of skeletal support owing to the contracture exerted by the healing flaps. Cartilaginous depressions are also seen following hematoma and abscess of the septum with destruction of the cartilage; this type of complication is not infrequent in childhood.

The dorsum of the nose may show a pseudohump due to depression of the cartilaginous dorsum, frequently accompanied by widening of the bony bridge and drooping of the tip. Satisfactory correction of this type of deformity can often be obtained by reducing the pseudohump, cartilage grafting of the dorsum, narrowing the nasal bridge by osteotomy of the lateral walls, and shortening the nose by excision of cartilage from the caudal border of the septum and from the alar cartilages.

Transplants and Implants for Repair of Saddle Nose Deformities. Various materials have been employed for nasal contour restoration. The author, however, prefers either autogenous bone or cartilage.

Cartilage allografts have been used extensively (Brown and McDowell, 1951). The work of Gibson, Curran, and Davis (1957) suggested the possibility of survival of fresh cartilage allografts. The latter have not been employed, because failure of maternal auricular cartilage allografts in the reconstruction of the microtic auricle has been observed. Bovine cartilage (Gillies and Kristensen, 1951) does not maintain its bulk and is progressively absorbed (see Chap. 17).

Allografts of sclera obtained from an eye bank have also been employed for the correction of minor nasal irregularities and depressions. According to Hadley (1975), Cottle used sclera in 1960, and the implant has been used in hundreds of cases and found to be useful to fill small defects. There has been no clinically observable local reaction after implantation. However, gradual absorption occurs and the sclera is replaced by fibrous tissue, hence the potential for contour irregularities.

Silicone rubber, acrylic, polyethylene, and other inorganic implants have also been used in the nose. It will be recalled that ivory was used as a nasal implant as late as the middle 1930's; this implant material was frequently extruded. Although inorganic materials may be tolerated in nasalplasty in Orientals or blacks, they are often extruded in the previously traumatized or operated nose. The rejected implant leaves a bed of dense fibrous tissue, complicating further reconstructive procedures. Lipschutz (1966) noted a rejection rate of 50 per cent for Silastic implants. Some of the most severe "crucified" noses are those seen following the extrusion of an alloplastic implant associated with suppuration.

Autogenous bone grafts, when placed in contact with living bone, consolidate with the host bone and become incorporated into the bony facial framework. Bone grafting is contraindicated only if contact between the bone graft and host bone cannot be achieved. Cartilage is the graft of preference in this situation.

Because bone autografts become consolidated with the underlying nasal bones, loosening or deviation of the graft is prevented. Consolidation with the nasal bones also maintains the projection of the lower part of the graft, thus achieving a cantilever effect. The bone graft may be fractured because of its rigidity, an unusual occurrence, but it usually consolidates uneventfully.

Costal cartilage autografts survive satisfactorily, do not require contact with the nasal bony framework (a requirement of bone grafts), and are specifically indicated when such contact cannot be established—e.g., in cases in which the nasal bones have been destroyed. Cartilage, however, tends to curl and bend, particularly in younger individuals; in older patients, who have partly calcified costal cartilage, the tendency for curling is lessened. Gibson and Davis (1958) described a technique in which the cartilage is cut according to a balanced cross section; this procedure reduces the tendency of the cartilage to curl. The technique is described in a later section devoted to costal cartilage grafts (see Fig. 35–164). For smaller nasal dorsal defects, septal and conchal cartilage (layered if necessary) can be used; curling is less of a problem with this type of cartilage (see Chap. 36).

ILIAC BONE GRAFT FOR NASAL CONTOUR RESTORATION

Iliac Bone Graft Removal. The technique of harvesting of iliac bone grafts has been described in Chapter 18. The bone graft is usually taken from the medial portion of the crest and inner table of the ilium, leaving the lateral portion of the crest for maintenance of the osseous contour. The author prefers the ilium as a donor since it provides a graft of optimal size and contour, as opposed to rib and calvaria.

Shaping the Graft (Fig. 35–157). In most cases, the piece of bone removed from the crest of the ilium is boat shaped, beveled at each end and on the undersurface. The convexity of the undersurface of the graft fits into and fills the concavity of the dorsum of the typical saddle nose; the graft should "sit" in a stable manner without any "rocking." This is a critical technical detail, for it is the fit of the graft within the concavity of the saddle deformity that ensures the stability of the transplant and its consolidation to the host bone. The graft should be wider in the middle and concave transversely in order to adapt to the nasal bones and frontal processes of the maxilla.

The graft should be shaped to reproduce the contour of a normal dorsum: it is narrow cephalad, becomes wider with rounded edges, and is narrowest caudad. First the graft is roughly shaped with large, double-jointed bone cutters; finally it is contoured with the aid of a Lindemann spiral bur activated by an air turbine drill under a constant stream of sterile cold saline. Some of the cortex should be left on the graft for rigidity and to avoid splintering during shaping. When the graft is extended into the tip of the nose, it is shaped in the form of the prow of a ship (see Fig. 35–157C).

Routes of Introduction of Bone Grafts. The incision for exposure should be placed distal to the area of the dorsum that requires the bone graft. The intercartilaginous incision can rarely be employed except for grafts placed over the bony dorsum near the root of the nose, since most grafts extend caudad over the cartilaginous portion of the nose.

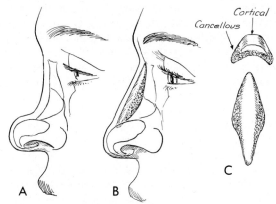

Figure 35–157. Shaping the bone graft. *A,* Diagram of a saddle nose. *B,* The bone graft in position. *C,* Frontal section of the bone graft *(above);* shape of the corticocancellous bone graft *(below).*

The danger of intranasal exposure of the graft through the intercartilaginous incisions should be avoided.

A *transcartilaginous incision* through the alar cartilage is preferred (Fig. 35–158). It extends from the medial crus medially to a predetermined point in the lateral crus laterally, the length of the incision depending on the size or width of the graft.

When the graft is to be introduced into the nasal tip, an incision extends along the cau-

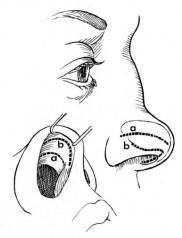

Figure 35–158. Intranasal incisions for the insertion of bone or cartilage grafts. *a,* Transcartilaginous incision through the alar cartilage. *b,* The rim incision along the caudal edge of the lateral and medial crura. When the shape of the tip of the nose requires modification and excision of alar cartilage, the rim incisions are made bilaterally. The transcartilaginous incision may also be made bilaterally to facilitate the elevation of the soft tissue over the dorsum of the nose and the placing of the graft in the midline of the nose.

dal margin of the lateral crus of the alar cartilage, around the point of junction of the lateral and medial crura, and downward along the caudal margin of the medial crus. The *rim incision* (Fig. 35–158), when done bilaterally, provides sufficient exposure of the nasal tip to enable the operation illustrated in Figures 35–160 and 35–161 to be performed.

Transplants over the nasal dorsum introduced through an intranasal incision are used almost exclusively. External incisions at the tip of the nose, either the butterfly or the midcolumellar splitting type, are only occasionally indicated. The vertical midcolumellar incision has proved superior to the horizontally placed butterfly or bird-in-flight incision, and in most cases leaves a barely discernible scar. A vertical midcolumellar incision extending from the root of the nose to the nasal tip is indicated in complicated congenital or traumatic deformities. Dermabrasion often removes the last vestiges of the scar. The presence of a preexisting post-traumatic scar over the dorsum necessitates the repair of the scar; the nasal pyramid can be approached through the area of scar excision and the graft introduced through the latter.

Preparation of Recipient Site and Introduction of Bone Graft. The nasal dorsum is approached through one of the incisions previously described. The soft tissues over the cartilaginous portion of the nose are raised with scissors (Fig. 35–159), the plane of dissection remaining close to the cartilages. If the bone graft is of moderate or large size,

it can be difficult to introduce it under the raised periosteum. As contact of the bone graft with the host bone is essential, the periosteum must be incised and reflected.

The soft tissues are dissected (Fig. 35–159A), the lower end of the incision being joined by two horizontal incisions along the lower border of the nasal bones to an inverted T (Fig. 35–159B). The periosteum is reflected from the bone (Fig. 35–159C). If the overlying nasal soft tissues are excessively tight and deficient, wide undermining is indicated (Wheeler, Kawamoto, and Zarem, 1982). It is often necessary to remove bone from the cephalic portion of the bony dorsum with an osteotome in order to flatten the host surface, reducing the projection of the host site so that the bone graft will "sit" on a flat surface and will not eliminate the nasofrontal angle. Bony irregularities are smoothed with a rasp.

In malunited comminuted fractures, it is particularly necessary to denude the bone of scar tissue in order to ensure intimate contact between the graft and the recipient bone. The bone graft from the ilium is shaped and introduced. The graft should rest in position without "rocking." "Rocking" is minimized by adequate shaping of the host bone, reducing the projection of the bone, smoothing irregularities caused by malunited fracture, and fitting the undersurface of the bone graft into the concavity of the dorsum.

Cantilever Bone Graft Wired to Nasal Bones. In saddle nose and flat nose deformities (Fig. 35–160A) the distal end of the bone graft should extend to the nasal tip in order

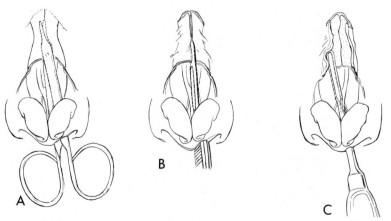

Figure 35–159. Preparation of the host site for a bone graft. *A,* Scissors have undermined the soft tissues over the cartilages. *B,* A vertical incision is made through the periosteum; a horizontal incision through the periosteum is made along the lower border of the nasal bones. *C,* The periosteum is raised from the bone. (From Converse J. M.: Technique of bone grafting for contour restoration of the face. Plast. Reconstr. Surg. *14*:332, 1954. Copyright © 1954. The Williams & Wilkins Company, Baltimore.)

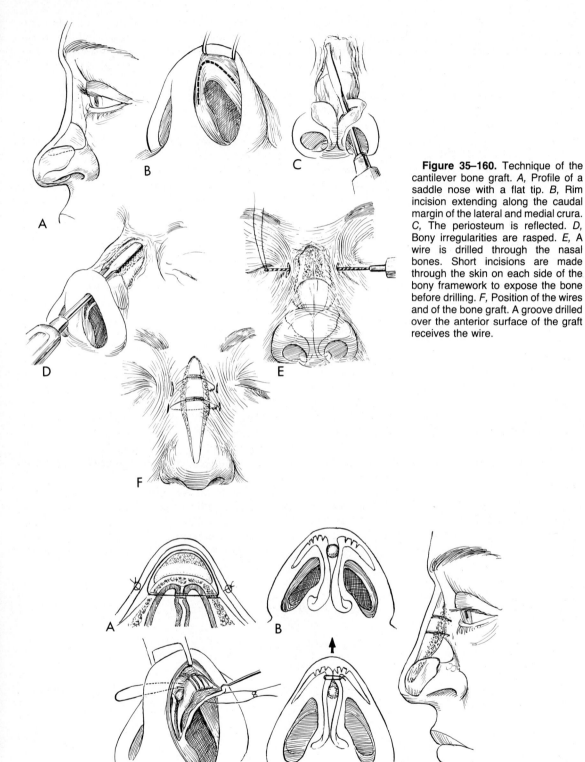

Figure 35–160. Technique of the cantilever bone graft. *A,* Profile of a saddle nose with a flat tip. *B,* Rim incision extending along the caudal margin of the lateral and medial crura. *C,* The periosteum is reflected. *D,* Bony irregularities are rasped. *E,* A wire is drilled through the nasal bones. Short incisions are made through the skin on each side of the bony framework to expose the bone before drilling. *F,* Position of the wires and of the bone graft. A groove drilled over the anterior surface of the graft receives the wire.

Figure 35–161. Technique of the cantilever bone graft (continued). *A,* Cross section showing the position of the wires and the bone graft. *B,* Position of the distal portion of the bone graft between the medial crura. In this technique, the domes and a portion of each lateral crus have been weakened by a series of partial-thickness incisions; this procedure is not always necessary. *C,* A mattress suture is placed through the domes of each alar cartilage. *D,* Position of the domes over the distal end of the bone graft. The cantilever graft thus elevates the tip of the nose. *E,* The cantilever bone graft wired to the nasal bones supports the alar cartilages.

to increase the projection of the tip. However, the distal end of the graft is subjected to a downward traction, causing a "rocking" movement of the graft and a protrusion of the cephalic end of the graft at the root of the nose. A technique to prevent the downward tilting of the graft and to maintain adequate projection of the nasal tip is to wire the graft to the nasal bones (*cantilever technique*). The dorsum is approached through a rim incision that extends downward to free the medial crura from the columellar soft tissue attachments (Fig. 35–160*B*). The periosteum is raised (Fig. 35–160*C*), and a burr or rasp removes any bony irregularities (Fig. 35–160*D*). Fixation with stainless steel wire is done through small incisions made on each side of the lateral nasal walls. A turbine driven drill (Fig. 35–160*E*) is employed to perforate the nasal cavity from one lateral wall to the other; a stainless steel wire is passed through the nasal cavity and looped over the bone graft (Fig. 35–160*F*). The wire passes into a groove especially made for it on the dorsal surface of the bone graft to avoid protrusion of the wire above the level of the graft. The wire is twisted and cut, and the remaining stump of wire is tucked into the drill hole. The edges of the skin incisions are approximated with fine sutures. Two wires placed at different levels are required to prevent lateral rotation of the graft (Fig. 35–160*F*).

The wires maintain firm fixation of the bone graft to the host bed (Fig. 35–161*A*). The distal portion of the graft is introduced between the medial crura immediately beneath the domes (Fig. 35–161*B*). Tip remodeling procedures may be carried out simultaneously. If necessary, partial-thickness incisions are made through the domes (Fig. 35–161*B*) to assist in obtaining increased projection of the tip (Fig. 35–161*C* to *E*). A nonabsorbable mattress suture joins the medial crura over the distal end of the graft, thus increasing the projection of the domes and camouflaging the tip of the graft (Fig. 35–161*C,D*).

If the bone graft is introduced through a dorsal nasal or bicoronal incision, the graft can be secured by two self-tapping screws passed through the graft and bony recipient site.

Bone Graft with a Columellar Strut. Downward tilting of the distal end of the bone graft can be prevented by use of a columellar strut that maintains the projection of the distal end of the graft. The columella is tunneled downward toward the nasal spine, and a bony strut is placed over the nasal spine after the latter has been stripped of periosteum. It is usually necessary to excise a small, V-shaped segment of bone from the lower end of the strut in order to fit it over the nasal spine; this procedure controls the tendency of the strut to shift. The junction between the strut and the dorsal graft is best achieved by the "tent pole" technique, which prevents the loss of contact between the two pieces of bone. A small hole is drilled through the caudal end of the bone graft, and the pointed end of the strut is introduced into the hole. After the desired degree of elevation of the tip is achieved, two shoulders are cut on the strut to prevent the pointed end of the strut from extending too far through the hole. The strut, wired to the nasal spine, is often progressively absorbed, but it serves as a support until the consolidation of the graft to the nasal bones is completed.

The use of a columellar strut presupposes a columella of good quality; generally it cannot be used in the reconstructed columella. The cantilever bone graft is a preferable and more reliable technique; it does not eliminate the suppleness and flexibility of the nasal tip area, an important esthetic consideration, and the chances of fracture are less.

Various Applications of Iliac Bone Grafts for Correction of Depressed Nasal Dorsum. A cosmetic rhinoplasty was the cause of the saddle nose deformity in the patient shown in Figure 35–162. Collapse of the nose following a rhinoplasty combined with an overzealous submucous resection of the septum was responsible for the deformity shown in Figure 35–163. In both cases a satisfactory improvement was obtained by iliac bone grafting.

Other Types of Bone Grafts. Tibial grafts were used successfully in the past but have been mostly discontinued because of the increased density of the bone and because of possible pathologic fracture due to weakening of the tibia. Other sources of bone grafts are the rib, the calvaria (McCarthy and Zide, 1984), the greater trochanter, the olecranon, and portions of the subcutaneous border of the ulna (Antia, 1974). As previously mentioned, the author considers that the alternative donor sites are inferior to the ilium because of the brittle character, inadequate

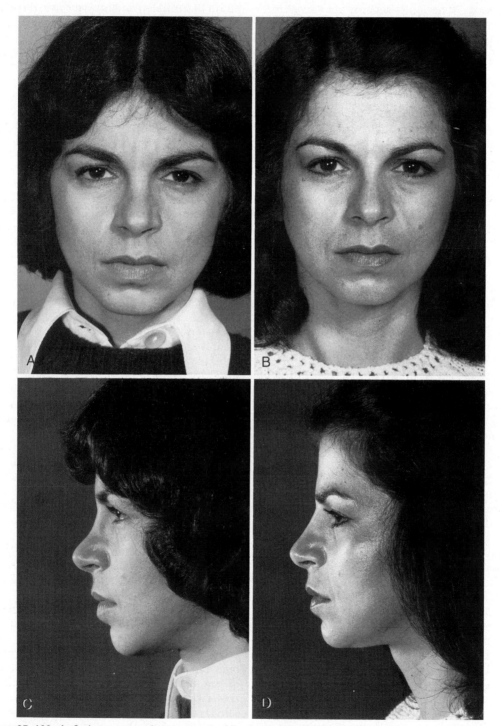

Figure 35–162. *A, C,* Appearance after a cosmetic rhinoplasty. Note the saddle deformity and supratip protrusion. *B, D,* Following iliac bone grafting of the nasal dorsum by the technique illustrated in Figure 35–160.

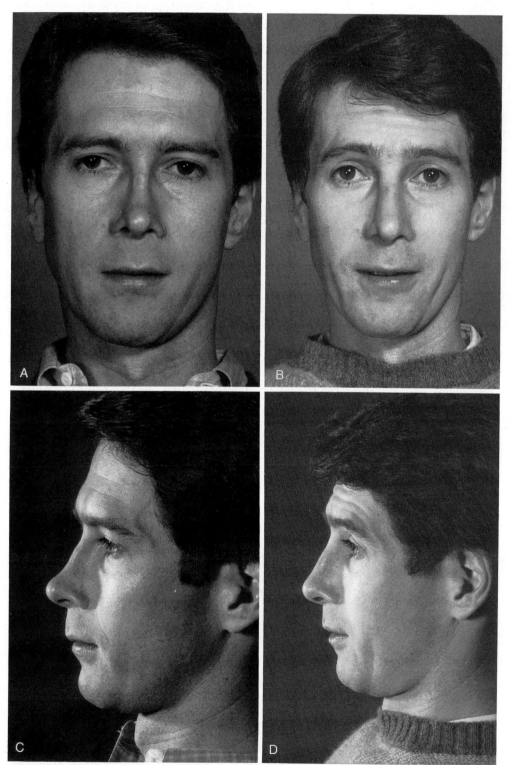

Figure 35–163. Saddle nose deformity resulting from esthetic rhinoplasty and submucous resection. *A, C,* Preoperative views. *B, D,* Appearance after insertion of an iliac bone graft.

contour, and decreased volume of the harvested bone.

COSTAL CARTILAGE GRAFT FOR NASAL CONTOUR RESTORATION

The technique of removal of costal cartilage has been described in Chapter 17. The cartilage graft is shaped by paring it with a knife and is introduced into the nose according to techniques similar to those already described for bone grafts. Certain precautions must be taken, however, to avoid curling and warping of the transplant. The tendency to warp is particularly noted in children's cartilage; older patients' cartilage (partly calcified) does not have this characteristic. Gillies (1920) noted that the graft, when denuded of perichondrium on one side, tends to curve toward that side. Mowlem (1938), reviewing a series of 35 cartilage grafts applied to the nasal bridge, reported that 17 became twisted; he subsequently advocated the use of iliac bone grafts for nasal transplants. New and Erich (1941) dipped the cartilage into boiling water for a few seconds, thus eliminating the curling tendency; no follow-up concerning the ultimate fate of these grafts has been reported. Gibson and Davis (1958) showed that not only the perichondrium but also the surface layer of the cartilage played a role in the warping when it was removed on one side. They advocated a technique that applied the principle of balanced cross section (Fig. 35–164). All the perichondrium surrounding a full-thickness section of a rib cartilage, as well as the cortical cartilage layer, should be removed.

The one-piece, L-shaped graft that extends over the dorsum and is angulated downward into the columella as far as the nasal spine is not recommended (Fig. 35–165). This type of graft produces a rigid lower nose, eliminates the natural resilience provided by the membranous septum, and can interfere with the normal physiology of the nose.

The costal cartilage graft also gives excellent results and has the advantage that it does not require contact with the underlying host bone for survival; a disadvantage is that the cartilage graft, because it is not consolidated with the underlying host bone, is occasionally subjected to the traction forces exerted by the soft tissues and may be displaced.

The use of septal and conchal cartilage grafts as single pieces or in layers to restore the nasal dorsum is discussed in detail in Chapter 36.

Bone and Cartilage Grafting in Conjunction with Osteotomy and Septal Framework Resection

Because many of the noses requiring restoration of contour by bone and cartilage grafts have been severely traumatized and may show, in addition to the saddle or flat appearance of the nose, widening of the bony dorsum or deviation, osteotomy of the lateral walls of the nose is required. Some severely

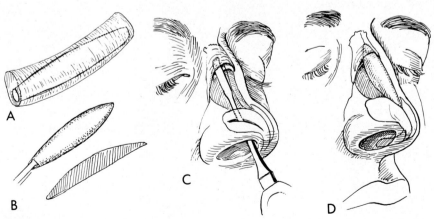

Figure 35–164. Costal cartilage graft. *A,* Gibson's technique (the principle of balanced cross section) to avoid warping of the cartilage graft. *B,* Shape of the graft, front and side views. The convex undersurface of the graft fits the concave surface of the nasal dorsum. *C,* Periosteal elevator, introduced through a transcartilaginous incision through the alar cartilage, raising the periosteum. *D,* The costal cartilage graft in position. Guide sutures inserted through the graft can be passed through the overlying skin to maintain graft position.

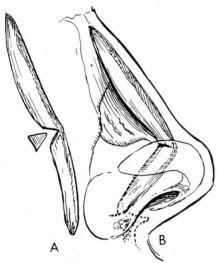

A   B

Figure 35–165. The hinged costal cartilage graft (after Gillies, 1920). The hinge is provided by the perichondrium, which is preserved on one side. A variant of this graft is the osteocartilaginous graft taken from the area of junction of the bone with the cartilaginous rib. The bony portion of the graft consolidates with the bony dorsum of the nose.

traumatized noses have a thickened deviated septum that also requires straightening by submucous resection of the septal framework. The question arises whether these procedures can be carried out in a single operative stage (see Fig. 35–162), or whether straightening of the framework of the nose and septum should be done in a preliminary stage.

The decision varies according to the magnitude of the overall septonasal deformity. In severely traumatized noses, septal surgery and lateral osteotomies should be performed in a preliminary stage because of the tedious surgery required for a successful submucous resection of the thickened septum and adherent flaps with underlying fibrosis. After a suitable interval, the bone or cartilage graft is performed; additional corrective nasal tip surgery can be carried out in the latter stage. Because in the more extensive surgery there is the danger of hematoma formation and communication between the nasal cavity and the recipient site of the graft, it is prudent that septal surgery, osteotomies, and tip surgery should be performed in a separate stage before insertion of a nasal dorsal transplant.

REFERENCES

Anderson, J. R.: A new approach to rhinoplasty. Trans. Am. Acad. Ophthalmol. Otolaryngol., 70:183, 1966.

Anderson, J. R., and Rubin, W.: Retrograde intramucosal

hump removal in rhinoplasty. A. M. A. Arch. Otolaryngol., 68:346, 1958.

Antia, N. H.: The scope of plastic surgery in leprosy: a ten-year progress report. Clin. Plast. Surg., 1:69, 1974.

Aufricht, G.: A few hints and surgical details in rhinoplasty. Laryngoscope, 53:317, 1943.

Aufricht, G.: Symposium on corrective rhinoplasty. Plast. Reconstr. Surg., 28:241, 1961.

Boo-Chai, K.: Augmentation of rhinoplasty in the orientals. Plast. Reconstr. Surg., 34:81, 1964.

Brown, J. B., and McDowell, F.: Plastic Surgery of the Nose. St. Louis, MO, C. V. Mosby Company, 1951.

Converse, J. M.: Corrective surgery of the nasal tip. Ann. Otol. Rhinol. Laryngol., 49:895, 1940.

Converse, J. M.: The cartilaginous structures of the nose. Ann. Otol. Rhinol. Laryngol., 64:220, 1955.

Converse, J. M.: Deformities of the nose (Fig. 21–60). *In* Converse, J. M. (Ed.): Reconstructive Plastic Surgery. Philadelphia, W. B. Saunders Company, 1964, p. 729.

Converse, J. M.: The deformity termed "pug nose" and its correction by a simple operation. John O. Roe, Rochester, NY. (Reprinted from the Medical Record, June 4, 1887.) Plast. Reconstr. Surg., 45:78, 1970.

Cottle, M. H.: Corrective surgery of the nasal septum and the external pyramid—study notes and laboratory manual. Chicago, American Rhinologic Society, 1960.

Courtiss, E. H., Goldwyn, R. M., and O'Brien, J. O.: Resection of obstructing inferior nasal turbinates. Plast. Reconstr. Surg., 62:249, 1978.

Daniel, R. K.: Rhinoplasty: creating an aesthetic tip. A preliminary report. Plast. Reconstr. Surg., 80:775, 1987.

Daniel, R. K., and Lessard, M. L.: Rhinoplasty—a graded aesthetic-anatomical approach. Ann. Plast. Surg., 13:436, 1984.

DeKleine, E. H.: Nasal tip reconstruction through external incisions. Plast. Reconstr. Surg., 15:502, 1955.

Dingman, R. O., and Walter, C.: Use of composite ear grafts in correction of short nose. Plast. Reconstr. Surg., 43:117, 1969.

Falces, E., Wesser, D., and Gorney, M.: Cosmetic surgery of the non-Caucasian nose. Plast. Reconstr. Surg., 45:317, 1970.

Firmin, F., and Le Pesteur, J.: Reflexions sur l'auvert cartilagineux nasal. Ann. Chir. Plast., 22:1, 1977.

Flowers, R. S., and Anderson, R.: Injury to the lacrimal apparatus during rhinoplasty. Plast. Reconstr. Surg., 42:577, 1968.

Fomon, S.: Cosmetic Surgery. Principles and Practice. Philadelphia, J. B. Lippincott Company, 1960.

Freer, O.: Deflection of the nasal septum; a critical review of the methods of their correction, with a report of 116 operations. Ann. Otol. Rhinol. Laryngol., 15:213, 1902.

Fry, H. J. H.: Judicious turbinectomy for nasal obstruction. Aust. N.Z. J. Surg., 42:291, 1973.

Fry, H. J. H., and Robertson, W. B.: Interlocked stresses in human septal cartilage. Br. J. Plast. Surg., 19:392, 1967.

Furukawa, M.: Oriental rhinoplasty. Clin. Plast. Surg., 1:129, 1974.

Gibson, T., Curran, R. C., and Davis, W. B.: The survival of living homograft cartilages in man. Transplant. Bull., 4:105, 1957.

Gibson, T., and Davis, W. B.: The distortion of autogenous cartilage grafts: its cause and prevention. Br. J. Plast. Surg., 10:257, 1958.

Gillies, H. D.: Plastic Surgery of the Face. London, Oxford University Press, 1920, p. 274.

Gillies, H. D., and Kristensen, H. K.: Ox cartilage in plastic surgery. Br. J. Plast. Surg., *4*:63, 1951.

Gruber, R. P.: Open rhinoplasty. Clin. Plast. Surg., *15*:95, 1988.

Hadley, R. C.: Personal communication, 1975.

Hilger, J. A.: The internal osteotomy in rhinoplasty. Arch. Otolaryngol., *88*:211, 1968.

Johnson, N. E.: Septal surgery and rhinoplasty. Trans. Am. Acad. Ophthalmol. Otolaryngol., *68*:869, 1964.

Joseph, J.: Nasenplastik und sonstige Gesichtplastik (nebst einem Anhang über Mammaplastik und einige weitere Operationen aus dem Gebiete ausseren Korperplastik: ein Atlas und Lehrbuch). Leipzig, Kabitzsch, 1931, pp. 498–842.

Jost, G., Vergnon, L., and Hadjean, E.: Les asymétries nasales postopératories. Ann. Chir. Plast., *20*:123, 1973.

Kaye, B. L.: Discussion of paper. Plast. Reconstr. Surg., *71*:38, 1983.

Killian, G.: Die submucose Fensterresektion der Nasenscheidewand. Arch. Laryngol. Rhinol. (Berl.), *16*:362, 1904.

Kirschner, J. A.: Traumatic nasal deformity in the newborn. A. M. A. Arch. Otolaryngol., *62*:139, 1955.

Kravits, H., Driessen, G., Gomberg, R., and Korach, A.: Accidental falls from elevated surfaces in infants from birth to one year of age. Pediatrics (Suppl), *44*:869, 1969.

Lipschutz, H.: A clinical evaluation of subdermal and subcutaneous silicone implants. Plast. Reconstr. Surg., *37*:249, 1966.

Lipsett, E. M.: A new approach to surgery of the lower cartilaginous vault. Arch. Otolaryngol., *70*:42, 1959.

Matory, W. E., Jr., and Falces, E.: Non-Caucasian rhinoplasty: a 16-year experience. Plast. Reconstr. Surg., *77*:239, 1986.

McCarthy, J. G., and Zide, B.: The spectrum of calvarial bone grafting: introduction of the vascularized bone flap. Plast. Reconstr. Surg., *74*:10, 1984.

McDowell, F., Valone, J. A., and Brown, J. B.: Bibliography and historical note on plastic surgery of nose. Plast. Reconstr. Surg., *10*:149, 1952.

McKinney, P., and Shively, R.: Straightening the twisted nose. Plast. Reconstr. Surg., *64*:176, 1979.

Meyer, R.: Nasal-septal perforation and nostril stenosis. *In* Goldwyn, R. M. (Ed.): The Unfavorable Result in Plastic Surgery. Boston, Little, Brown & Company, 1972.

Millard, D. R., Jr.: Alar margin sculpturing. Plast. Reconstr. Surg., *40*:337, 1967.

Millard, D. R., Jr.: Lengthening the columella. *In* Georgiade, N. G., and Hagerty, R. F. (Eds.): Symposium on Management of Cleft Lip and Palate and Associated Deformities. St. Louis, C. V. Mosby Company, 1974.

Millard, D. R., Jr.: The alar cinch in the flat, flaring nose. Plast. Reconstr. Surg., *65*:669, 1980.

Mink, P. J.: Physiologie der oberen Luftwege. Leipzig, Vogel, 1920.

Mowlem, R.: The use and behavior of iliac bone grafts in the restoration of nasal contour. Clinical and radiographic observations. Rev. Chir. Structive, *8*:23, 1938.

Natvig, P.: Jacques Joseph: Surgical Sculptor. Philadelphia, W. B. Saunders, 1982.

Natvig, P., Sether, L. A., Gingrass, R. P., and Gardner, W. D.: Anatomical details of the osseous-cartilaginous framework of the nose. Plast. Reconstr. Surg., *48*:528, 1971.

Nélaton, C., and Ombrédanne, L.: La Rhinoplastie. Paris, G. Steinheil, 1904.

New, G. B., and Erich, J. B.: A method to prevent fresh costal cartilage grafts from warping. Am. J. Surg., *54*:435, 1941.

Ortiz-Monasterio, F.: Personal communication, 1975.

Parkes, M. L., and Brennan, H. G.: High septal transfixion to shorten the nose. Plast. Reconstr. Surg., *45*:487, 1970.

Peck, G. C.: The onlay graft for nasal tip projection. Plast. Reconstr. Surg., *71*:27, 1983.

Rees, T. D.: Nasal plastic surgery in the Negro. Plast. Reconstr. Surg., *43*:13, 1969.

Rees, T. D.: Aesthetic Plastic Surgery. Philadelphia, W. B. Saunders, 1980.

Rees, T. D.: Surgical correction of the severely deviated nose by extramucosal excision of the osseocartilaginous septum and replacement as a free graft. Plast. Reconstr. Surg., *78*:320, 1986.

Rees, T. D., and Wood-Smith, D.: Cosmetic Facial Surgery. Philadelphia, W. B. Saunders Company, 1972.

Rethi, A.: Raccourcissement du nez trop long. Rev. Chir. Plast., *2*:85, 1934.

Robin, J. L.: Réduction extra-muqueuse contrôlée de l'arête nasale. Proceedings of the Ninth International Congress of Otolaryngology, Mexico. Amsterdam, Excerpta Medica International Series No. 206, 711, 1969.

Rogers, B. O.: The role of physical anthropology in plastic surgery today. Clin. Plast. Surg., *1*:439, 1974.

Rogers, B. O.: John Orlando Roe—not Jacques Joseph—the father of aesthetic rhinoplasty. Aesthetic Plast. Surg., *10*:63, 1986.

Safian, J.: Corrective Rhinoplastic Surgery. New York, Paul B. Hoeber, 1934.

Sheen, J. H.: Achieving more nasal tip projection by the use of a small autogenous vomer or septal cartilage graft. Plast. Reconstr. Surg., *56*:35, 1975a.

Sheen, J. H.: Secondary rhinoplasty. Plast. Reconstr. Surg., *56*:137, 1975b.

Sheen, J. H.: Aesthetic Rhinoplasty. St. Louis, C. V. Mosby Company, 1978.

Sheen, J. H., and Sheen, A. P.: Aesthetic Rhinoplasty. St. Louis, C. V. Mosby Company, 1987.

Skoog, T.: Plastic Surgery—New Methods and Refinements. Philadelphia, W. B. Saunders Company, 1974.

Straatsma, B. R., and Straatsma, C. R.: The anatomical relationship of the lateral nasal cartilage to the nasal bone and the cartilaginous nasal septum. Plast. Reconstr. Surg., *8*:443, 1951.

Testut, L., and Jacob, O.: Traité d'Anatomie Topographique avec Applications Médico-chirurgicales. Paris, Octave Doin & Cie, 1929.

Uchida, J.: The Practice of Plastic Surgery. Tokyo, Kinbara, 1958.

Van Dishoek, H. A. E.: Elektograms der Nasenflugelmuskein und Nasenwiderstandskurve. Acta Otolaryngol., *25*:285, 1937.

Weir, R. R.: On restoring sunken noses without scarring the face. N.Y. Med. J., *56*:499, 1892.

Wen, I. C.: Ontogeny and phylogeny of the nasal cartilages. Cont. Embryol., Carnegie Institution, *414*:109, 1921.

Wheeler, E. S., Kawamoto, H. K., and Zarem, H. A.: Bone grafts for nasal reconstruction. Plast. Reconstr. Surg., *69*:9, 1982.

Zelnick, J., and Gingrass, R. P.: Anatomy of the alar cartilage. Plast. Reconstr. Surg., *64*:650, 1979.

Zide, B. M.: Nasal anatomy: the muscles and tip sensation. Aesth. Plast. Surg., *9*:193, 1985.

Zukerhandl, E.: Normal u. Pathol. Anat. der Nasenhohlen. Wien, Braumuller, 1892.

36

Jack H. Sheen

Secondary Rhinoplasty

Secondary rhinoplasty involves a wide and complex span of problems requiring solutions that are sometimes subtle, occasionally heroic, but always demanding of judgment and careful technique. The margin for error is small and the effects of error are often permanent. Scarring and tissue deficit are cumulative and may result in nasal disfigurement and dysfunction. Because the surgeon is faced with insufficient tissues, damaged blood supply, and altered anatomy, secondary procedures differ significantly from primary operations, both in the diagnostic and technical skills required and in the limitations built into the expected outcome.

THE CONSULTATION

Whereas a patient seeking a primary rhinoplasty is generally happy and filled with hope at the time of consultation, a patient at consultation for secondary procedures is always dissatisfied, and often disillusioned and angry. The latter individual requires a more compassionate and understanding surgeon—one who is supportive and patient and one who listens.

To establish credibility, the surgeon must be completely honest. Problems cannot be denied. All anatomic problems are candidly pointed out and the potential for improvement or correction is discussed. Septal fistulas, collapsed alae, vestibular stenosis, and supratip deformity are mentioned if present, and the surgical plans are discussed along with an estimation of the final outcome. The problems that cannot be changed or improved are specifially identified, such as telangiectasia, dermal scars, and the foreshortened nose.

Any special problems, such as thick or thin skin or disproportions, are noted and discussed with the patient. The presence of vestibular scars and septal fistulas and the configurations of the internal valves are noted. The septum is carefully examined after desensitization of the mucosa with 2 per cent tetracaine (Pontocaine). If possible, the internal examination must include the posterior parts in order to detect whether there are significant bone deformities that might result in decreased function. The quality and amount of the available material is assessed so as to determine whether reconstruction is likely to be accomplished with available materials or whether an additional donor site will be necessary. Permission should be obtained to harvest graft material from a secondary donor site.

GROUND RULES

The following guidelines or ground rules should be generally applied in the management of problem noses:
1. Establish realistic patient expectations.
2. Defer surgery for at least one year.
3. Use *only* autogenous materials.
4. Limit the dissection (*no* unnecessary incisions).
5. Have a specific esthetic goal.
6. Make a proper diagnosis with an appropriate surgical plan.

Establish Realistic Patient Expectations

A detailed discussion of expected results helps to establish realistic patient expectations. The nose that is displaced off the midline is noted and the patient is told that it will remain so. Asymmetric or deviated noses that are improved by camouflage techniques will always be wider than they were before surgery and the patients must accept this fact (Fig. 36–1). Tip grafts may be asymmetric, but the slight asymmetry is a worthwhile trade-off for a more desirable position of the tip. Late adjustments can also be made. These

problems are not the result of surgical errors, but they should be anticipated from the formation of a new framework. They often depend on the type of graft material used, the character of the patient's tisses, and the degree to which tissue contour or position is changed.

Defer Surgery

Extreme patient anxiety and the surgeon's eagerness to please are elements that may force a decision for an early surgical revision. Early surgery unfortunately compounds the problem. The patient who "cannot live with the present result" must be made to understand that a premature secondary assault on the nasal tissues could jeopardize any potential for improvement and could make the final result even worse. Consultation with an experienced colleague is helpful to reinforce the recommendation to defer surgery. Tissues must have time to heal so that an accurate assessment of the secondary procedure is made possible. The minimal time of one year is recommended for patients with only one previous operation. For those who have undergone multiple operations, the time must often be extended for two years or longer until the tissues have softened and there is no evidence of further resolution. There are exceptions to this rule. When there is a gross malposition of a graft or an obvious and distorting skeletal part, a limited approach to correct the specific problem may be made.

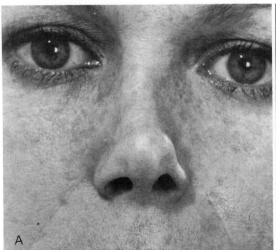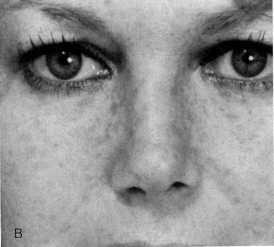

Figure 36–1. Augmentation to camouflage the deviated nose. Patients must understand before surgery that correction by augmentation makes the nose wider. *A*, Preoperative view. *B*, Postoperative view.

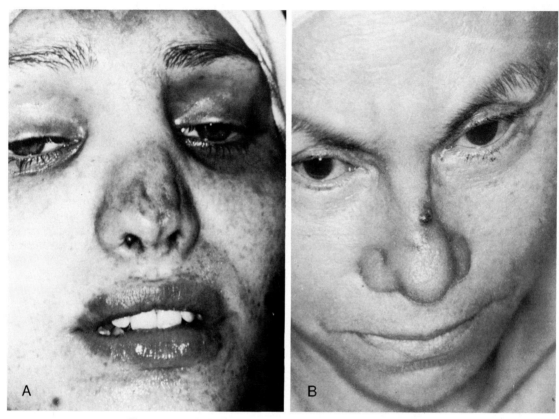

Figure 36–2. *A, B,* Extrusion of alloplastic material in two patients.

Use Only Autogenous Materials

The following is a list of the autogenous materials available to the plastic surgeon, listed in the author's order of preference and frequency of use:

1. Septum—cartilage and bone.
2. Ears—cartilage, and cartilage with skin as a composite graft.
3. Cranial bone—outer table (including "curls").
4. Rib cartilage and bone.
5. Temporal fascia.
6. Dermal grafts.
7. Iliac bone grafts.

In view of the availability, variety, and quality of autogenous materials, it is impossible to recommend anything but autogenous materials for nasal reconstruction. This view is reinforced by the excellent long-term survival rate as compared with the debatable longevity of other forms of specially treated human or animal materials.

The use of alloplastic materials is mentioned only to be condemned for the purposes of secondary rhinoplasty. The failure and complication rates are high, and the complications frequently result in distortions that are permanent and irreparable (Fig. 36–2).

Limit the Dissection

In secondary rhinoplasty, in particular, the integrity of the tissues must be preserved. The concept of "exploration" in secondary rhinoplasty should be abandoned. There is no need to "explore" a nasal tip to find remnants of lateral crura embedded in dense scar tissue; nothing is gained and the final result may be compromised. Furthermore, healing is prolonged, and tissue vascularity is unnecessarily disturbed.

Separate pockets should be made for dorsal and lateral grafts. A separate intercartilaginous incision for lateral wall grafting preserves the dorsal pocket and ensures a stable and secure dorsal graft. A hemitransfixion incision to reduce the caudal septum for columellar-alar rim adjustments is preferable to the usual transfixion incision as practiced during primary rhinoplasty (see Fig. 35–54, p. 1820).

Have a Specific Esthetic Goal

The surgeon must have an understanding of normal anatomy and nasofacial esthetics as a reference base for the planned reconstruction. In addition, an understanding of the patient's esthetic sense contributes to the formulation of the surgical plan. Specific esthetic points, which can be varied, are brought into focus for the patient's evaluation and selection: the position of the tip relative to the dorsum; the character of the tip, whether sharply faceted or softly rounded; the height and character of the new dorsal line; and the width of the nasal base. The patient is told that *these are points of direction, that success certainly cannot be guaranteed,* and that it is not possible to produce an exact "ideal" nose.

The patient's esthetic sense must be considered in all surgical plans for secondary rhinoplasty. For example, to ask the patient for specific information regarding the type of nasal tip can be helpful in obtaining a result that is closer to the hoped-for ideal. The two patients shown in Figure 36–3, with approximately similar skin sleeves, differed in their request for tip contour. The first patient (Fig. 36–3*A, B*) asked for a sharply angled tip slightly higher than the dorsum (slightly retroussé). The second patient (Fig. 36–3*C, D*) requested the softest, roundest tip possible. The first patient obtained solid cartilage grafts to form an angled, more faceted tip. The second received crushed cartilage grafts to soften the tip contour in order to provide an almost bulbous appearance.

Make a Proper Diagnosis

A proper diagnosis includes a correct analysis of the underlying causes of the

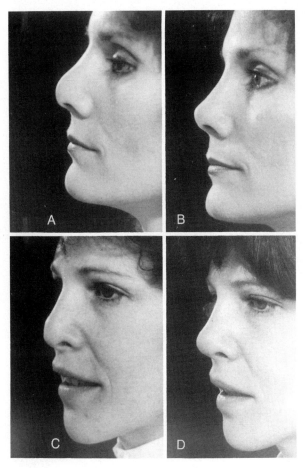

Figure 36–3. These two patients had specific and differing requests for their "ideal" tip configuration. The top patient *(A, B)* wanted the tip as sharply defined as possible; the lower patient *(C, D)* requested the roundest, softest contour possible.

secondary deformities. The surgeon must decide whether a supratip deformity is a reflection of inadequate resection of skeletal parts or whether it reflects superfluous soft tissues. If the correct diagnosis is the latter, further skeletal reduction will not be helpful, whereas further attempts to reduce the skin volume by subdermal dissection could result in an irreparable deformity.

The diagnosis of supratip deformity is no more than a recognition of a convexity cephalad to the tip; the determination of etiology is essential for successful treatment. The patients shown in Figure 36–4 illustrate clas-

sical supratip deformity. The diagnosis can often be confirmed by compressing the redundant arch of tissues over the supratip onto the anterior edge of the septum (Fig. 36–5).

Figure 36–6 shows an example of a supratip deformity that is caused mainly by an unresected anterior edge of the septum. The tissues are thin, and the deformity is continuous with the anterior edge of the septum. Palpation usually confirms the edge of the septum as the cause of the deformity.

The loss of tip projection is often a major cause of apparent supratip deformity. With a loss of tip projection, the supratip area ap-

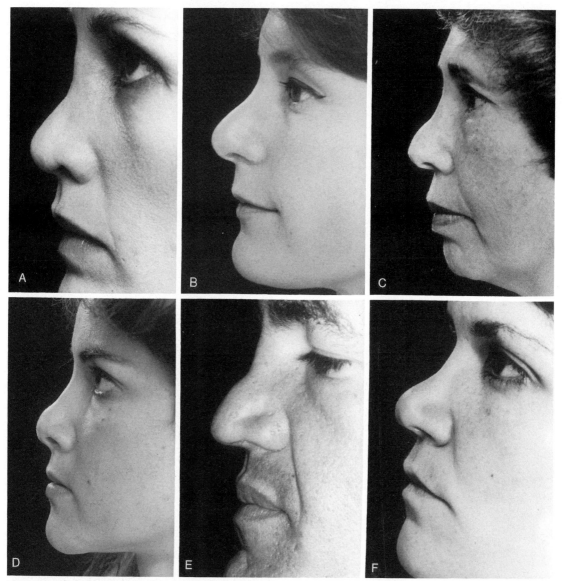

Figure 36–4. *A* to *F,* Classic examples of supratip deformity. There is a redundant skin sleeve over the caudal third as a result of excess resection of skeletal parts.

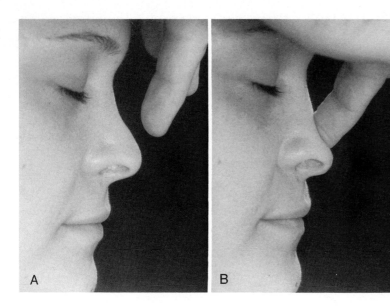

Figure 36–5. *A, B,* The diagnosis of patients with a redundant skin sleeve can be established by palpation, as illustrated.

Figure 36–6. Supratip deformity caused by inadequate resection of the anterior septum. The deformity is confirmed by palpation. *A, C,* Preoperative views. *B, D,* After septal resection.

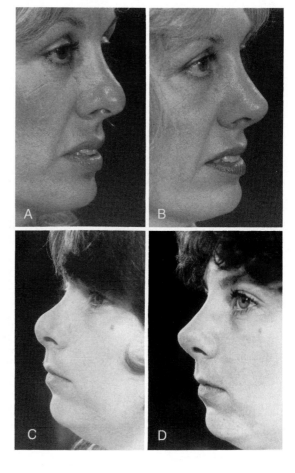

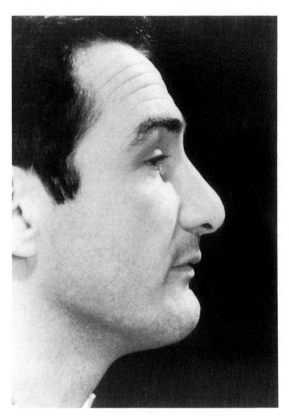

Figure 36–7. Apparent supratip deformity caused by an inadequately projecting tip. Treatment must include some form of tip augmentation (see Fig. 36–43).

pears inordinately high. Treatment must be directed at increasing the projection of the tip (Fig. 36–7).

Patients do not always analyze their unsatisfactory result: they know only that they are unhappy with how they look. They view their problem as though it were a contour on a computer imaging device, being convinced that all that the surgeon needs to do in order to obtain an "ideal result" is to draw lines through those parts not wanted, or simply remove parts that seem redundant. They do not consider the behavior of tissue, the limitations of wound healing, or the importance of balance of parts of the nose to each other and to the remaining face.

The patient illustrated in Figure 36–8A was dissatisfied with his nasal contour. His primary complaint was that the surgeon had not made the bridge of the nose straight. He wanted a strong, straight, masculine nose and specifically requested that the bridge be lowered further to obtain the contour he desired. However, if this were done, the nasofrontal

angle would be too wide, and the nose would appear almost triangular and disproportionate. The tip also does not have (at this time) the necessary skeletal structure to hold it at or above the dorsum.

The correct diagnosis for this patient is over-reduction of skeletal parts (the dorsum, as well as the alar cartilages), a tip that lacks skeletal support, a nasofrontal angle excessively wide, and a nasal contour that appears too short.

One year after revision (Fig. 36–8B) he was pleased with the result, but his initial reaction to the proposed surgical plan had been one of disbelief. The result was obtained by dorsal augmentation (septal cartilage) and tip augmentation (multiple solid and crushed septal cartilage grafts).

The patient shown in Figure 36–9A, C had had three previous nasal procedures, all designed to make her nose appear as "pert" as possible. At the time of consultation, she was determined and presented her own surgical plan, which had obviously been followed three times. Each time the surgeon tried to reduce the base of her nose to give her the "pert" look, without success.

The following problems went undiagnosed:

1. The nasofacial angle was flat. The nasal contour appeared to hang from the glabella.

2. The base of the nose could not be reduced further. Attempts to do so would result in irreparable distortion and scarring.

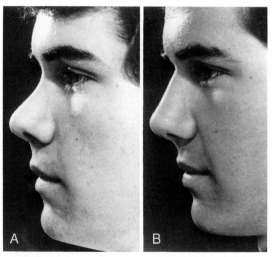

Figure 36—8. A, The patient after a primary rhinoplasty requested further reduction of the dorsum to obtain a straight, masculine nose. B, One year later after dorsal and tip augmentation (cartilage).

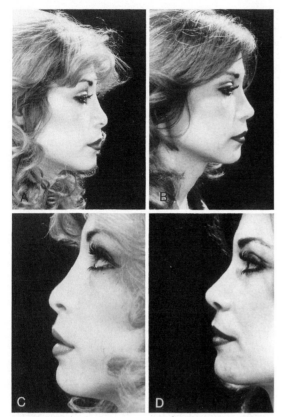

Figure 36–9. *A, C,* A patient after three attempts to produce a "pert" look. *B, D,* The result two years after surgery, which included reduction of the radix, dorsal augmentation, and tip augmentation.

The surgical procedure recommended was as follows:

1. Reduction of the radix. This maneuver would serve to reduce the length of her nose (a high priority with this patient).

2. Augmentation of the dorsum to bring the caudal third to a more appropriate height and to improve the nasofacial angle.

3. Augmentation of the tip and placing it above the new dorsal line.

4. Maxillary augmentation.

The patient's response to the plan was a combination of exasperation, horror, and anger. After much consideration, however, she relented but declined the maxillary augmentation. She is shown approximately two years after secondary rhinoplasty (Fig. 36–9*B, D*).

When the patient complains of an unacceptably wide nasal base, the correct diagnosis may relate to the overly narrow middle and bony vaults. Surgical corection of the disproportion visually brings the base into

better balance with the other parts of the nose. The patients illustrated in Figure 36–10 complained of an inordinately wide base and a nasal bridge that was excessively narrow. They were pleased with the ultimate improvement in the balance of the nose and are shown over four years after surgical correction.

GRAFT MATERIALS

The Septum

Septal cartilage and bone are by far the most accessible and superior materials for nasal reconstruction. In addition, septoplasty can provide the double benefit of improved airway function. The surgeon must therefore become expert at the extraction of septal cartilage and the treatment of skeletal deformities of the septum. He must know what can be sacrificed and what must be preserved to maintain skeletal support for the nose (see Chap. 35). Familiarity with the techniques for resection of the vomer and the posterior bony parts is essential to successful nasal surgery in general. However, it is especially useful in secondary rhinoplasty because of the additional graft material that is made available.

In general, septal cartilage is the material of choice in secondary rhinoplasty. There is no other autogenous material that can be as effectively used in so large a variety of circumstances. It can be used for support, for contouring, or for fill. Since it is malleable, it can also be crushed to a large variety of thickness. It can also be used "as is" to provide a sturdy recontouring material as in tip grafts. It does not warp or curl if the surfaces are not unilaterally scored or cut. Its clinical record of survival in the author's practice (over 20 years) has been excellent and it is, for the most part, accepted by the majority of clinicans as being a permanent reconstructive material.

The area outlined in Figure 36–11 indicates the portions of septal cartilage, ethmoid, and vomer available for graft harvesting. Preservation of anterior and caudal struts ensures adequate support. The surgeon must determine before the harvesting, however, whether or not the remaining 1.5 cm of anterior strut has sufficient bony attachment to provide the necessary support. An impressive

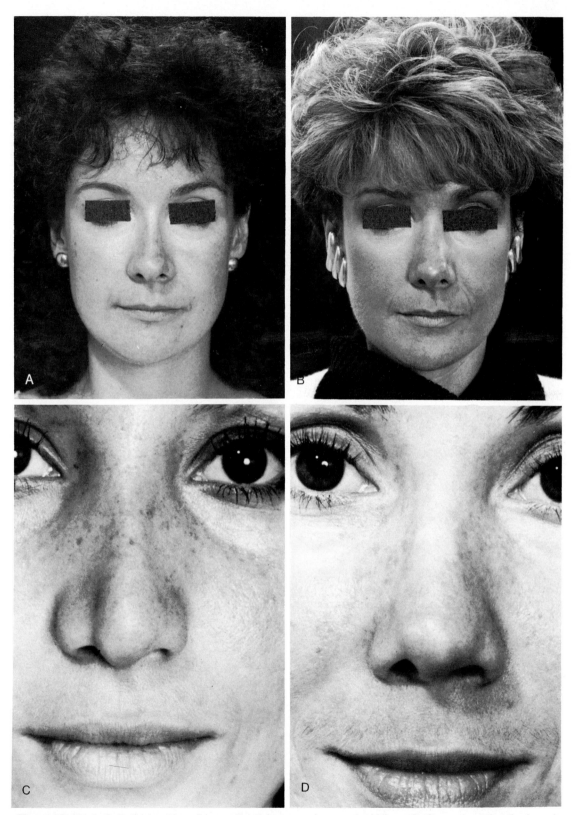

Figure 36–10. *A, C,* Patients with a disproportionately narrow bony and middle vault often request that the base be narrowed. *B, D,* If this is not possible, balance can be improved by insertion of lateral grafts, as shown in the two patients at least four years after surgery.

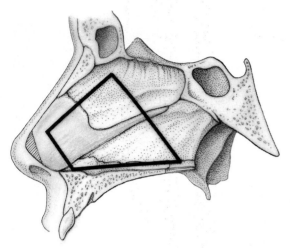

Figure 36–11. Cross section of the septum illustrating the location and amounts of available bone and cartilage for grafting. Preservation of anterior and caudal struts is critical for support.

amount of graft material can be harvested (Fig. 36–12) and a single piece of sufficient size and contour can restore the nasal dorsum (Fig. 36–13).

Septal cartilage grafts can be multilayered (Fig. 36–14) and appropriately crushed to provide a smooth contour (Figs. 36–15, 36–16). Spreader grafts (Fig. 36–17) are used to reposition the lateral wall and open the internal valve.

Grafts harvested from the ethmoid and vomer suffer the disadvantage of being rigid and difficult to mold. However, they can be appropriately shaped.

Ear Cartilage

Conchal cartilage has become popular as graft material in nasal reconstruction over

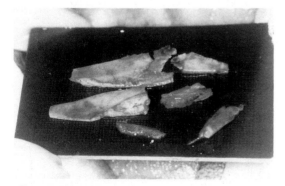

Figure 36–12. The average yield of cartilage and bone harvested from the septum. Unused pieces can be crushed and returned to the septum.

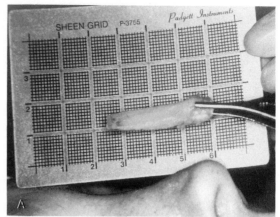

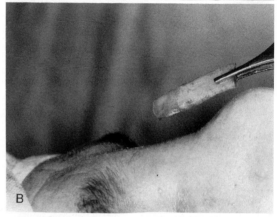

Figure 36–13. *A,* Septal cartilage graft before insertion for dorsal augmentation. *B,* The solid, recontoured dorsal graft can eliminate the inverted V deformity, provide smooth contour lines from the root to the base, elevate the dorsum to a proper level relative to the tip, and often correct the greatest cause of supratip deformity—a loss of skeletal support.

the past several years (Figs. 36–18, 36–19). Although ear cartilage is a more sturdy material and is superior to septal cartilage in areas of reduced vascularity, there are some inherent problems. It is not malleable and does not thin with crushing; it just breaks (Fig. 36–20). It is most predictable when used as an unmodified unit (no cuts or scoring). When used as a circumferentially wrapped graft, ear cartilage can improve dorsal contour but may result in late irregularities (Fig. 36–21). Attempts to modify such irregularities may result in a greater deformity consequent upon the internal stresses present with curled and wrapped ear cartilage (Fig. 36–22). In general, therefore, "minor" surgical refinements of ear cartilage grafts should not be undertaken. If the surgeon does attempt to modify ear cartilage grafts, he must be prepared to resect completely the errant part

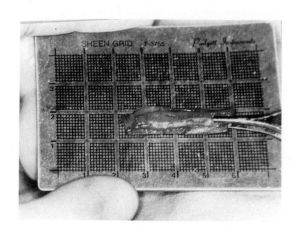

Figure 36–14. Multilayered cartilage grafts before insertion. The posterior graft is placed to correspond to the deformity. The anterior graft must be the optimal material with edges feathered and contoured to reproduce a natural dorsal line.

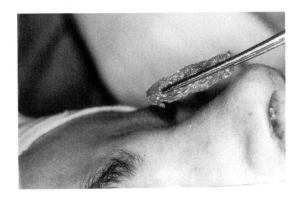

Figure 36–15. Crushed cartilage provides an excellent smooth cover to tie in all edges of the middle and bony vaults while slightly augmenting the dorsal height.

Figure 36–16. Solid *(lower)* and crushed *(upper)* grafts used in tip recontouring. The crushed cartilage grafts are used when a softer tip is desired.

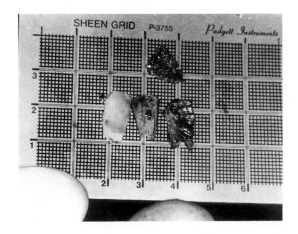

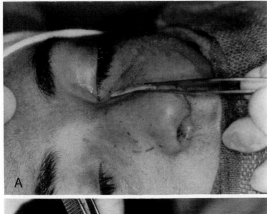
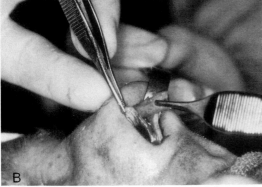

Figure 36–17. *A,* Spreader graft before insertion. *B,* Spreader graft being inserted into a pocket along the anterior or dorsal edge of the septum in order to reposition the lateral wall and open the internal valve.

Figure 36–18. A rolled and tied dorsal graft of ear cartilage. The posterior nasal concavity is filled with autogenous cartilage and bony debris.

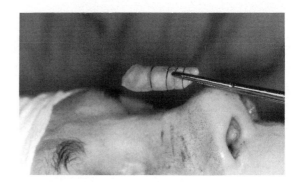

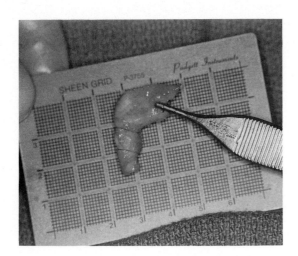

Figure 36–19. Shaped into a right angle, conchal cartilage is unsurpassed as a caudal support when the caudal septum has been lost.

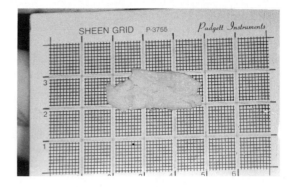

Figure 36–20. Ear cartilage does not crush well and is not malleable. Crushing generally produces a broken and disconnected mass of cartilage that frequently becomes unusable.

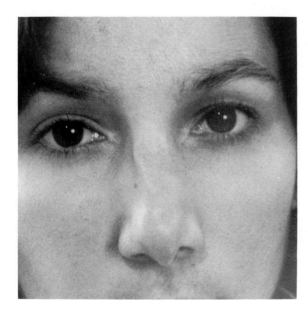

Figure 36–21. Ear cartilage that has not been properly folded and secured may cause late dorsal irregularity as attachments cause a distortion of the original smooth dorsal contour.

Figure 36–22. Attempts to trim the slightest irregularity may result in worse deformity as the cartilage flares at the area of resection.

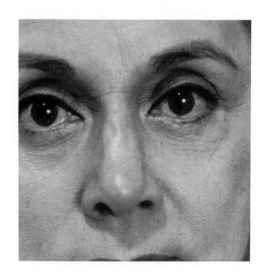

and start again with an entirely new donor specimen.

Cranial Bone

Over the past several years, there has been growing interest in the use of the outer table of the calvarium for nasal reconstruction, spurred by the work of Tessier (1982), McCarthy and Zide (1984), and others. There is evidence that cranial bone (Fig. 36–23) is superior to iliac bone in its revascularization and in its survival (Zins and Whitaker, 1983). The surgeon who attempts to harvest cranial bone should become familiar with its texture, anatomy, and resistance to surgical manipulation. Only with experience can the surgeon fully appreciate the wide variety of thicknesses (Pensler and McCarthy, 1985) and textures of calvarial bone, which make its harvesting sometimes difficult and hazardous (see Chap. 18).

Penetration of the inner table, dura, and brain has occurred during harvesting of cranial bone. Each tap of the chisel or progres-

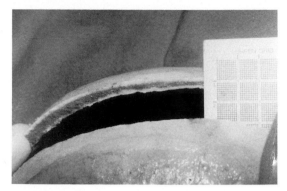

Figure 36–23. Cross section of calvarial bone at the approximate donor site in a 35 year old male cadaver. Note the thickness of the diploë and the variations in thickness of the outer and inner tables.

sion of the cutting bur should be made with the strictest attention to instrument position and the application of force to the mallet or bur (Fig. 36–24). The area of resection should be more posterior in the male to ensure there is no visible scar in case of the development of pattern baldness.

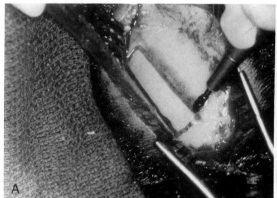

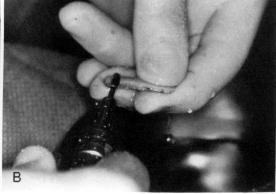

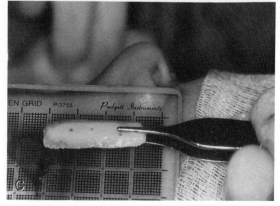

Figure 36–24. *A,* Graft outlines, and the lateral bone smoothed before removal with an osteotome. *B,* The edges of the graft are smoothed with a low rpm bur while being irrigated with saline. *C,* Remodeled graft ready for insertion.

Rib Cartilage and Bone

Rib cartilage and bone are excellent graft materials with a wide variety of sizes and shapes. The recommended donor site is low on the rib cage. Although the operative donor site leaves a visible scar, the trade-off is worth the improved graft material obtained from the distal ends of the eighth, ninth, or tenth ribs. When cartilage from the fifth or sixth ribs is harvested, the incision may be camouflaged in the inframammary crease, but the thick rib obtained must be trimmed to size. This can lead to late distortion as the internal stresses settle into a new equilibrium, changing the graft contour (Fig. 36–25). Use of the seventh, eighth, or ninth ribs (Fig. 36–26) makes available a wide variety of graft sizes applicable to most reconstructive needs, with segments of small diameters, perichondrially wrapped to ensure survival without contour changes (Fig. 36–27).

Although rib cartilage does not crush well, it can be used effectively as filler or augmentation material by thinly slicing cross sections of cartilage, as shown in Figure 36–28.

Temporal Fascia

Temporal fascia may be harvested in fairly large amounts and its use has been popularized by Guerrerosantos (1984) as a cover for grafts that are irregular in shape (Fig. 36–29). There are two layers of temporal fascia, one superficial, which represents an extension of the Superficial Musculo Aponeurotic

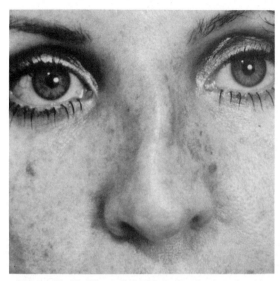

Figure 36–25. Rib cartilage always curls when there is a disturbance of the internal stresses consequent upon graft trimming.

System (SMAS), and a deep one, which is intimate with the temporalis muscle (Cutting, McCarthy, and Berenstein, 1984). The graft material is flimsy, and the late results in the author's experience have not been favorable. Most patients who received a double layer of temporal fascia to soften dorsal irregularities were not significantly improved.

It is possible that this material could be used as a suitable filler material, but handling it can be frustrating. It is much less controllable than successive layers of crushed cartilage.

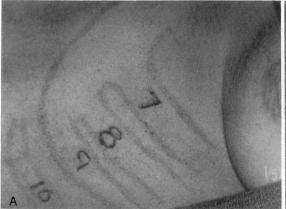
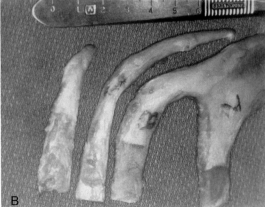

Figure 36–26. *A,* Outline of available sites for harvesting rib cartilage. *B,* Shape and size of various rib cartilages useful in nasal reconstruction.

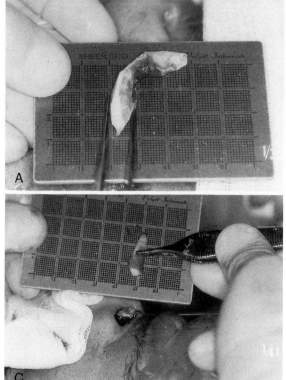

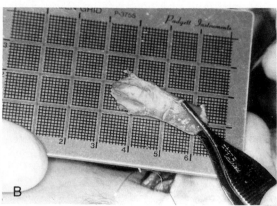

Figure 36–27. *A,* Material from the eighth rib used in maxillary augmentation. *B,* Prepared dorsal graft harvested from the seventh rib. *C,* Small columellar strut harvested from the ninth rib.

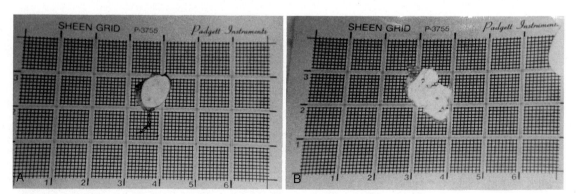

Figure 36–28. *A,* Cross section of the ninth rib before crushing. *B,* Although rib cartilage does not crush well, it can be effectively used for fill even though it "breaks up" after crushing.

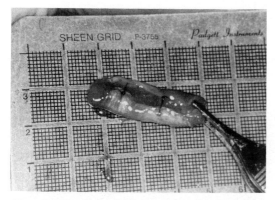

Figure 36–29. Bone graft covered with a double layer of temporal fascia and secured with nonabsorbable sutures.

Iliac Bone Graft

Because the author's experience with iliac bone graft is limited, it will not be discussed here (see Chap. 35, p. 1886).

INDIVIDUAL DEFORMITIES

Supratip Deformity

Supratip deformity is an unesthetic, permanent postsurgical convexity located just cephalad to the tip (see Fig. 36–4). There is disagreement as to its cause.

In 1976 the author challenged the traditional view that the cause of supratip deformity was inadequate resection of parts (Sheen, 1976). It was proposed instead that the deformity was the result of *excessive* resection of skeletal parts. It has been the author's experience over the past ten years that more than 90 per cent of patients with supratip deformity have had an over-resection of skeletal parts.

If over-resection were accepted as the major etiologic factor, the correction in most cases of supratip deformity should be directed toward augmentation. During the past ten years, in the author's series of supratip deformities (over 1000 cases), 90 per cent of patients have undergone some type of dorsal augmentation in combination with reduction of the anterior caudal septal part, or in combination with an external excision of soft tissues. With this surgical protocol, supratip deformities have been corrected in all patients so treated and the correction has lasted over the years.

Patients with a supratip deformity can be positively diagnosed as having an over-resection of skeletal parts by palpation. If the arch of soft tissue compresses to the lowered skeleton, as shown in Figure 36–30, further resection of soft tissues would be counterproductive and potentially dangerous, whereas augmentation could be corrective.

There continues to be an erroneous surgical

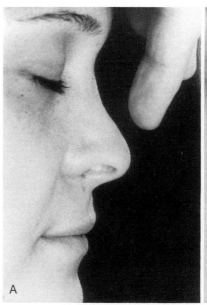 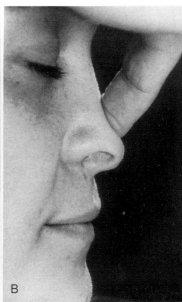

Figure 36–30. *A, B,* In the diagnosis of supratip deformity, compression of the area can positively identify the etiology as being an over-resection of skeletal parts.

A

B

concept that the convexity can be symmetrically reduced by subdermal thinning. The basal arch of tissues cannot be reduced beyond its limit without permanent disfigurement (Fig. 36–31).

A young adult male presented with a history of one previous rhinoplasty. His major complaints concerned the dorsal convexity and an inability to breathe. He felt that the nose had a "pinched" look on the frontal view,

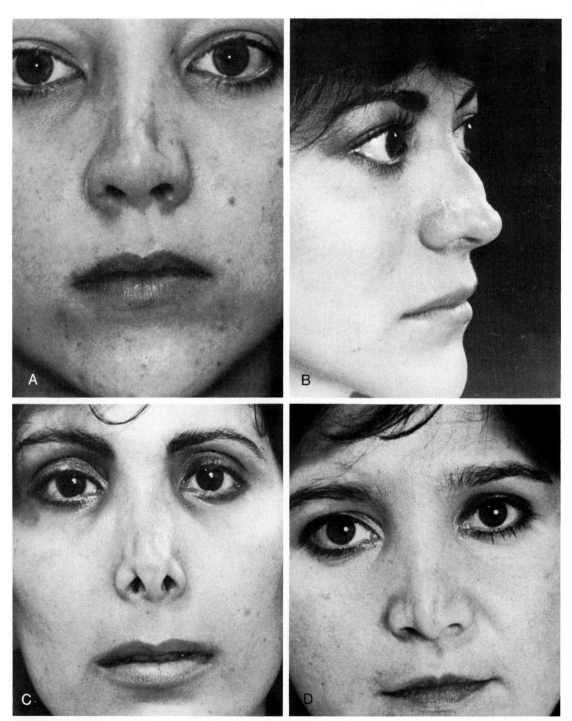

Figure 36–31. *A* to *D,* Patients on whom further subdermal dissection was performed to decrease the arch of soft tissues. This may result in irreparable damage to the soft tissues, as illustrated here.

was generally too small, and had an "ugly hump" on the lateral view. His hope was for a straight, "nonsurgical"-appearing male nose.

On frontal view (Fig. 36–32A), the nasal length is adequate for the face. There is an inverted V deformity from middle vault collapse. The central third of the nose appears somewhat broader, a normal consequence of the reduced height. The tip of the nose appears "pinched" owing to its narrow configuration, set off by parenthesis, a consequence of alar collapse. The general contour is elliptic, the root and the tip being the narrowest parts, and the central third the widest. The columella is low relative to the alae. On internal examination, both internal valves are narrowed. The septal partition is firm and shifted to the left side, which is virtually impacted.

On lateral view (Fig. 36–32B), the nose is small for the face. The dorsum has been overresected, the supratip forming an unattractive convexity, ending in a tip without projection.

The question of whether the convexity is soft tissue or inadequate resection is a moot one. Nasal proportion and size are at issue. The nose is already too small for a man and certainly small relative to his face. The issue of etiology would not alter the surgical plan. To bring the nose into satisfactory balance with the face and with its vaults, augmentation is key.

On frontal view, to obtain divergent lines from root to tip, the tip must be augmented both anteriorly and laterally.

The inverted V deformity (collapse of the middle vault) should be corrected by a substantial dorsal graft. A suitable graft would increase the height of the dorsum, smooth out the lines from root to base, and laterally distract the tissues of the middle vault, acting as spreader grafts as well.

The surgical plan was as follows:

1. Skeletonize through a left *intra*cartilaginous incision, making a dorsal pocket to the root sufficiently large to accommodate a substantial dorsal graft.
2. Make a hemitransfixion incision to the posterior third of the septum.
3. Resect 2 mm of caudal septum.
4. Rasp the dorsum to prepare for grafting and trim dorsal parts.
5. Perform submucous resection of the septum.
6. Prepare the dorsal graft and insert.
7. Perform additional caudal augmentation using ethmoid bone.
8. Create alar rim grafts, bilateral.
9. Create tip grafts (solid and crushed).

On frontal view, the inverted V deformity has been eliminated (Fig. 36–33). The lateral lines are symmetric and diverge to a tip that is well delineated from the dorsum and is viewed as a separate anatomic part. The relationship of columella to alae has been improved, and elevation of the columella has improved the base to an ideal "gull-in-flight" configuration. The nasal length has been reduced slightly by the trim of the caudal septum, but has been visually increased by more sharply delineating the root and tip.

On lateral view (Fig. 36–34), the nose has

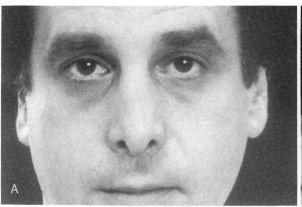 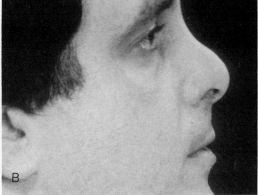

Figure 36–32. *A,* Frontal view of a patient after a rhinoplasty. The nose appears broad in the central third, with the tip and the root narrow. This results in an elliptic contour to the nose. The columella is low relative to the alae. On internal examination, the internal valves are narrow, as would be expected from the collapse of the middle vault. *B,* On lateral view, the patient presents with a classic supratip deformity, ending in a rounded tip without definition. The overall size of the nose is small relative to the face.

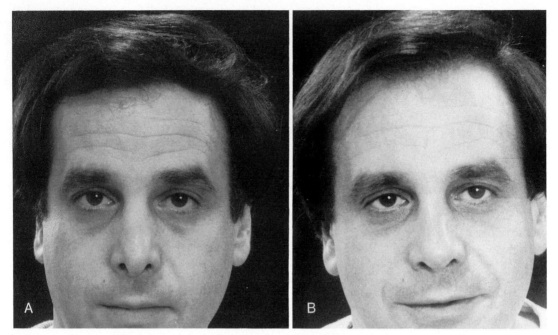

Figure 36–33. On frontal view there is an improved balance to the nose, with the lateral lines diverging at the base. The columellar-alar relationship has improved; the base has the "gull-in-flight" configuration. The central depression has been eliminated by the dorsal graft. *A,* Preoperative view. *B,* Postoperative view.

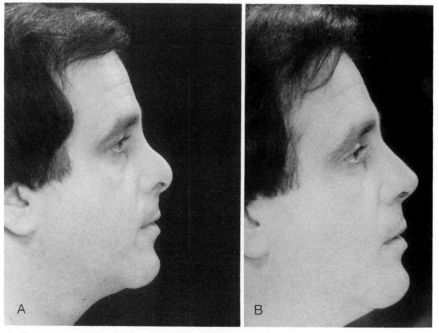

Figure 36–34. Despite the generalized augmentation of the nose, it remains small relative to the face. The dorsum is straight, ending in a tip that is well defined and in line with the dorsum. *A,* Preoperative view. *B,* Postoperative view.

a much more natural appearance with a stronger dorsum, in line with a projecting nasal tip. Because the tip has greater projection and the root is better defined, there is a visual lengthening of the nose even though it has been slightly shortened. The relationship of columella to alar rim has been improved.

The oblique views (Fig. 36–35) demonstrate the symmetry of the nasal walls and the tip.

Although the author believes that overresection represents the etiology in the overwhelming majority of supratip deformities, it is not the sole cause of this deformity. Figure 36–36 shows a patient with a supratip deformity caused by an inadequate trim of the anterior (dorsal) edge of the septum. Correction was accomplished by trimming the errant part, augmenting the dorsum, and placing appropriate tip grafts.

Regardless of the thickness of the soft tissues, augmentation can correct the supratip deformity, which is more likely to result in these patients than in those with soft tissues that are more apt to drape properly. The patient in Figure 36–37 is a male with thick nasal skin cover treated successfully by augmentation. A large nose with balance is far more desirable than a small nose that has an "operative" appearance.

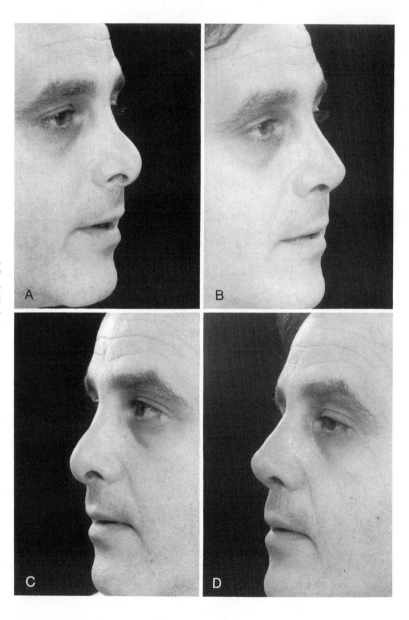

Figure 36–35. Oblique views are the absolute test for evaluation of dorsal and tip symmetry. The slightly higher projection of the left side of the nasal tip is manifest as a slightly more projecting part in comparison with the opposite view. *A, C,* Preoperative views. *B, D,* Postoperative views.

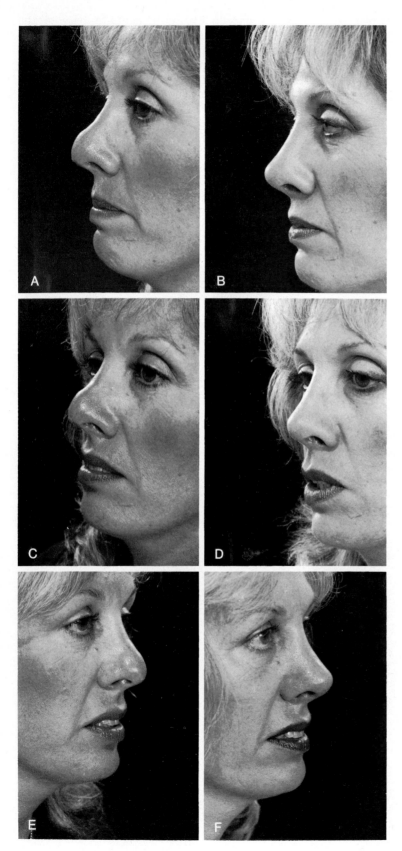

Figure 36–36. An inadequately re-sected anterior (dorsal) edge of the septum. At surgery, the errant edge was resected, a new dorsum created by septal cartilage graft, and the tip re-formed by tip grafting. *A, C, E,* Preoperative views. *B, D, F,* Postop-erative views.

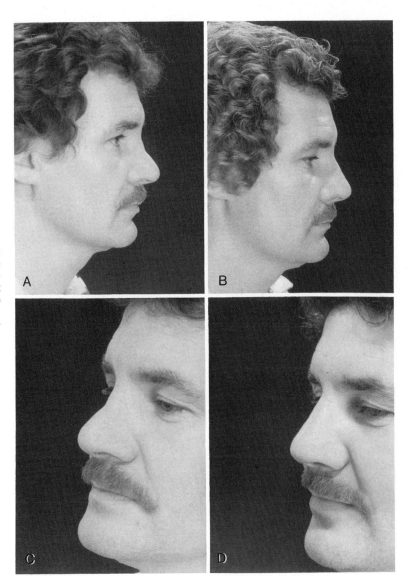

Figure 36–37. In patients with exceedingly thick skin, the same techniques of correction by augmentation apply. The tissues must have sufficient skeletal support to provide a natural contour. *A, C,* Preoperative views. *B, D,* Postoperative views.

Middle Vault Problems

Middle vault collapse is a natural consequence of dorsal resection. The roof of the middle vault is "T" shaped. Its function is to hold the lateral walls of the middle vault in appropriate alignment with the caudal edges of the bony vault, and to maintain a suitable position for an effectively functioning internal valve. Following resection of the roof and ablation of the "T," there is often middle vault collapse, creating three distinct problems (Fig. 36–38): (1) an inverted V deformity visible on frontal view, creating a distortion of the natural lines from root to tip; (2) on oblique view, a notch at the junction of the

middle and bony vaults, which the patient misconstrues as a "hump" but which causes a distinct break in the smooth line from root to base; (3) a narrowing of the internal valve, which makes breathing difficult to impossible since air can be exhaled through the nose, but on inspiration the internal valves collapse with obstruction of the airway.

Treatment is to support internally the middle vault by spreader grafts whenever possible, or to "reroof" the dorsum, thereby creating a new "T" to reposition the middle vault.

Four patients who illustrate the inverted V deformity following resection of the roof of the middle vault are shown in Figure 36–38. The degree of visibility depends on skin thick-

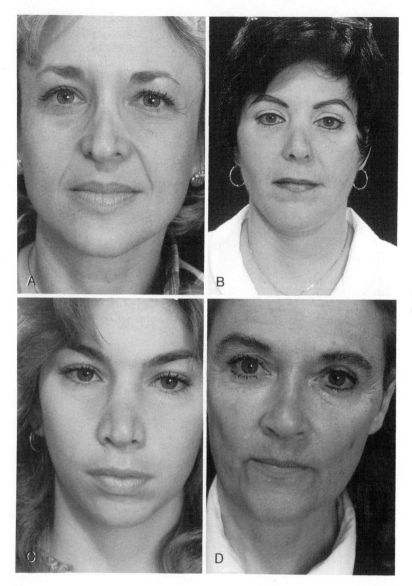

Figure 36–38. *A* to *D,* The inverted V deformity associated wtih middle vault problems.

ness, the size and position of the bony arch, and the effectiveness of the osteotomy in realigning the caudal arch of the bony pyramid. The effect of lateral wall collapse after roof resection is illustrated in Figure 36–39. These patients have straight dorsal contours on lateral view but on oblique view appear to have a dorsal hump. They also complain frequently of nasal airway obstruction, but on examination, if the nasal speculum spreads the internal valve laterally, there may be no evidence of the obstruction. The diagnosis can be made by observing the internal valve during nasal respiration with the patient's head tilted back and without a speculum in place.

The Spreader Graft. The spreader graft (Fig. 36–40 and see Fig. 36–17) was introduced to counter the effects of an excessive dorsal resection (Sheen, 1987). Although it was originally designed for use in primary rhinoplasty whenever the roof of the middle vault was resected, it is also useful in secondary rhinoplasty for patients with curves or middle vault collapse who have adequate dorsal height. However, it should be attempted only if there is adequate tissue along the anterior (dorsal) septal edge to allow dissection of an appropriate pocket, and only if there is sufficient autogenous material to use for the grafts.

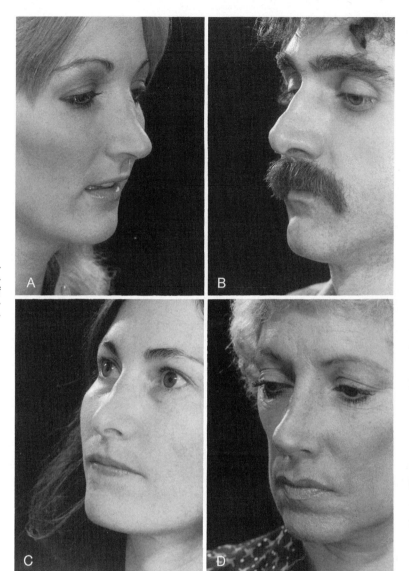

Figure 36–39. *A* to *D,* Four patients who have had a primary rhinoplasty with resection of the roof of the middle vault, and demonstrate the inverted V deformity consequent upon loss of roof support.

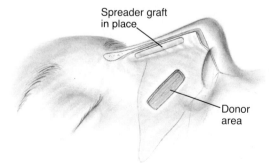

Spreader graft
in place

Donor
area

Figure 36–40. The spreader graft: donor site and its placement. Septal cartilage from the vomerian groove makes an ideal spreader graft.

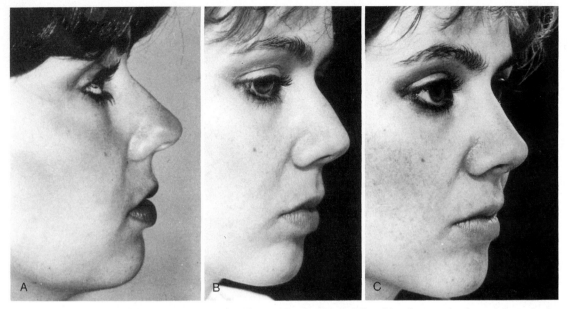

Figure 36–41. *A,* The patient before surgery. *B,* The result of a conservative rhinoplasty and a loss of tip projection following a trim of the alar cartilages. *C,* After a crushed cartilage graft to the radix and grafting of the tip. (See Fig. 36–42.)

Loss of Tip Definition/Projection

Although the many techniques of alar modification (see Chap. 35) are designed to improve tip definition, often in conjunction with partial alar cartilage resection, there is a loss of both projection and definition. This is especially true when the surgeon combines a more aggressive handling of the alar carti-lages with a conservative rhinoplasty. The latter combination of techniques is illlustrated in Figure 36–41. The primary surgeon had planned a "finesse" type of rhinoplasty with only minimal changes. The patient was unhappy with the radical change that resulted from the loss of tip projection and definition.

The postoperative result (Fig. 36–41*C*) is

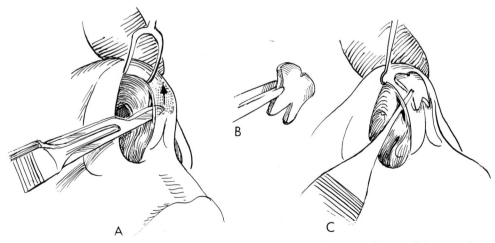

Figure 36–42. Placement of the cartilage graft. *A,* Incision along the caudal edge of the medial crus and preparation of the subcutaneous pocket. *B,* Sculptured cartilage graft. *C,* The cartilage graft is embedded.

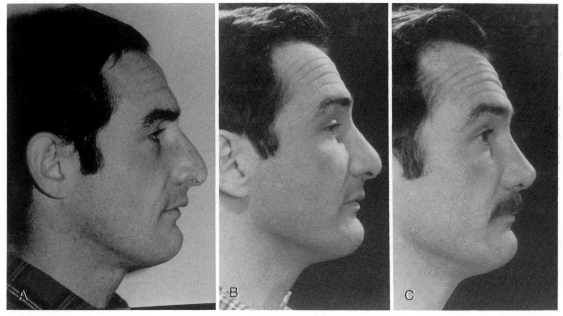

Figure 36–43. The effect of a conservative rhinoplasty on a patient with an inadequately projecting tip. *A,* Appearance before any surgery. *B,* The result following a conservative rhinoplasty. *C,* The result three years after dorsal grafting and tip (cartilage graft) augmentation.

shown after insertion of a radix graft of crushed cartilage in addition to grafting of the tip (Fig. 36–42 and see Figs. 36–3, 36–16).

The Conservative Tip-plasty. When a patient presents with an inadequately projecting tip, any modification of the alar cartilages increases the problem by making the tip even less projecting. Diagnosis of the tip with inadequate projection is important before any surgery of the alar cartilages is performed. In secondary rhinoplasty, when the surgeon attempts to correct the inadequately projecting tip, a working knowledge of tip grafting techniques is mandatory in order to reposition the tip for proper balance.

The male patient in Figure 36–43, who requested a rhinoplasty, demonstrates a tip that is clearly lacking in adequate projection. This result followed a most conservative primary rhinoplasty and tip-plasty. If the surgeon had been more aggressive in the reduction of the dorsum, a supratip deformity would likely have developed. The correct management of this nose would have included tip grafting to bring the tip into an appropriate position relative to the dorsum. The author would not have resected any of the alar cartilage in this patient but would have simply liberated the overlying soft tissues, placing appropriate tip grafts to recontour and project the tip.

The patient is shown (Fig. 36–43*C*) two years after a single cartilage graft to the dorsum, and multiple tip grafts to realign and project it to the new dorsal line.

REFERENCES

Anderson, R., Sprinkle, P. M., Bouquot, J., and Hyams, V.: Complications of septorhinoplasty. Benign or malignant? Arch. Otolaryngol., *109*:489, 1983.

Barton, F. E., Jr.: Aesthetic aspects of partial nasal reconstruction. Clin. Plast. Surg., *8*:77, 1981.

Beekhuis, G. J.: Surgical correction of saddle nose deformity. Trans. Am. Acad. Ophthalmol. Otolaryngol., *80*:596, 1975.

Berman, W. E.: Secondary rhinoplasties and composite grafts. Trans. Am. Acad. Ophthalmol. Otolaryngol., *84*:952, 1977.

Brown, J. B., and McDowell, F.: Plastic Surgery of the Nose. St. Louis, MO, C. V. Mosby Company, 1965.

Chait, L. A., Becker, H., and Cort, A.: The versatile costal osteochondrial graft in nasal reconstruction. Br. J. Plast. Surg., *33*:179, 1969.

Cinelli, J. A.: Lengthening of the nose by a septal flap. Plast. Reconstr. Surg. *43*:99, 1969.

Cohen, S.: Complications following rhinoplasty. Plast. Reconstr. Surg., *18*:213, 1956.

Conley, J.: Intranasal composite grafts for dorsal support. Arch. Otolaryngol., *111*:241, 1985.

Converse, J. M.: Corrective rhinoplasty. *In* Converse, J. M. (Ed.): Reconstructive Plastic Surgery. Philadephia, W. B. Saunders Company, 1977, Vol. 2, pp. 1040–1163.

Cutting, C. B., McCarthy, J. G., and Berenstein, A.: Blood supply of the upper craniofacial skeleton: the search for composite calvarial bone flaps. Plast. Reconstr. Surg., *74*:603, 1984.

daSilva, G.: A new method of reconstructing the columella with a naso-labial flap. Plast. Reconstr. Surg., *34*:63, 1964.

Davis, P. K., and Jones, S. M.: The complications of Silastic implants: experience with 137 consecutive cases. Br. J. Plast. Surg., *24*:405, 1971.

Denecke, H. J., and Meyer, R.: Plastic Surgery of Head and Neck. New York, Springer-Verlag, 1967.

Dingman, R. O., and Walter, C.: Use of composite ear grafts in correction of the short nose. Plast. Reconstr. Surg., *43*:117, 1969.

Drumbellar, G. H.: Septal reconstruction in the deficient nose. Rhinology, *14*:189, 1976.

Elliott, R. A., Jr.: Rotation flaps to the nose. Plast. Reconstr. Surg., *44*:147, 1969.

Elsahy, N. I.: Prevention of parrot's beak deformity after reduction rhinoplasty. Acta. Chir. Plast. (Prague), *19*:63, 1977.

Fahoun, K.: Secondary correction of tip of nose. Acta Chir. Plast. (Prague), *23*:221, 1981.

Fanous, N., and Webster, R. C.: Revision rhinoplasty. A decision dilemma. Arch. Otolaryngol., *110*:359, 1984.

Farina, R., Cury, E., and Ackel, I. A.: Traumatic nasal deformities. Aesthetic Plast. Surg., *7*:233, 1983.

Farina, R., and Villano, J. B.: Follow-up of bone grafts to the nose. Plast. Reconstr. Surg., *48*:251, 1971.

Fomon, S., and Bell, J. W.: Rhinoplasty—New Concepts: Evaluation and Application. Springfield, IL, Charles C Thomas, 1970.

Gerow, R. J., Stal, S., and Spira, M.: The totem pole rib graft reconstruction of the nose. Ann. Plast. Surg., *11*:273, 1983.

Goode, R. L.: Surgery of the incompetent nasal valve. Laryngoscope, *95*:546, 1985.

Guerrerosantos, J.: Temporoparietal free fascia grafts in rhinoplasty. Plast. Reconstr. Surg., *74*:465, 1984.

Hagan, W. E.: Collapse of the nasal dorsum: a method for intraoperative reconstruction. Laryngoscope, *94*:409, 1984.

Hallock, G. G., and Trier, W. C.: Cerebrospinal fluid rhinorrhea following rhinoplasty. Plast. Reconstr. Surg., *71*:109, 1983.

Hardin, J. C., Jr.: Alar rim reconstruction by a dorsal nasal flap. Plast. Reconstr. Surg., *66*:293, 1980.

Hirshowitz, B., Kaufman, T., and Ullman, J.: Reconstruction of the tip of the nose and ala by load cycling of the nasal skin and harnessing of extra skin. Plast. Reconstr. Surg., *77*:316, 1986.

Jackson, I. T., Smith, J., and Mixter, R. C.: Nasal bone grafting using split skull grafts. Ann. Plast. Surg., *11*:533, 1983.

Juri, J., Juri, C., Belmont, J. A., Grili, D. A., and Angrigiani, C.: Neighboring flaps and cartilage grafts for correction of serious secondary nasal deformities. Plast. Reconstr. Surg., *76*:876, 1985.

Juri, J., Juri, C., Grilli, D. A., Zeaiter, M. C., and Belmont, J.: Correction of the secondary nasal tip. Ann. Plast. Surg., *16*:322, 1986.

Karlan, M. S., Ossoff, R. H., and Sisson, G. A.: A compendium of intranasal flaps. Laryngoscope, *92*:774, 1982.

Kazanjian, V. H., and Converse, J. M.: Deformities of the nose. *In* Converse, J. M. (Ed.): Kazanjian and Converse's Surgical Treatment of Facial Injuries. 3rd Ed. Baltimore, Williams & Wilkins Company, 1974.

Kerth, J. D., and Bytell, D. E.: Revision in unsuccessful rhinoplasty. Otolaryngol. Clin. North Am., *7*:65, 1974.

Klabunde, E. H., and Falces, E.: Incidence of complications in cosmetic rhinoplasties. Plast. Reconstr. Surg., *34*:192, 1964.

Lewis, M. L.: Prevention and correction of cicatricial intranasal adhesions in rhinoplastic surgery. Arch. Otolaryngol., *60*:215, 1954.

Marshall, D. R., and Slattery, P. G.: Intracranial complications of rhinoplasty. Br. J. Plast. Surg., *36*:342, 1983.

McCabe, B. F.: The problem of the collapsing upper lateral cartilage. Ann. Otol. Rhinol. Laryngol., *88*:524, 1979.

McCarthy, J. G., and Zide, B. M.: The spectrum of calvarial bone grafting: introduction of the vascularized calvarial bone flap. Plast. Reconstr. Surg., *74*:10, 1984.

McGlynn, M. J., and Sharpe, D. T.: Cialit preserved homograft cartilage in nasal augmentation: a long-term review. Br. J. Plast. Surg., *34*:53, 1981.

Millard, D. R., Jr.: Secondary corrective rhinoplasty. Plast. Reconstr. Surg., *44*:545, 1969.

Millard, D. R., Jr.: Reconstructive rhinoplasty for the lower two-thirds of the nose. Plast. Reconstr. Surg., *57*:722, 1976a.

Millard, D. R., Jr. (Ed.): Symposium on Corrective Rhinoplasty. St. Louis, MO, C. V. Mosby Company, 1976b.

O'Connor, G. B., and McGregor, M. W.: Secondary rhinoplasties: their cause and prevention. Plast. Reconstr. Surg., *15*:404, 1955.

Olbourne, N. A., and Kraaijenhagen, J. H.: Rotation flap for distal nasal defects. Br. J. Plast. Surg., *28*:64, 1975.

Orticochea, M.: A new method for reconstruction of the nose: the ears as donor areas. Br. J. Plast. Surg., *24*:225, 1971.

Orticochea, M.: Refined technique for reconstructing the whole nose with the conchas of the ears. Br. J. Plast. Surg., *33*:68, 1980.

Ortiz-Monasterio, F., and Olmedo, A.: Reconstruction of major nasal defects. Clin. Plast. Surg., *8*:565, 1981.

Pardina, A. J., and Vaca, J. F.: Evaluation of the different methods used in the treatment of rhinoplastic sequelae. Aesthetic Plast. Surg., *7*:237, 1983.

Parkes, M. L., and Kanodia, R.: Avulsion of the upper lateral cartilage: etiology, diagnosis, surgical anatomy and management. Laryngoscope, *91*:758, 1981.

Peck, G. C.: Techniques in Aesthetic Rhinoplasty. New York, Gower Medical Publishing Company, 1984.

Pensler, J., and McCarthy, J. G.: The calvarial donor site: an anatomic study in cadavers. Plast. Reconstr. Surg., *75*:648, 1985.

Pitanguy, I., and Ceravolo, M. P.: Secondary rhinoplasty. Aesthetic Plast. Surg., *6*:47, 1982.

Pollet, J., and Weikel, A. M.: Revision rhinoplasty. Clin. Plast. Surg., *4*:47, 1977.

Rees, T. D.: An aid to the treatment of supratip swelling after rhinoplasty. Laryngoscope, *81*:308, 1971.

Rees, T. D.: Aesthetic Plastic Surgery. Philadelphia, W. B. Saunders Company, 1980.

Rees, T. D., Guy, C., Wood-Smith, D., and Converse, J. M.: Composite grafts. *In* Transactions of the Third International Congress of Plastic Surgery. Washington, DC, Excerpta Medica, 1963, p. 821.

Rees, T. D., Krupp, S., and Wood-Smith, D.: Secondary rhinoplasty. Plast. Reconstr. Surg., 46:322, 1970.

Regnault, P., and Daniel, R. K. (Eds.): Aesthetic Plastic Surgery. Principles and Techniques. Boston, Little, Brown & Company, 1984.

Rigg, B. M.: The dorsal nasal flap. Plast. Reconstr. Surg., 52:361, 1973.

Rogers, B. O.: The importance of "delay" in timing secondary and tertiary rhinoplastic deformities. *In* Transactions of the Fourth International Congress of Plastic and Reconstructive Surgery. Amsterdam, Excerpta Medica, 1969, p. 1065.

Rogers, B. O.: Secondary and tertiary correction of post-rhinoplastic deformities: some dos and don'ts. *In* Millard, D. R., Jr. (Ed.): Symposium on Corrective Rhinoplasty. St. Louis, MO, C. V. Mosby Company, 1976, p. 23.

Safian, J.: Corrective Rhinoplastic Surgery. New York, Hoeber Company, 1935.

Sheen, J. H.: Secondary rhinoplasty. Plast. Reconstr. Surg., 56:137, 1975.

Sheen, J. H.: Secondary rhinoplasty surgery. *In* Millard, D. R., Jr. (Ed.): Symposium on Corrective Rhinoplasty. St Louis, MO, C. V. Mosby Company, 1976, p. 133.

Sheen, J. H.: Aesthetic Rhinoplasty. St. Louis, MO, C. V. Mosby Company, 1978.

Sheen, J. H.: A new look at supratip deformity. Ann. Plast. Surg., 3:498, 1979.

Sheen, J. H.: Aesthetic aspects of post-traumatic nasal reconstruction. A case study. Clin. Plast. Surg., 8:193, 1981.

Sheen, J. H.: Aesthetic Rhinoplasty. 2nd Ed. St. Louis, MO, C. V. Mosby Company, 1987.

Shirakabe, Y., Shirakabe, T., and Kishimoto, T.: The classification of complications after augmentation rhinoplasty. Aesthetic Plast. Surg., 9:185, 1985.

Steiss, C. F.: Errors in rhinoplasty and their correction. Plast. Reconstr. Surg., 28:276, 1961.

Stoksted, P., and Gutierrez, C.: The nasal passage following rhinoplastic surgery. J. Laryngol. Otol., 97:49, 1983.

Tessier, P.: Autogenous bone grafts taken from the calvarium for facial and cranial applications. Clin. Plast. Surg., 9:531, 1982.

Thomas, J. R., and Tardy, M. E., Jr.: Complications of rhinoplasty. Ear Nose Throat J., 65:19, 1986.

Tobin, H. A., and Webster, R. C.: The less-than-satisfactory rhinoplasty: comparison of patient and surgeon satisfaction. Otolaryngol. Head Neck Surg., 94:86, 1986.

Walter, C. D.: Composite grafts in nasal surgery. Arch. Otolaryngol., 90:622, 1969.

Walter, C. D.: Secondary nasal revisions after rhinoplasties. Trans. Am. Acad. Ophthalmol. Otolaryngol., 80:519, 1975.

Webster, R. C.: Revisional rhinoplasty. Otolaryngol. Clin. North Am., 8:753, 1975.

Webster, R. C., Hamdan, U. S., Gaunt, J. M., Fuleihan, N. S., and Smith, R. C.: Rhinoplastic revisions with injectable silicone. Arch. Otolaryngol. Head Neck Surg., 112:269, 1986.

Wheeler, E. S., Kawamoto, H. K., and Zarem, H. A.: Bone grafts for nasal reconstruction. Plast. Reconstr. Surg., 69:9, 1982.

Williams, J. E.: The pinched nasal tip. Clin. Plast. Surg., 4:41, 1977.

Wright, W. K.: Symposium: the supratip in rhinoplasty: a dilemma. II. Influence of surrounding structure and prevention. Laryngoscope, 86:50, 1976.

Zins, J. E., and Whitaker, L. A.: Membranous versus endochondral bone: implications for craniofacial reconstruction. Plast. Reconstr. Surg., 72:778, 1983.

Fritz E. Barton, Jr.
H. Steve Byrd

Acquired Deformities of the Nose

ANATOMY

The nose is traditionally divided into thirds on the basis of the underlying skeletal structure. The proximal third rests on the nasal bones; the middle third rests on the upper lateral cartilages. The skin over both of these areas is relatively thin and nonsebaceous, and is separated from the underlying skeleton by a loose areolar plane that allows free sliding. The skin of the distal third of the nose overlies the domes and lateral crura of the lower lateral (alar) cartilages medially, and the sesamoid cartilages surrounded by fibrofatty connective tissue laterally. The skin of the nasal tip has a thick dermal layer and prominent sebaceous glands, and is firmly adherent to the underlying cartilages so as to prohibit any sliding.

The mobile lower portion of the nose is collectively referred to as the *lobule* and is divided into the *tip*, the *alae*, the *columella*, and the *membranous septum*. The floor of the entrance to the vestibule is the *nostril sill*. The *soft triangle* spans the junction of the ala with the columella (Fig. 37–1).

Special emphasis must be drawn to the relationship between the lateral crus of the alar cartilage and the alar rim. This relationship is often illustrated incorrectly in texts that show the cartilage to lie within and parallel to the soft tissue rim. In fact, the cartilage courses obliquely upward within the nasal tip, and its caudal (lateral) border forms the medial portion of the crease that separates the alar wing from the tip (Fig. 37–1). In the lateral alar rim the external nasal skin abuts the vestibular skin, with only a thin layer of connective tissue in between (Fig. 37–2) (Natvig, Sether, and Dingman, 1979).

Figure 37–1. Anatomy of the nasal lobule.

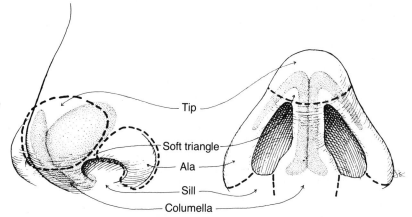

There are two points concerning the circumference of the nostril that merit special attention. First, the *soft triangle* at the nostril apex is especially susceptible either to grooving into an angular slit or to webbing into stenosis of the nostril from scars that pass through this delicate skin fold. Second, the *junction of the alar wing with the side of the tip* is a location of possible collapse. In this area the fibrofatty tissue of the ala attaches to the caudal border of the lower lateral cartilage. This attachment is fragile and, once divided, cannot easily be restored. It is frequently necessary to splint the nostril border with a cartilage graft to avoid buckling. Specific application of this principle will be discussed under the subject of skeletal support.

In considering nasal anatomy, one must not become so preoccupied with the graceful external curves and prominences that the internal airway is overlooked. Within the nostril orifice lies the *vestibule*, which is lined by keratinized squamous epithelium with hair called vibrissae. The hair filaments serve to collect dust and particulate matter to prevent its entry into the internal airway.

Inspired air passes from the vestibule into the nasal cavity through the *internal nasal valve*. The area of the internal nasal valve is a triangular space bounded medially by the nasal septum, superolaterally by the upper lateral cartilage, and inferiorly by the floor of the vestibule. This anatomic point is not a true valve but rather a constriction in the airway that serves functionally as a valve. It is important in reconstruction from two aspects: caliber and stability. Air flow may become obstructed, even with normal airway caliber, by instability of the superolateral wall.

Finally, it is not sufficient merely to be familiar with the idealized "normal" nose

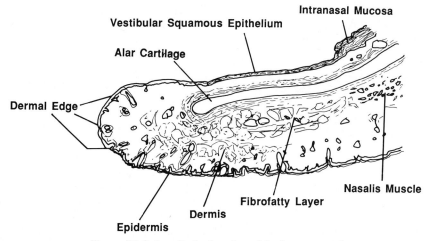

Figure 37–2. Longitudinal section of the human nostril.

form. One only has to glance casually around any group of people to see that there are many different shapes and sizes of noses. For example, anthropometric studies have demonstrated that there are at least seven types of nostril shape (Fig. 37–3) (Farkas, Hreczko, and Deutsch, 1983). Most significant in relation to reconstruction are the ethnic variations that occur in the nasal lobule.

Using the basal or "worm's eye" view, the angle of inclination of the axis of the nostril can be measured and classified. Farkas, Kolar, and Munro (1986) correlated these patterns with racial background. Most *Caucasians* showed Type I or II noses with angles of inclination between 55 and 90 degrees. In Caucasians also the height of the columella was approximately 60 per cent of the total height of the lobule. The average total height of the lobule was approximately 20 mm, and the average total width across the alae at their widest points was 35 mm, so that the ratio of height to width of the lobule was 0.57 to 1.

Asians demonstrated mainly Type III or V, with angles of inclination between 25 and 54 degrees. An occasional Asian had round nostrils, which precluded measurement of the angle. Overall, Asians had less lobule projection and greater alar width than Caucasians.

Blacks tended to have Type VI or VII nostrils, but a few had Type IV. The height of

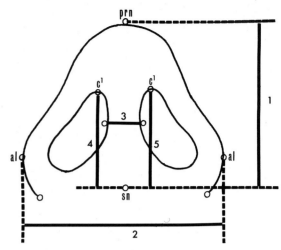

Figure 37–4. Surface measurements of the soft nose. 1 = protrusion of nasal tip (sn-prn); 2 = width of the nose (al-al); 3 = width of the columella; 4 and 5 = length of the columella rim (sn-c'). (From Farkas, L. G., Hreczko, T. A., and Deutsch, C. K.: Objective assessment of standard nostril types—a morphometric study. Ann. Plast. Surg., *11*:381, 1983.)

the lobule tended to be the same as that of the Asian nose, although the width of the nose was slightly greater. Specific measurements are illustrated in Figure 37–4 and Table 37–1.

The true artist of nasal reconstruction must keep these racial and ethnic variances in mind. When sufficient shape of the nose remains to serve as a guide, the surgeon need only match it. However, if the entire lobule is missing, these subtle differences must be taken into account when formulating the reconstructive design.

PLANNING

The lower two-thirds of the nose is mobile, soft, and easily severed. It is the part most commonly amputated, whether by accident or intent, and its reconstruction is termed "subtotal."

The upper one-third of the nose overlying the nasal bones serves as the skeletal platform upon which reconstruction of the more distal nose can be based. When the bony portion of the nose is also absent, the reconstruction becomes very much more complex and is termed "total" (Millard, 1966).

As for any reconstruction, the operative plan begins with evaluation of the defect. It is helpful to think first in terms of the *layers*

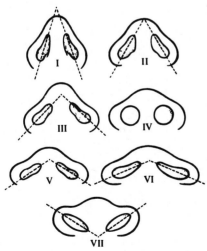

Figure 37–3. Nostril Types I through VII showing the average inclination of the medial longitudinal axis, the average width of the alar base, and the average width and height of the columella for each type. (From Farkas, L. G., Hreczko, T. A., and Deutsch, C. K.: Objective assessment of standard nostril types—a morphometric study. Ann. Plast. Surg., *11*:381, 1983.)

Table 37–1. Nostril Types in Young Adult North American Caucasians, Asians, and Blacks

Nostril Type	Inclination (degrees)	Caucasians (N = 125)		Asians (N = 53)		Blacks (N = 32)	
		N	%	N	%	N	%
I	70–90	53	42.4	0	0	0	0
II	55–69	66	52.8	10	18.9	1	3.1
III	40–54	6	4.8	28	52.8	5	15.6
IV	0	0	0	3	5.7	2	6.3
V	25–39	0	0	10	18.9	1	3.1
VI	10–24	0	0	2	3.8	16	50.0
VII	(−50)–(−20)	0	0	0	0	7	21.9

From Farkas, L. G.: Geography of the nose: a morphometric study. Aesth. Plast. Surg., *10*:191, 1986. Copyright 1986, Springer-Verlag.

of the nose requiring restoration—i.e., lining, skeleton, and skin cover. In general, lining and skeletal support should be provided at the time of delivery of skin cover, because the external envelope will never be more expansile. After the skin surface has contracted, it is extremely difficult to regain its original dimension.

Techniques for replacement of lining and skeletal framework are discussed later in the text. The surface skin is the most visible portion of the surgical result, so it is not surprising that procedures have historically focused on methods to replace the external nasal skin.

Mechanism of Closure

As for any wound, the hierarchy of techniques must be (1) primary closure, (2) healing by secondary intention, (3) skin graft, and (4) skin flap. Influencing the method of choice are the laxity in the surrounding skin, the adequacy of the wound bed vascularity to support a graft, and the later need for skeletal support to be introduced between the layers.

Quality of Coverage

The need for *color* match influences the choice between the white skin of a split-thickness skin graft or distant flap and the redder tint of a full-thickness skin graft or flap taken from the actinically exposed skin above the clavicles.

The desired *texture* dictates the choice of rough sebaceous skin (for the tip of a male nose) or smooth thin skin (for a female nasal dorsum).

The physical *contour* of the wound—a deep depression from loss of skin plus subcuta-

neous fat versus a shallow wound with only skin missing—also influences whether thin grafts or thicker flaps should be used.

Quantity of Coverage

In order to avoid a patchwork appearance to the reconstructed nose, one must consider where to place the seams between the normal nasal skin and the new skin. González-Ulloa (1956), in his classic article on regional esthetics of the face, considered the entire nasal dorsum as a single esthetic unit. This is especially true when only a small portion of external skin remains on the ala.

More limited subunits of the nose have been proposed (Millard, 1981; Burget, 1985). These lines coincide with topographic points that influence different light reflections and serve as ideal locations for the placement of suture lines (Fig. 37–5).

The early attempts at nasal reconstruction

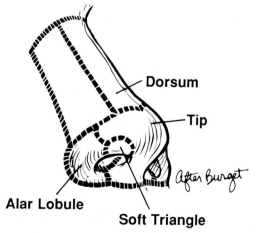

Figure 37–5. Esthetic subunits of the nose.

frequently underestimated the surface area of the defect, so that when transferred the flap was insufficient for a satisfactory esthetic result. Limberg (1963) is credited with popularizing the concept of constructing a preoperative pattern to enhance accuracy (Fig. 37–6).

While Limberg's pattern was a great contribution to nasal reconstruction, close inspection reveals subtle deficiencies of detail: from the basal perspective, the nostrils occupy almost the entire height of the lobule, producing a "gun-barrel" appearance. Limberg did, however, establish standardized dimensions required to form a complete lobule, i.e., 8 cm across the lobule from alar crease to alar crease, and a 2.5 cm tall lobule at the columella.

In 1921 Blair (1922) added his modifications to the total nasal pattern, using the same general measurements as Limberg, and popularized them in the United States. Little new was added to the designs for nasal repair until Millard (1974), under the influence of

Gillies, conceived the "gull-wing" flap to produce a more gracefully curved ala.

A number of materials have been used for making patterns in nasal reconstruction, among them wax, plaster of paris (Ivy, 1925), aluminum, and flannel. Microfoam tape (DiGeronimo, 1984) seems to be an effective modern substitute.

SKIN CLOSURE

Cutaneous Scars

As is true in other areas of the face, the skin of the nose is capable of healing with a barely visible scar. Simple lacerations without tissue loss usually can be approximated in a tension-free closure, making dermal dehiscence and resultant wide scars an uncommon phenomenon. The thick dermis and curving planes of the nostril, however, are prone to depressed scars unless the skin edges are meticulously everted; the alar rim, in partic-

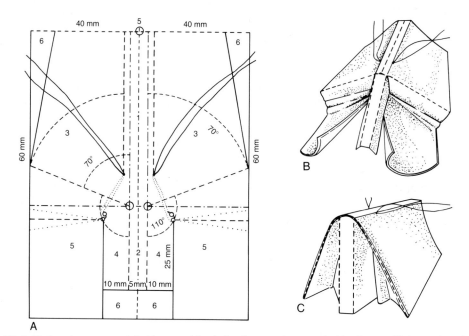

Figure 37–6. Limberg's paper model of two combined standing cones separated by 5 mm with two external sectors of 70 degrees and two inner-lying cones from sectors of 110 degrees. (From Limberg, A. A.: The Planning of Local Plastic Operations on the Body Surface. Theory and Practice. Translated by Wolfe, S. A. Lexington, MA, D. C. Heath and Company, 1984.)

ular, tends to notch after a through and through incision.

Dermabrasion can be helpful in slightly depressed scars of the nose, especially near the tip where the dermis is thick. More depressed nasal scars are best corrected by excision and re-eversion, Z-plasty, or W-plasty (see Chap. 1). Each of the revisional methods, while improving the scar, does so through further excision and advancement of adjacent tissues. However, scar excision and edge advancements may decrease the circumference of the nostril and distort the nostril rim.

Healing by Secondary Intention

In planning the repair of a nasal defect, one must not forget the possibility of allowing the wound to heal by secondary intention (Goldwyn and Rueckert, 1977). Acute defects in the medial canthus, alar crease, and nasal dorsum heal quite well without surgical intervention. Small defects of the nasal tip less than 1 cm in diameter may also be allowed to heal spontaneously. Larger defects distort the alar rims if left to heal by secondary intention.

Exposed cartilages, if bare of perichondrium, desiccate and extrude, with resultant loss of skeletal support to the nose. In contrast, the nasal bones are membranous in origin and, if kept moist with a nondesiccating dressing, granulate sufficiently to support a skin graft. This latter approach may be useful in debilitated patients who cannot tolerate complicated surgical repairs.

SKIN GRAFTS

Split-Thickness Skin Grafts

Split-thickness skin grafts are used primarily in compromise situations, since they result in pale shiny skin and contracture distortion. Such grafts are most useful to cover large wounds in debilitated patients, where they heal rapidly to form a stable base for a prosthesis.

Full-Thickness Skin Grafts

Surface wounds with satisfactory vascular beds may be repaired by full-thickness skin grafts. The source of the graft is adjusted according to the reconstructive needs, i.e., the desired thickness of the dermis for the repair.

The thickness of the dermis varies from one area of the body to another (González-Ulloa, 1956). The skin of the nasal dorsum of the normal male measures approximately 1300 microns (0.050 inch), while the skin of the lobule measures approximately 2400 microns (0.096 inch). Female skin may be significantly thinner. The skin thickness of the usual sources of a full-thickness skin graft for nasal reconstruction varies:

Cheek (nasolabial):	2900 microns
Mental (submental):	2500 microns
Neck (supraclavicular):	1800 microns
Postauricular:	800 microns

If skin of adequate thickness cannot be obtained from one of these sources, a thin layer of fat can be left on the underside of the graft to increase its bulk. One should note however, that as the thickness of the graft increases, the likelihood of a complete "take" decreases. This is especially true in the case of a composite skin-fat graft.

The most common donor site of full-thickness skin to be used for nasal reconstruction is the postauricular area. A graft 4 to 5 cm in diameter can be harvested from behind the adult ear, and yet the donor site can be closed primarily by advancing the mastoid skin. Even larger grafts extending from the helical rim to the hairline can be harvested from behind the ear, provided that the donor defect is closed by a separate split-thickness skin graft. When raised bilaterally, sufficient skin can be obtained from the postauricular area to resurface almost the whole surface of the nose.

The preauricular (Breach, 1978), nasolabial (Beare and Bennett, 1972), and submental areas can yield full-thickness grafts up to 2 cm in diameter, and they can still be closed primarily. When the size requirement of the defect is met by a graft from one of these areas, they offer the added attraction of skin that has been subjected to the same actinic exposure as the nose, for an excellent color match.

The supraclavicular area is the source of the largest potential graft of appropriate texture and pigment for use in nasal reconstruction. The entire nasal dorsum can be resurfaced with skin from the supraclavicular area, while the edges of the donor defect can be reapproximated (Fig. 37–7).

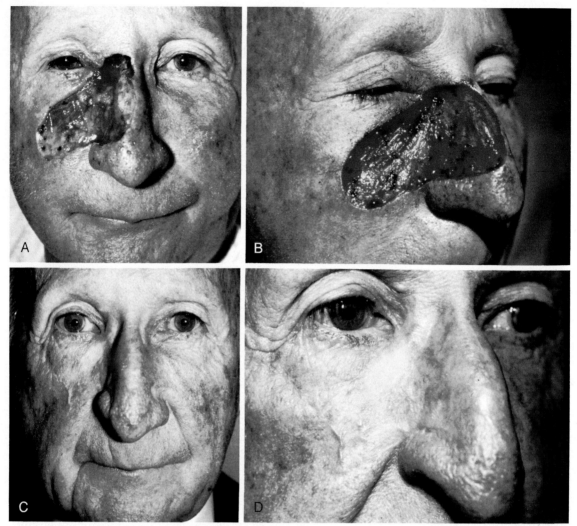

Figure 37–7. An 88 year old man with a skin defect secondary to removal of a basal cell carcinoma by histographic (Mohs) surgery. *A, B,* The patient preoperatively. *C, D,* Result after repair of the nasofacial wound with a supraclavicular full-thickness skin graft.

Unlike split-thickness skin grafts, the recipient bed of any full-thickness graft must be vascular and hemostasis must be complete. The graft is held in place by an external nasal splint or tie-over bolster dressing combined with intranasal packing for extra compression and adherence. The dressing is usually removed after five days, although complete vascularization of a thick full-thickness skin graft may take 10 to 14 days. Fresh grafts should be protected from the sun for six to 12 weeks to avoid hyperpigmentation.

When full-thickness replacement of the nose is necessary, intranasal lining may be achieved by the application of a graft to the undersurface of the flap used for the external nasal form (Lössen, 1898). Gillies (1943) ex-panded this concept by grafting a composite of skin and cartilage from the ear to the underside of a forehead flap.

COMPOSITE GRAFTS

Skin and Cartilage

The first record of composite grafts in nasal reconstruction is traced to Koenig in 1902. Over the next half-century there were sporadic reports in Europe of the use of grafts of skin and cartilage to repair nasal defects, most notably from Makara (1908), Haberer (1917), and Limberg (1935). Nevertheless, because of the pessimistic view held by Lexer

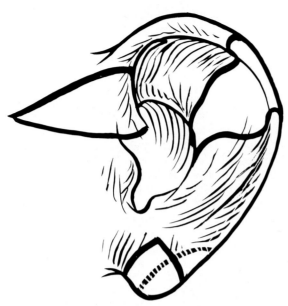

Figure 37–8. Sources of auricular composite grafts.

and Joseph, the foremost plastic surgeons of their day, the method did not receive much attention.

As a by-product of the resurgence of reconstructive surgery during World War II, a renewed interest developed in composite grafts. In Europe, Gillies (1943) described lining a forehead flap with a composite graft of auricular skin and cartilage. In America, Brown and Cannon (1946) and Dupertuis (1946) popularized the method.

Both the nasal lobule and auricle are essentially frameworks of cartilage covered by tightly adherent skin, attributes that make the ear a logical choice of donor tissue for nasal reconstruction. Chondrocutaneous grafts are commonly harvested from the anterior root of the helix, the helical rim, or the concha (Fig. 37–8).

For small defects of the alar rim, the most useful donor site is the root of the helix, as described by Argamaso (1975). A preauricular graft of up to 2 cm can be harvested from the non–hair-bearing skin behind the sideburn. Primary closure can be facilitated by upward advancement of the cheek skin (Fig. 37–9).

A considerable amount of experimental evidence has accumulated on the mode of revascularization of composite grafts. An experimental model was designed by Ballantyne and Converse (1958). A composite graft consisting of cartilage from the rabbit's ear with skin attached on one side was placed over the chorioallantois of the chick embryo, and the revascularization of the composite graft was studied by histologic examination of sections removed on the fourth and fifth days after transplantation. The difference in structure between the avian nucleated erythrocytes and the non-nucleated erythrocytes facilitated the study. The avian vessels, unable to penetrate the cartilage portion of the graft, were seen to extend along the undersurface of the cartilage until the dermis of the attached skin was reached; at this point the vessels penetrated the dermis of the composite graft.

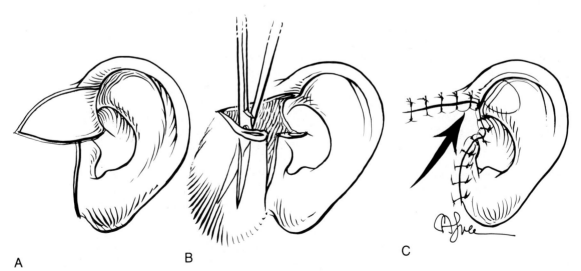

A   B   C

Figure 37–9. *A* to *C*, Composite graft of the root of the helix and cheek skin with closure of the defect by a cheek advancement flap.

Studies have shown that the revascularization process of skin grafts is particularly active at the junction of the graft with the edge of the skin of the recipient site (Ballantyne, Uhlschmid, and Converse, 1969). Revascularization appeared to be more active in this area than in the bed of the graft, at least in the rodent model.

Present concepts to explain the surprising success of composite grafts can be summarized as follows. Highly vascularized tissues, such as the nose and the auricle, contain a proportionally denser network of endothelial channels than other tissues. This characteristic facilitates the imbibition of fluids from the recipient tissues, a phenomenon that maintains the moisture of the graft until vascular connections and ingrowth from the host establish the final revascularization of the graft.

Stereomicroscopic observations in man detected vascular flow in composite grafts after 48 hours (Rees and associates, 1963). Blood flow is established initially in the area adjacent to the site of junction with the host bed; active flow is gradually propagated toward the center of the graft during subsequent days.

McLaughlin (1954) described the clinical appearance of a composite graft during its first days of revascularization. The initial dead white color is replaced some six to 24 hours later by the pale pink tinge representing erythrocyte invasion. At approximately 24 hours the graft becomes cyanotic from venous congestion, but if the graft is destined to survive the cyanosis gradually turns into a healthy pink color in three to seven days.

Medawar (1942) hypothesized that reducing the temperature of a graft would lower its metabolic activity and catabolism during the period of revascularization. Conley and von Fraenkel (1956) followed with a recommendation to cool grafts in the clinical setting to enhance "take" (the scientific validity of this premise has not been established, and to date cooling of grafts is routinely performed on an empiric basis). Rees and associates (1963) noted 94 per cent survival of composite grafts that had been cooled to 5° to 10°C for 72 hours.

The maximal size of a composite graft is still a matter of conjecture. As a rule of thumb for all soft tissue transplants, tissues that are to survive must be no farther than 5 mm distant from the point of vascular contact; thus, the upper limit of a composite graft, which will predictably survive only by perfusion from its peripheral edge, is 1 cm. Although Rees and associates (1963) and others successfully transferred composite grafts up to 3 cm in diameter, the practical diameter maximum for revascularization is probably no greater than 1.5 cm, and the graft shrinkage commonly seen undoubtedly represents central necrosis.

Survival of large composite grafts can be enhanced by increasing the available raw surface in the recipient bed to promote neovascularization. "Hinge" flaps of normal skin turned down from the edge of a healed wound effectively enlarge the contact area between graft and host, instead of depending merely on edge to edge contact.

Larger grafts are made possible by manipulating the relative proportions of the various layers of the graft, i.e., transferring more skin than cartilage. For instance, a small defect of the alar rim associated with a larger deficit of dorsal skin can be managed with a large full-thickness skin graft *and* a smaller multilayer composite graft attached at one edge (Fig. 37–10).

Skin and Adipose Tissue

The postoperative shrinkage of skin-fat grafts must be considered when planning the reconstructive procedure. Grafts of skin and fat removed from the lobe of the ear (Dupertuis, 1946) are used to repair small defects of the nasal tip, the medial portion of the ala, and the columella. Grafts taken from the base of the ala may also be transplanted to repair defects on the contralateral side.

Observations made over a period of ten years showed that composite grafts in young children grow in proportion to the remainder of the nose, thus maintaining symmetry between the alae.

SKIN FLAPS

Nasal reconstruction was apparently born in India around 3000 B.C. In Indian culture the nose was considered to be the organ of respect and reputation, so nasal mutilation or amputation was often used to humiliate social offenders. The first description of the repair of an amputated nose is found in the Sushruta Samhida (circa 600 B.C.), one of the Brahmin holy books (Nichter, Morgan, and

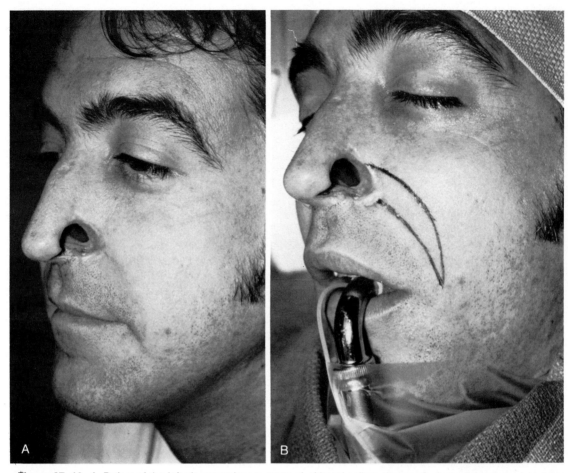

Figure 37–10. *A,* Defect of the left ala secondary to removal of basal cell carcinoma. *B,* An ipsilateral nasolabial flap has been marked for the reconstruction.

Illustration continued on the following page

Nichter, 1983). How knowledge of these Indian nasal reconstructive procedures spread to the European culture is unclear from recorded accounts. Apparently Buddhist missionaries carried the knowledge to Greece during the Golden Age, since by A.D. 25 Celsius, the celebrated Roman physician, was known to have tried portions of the Indian techniques.

After a long silent period in the history of recorded nasal reconstruction, reports began to surface in the mid-fifteenth century that the Brancas of Sicily had adopted the Indian method of reconstruction of the nose. The Brancas went on to use an arm flap in nasal surgery for the first time, although a written record apparently does not exist until 1597, when a report by Gaspare Tagliacozzi disclosed that he had adopted the method and popularized it.

In 1794 a letter appeared in the "Gentlemen's Magazine" of London describing the reconstruction of a mutilated nose with a flap from the central forehead. The author of the article was listed as B.L., who apparently was a Mr. Lucas, an English surgeon then residing in Madras, India. This now-famous story recounts the fate of Cowasjee (Fig. 37–11), a bullock driver with the English Army in India, who as a penalty of war had his nose and one of his hands amputated. The description of the reconstructive surgery of Cowasjee's deformity effectively introduced the Indian method to the English-speaking world.

Many eminent European surgeons then adopted the midline forehead flap method. Among them was Joseph Carpue, who in 1816 reported his experience with two successful procedures in the English literature.

Von Graefe in 1818 performed a nasal reconstruction in Berlin using the method of Tagliacozzi, and the next year he employed the Indian method. Reiner (1817), after a voyage to England where he had seen Carpue operate, also employed the Indian method in Munich. In France the Indian rhinoplastic

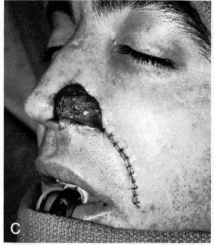

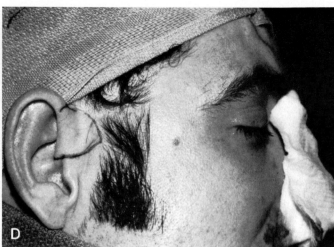

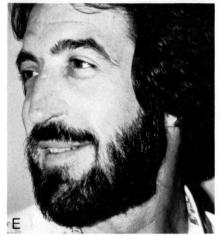

Figure 37–10 *Continued C*, The nasolabial flap has been transferred to the nose to restore lining and to provide a vascular bed to receive the chondrocutaneous auricular graft. *D*, Design of the helical root composite graft. This will be applied to the raw surface of the previously transferred nasolabial flap on the nose to give external cover and cartilginous support to the nostril wing. *E*, Postoperative result.

operation was practiced by Delpech and Montpelier in 1823 (Delpech, 1824), and within the next few years by Lisfranc (1827), Labat (1834), and Jobert (1849). Dieffenbach as early as 1829 began to classify procedures and improvements in the technique of forehead flap rhinoplasty, and described them in his 1845 book. The history of the evolution of nasal reconstruction techniques is also discussed in Chapter 1.

Thus, the evolution of nasal reconstructive procedures followed three basic lines: (1) the Indian method employing a midline forehead flap, (2) the French method using lateral cheek flaps, and (3) the Italian method involving the brachial or arm flap. The modern procedures currently used for nasal reconstruction are modifications and descendants of these three basic conceptual pathways.

Local Nasal Flaps

The most readily available tissue for the repair of nasal defects is that of the nose itself. Almost all procedures that use local nasal tissue are designed to take advantage of the skin laxity in the upper nose and lateral nasal walls. This loose skin can be advanced inferiorly to cover defects of the lobule or horizontally to close the donor sites of small flaps that are then rotated to cover adjacent defects. For practical purposes, defects up to 2 cm in diameter, except in the columella, may be repaired with flaps of nasal skin.

There are two categories of local nasal flaps: those designed to cover defects of the nasal dorsum and those designed to restore the alar rim.

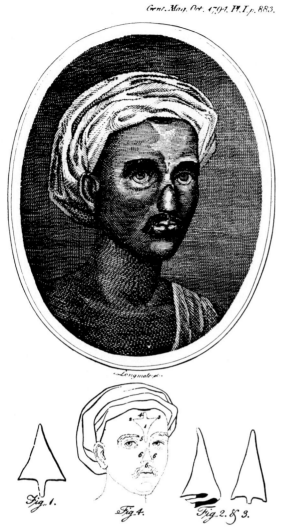

Gent.Mag. Oct. 1794. Pl.I.p. 883.

Figure 37–11. The Indian midline rhinoplasty (circa 600 B.C.).

NASAL DORSUM

A number of small flaps designed from areas adjacent to dorsal nasal defects have achieved popularity. Each takes advantage of the laxity in the dorsal nasal skin, mostly in a vertical direction, to provide small flaps that can be transposed downward while achieving primary closure of the donor site defect (Fig. 37–12).

Perhaps the simplest of these flaps is the "banner" flap (Fig. 37–12*A*), which is a narrow triangle designed along the tangent of the defect to be closed. Elliott (1969) suffered only one partial loss in 70 flaps transferred for reconstruction of nasal wounds measuring 0.7 to 1.2 cm in diameter. By extending the banner flap to cross over onto the opposite nasal dorsum, the size and reach can be

increased (Masson and Mendelson, 1977). The modification allows closure of defects up to 2 cm in diameter.

Similar transposition flaps can be achieved by the geometric patterns of Limberg (1963) (Fig. 37–12*B*) and Dufourmentel and Talaat (1971). The disadvantage of these flaps from the nasal dorsum is that closure of the donor site results in elevation and distortion of the nostril rim.

In an effort to rotate local tissues while avoiding distortion from closure of the donor site, Esser (1918) described the bilobed flap (Fig. 37–12*C*). The design of the bilobed flap was elucidated and popularized by Zimany (1953), who also modified it to make the second lobe narrower than the first. Theoret-

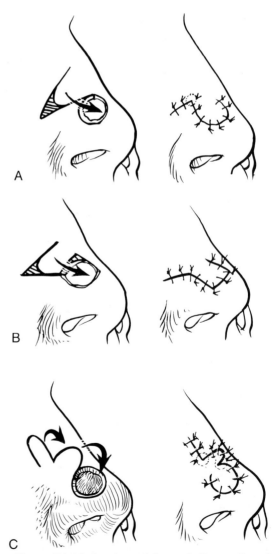

Figure 37–12. Local nasal flaps. *A*, Banner flap. *B*, Limberg flap. *C*, Bilobed flap.

ically, the bilobed flap spreads the tension resulting from donor site closure over a larger area, thus reducing the distortion in any one site. This advantage is counterbalanced by a significantly longer scar.

In larger defects of the dorsum of the nasal lobule, it is perhaps wiser to utilize a large rotation-advancement flap of the skin of the entire nasal dorsum. Stimulated by Mc-Gregor's (1960) description of the glabellar flap, which took advantage of the redundant skin of the glabella for closure of nasal defects, the dorsal nasal rotation-advancement flap was developed (Rieger, 1967; Rigg, 1973). The flap is based on branches of the angular artery as it descends along the base of the nasal wall to approach the medial canthal area (Fig. 37–13) (Hardin, 1980).

Whereas the skin of the entire nasal dorsum can be undermined to allow freedom of downward movement, care must be taken not to sever the attachments of the cutaneous branches of the angular artery, for the distal portion of the flap is unreliable on the basis of dermal circulation alone. The flap can be back-cut, however, to be supplied only by the cutaneous arterial branch that exits from the angular artery near the medial canthus (Marchac and Toth, 1985).

The circumference of the flap is outlined so as to fall within the appropriate esthetic units. It is often helpful to base the flap contralateral to the defect in order to achieve more downward mobility. Defects of up to 2 cm on the nasal dorsum and lobule may be successfully managed by this procedure (Fig. 37–14).

The disadvantage of the dorsal nasal flap is that it does not seem to achieve as much downward migration of tissue as one would initially anticipate on the basis of the laxity of the dorsal nasal skin. One must also be careful not to create torsion and secondary asymmetry of the alar rims by uneven distribution of the tension at closure. The flap's primary use is in defects in the plane of the dorsum of the nose. It will not comfortably reach around the nasal tip into the columella.

ALAR RIM

From a planning standpoint, defects of the lobule are most critical when they also involve loss or irregularity of the alar rim. A variety of procedures have been designed that use the skin of the nasal dorsum and lateral nasal wall to reconstitute the alar rim.

For the slightly retracted ala, Kazanjian (1948) used a bipedicle flap procedure that lowered the skin of the caudal border of the defect (Fig. 37–15A). The lining was advanced by undermining inside the lateral nasal wall, and the external defect was closed with a full-thickness skin graft.

A Z-plasty type of closure was originated by Denonvilliers (1854). The caudal border of the nasal defect was transposed downward to its appropriate position, and the superior defect was filled by a dorsal nasal skin flap transposed as a Z-plasty (Fig. 37–15B). Re-

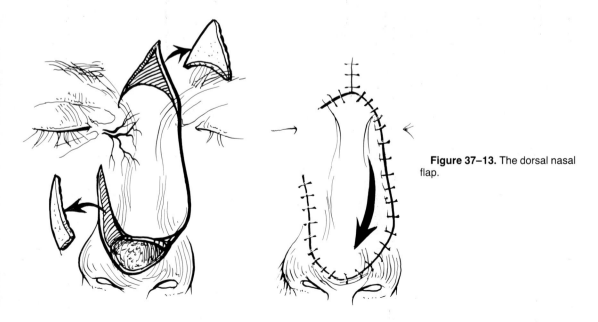

Figure 37–13. The dorsal nasal flap.

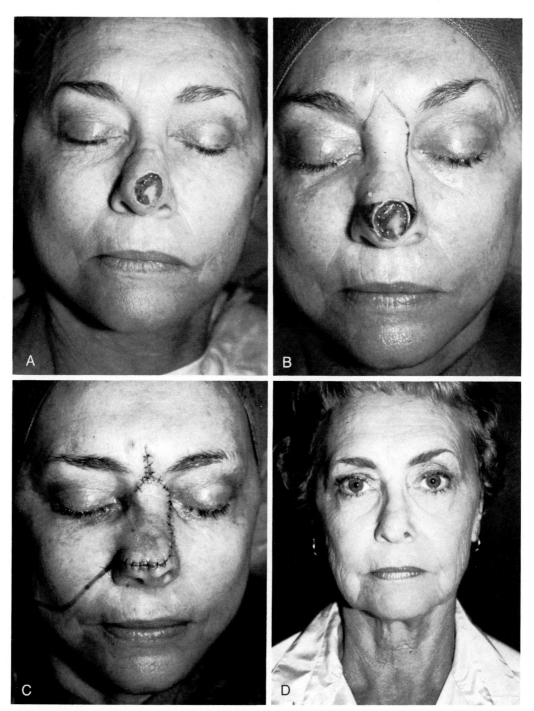

Figure 37–14. *A*, Patient with a 2 cm skin defect of the midline of the nasal lobule. The alar cartilages are intact. *B*, Outline of the dorsal nasal flap. The skin to be excised is outlined in ink. *C*, Flap sutured in place. Note the "butterfly" drain. *D*, Final result.

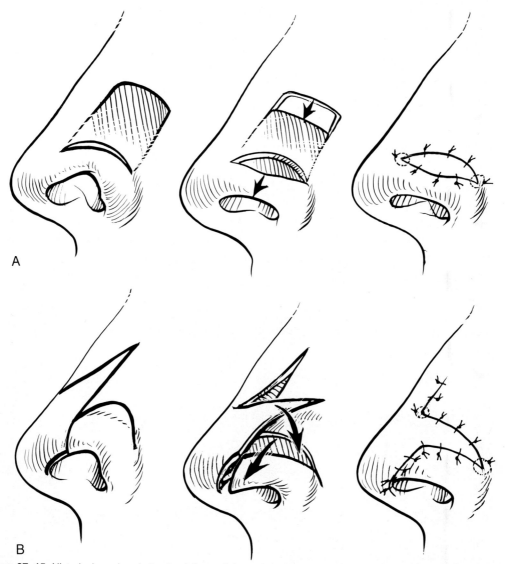

Figure 37–15. Historical repairs of alar rim defects. *A,* Lowering of the rim with advancement of the undermined nasal lining *(upper arrow)* and application of a full-thickness skin graft to the external skin defect. *B,* Z-plasty of the nasal rim.

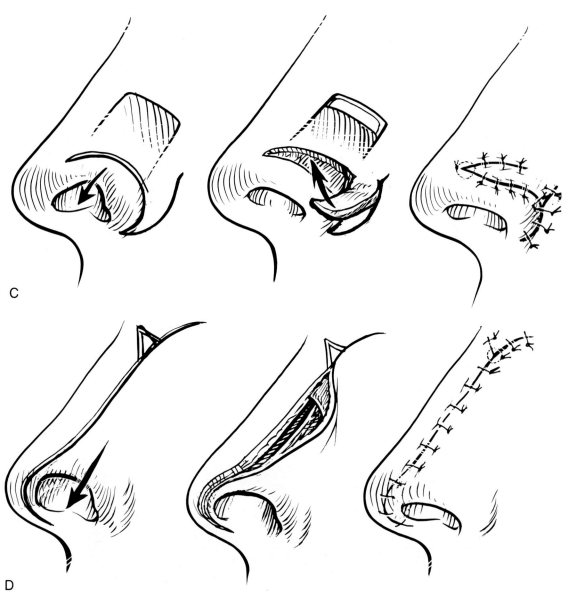

Figure 37–15 *Continued C*, Perialar transposition flap with advancement of the nasal lining. *D*, Laterally based dorsal nasal advancement.

placement of the lining required either advancement of the remaining intranasal lining or grafting inside the nasal cavity.

In defects with lateral alar base retraction, Joseph's (1931) modification of Denonvilliers' alar rim Z-plasty advancement can be carried out to lower the lateral portion, in a manner similar to that described for lowering the medial nostril rim. The secondary defect of the lateral nasal skin is filled by a transposition flap from the nasolabial crease. Lining is supplied by undermining and advancement (Fig. 37–15*C*).

Denecke and Meyer (1967) described using the lateral nasal skin as a dorsal nasal advancement, carrying the caudal border of the alar rim down to its appropriate level (Fig. 37–15*D*). Lining is achieved by advancement of the nasal mucosa.

Most of these nasal rim advancements were designed for problems in which retraction of the alar rim originated from loss of external nasal skin (Fig. 37–16). The design presupposed that adequate lining remained to be readvanced to normal length.

Nasolabial Cheek Flaps

Nineteenth century European surgeons, primarily from France and Germany, pioneered a variety of techniques in which tissues from the paranasal cheek area were transferred to repair nasal deformities.

By undermining the cheek in the subcutaneous plane, approximately 2 to 3 cm of skin can be mobilized for use in nasal repair; 3 cm is usually the practical upper margin of donor skin that can be taken while achieving primary closure of the nasofacial donor site without noticeable facial distortion. The nasolabial cheek tissue can be delivered to the nose by a variety of methods.

SUBCUTANEOUS PEDICLE FLAPS

The vascular anatomy of the paranasal cheek area has been studied by Hagerty and Smith (1958), McLaren (1963), and Herbert and Harrison (1975). The area is supplied medially by the angular artery and its perforating branches. The central cheek is supplied by perforating branches from the internal maxillary artery as well as by the extensions of the transverse facial branch from the superficial temporal artery. This relatively rich vascular supply to the subcutaneous tissue of the cheek makes it quite amenable to subcutaneously based flaps.

These flaps are especially useful in reconstruction of the lateral nasal wall or alar wing, and may be mobilized either by direct advancement in a V-Y manner (Fig. 37–17*A*) or by constructing a subcutaneous pedicle based laterally, which allows superior mobilization of the overlying skin (Figs. 37–17*B*, 37–18). In addition, the nasolabial skin can be turned upon itself at the edge of the piriform aperture to provide internal nasal lining, and then folded back externally to supply external nasal coverage (Fig. 37–19).

The subcutaneous pedicle flap method was popularized by Bouisson (1864), Hacker (1897), Preindelberger (1898), Barron and Emmett (1965), Pers (1967), Dufourmentel

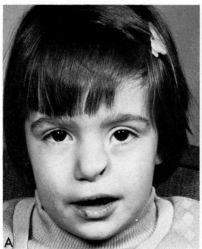
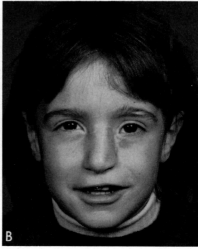

Figure 37–16. Retracted ala due to a facial cleft. *A,* The patient at 5 years of age. *B,* Three years later, after correction by advancing the upper lateral nasal wall downward and skin grafting the donor defect at the radix.

Figure 37–17. Subcutaneous pedicle cheek flaps. *A*, V-Y advancement for external coverage. *B*, Lateral subcutaneous pedicle for external coverage.

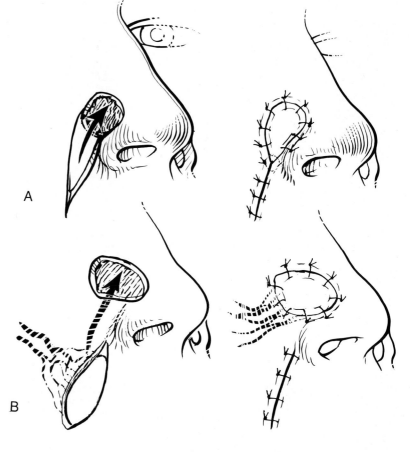

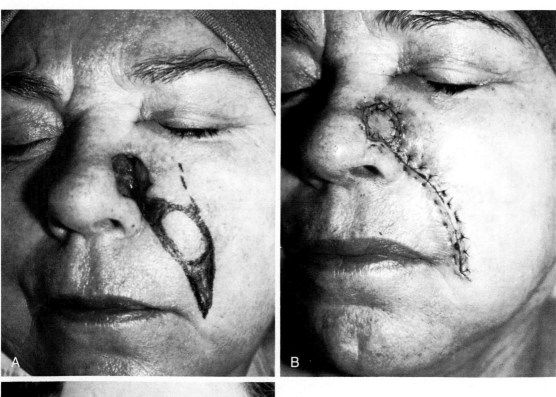

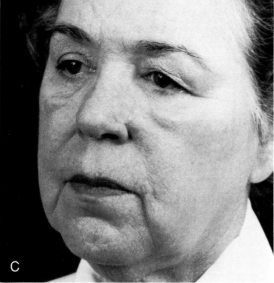

Figure 37–18. *A,* Patient with a lateral nasal defect to be repaired by a superiorly based nasolabial island flap raised on a subcutaneous pedicle. *B,* Flap transposed and the donor site closed. *C,* Final result.

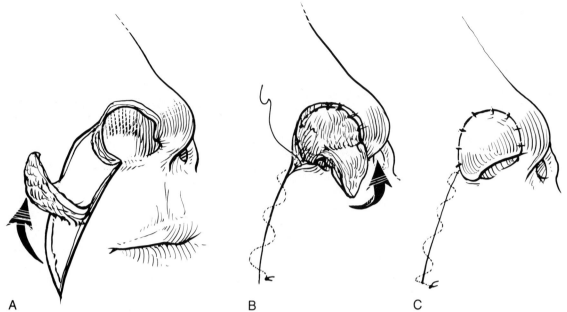

Figure 37–19. A 78 year old male with a full-thickness alar defect. *A* to *C*, Design of turned back nasolabial flap.
Illustration continued on following page

and Talaat (1971), Herbert and Harrison (1975), and Spear, Kroll, and Romm (1987).

NASOLABIAL TRANSPOSITION FLAPS

The use of nasolabial tissue as a transposition flap was popularized by Dieffenbach (1845). The pedicle can be based inferiorly or superiorly; the superior pedicle technique allows the use of the cheek tissue adjacent to the upper lip from which a larger flap can be harvested (Figs. 37–20, 37–21).

When the defect to be reconstructed is on the lateral lobule and does not cross the midline, the flap may be raised and transferred at a single stage based only on dermal blood supply. The medial border of the flap should be drawn from the tangent at the edge of the defect so as to leave the lateral alar crease intact. The flap is then back-cut to approximately the same level and a Burow's triangle is removed from the upper lateral nasal skin.

The cheek skin over the malar and buccal areas is then elevated in a subcutaneous plane, so that the transposition flap becomes a secondary extension from the edge of the cheek advancement flap. The nasolabial transposition flap can be defatted to the appropriate thickness at the time of transfer; secondary revision should be unnecessary. Cartilage strips may be placed underneath the flap to support the alar rim at the time

of transfer (Ohtsuka, Shioya, and Asano, 1981).

If the flap is to be folded upon itself for nasal lining, or if it is to be extended past the midline, consideration may be given either to delay of the flap or to maintaining a direct communication with the subcutaneous portion of the pedicle and its branches from the angular artery.

CHEEK ADVANCEMENT FLAPS

In 1940 Twyman rekindled interest in the sliding flap method for partial nasal reconstruction, which had originally been utilized by French surgeons in the nineteenth century. The operation consists of elevating the dorsal nasal skin and advancing the paranasal cheek tissue onto the nose (Figs. 37–22, 37–23).

For defects of the nasal domes, the incision may be carried along the alar rim so as to elevate the external alar skin for transfer onto the nose. The skin of the ala, however, is fibrofatty and seems to have poor dermal circulation; often the transferred skin does not provide healthy primary healing. It is thus preferable to design the flap with its inferior border falling in the alar crease, and to transfer the paranasal skin above the alar wing inferiorly and medially. A Burow's triangle can be excised along the nasolabial fold to complete the closure.

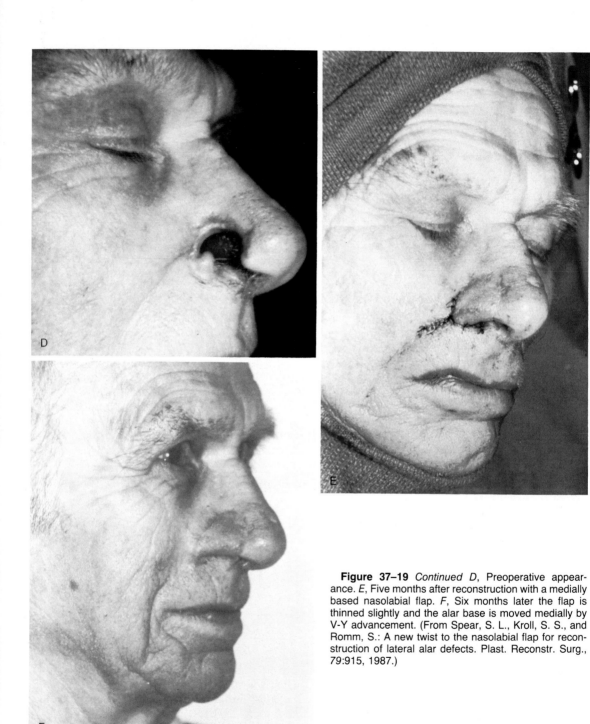

Figure 37–19 *Continued D*, Preoperative appearance. *E*, Five months after reconstruction with a medially based nasolabial flap. *F*, Six months later the flap is thinned slightly and the alar base is moved medially by V-Y advancement. (From Spear, S. L., Kroll, S. S., and Romm, S.: A new twist to the nasolabial flap for reconstruction of lateral alar defects. Plast. Reconstr. Surg., 79:915, 1987.)

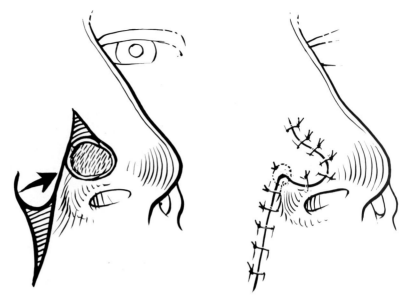

Figure 37–20. A superiorly based nasolabial transposition flap.

Forehead Flaps

The nineteenth century literature was compiled and classified by Nélaton and Ombrédanne in 1904, in a treatise that remains one of the most reliable sources of reference material for the nasal reconstructive surgeon. Joseph's 1931 book includes his modifications of the known procedures of the time. Historical reviews by Davis (1919, 1941), Fomon (1939), Mazzola and Marcus (1983), and Nichter, Morgan, and Nichter (1983) are well-researched discussions of the various therapeutic approaches through the ages to the problem of acquired nasal defects.

It is important to realize that all flaps used in nasal reconstruction were designed to provide external nasal coverage. There was a delay in recognizing the need to replace intranasal lining, and these early attempts at reconstituting nasal form frequently resulted in constricted, distorted nostrils. Ivy (1925) credits Labat (1834) with the first attempt to improve the shape of the reconstructed nostril by supplying lining. Subsequently, lining was provided by a turn-down flap from the edge of the nasal defect (Volkmann, 1874), flaps from the adjacent facial area (Thiersch, 1879), or split-thickness skin grafts (Lössen, 1898).

Blair in 1925 reviewed the various techniques available for restoration of the nose and concluded that the midline forehead flap method was the most effective in major nasal defects. He is credited with establishing the dominance of the midline forehead flap method for nasal reconstruction in America.

MIDLINE FOREHEAD FLAPS

The classic Indian design of the midline forehead flap was along a straight vertical axis extending from the glabella to the hairline. In patients with high hairlines, adequate length can be achieved to reach the tip of the nose; however, in patients with low hairlines additional length must be obtained, preferably without including hair-bearing skin. Additional length on the midline forehead flap is achieved by one of two variations: (1) tilting the axis of the flap to a more oblique position or (2) lowering the point of rotation by back-cutting the pedicle in the glabella.

The concept of reorienting the midline forehead flap to an oblique position (Fig. 37–24) can be traced to Auvert (1856), a French surgeon of the 1800's. Since that time Millard (1967), Dhawan, Aggarwal, and Hariharan (1974), Sawhney (1976), and Barton (1981) have amplified their experiences in variations of the technique.

The second means of increasing the effective length of the midline forehead flap is to back-cut the pedicle in the area of the glabella. The blood supply to the midline forehead flap is from the supratrochlear extension of the angular artery, which collateralizes with the ophthalmic artery in the medial portion of the orbit near the medial canthal

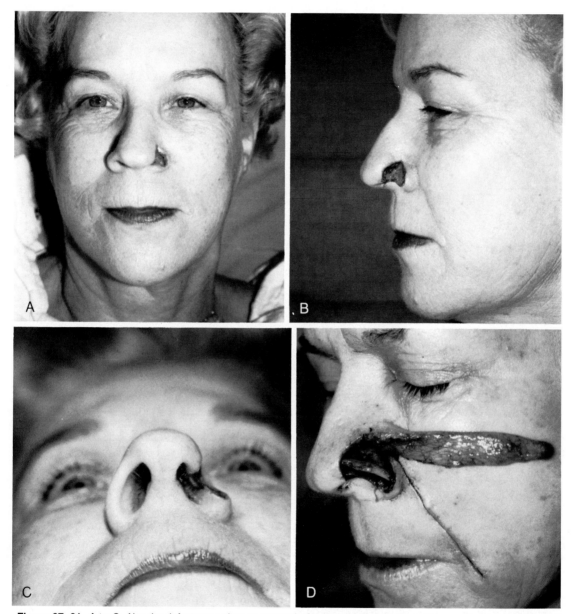

Figure 37–21. *A* to *C*, Alar rim defect secondary to removal of a basal cell carcinoma. The vestibular lining is intact. *D*, A superiorly based nasolabial transposition flap has been elevated and the donor site has been closed primarily. Note the auricular cartilage graft, which has been placed nonanatomically to splint the alar rim.

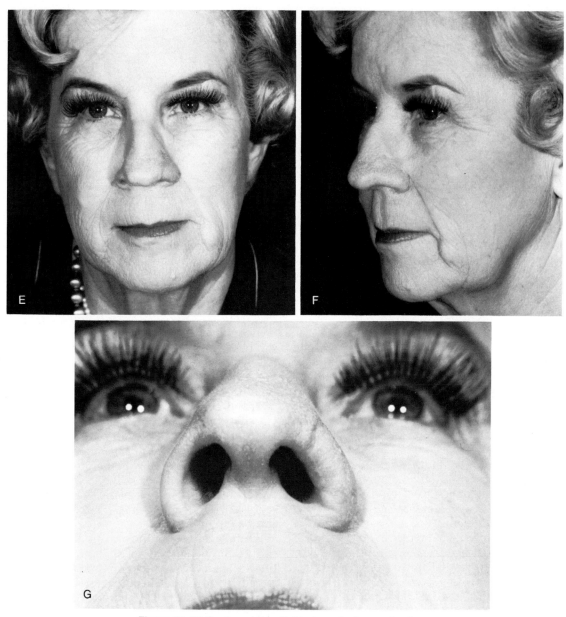

Figure 37–21 *Continued E* to *G*, Final result of reconstruction.

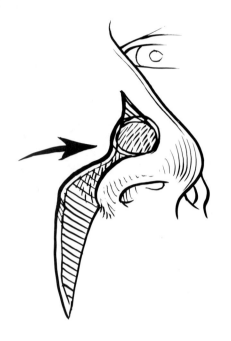
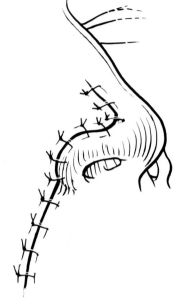

Figure 37–22. The cheek advancement flap.

tendon. Only one supratrochlear vessel is required to carry the entire flap, and if the angular artery is intact, the pedicle can be back-cut inferiorly into the medial canthus to achieve additional flap length (McCarthy and associates, 1985).

The effective length of the flap can also be increased by modifying the pattern of the pedicular base. Since the dermis and galea in this area are quite thick, folding the pedicle upon itself to rotate the flap 180 degrees uses up much of its length. A variety of geometric incisions have been designed to minimize the loss of length when folding the pedicle (Fig. 37–25).

The width of the midline forehead flap that can be taken while still achieving primary closure of the donor site is approximately 2.5 to 3 cm (Peet and Patterson, 1964). This width is usually sufficient to reconstruct half of the surface of the nasal lobule. Wider flaps capable of providing essentially total nasal coverage can be carried on a single supratrochlear vessel.

The design of the paddle when the flap is to be used for alar reconstruction has evolved from a blunt trapezoidal shape into a "gull-wing" shape that provides a more graceful alar contour. The gull-wing modification was described by Gillies in 1920 and refined by Millard in 1974. The pedicle can be kept relatively narrow while the wings are extended to provide nasal coverage. The donor defect is closed primarily (Fig. 37–26).

Closure of the donor defect usually requires extensive mobilization of the forehead and scalp. Approximately 2 cm of additional scalp laxity can be achieved by scoring the undersurface of the forehead to release the galea and frontalis (Fig. 37–27A). If additional mobilization to close a larger defect is needed, bilateral forehead advancement flaps (Fig. 37–27B) or temporal rotation-advancement flaps (Fig. 37–27C) as described by Schimmelbusch (1895) can be used.

The greater part of a donor defect can be closed primarily while the remainder is allowed to heal by secondary intention. This avoids extensive secondary procedures (Millard, 1967). It may also be helpful to place a counterincision in the scalp to allow immediate closure of the exposed forehead. The scalp portion can then be left to heal by secondary intention.

When adequate lining and skeletal support can be provided from local tissues, the midline forehead flap can be immediately transferred for external nasal cover (Fig. 37–28). For practical purposes, the entire nasal contour can be carried on a midline forehead flap without the need for delay; this is true even with the oblique orientation. Although early venous congestion will be present, the flap is durable and sturdy, and complete healing is the rule (Fig. 37–29).

In a full-thickness defect of the nasal lobule, if adequate lining cannot be mobilized from local tissues, preparatory lining of the

Text continued on page 1957

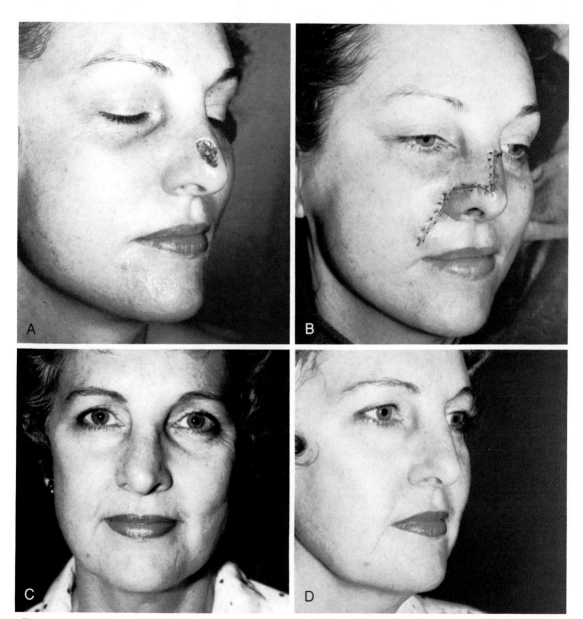

Figure 37–23. *A*, Paramidline defect of the nasal dorsum secondary to removal of a basal cell carcinoma. *B*, Closure with a cheek advancement flap. *C, D*, Postoperative result.

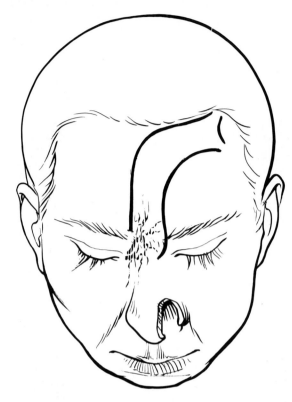

Figure 37–24. A midline forehead flap oriented obliquely to provide greater length.

Figure 37–25. Modifications of the base of the midline forehead flap for greater flap mobility. *A,* Indian rhinoplasty. *B,* Lisfranc's modification. *C, D,* Labat's modifications. *E,* Dieffenbach's modification.

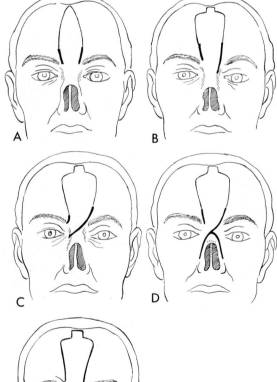

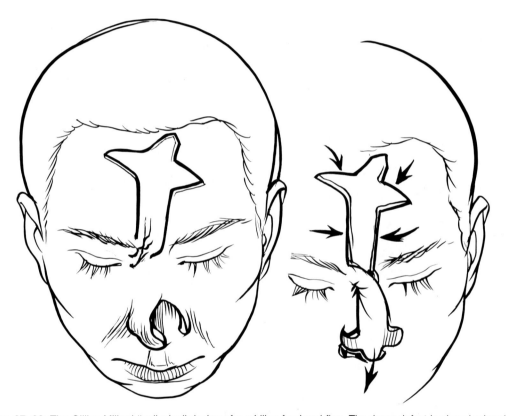

Figure 37–26. The Gillies-Millard "gull-wing" design of a midline forehead flap. The donor defect is closed primarily.

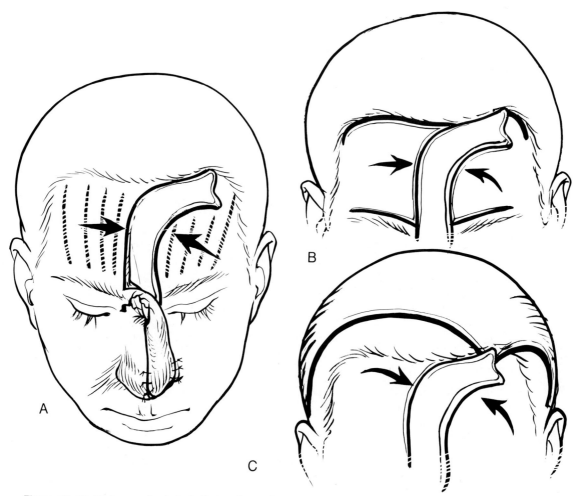

Figure 37–27. Various methods to facilitate primary closure of the midline forehead flap defect. *A,* Scoring the galea. *B,* Bilateral forehead advancement flaps. *C,* Bilateral temporal rotation-advancement flaps.

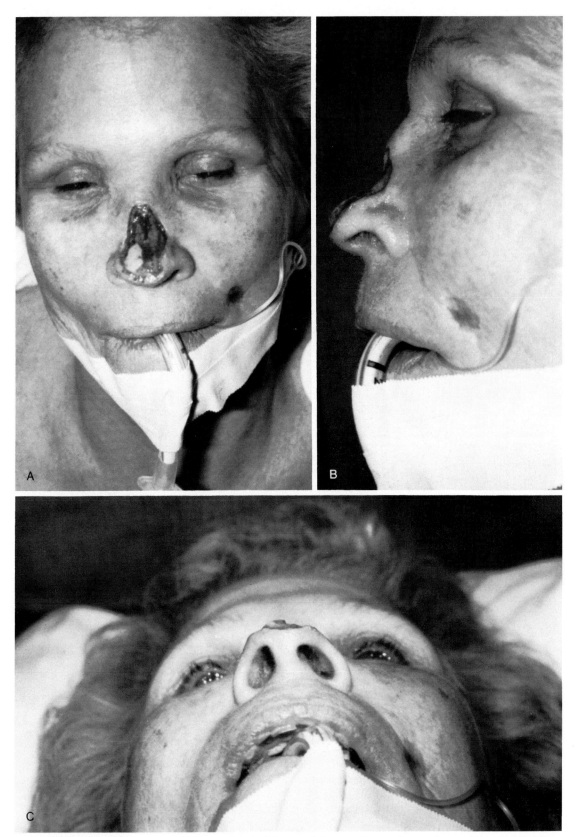

Figure 37–28. *A* to *C*, Large full-thickness defect of the nasal dorsum. The septum and upper lateral cartilages are exposed but mostly intact.

Illustration continued on following page

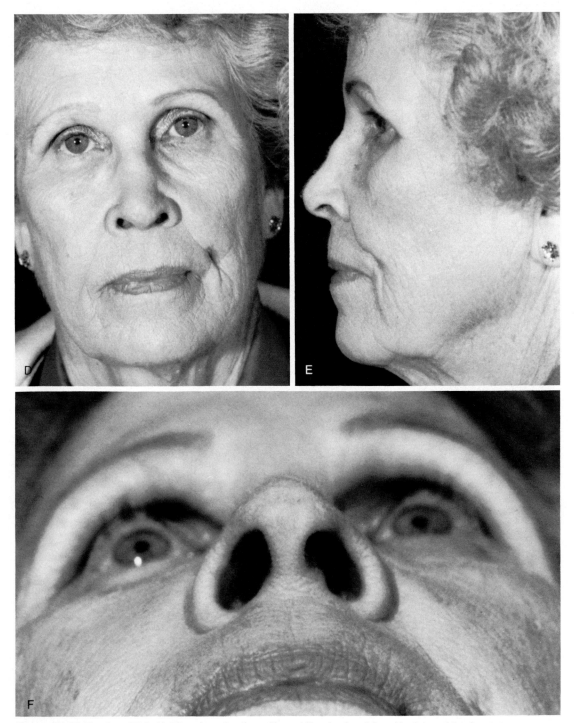

Figure 37–28 *Continued D to F,* After reconstruction with a midline forehead flap. No delay of the flap was necessary.

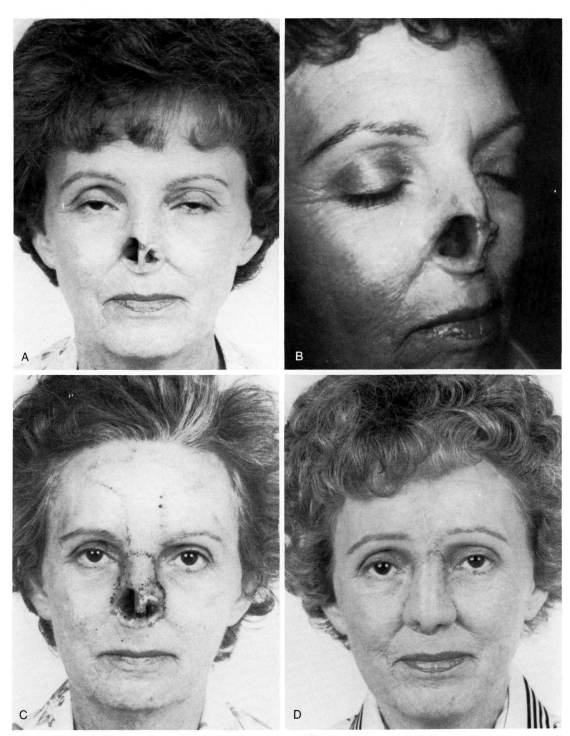

Figure 37–29. A 47 year old woman with a defect of the distal half of the nose. *A, B,* Preoperative appearance. *C,* After delay of the "gull-wing" forehead flap and the skin of the dorsal nose to be used in lining. An L-shaped flap of septum hinged on the nasal bones has been rotated outward for tip support. *D,* The flap has been transferred to the nose and the pedicle has been divided.

Illustration continued on following page

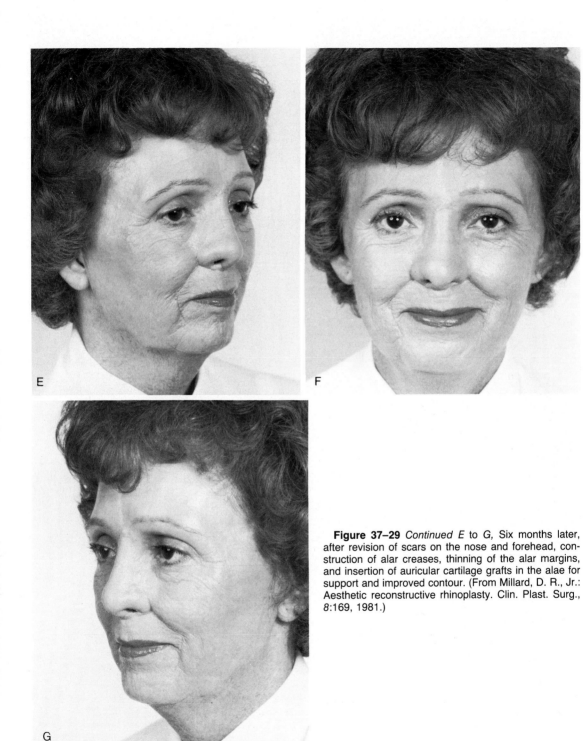

Figure 37–29 *Continued E* to *G,* Six months later, after revision of scars on the nose and forehead, construction of alar creases, thinning of the alar margins, and insertion of auricular cartilage grafts in the alae for support and improved contour. (From Millard, D. R., Jr.: Aesthetic reconstructive rhinoplasty. Clin. Plast. Surg., 8:169, 1981.)

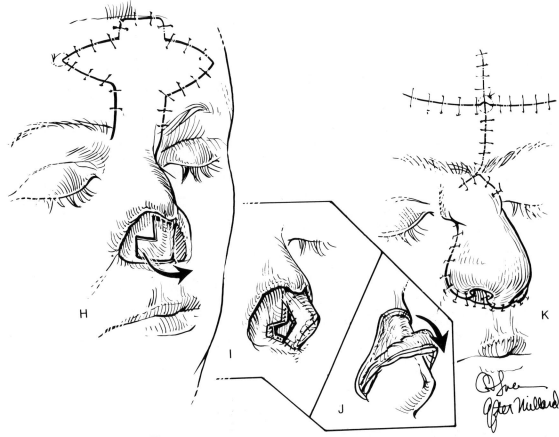

Figure 37–29 *Continued H* to *K*, The operative sequence.

undersurface of the midline forehead flap with a chondrocutaneous composite graft may be helpful. Thin auricular skin and auricular cartilage may be harvested in a variety of ways. The skin and cartilage need not be attached to each other. It is usually convenient to harvest a full-thickness postauricular skin graft from the auriculocephalic sulcus and take a strip of vertical conchal wall cartilage through the same wound (Fig. 37–30A). The cartilage strip should be approximately 3 to 4 mm in width and 3.5 cm in length.

When lining the undersurface of a midline forehead flap with a chondrocutaneous composite graft, it is usually safer to allow the composite graft to heal to the undersurface of the forehead flap while still on the forehead. The appropriate thickness of the tip of the forehead flap can be achieved by removing the undersurface frontalis muscle and subcutaneous tissue and laminating an ala of appropriate dimension in the forehead (Fig. 37–30B). If the "take" of the composite graft is inadequate, it may be repeated until a satisfactory healed unit is ready for transfer.

If one attempted to place the composite graft on the undersurface of the midline forehead flap at the time of transfer, and if partial loss of the composite graft occurred, the resultant cicatricial distortion would be difficult to correct secondarily.

An interval of approximately four weeks is usually necessary to allow complete healing of the chondrocutaneous graft to the underside of the midline forehead flap. Most of the edema in the flap should resolve by this time.

Every attempt should be made at the time of flap transfer to sculpt the alar rim in its final form so as to avoid secondary defatting and shaping procedures. It is important to step the closure of the layers of the flap to avoid grooving (Fig. 37–31). The conchal cartilage should span the arch of the ala, resting on the residual portion of the medial crus or dome remnant medially and the soft tissue at the piriform aperture laterally (Figs. 37–32, 37–33).

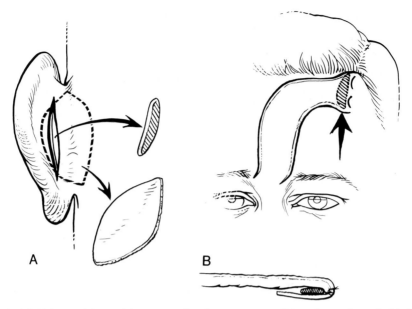

Figure 37–30. In full-thickness defects of the nose, a chondrocutaneous graft from the ear is applied to the undersurface of the main reconstructive flap and laminated on the forehead before transfer. *A,* A vertical strip of cartilage from the conchal wall is obtained through a postauricular incision as outlined. The cartilage should be approximately 3 to 4 mm wide and 3.5 cm long. The postauricular skin is harvested full thickness and the resultant defect is closed primarily. *B,* The chondrocutaneous graft is sutured to the reconstructive flap while still on the forehead. The skin will serve as lining for the nose and the cartilage will provide lateral alar support.

The management of the pedicle of the midline forehead flap is somewhat controversial. Millard (1974) recalled Gillies' admonition that the "forehead flap noses never look quite as fine after the pedicle has been divided," and suggested that the neurovascular pedicle be permanently inset in the nasal radix to avoid secondary lymphedema. However, if adequate resolution of the edema is allowed to occur after transfer and attachment of the flap to the nose—approximately four weeks, division of the pedicle can be carried out without concern for lymphedema. If the lam-

ination of the alar rim has been accurate at the time of construction, secondary defatting and shaping procedures should be unnecessary.

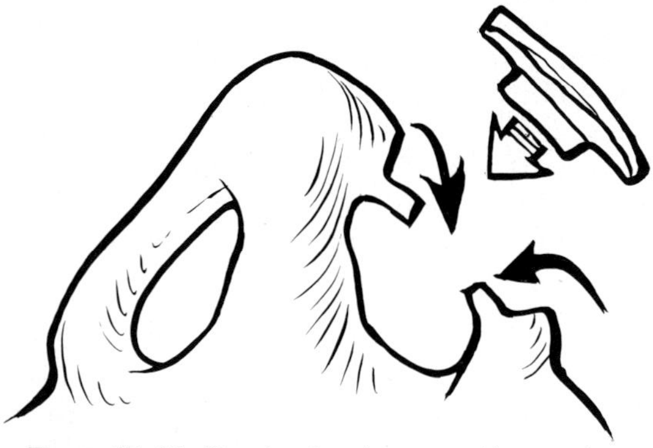

It is frequently helpful to reinset a small triangular portion of the pedicle of the midline forehead flap into the glabella in order to restore the medial portions of the brows to their normal positions.

The *island midline forehead flap*, based on a subcutaneous neurovascular pedicle, was described by Converse and Wood-Smith in 1963. This modification was developed in an attempt to avoid the need for secondary division and inset of the cutaneous pedicle. The design of the flap is essentially the same as for a standard midline forehead flap, except that the glabellar portion is dissected beneath an intact skin, leaving the frontalis and the neurovascular pedicle in a subcutaneous base. It is rotated 180 degrees into the nose for final inset.

The procedure, however, has not achieved significant popularity owing to its tendency to cause venous congestion. If the pedicle is left bulky enough to provide adequate venous outflow, secondary defatting of the radix is necessary, thus precluding its advantage as a one-stage procedure.

Figure 37–31. Stepping the closure avoids grooving at the junctions.

Text continued on page 1965

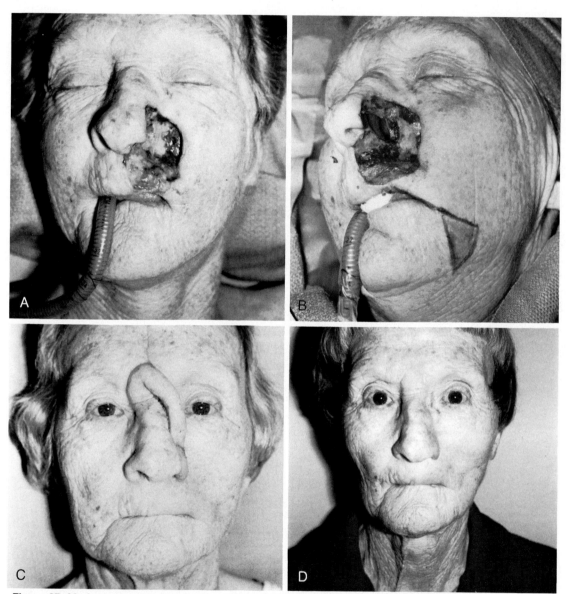

Figure 37–32. A 69 year old woman with a defect of the left ala, cheek, and lip. *A, B,* Cheek advancement flap to resurface the upper lip and provide a platform on which to erect the ala. *C,* An extended midline forehead flap to resurface the ala. Full-thickness skin and cartilage were harvested from the concha and placed under the distal aspect of the forehead flap. Four weeks later, the forehead flap pedicle was divided and inset in the glabella. *D to G,* One year after the reconstruction was completed.

Illustration continued on following page

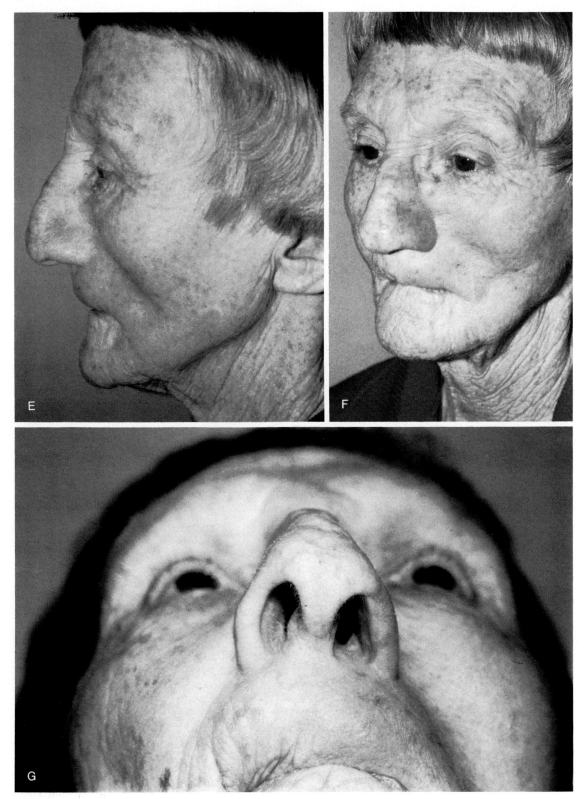

Figure 37–32 *Continued*

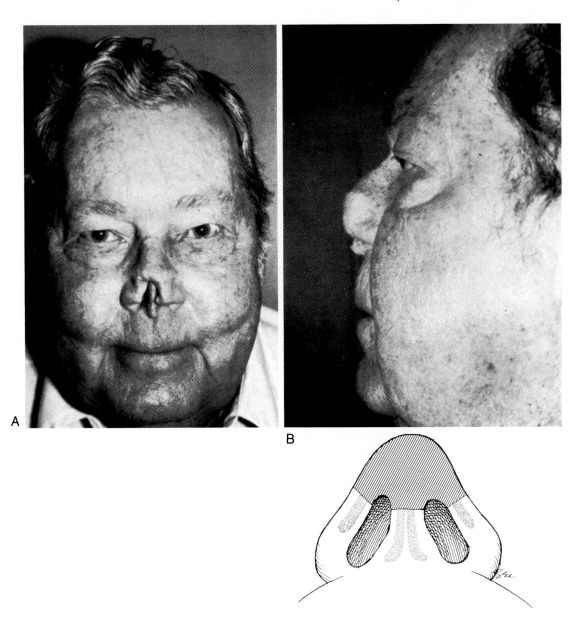

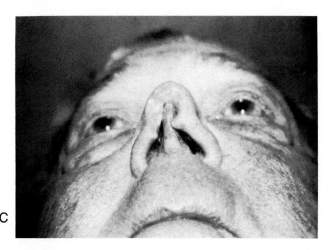

Figure 37–33. *A* to *C,* A 77 year old man with a healed defect of the nasal tip.
Illustration continued on following page

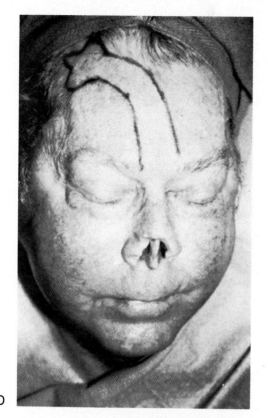

D

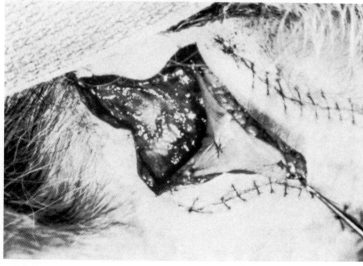

E

Figure 37–33 *Continued D,* Design of the extended midline forehead flap. *E,* A split-thickness skin graft applied to the tip of the delayed flap for nasal lining.

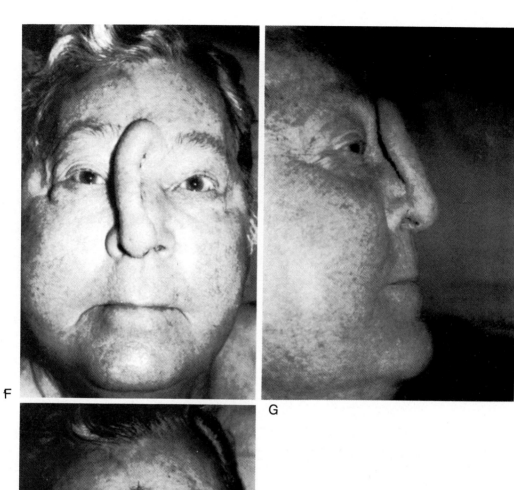

F

G

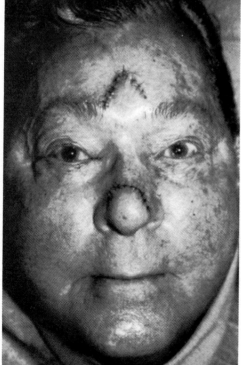

H

Figure 37–33 *Continued F, G,* The forehead flap transferred to the nose. *H,* After division of the pedicle, insert of the base between the brows, and defatting of the tip.

Illustration continued on following page

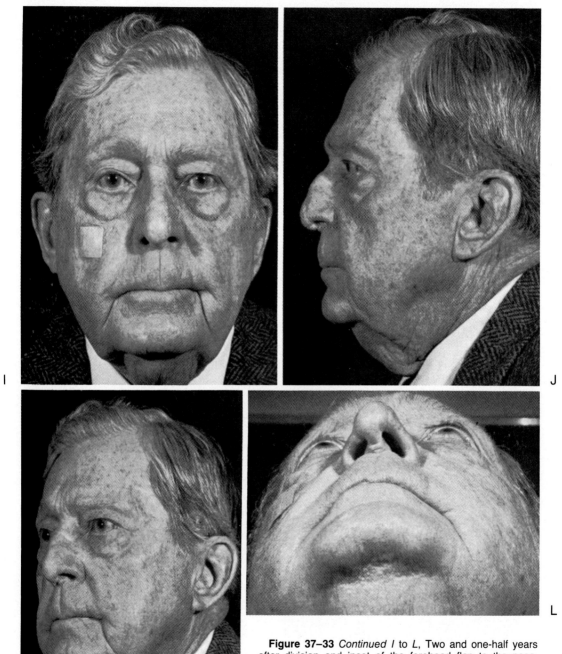

Figure 37–33 *Continued* I to L, Two and one-half years after division and inset of the forehead flap to the nose. (From Barton, F. E., Jr.: Aesthetic aspects of partial nasal reconstruction. Clin. Plast. Surg., *8*:177, 1981.)

FRONTOTEMPORAL FLAPS

In 1952 Schmid described the frontotemporal flap. Also based on the supratrochlear vessels, the pedicle is oriented horizontally across the lower forehead just above the brow. This pedicle thus carries temporal skin that can be transferred to the nose.

The disadvantage of the procedure is the need for delay, since there is not a true axial vessel pattern in the flap. In addition, it creates noticeable scarring and potential elevation of the brow. It may be a procedure to bear in mind, however, for patients with forehead scarring or exceedingly low hairlines.

UP-AND-DOWN FLAPS

Because the midline forehead flap was limited by its central scar, size, and maximum length, alternative means of bringing forehead skin to the nasal area evolved. Gillies (1935a) described the up-and-down flap, which increased the length of the flap and allowed for a wider skin paddle. While a total lobule could be reconstructed with reliable blood supply based on the supratrochlear and supraorbital vessels, the donor defect could not be closed primarily, and significant central forehead scarring resulted.

SCALPING FLAPS

In response to the apparent scar deformities in the central forehead, procedures shifted toward carrying high lateral temporal skin with the pedicle concealed in the hair-bearing scalp and based on the superficial temporal vessels. The two most recognized variations of these methods were the scalping flap described and popularized by Converse (1942, 1959, 1969) and the sickle flap described by New in 1945. Owing to its better vascular reliability, the scalping flap technique gained dominance.

The scalping flap has several potential advantages in large nasal reconstructions. First, the area of skin to be transferred to the nose, i.e., the high temporal portion of the forehead, is in fact the same skin carried on an oblique forehead flap. When the amount of skin to be carried is small, as in a heminasal reconstruction, primary closure is simple and the midline forehead pedicle is more convenient. One should note, however, that the scarring from the pedicle remains in the central forehead when the midline forehead flap method is used. In contrast, the scalping flap technique leaves only the scar resulting from the skin paddle that has been transferred to the nose. The vascular pedicle incisions are well concealed within the scalp.

Second, in patients with low hairlines the scalping flap technique provides more mobility to achieve adequate flap length to reach the nasal tip. Finally, when large areas of tissue are to be covered, such as in a subtotal nasal reconstruction, the vascular supply and especially the venous drainage from the scalping flap are superior to that of the midline forehead flap. Thus, there is more predictable healing.

In conclusion, when a large skin paddle from the forehead is needed so that primary closure of the donor defect cannot be achieved, it is both safer and less disfiguring to use the scalping flap pedicle as the method of delivery of the frontotemporal skin.

The planning of a scalping flap is similar to that for other flap coverage methods. Lining as well as skeletal support must be included in the plan. The same methods of achieving lining already described apply to the scalping flap. Chondrocutaneous composites may be initially implanted beneath its surface while the flap is still on the forehead, turn-in flaps from the nasal area may serve as lining when available, and the flap may be turned upon itself to provide a columella and alar rims when necessary. The latter method, although the traditional way of providing lining of the vestibules, produces a thick ala with constricted airway.

The pattern required for nasal reconstruction is applied to the frontotemporal skin on the side opposite the superficial temporal artery that serves as the vascular base. If no preparatory lining grafts are necessary, the flap may be raised undelayed. The portion of skin to serve as nasal cover is raised superficial to the frontalis muscle, leaving only skin and a thin layer of subcutaneous tissue (Fig. 37–34). At the level of the hairline the plane of dissection is deepened, penetrating the galea to raise the remainder of the pedicle of the flap in the subgaleal plane.

Care must be taken in designing the pedicle not to design the arc of the coronal portion of the pedicle too far anteriorly, otherwise the base of the attachment to the frontal skin will be too narrow. A minimum of 4 cm of pedicle width is advised.

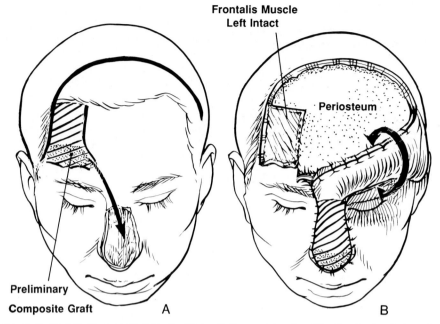

Frontalis Muscle Left Intact

Periosteum

Preliminary

Composite Graft   A   B

Figure 37–34. *A, B,* Technique of nasal reconstruction with the scalping flap. The flap is elevated contralateral to the donor vessels. Preliminary grafting of the undersurface can be done as needed.

The hair need not be completely shaved, but can be clipped in the area of the incision and cut short in the frontal area so as not to hang down offensively onto the face.

The donor site on the scalp may be either temporarily grafted with split-thickness skin or left open to be treated by nondesiccating dressings, depending on the convenience of the patient.

As with other flaps, the nasal attachment is left for three to four weeks, after which it is divided and the scalp portion of the pedicle is returned to its previous site. Traditionally a full-thickness skin graft, usually from the supraclavicular area, is applied over the frontalis muscle in the area where the frontal skin paddle has been removed. The full-thickness skin graft is usually subtle in appearance and requires no revision; however, serial excision with the aid of temporary skin expansion can be used to excise secondarily the donor graft area.

In balding patients with receding hairlines, the high (cephalic) placement of the skin paddle may make it difficult to unfurl the flap adequately to reach the nose. In such a case a vertical back cut in the forehead (Fig. 37–35) extends the reach of the flap and it can be secondarily closed at the time when the pedicle is returned to the forehead (Fig. 37–36).

Retroauricular Flaps

WASHIO FLAPS

Inspired by the reliability of the superficial temporal vessels as a vascular source for the scalping flap but disenchanted with the forehead scarring from the skin paddle, Washio

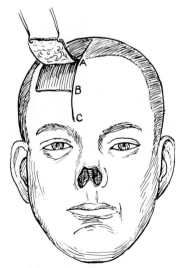

Figure 37–35. When only the upper portion of the forehead is required for the reconstruction, particularly in balding patients with a recessed hairline, additional flap length is obtained by a vertical incision extending downward (A, B, C,) toward the eyebrow.

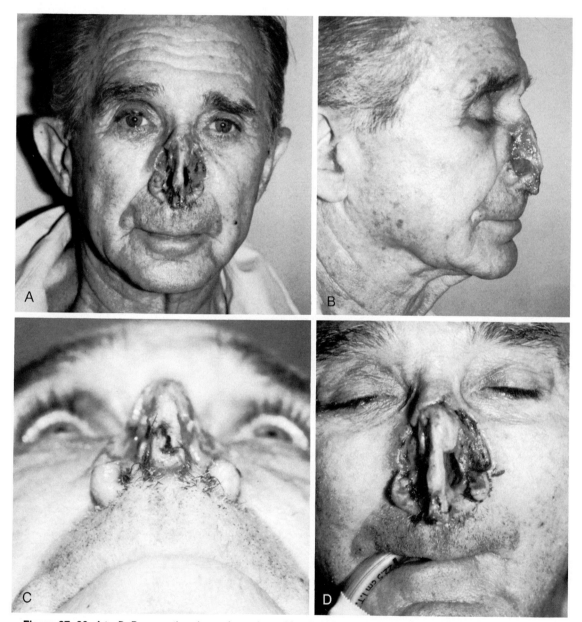

Figure 37–36. *A* to *D,* Preoperative views of a patient with subtotal loss of most of the nasal dorsum and lobule.

Illustration continued on following page

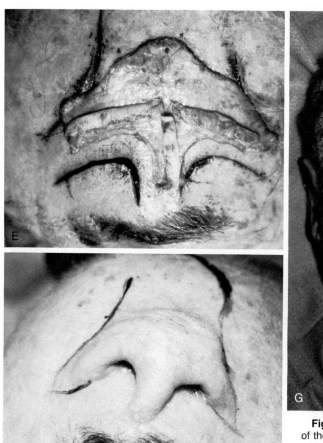

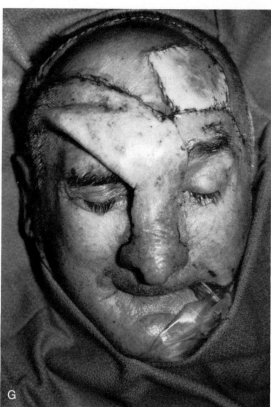

Figure 37–36 *Continued E,* Delay of forehead paddle of the scalping flap, showing the conchal cartilage graft and full-thickness skin graft that will be applied to the undersurface. *F,* Four weeks later the grafts have healed into the flap and the new nose has been molded on the forehead. *G,* The scalping flap has been transferred to the nose. The scalp defect has been covered with a split-thickness skin graft and the forehead defect resurfaced with a full-thickness skin graft.

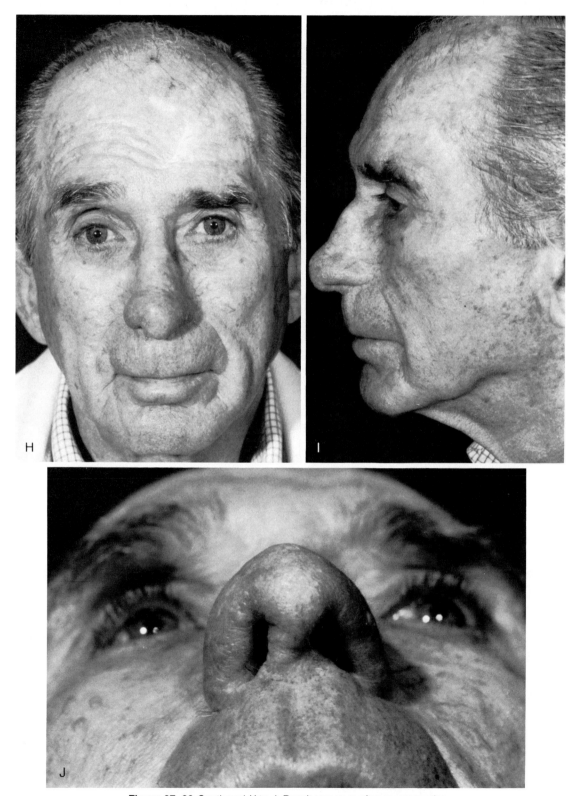

Figure 37–36 *Continued H* to *J,* Result one year after reconstruction.

(1969) developed the retroauricular-temporal flap. Loeb is credited with originally describing a temporomastoid flap in 1962, which seven years later Washio adapted for use in nasal reconstruction. Experiences with this flap method have been reported by Washio (1972), Orticochea (1971, 1980), and Maillard and Montandon (1982).

The vascular basis for the flap is the communication between the branches of the superficial temporal artery and those of the retroauricular (postauricular) artery. By including this vascular loop, an up-and-down type of flap can be designed to carry postauricular as well as mastoid skin for nasal reconstruction.

The flap can be elevated and transferred without delay. Although lining could be achieved by infolding the flap upon itself, Maillard and Montandon (1982) believed it preferable to use local turn-in flaps for more reliable healing. A strip of conchal cartilage, however, can be carried with the flap to provide skeletonization. Furthermore, the thickness in the flap skin can be altered, depending on whether mastoid or retroauricular skin is used.

The advantage of this method is the absence of scar in the forehead donor site from which the skin for nasal reconstruction is taken. While the skin match may not quite equal that of the forehead, the avoidance of a prominent forehead scar is a distinct advantage, especially in young patients.

The technique of the design and transfer of the retroauricular-temporal flap is illustrated in Figures 37–37 and 37–38. Flap length for unfurling of the pedicle is achieved by a vertical back cut in the center of the paddle; the incision must be made with care so as not to extend it vertically to the point of interrupting the vascular loop. Washio (1972) recommended that the back cut be done from the undersurface of the flap where the supplying vessels can be directly visualized. The care of the donor site and the timing of division and inset are essentially the same as those for a scalping flap. The donor site may be temporarily grafted or treated with a nondesiccating dressing. The pedicle is divided and returned to its position in the scalp two to four weeks after transfer.

CONTRALATERAL POSTAURICULAR FLAPS

A variation on the postauricular flap has been described by Galvao (1981) in which the superficial temporal vessels and scalp from one side are extended to carry the opposite postauricular skin for nasal reconstruction. With Galvao's technique the procedure requires a delay and offers little advantage over the ipsilateral method of Washio. It may be

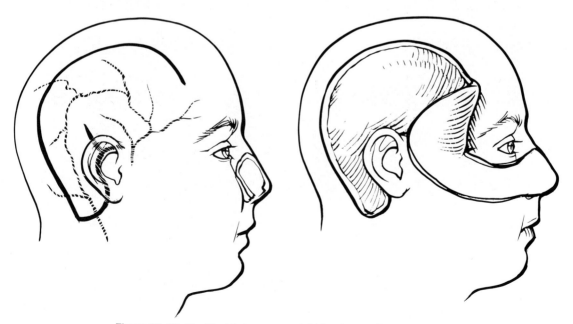

Figure 37–37. The Washio temporomastoid flap for nasal reconstruction.

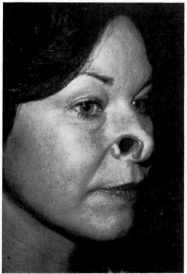
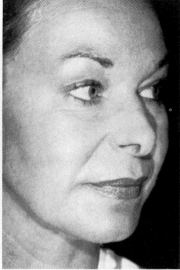
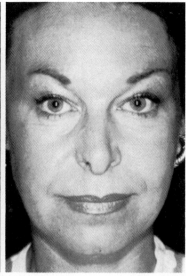

Figure 37–38. Reconstruction of the ala by a Washio flap in a young woman to avoid a scar on the face. (From Maillard, G. F., and Montandon, D.: The Washio tempororetroauricular flap: its use in 20 patients. Plast. Reconstr. Surg., 70:550, 1982.)

of use, however, when the ipsilateral post-auricular area has been previously damaged.

Distant Flaps

Occasionally the extent of injury to a patient with a nasal deformity is so great that all the facial and postauricular sources of skin for nasal reconstruction are unavailable. In such a situation, cover must be brought from a distant site. The techniques fall into two categories: standard flaps and free tissue transfers.

REMOTE FLAPS

Primarily of historical interest today, flaps for nasal reconstruction have been described as taken from the arm (the Tagliacozzi method, 1597); the neck (Gillies, 1935a; Kilner, 1937; Song, Wise, and Bromberg, 1973); the abdomen (Chitrov, 1954; Krauss, 1964); the chest as either skin (Song, Wise, and Bromberg, 1973) or myocutaneous flaps (Morgan, Sargent, and Hoopes, 1984); and the shoulder (Panje, 1982).

The original Tagliacozzi method (Fig. 37–39) used a distally based pedicle to facilitate transfer and was delayed to enhance blood supply (Fig. 37–40) (Gan, 1981; Miller, 1985). Mendelson and co-workers (1979) suggested using a proximally based flap that included the direct cutaneous vessel to the upper arm

(Daniel, Terzis, and Schwarz, 1975; Dolmans, Guimberteau, and Baudet, 1979; Kaplan and Pearl, 1980; Newsom, 1981; Song and associates, 1982) in the pedicle base to enhance flap reliability.

FREE FLAPS

The second method of transfer of distant tissue is by means of microvascular anastomoses (Fujino, Harashina, and Nakajima, 1976; Ohmori, Sekiguchi, and Ohmori, 1979; Shaw, 1981). The most popular of the methods for free tissue transfer in nasal reconstruction involves the *free dorsalis pedis flap* with the

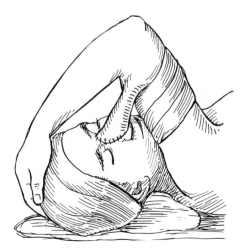

Figure 37–39. The Italian (Tagliacozzi) rhinoplasty.

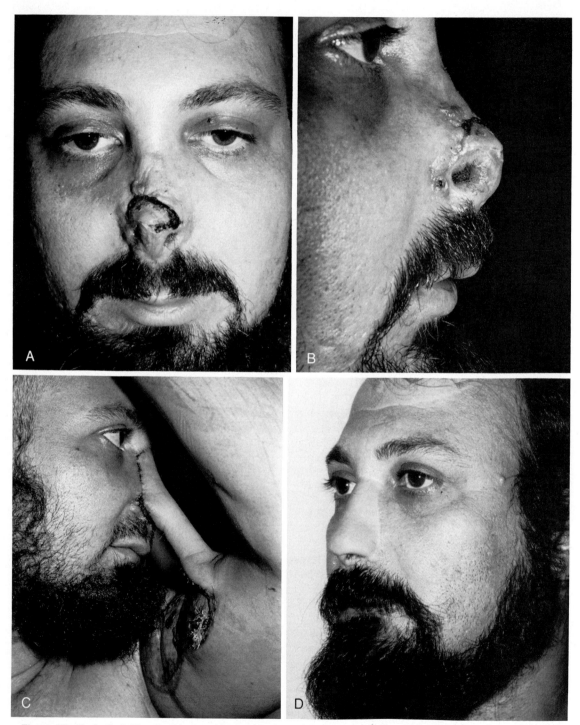

Figure 37–40. *A, B,* A 36 year old man with complete loss of the skin and cartilaginous structures of the nasal tip. *C,* The distally based upper arm flap in position. An iliac bone graft was used to augment the nasal dorsum. *D,* The color disparity between the nose and the rest of the face is evident.

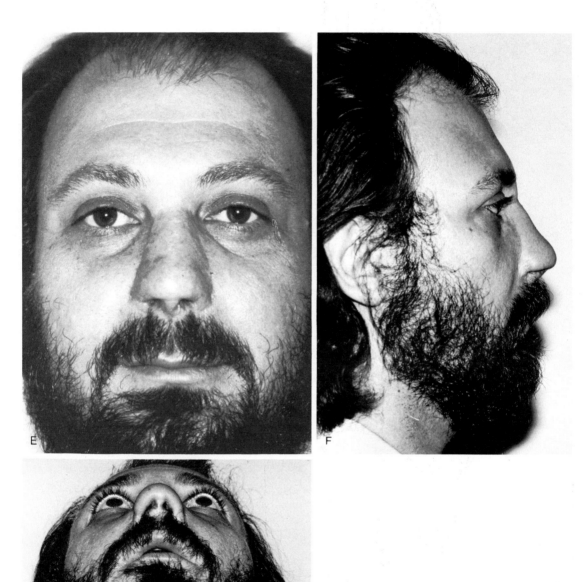

Figure 37–40 *Continued E to G,* Final result after replacing the flap skin with a full-thickness skin graft from the supraclavicular area. (From Miller, T. A.: The Tagliacozzi flap as a method of nasal and palatal reconstruction. Plast. Reconstr. Surg., *76:*870, 1985.)

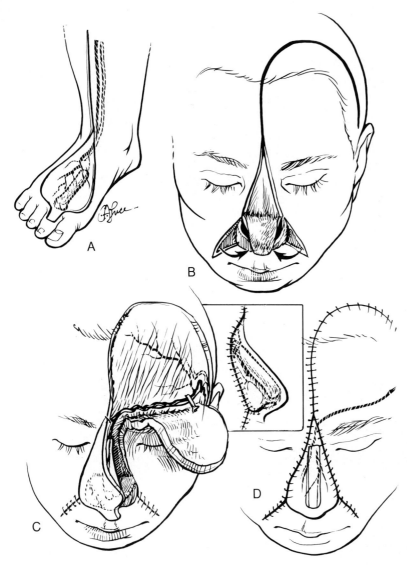

Figure 37–41. Technique of free dorsalis pedis–second metatarsal osteomyocutaneous flap transfer for nasal reconstruction. A, Outline of the flap. B, Turndown flaps provide the nasal lining. C, Anastomosis of the flap vessels to the superficial temporal vessels. D, Closure of all incisions. Note the metatarsal bone strut.

accompanying second metatarsal (Fig. 37–41) (Ohmori, Sekiguchi, and Ohmori, 1979).

The recipient vessels available for nasal reconstruction are principally those of the facial and labial arteries. The supratrochlear or superficial temporal vessels can also be used, but the former are small and the latter are somewhat distant for convenient use.

TISSUE EXPANSION

With the recent development of skin expansion techniques, there is the intriguing possibility of transferring initially expanded skin for nasal reconstruction and being able to close the donor defect primarily. Certainly this would make the forehead defect less disfiguring, although the expanded skin is stiff and indelicate when the underlying capsule is left attached.

Potential problems with skin expansion include the following: (1) removal of the capsule at the time of transfer may jeopardize the vascular supply to the transferred skin; (2) lamination of the flap with a lining composite graft, if needed, is difficult to control with an expander beneath; and (3) the extent of late retraction of expanded skin is not yet clear. Since nasal dimensions are critical, even slight late contraction would distort the result.

The concept of skin expansion is attractive, but its ultimate place in nasal reconstruction is undetermined.

LINING DEFORMITIES

Loss of lining of the nose can occur after injury, infection, irradiation, or tumor ablation. The condition is more complicated when the supporting framework of the nose has been fractured or partially destroyed. The external contour of the nose is not usually altered by adhesions of moderate degree within the nose; however, extensive loss of nasal lining may alter the contour of the lobule.

The surgical plan depends on whether there is merely a cicatricial band of stenosis or whether a substantial surface area of nasal lining is missing. In the former case it may be sufficient to rearrange the intranasal tissues to interrupt scar banding, but in the latter the nasal lining must be replaced.

The nasal lining is thin and directly adjacent to the undersurface of the cartilaginous and bony vault. Lining is best replaced by tissues of like thickness: either with remaining internal mucoperichondrial linings or with skin grafts. Turn-over flaps of nasal skin can also be used, since they contain minimal subcutaneous bulk.

Cheek or forehead flap tissue used for lining often causes some degree of airway compromise. These methods allow the secondary introduction of skeletal support, but the reconstructive surgeon must make every effort not to neglect the normal caliber of the nasal airway.

Z-Plasty for Linear Scar Contracture

When the air passages are reduced by a ring of scar tissue, the repair is accomplished by Z-plasty transposition flaps. These procedures are indicated when the web is limited to the vestibule, where incisions for the transposition of flaps are feasible.

The two layers of the ring of the stenosed area are separated by an incision along the border of the constriction. A vertical incision is made through the caudal portion of the vestibular lining, beginning at the roof of the nostril close to the septum and extending down to the edge of the ring. A second triangular flap is raised from the cephalic lining of the contracted ring by incising along the lateral wall, and the contracture is relieved by transposing the two flaps from either side of the stenosed area (Fig. 37–42).

Petrolatum gauze packing is maintained in the vestibule for several days. If recurrence of the contracture is feared, an impression of the vestibule can be taken with soft dental compound and a permanent acrylic mold fabricated to be worn by the patient for several months. The use of molds is also routine whenever an intranasal skin graft is applied.

Skin Grafting Within the Nose

Small defects within the nasal vestibule comprising less than 30 per cent of the circumference may be left to epithelize without significant secondary stenosis. However, if more than 30 per cent of the circumference is bare of epithelium, replacement by full-thickness skin is indicated.

The most common source of full-thickness graft for nasal lining is the thin, yet keratinized retroauricular skin. Petrolatum gauze left for a period of five days is usually all that is needed to provide coaptation of the graft. A permanent acrylic splint is indicated only for near-circumferential grafted defects (Fig. 37–43).

Nasomaxillary Skin Graft Inlay

A severe deformity results when the nasal bones and the middle portion of the maxilla have been destroyed or are underdeveloped as a result of trauma in childhood. The condition is called a "dish-face" deformity. Gillies (1943) developed a technique that frees the nose and the adjacent soft tissues from the atrophied or underdeveloped skeletal structures, and lines the cavity with a skin graft and a prosthetic appliance. The technique was applied to the treatment of the syphilitic nasomaxillary deformity, nowadays a rare condition.

Antia (1974) reported excellent results in correcting the saddle nose deformity of leprosy by the nasomaxillary skin graft technique. The nasal lining becomes progressively necrotic in leprosy, and the process spreads to the cartilages and bones of the

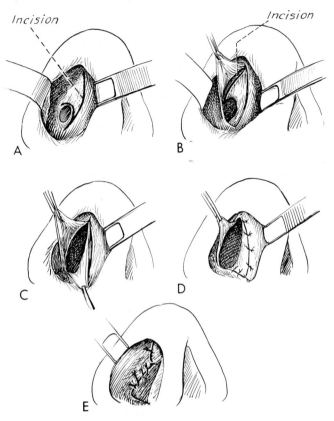

Figure 37–42. Correction of nasal stenosis. *A,* The septal mucoperichondrium incision is extended around the opening of the stenosed area. *B,* The lining is carefully dissected to form an anterior flap, which is outlined. *C,* The posterior flap is raised. *D,* The posterior flap covers the defect on the septum, and the anterior flap covers the raw area over the lateral wall.

nose. The nasomaxillary area, thus freed from its constricted state, is supported by a prosthesis. The technique carries the inconvenience that the patient must continuously wear, clean, and replace the appliance, and it is best suited for edentulous individuals, since the prosthetic support for the nose is an extension of the denture.

The nasal skin graft inlay technique is illustrated in Figures 37–44 and 37–45. The operative procedure consists of an incision in the upper buccal sulcus, entering the nasal fossa and freeing any adhesions. After removing the nasal spine, a dental compound mold with the apex pointing upward is constructed to fit the pyramidal cavity. A large split-

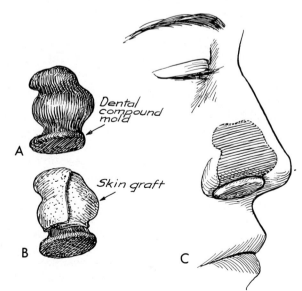

Figure 37–43. Skin grafting inlay technique for the correction of intranasal stenosis. *A,* Acrylic mold fabricated from an impression of the nasal airway after resection of the scar tissue causing the intranasal contracture. *B,* The mold covered by the skin graft. *C,* Outline of the mold inside the nasal cavity.

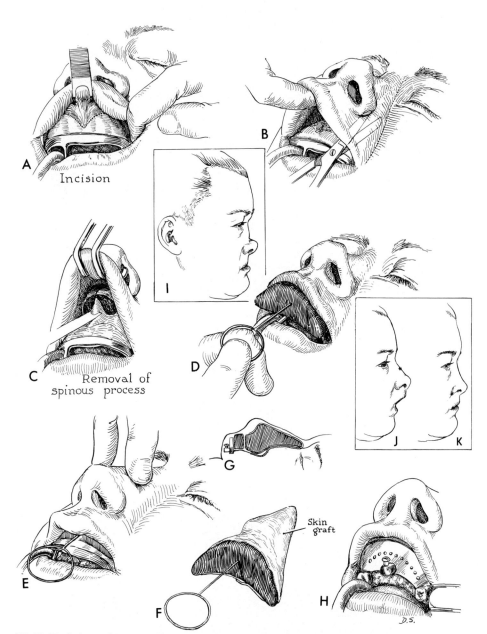

Figure 37–44. Technique of nasomaxillary skin graft inlay. *A,* Outline of the intraoral incision. *B,* The nasal cavity is entered through the mouth. *C,* The nasal spine is resected. *D,* A dental compound mold is fitted to the nasomaxillary cavity. *E,* The softened mold is molded to the contour of the cavity by external digital pressure. *F,* The mold is covered with a split-thickness skin graft, raw surface outward. *G,* The mold carrying the skin graft is placed inside the maxillary cavity and held in position by a splint anchored to the upper molars. *H,* The dental appliance maintaining the mold in the nasomaxillary cavity. *I* to *K,* Appearance of the patient before, during, and after the skin graft inlay procedure.

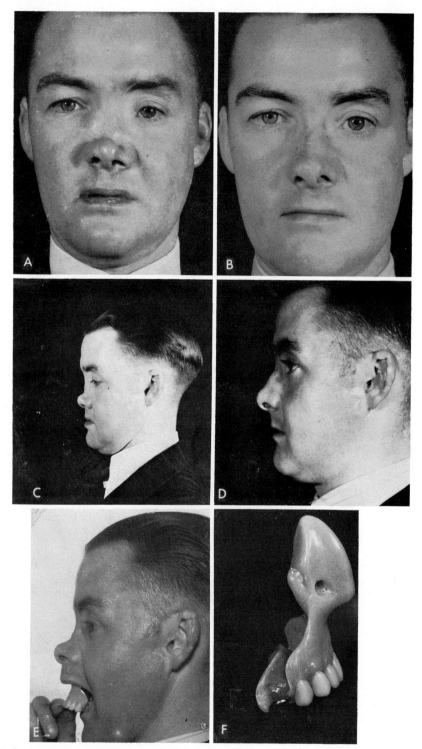

Figure 37–45. Contour restoration of the nasomaxillary area by the skin graft inlay technique. *A,* The deformity of the nasomaxillary area, consisting of destroyed nasal bone, superior alveolar process, and adjacent maxilla, nasal septum, and nasal lining, with retrusion of the midface. *B,* Result after reconstruction by the nasomaxillary skin graft inlay technique illustrated in Figure 37–44. *C, D,* Profile view of the patient before and after the operation. *E,* The patient introducing the prosthesis. *F,* The nasomaxillary appliance.

thickness skin graft from a hairless donor site is spread over the mold with the raw surface outward, and inserted into the nasal cavity. The skin graft is maintained by a splint attached to the molar teeth. Distention of the tissues by the mold ensures close coaptation of the graft and counteracts the tendency to contract. After two weeks the mold is removed so that the cavity can be examined and cleaned. At regular intervals in subsequent weeks the size of the mold is decreased until it is time for insertion of a permanent acrylic prosthesis.

The nasomaxillary inlay skin graft technique is indicated as a last resort in certain types of nasomaxillary deformity when no other solution can be found. It has also been employed in patients who receive radiation early in life and in whom the nose fails to develop.

Restoration with Intranasal Lining Remnants

When available, the residual intranasal lining provides the best source of replacement of the lobular lining. Kazanjian (1937) emphasized the benefit of mobilizing the mucoperichondrium and mucoperiosteum of the lateral nasal vault to allow downward sleeved advancement. If necessary, a raw surface can be left under the bony portion of the nasal cavity in an area where secondary epithelization will not lead to distortion or contraction of the mobile lobule.

The Kazanjian technique has been adopted in the form of a bipedicle flap of nasal mucosa from the caudal border of the defect (Burget and Menick, 1986). These authors base the bipedicle flap at the nasal septum and the lateral alar wall; the flap is lowered to form the lining of the alar rim and to support a graft. Although small, the flap is well vascularized. The defect secondarily produced in the area of the upper lateral cartilage can be repaired with either a septal chondromucosal flap or a skin graft (Fig. 37–46C).

Nasal Turn-In Flaps

According to Ivy (1925), Keegan was the first to turn over local tissues bordering nasal defects to line the nose. The skin is hinged on the cicatricial edge of the wound and rotated 180 degrees to serve as internal lining (Fig. 37–46A). This method is most useful when another major flap is used for external coverage. Its advantage is its local availability, while the donor site can be incorporated into the defect to be covered by the larger external flap.

The deficiency of this technique lies in the fact that the turn-in flaps may not be well vascularized through their cicatricial base, and thus behave more like full-thickness skin grafts. In addition, when one uses only the border of the contracted healed wound to serve as lining, by definition the intranasal vault has been constricted. The amount of lining replaced, therefore, is less than the size of the original defect, and this "collapsing principle" may yield deficient airway caliber.

Folded Flaps for Nasal Lining

Delpech (1824) originated the concept of folding a flap upon itself to achieve both internal lining and outer nasal coverage. Labat (1834) popularized the method in Europe and Blair (1925) introduced it to America years later.

Although flaps folded upon themselves may provide lining of the vestibular portion of the nose (Fig. 37–46E), they risk causing ischemic necrosis of the distal tip. When a flap is to be folded upon itself for such purposes, a preliminary delay may be advisable.

Nasolabial Flaps for Relining the Nose

In 1950 Gillies introduced the principle of bilateral nasolabial flaps turned inward on the piriform aperture for lining of the nasal vestibule and columella (Fig. 37–46B). The method has also been used by Antia (1974) to line the entire undersurface of the nose in patients with leprosy. By hinging the flaps on their subcutaneous bases at the piriform aperture, the donor site can be closed primarily.

The deficiency of this method of lining is its bulk—subcutaneous tissue must be carried with the flap to preserve vascularity. Such a thick flap is excessively bulky relative to the critical diameter of the vestibular passage.

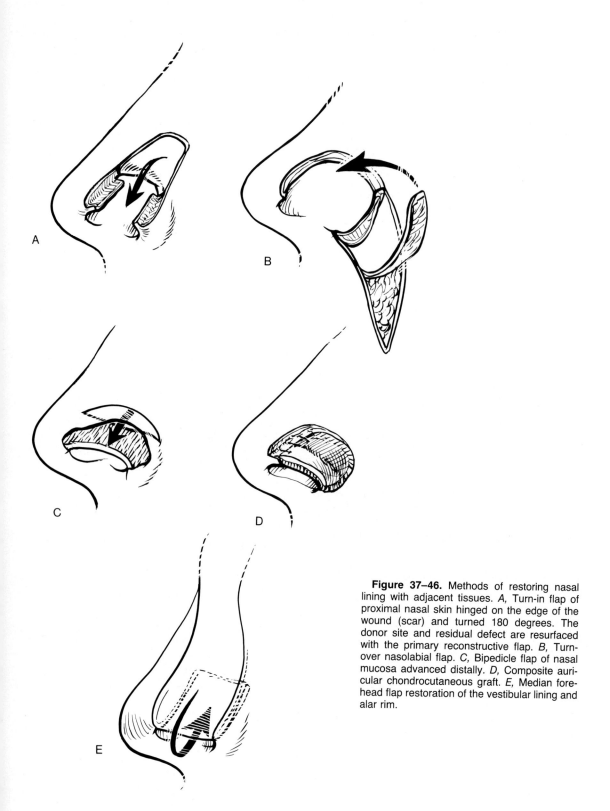

Figure 37–46. Methods of restoring nasal lining with adjacent tissues. *A,* Turn-in flap of proximal nasal skin hinged on the edge of the wound (scar) and turned 180 degrees. The donor site and residual defect are resurfaced with the primary reconstructive flap. *B,* Turn-over nasolabial flap. *C,* Bipedicle flap of nasal mucosa advanced distally. *D,* Composite auricular chondrocutaneous graft. *E,* Median forehead flap restoration of the vestibular lining and alar rim.

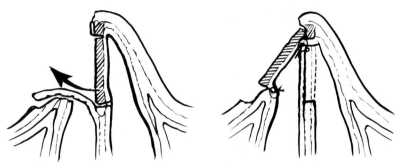

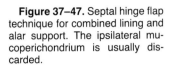

Figure 37–47. Septal hinge flap technique for combined lining and alar support. The ipsilateral mucoperichondrium is usually discarded.

Septal Flap Technique

The first use of a chondromucosal flap from the nasal septum for lining was reported by de Quervain in 1902. Subsequently, Kazanjian (1937), Millard (1967), Rawat and Sharma (1975), and Young and Weeks (1978) reported experience with this flap. The septal flap technique is most useful for lining defects of the lateral nasal wall in the area of the upper lateral cartilage. It does not easily extend to the alar rim.

In designing the flap, the ipsilateral mucoperichondrium is elevated from the septal cartilage and discarded (it can be repositioned in the midline to simulate a septum, but this often results in perforation). A rectangular portion of septum is divided and hinged on the contralateral dorsal mucoperichondrial attachment. It is important to leave a dorsal strut of septum caudally to prevent collapse of the tip (Fig. 37–47). Internal nasal lining as well as cartilaginous support of the lateral nasal wall may thus be accomplished in one step. A large septal window can be left beneath the hinge without undue hazard, and may even improve air flow in case of a constricted airway.

Preliminary Lining Graft

When full-thickness replacement of the nose is necessary, intranasal lining may be achieved by the application of a graft to the undersurface of the flap used to achieve external nasal coverage (Fig. 37–48). Millard (1966) traced the use of a preliminary skin graft to the undersurface of a reconstructive flap to Lössen in 1898. Gillies expanded this concept in 1943 by free-grafting a composite of skin and cartilage from the ear to the underside of an up-and-down flap. Converse (1956) reported a variation of the procedure

in which he grafted a chondromucosal segment from the nasal septum onto the tip of a forehead flap that was used in nasal reconstruction. The principle of preliminary skin grafting for lining the undersurface of the reconstructive flap has been widely adopted since that time.

Median Forehead Flap for Nasal Lining

Kazanjian in 1948 popularized the use of the median forehead flap for lining the nasal cavity in patients with major nasal defects. While the median forehead flap provides bulky coverage that may partially obstruct the nasal vault, it does yield immediate well-vascularized tissue, and is especially useful when bone grafting is necessary to restore the skeletal framework of the nose (discussed later under Total Nasal Reconstruction).

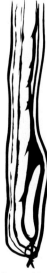

Figure 37–48. Preliminary skin grafting of the reconstructive flap for nasal lining. Cartilage may be integrated into the tip if needed for alar support.

RESTORATION OF NASAL SKELETON

Dating to 1861, Ollier is credited with including a piece of frontal bone attached by periosteum to a forehead flap used for nasal reconstruction. Around the turn of the century, Israel (1896) performed the first autogenous bone grafts for nasal support, while von Mangoldt (1900) transplanted costal cartilage for the same purpose.

From a skeletal standpoint, the nose can be divided into two elements: a rigid *midline scaffold* and flexible *lateral nasal walls*. The former helps to maintain tip elevation and nasal projection from the facial plane; the latter are responsible for restraining collapse of the nasal airway, while still being sufficiently malleable to withstand manipulation without fracture.

The need for rigid midline skeletal support is generally recognized, although opinions differ on how best to achieve it. From a planning standpoint, skeletal replacement is divided into subtotal defects and total defects, depending on the presence or absence of the nasal bones (Millard, 1966). In planning subtotal nasal skeletal restorations, one should initially assess the dorsal profile contour of the remaining nasal bones. Not uncommonly a prominent nasal hump is present and should be reduced to appropriate size in the early stages of reconstruction, while it is easily accessible (Fig. 37–49).

The appropriate timing for introduction of nasal support has been a controversial point in the development of nasal surgery. Both Blair (1925) and Ivy (1925) recommended waiting until soft tissue reconstruction was complete before inserting the skeletal support, but most authors now disagree with the delayed approach to providing skeletonization of the nose. It is far better to insert the skeletal support at the time of the application of the soft tissue draping; if the soft tissue is allowed to heal in a contracted position, it is much more difficult to ever recapture its original dimension and pliability.

Midline Support

From a practical standpoint, there are three common approaches to restoring the midline dorsal support of the nose: (1) rotations of the septal remnants, (2) an L-strut, and (3) a cantilever bone graft. Since the lobule is the most mobile portion of the nose and therefore the most commonly amputated, the root of the nasal septum is often left intact.

Outward Septal Rotation. The septal remnant can be rotated into greater projection to restore the absent septal angle by one of two methods. In 1920 Gillies described pivoting the septal remnant *on its attachment to the anterior nasal spine* (Fig. 37–50*B*). Millard (1967, 1974) later modified the technique to hinge the septum *at the caudal end of the nasal bones* (Fig. 37–50*A*). In either case the cartilaginous and bony attachments must be completely freed. These techniques may be utilized when a significant septal remnant remains.

L-Strut. The use of an L-strut, most commonly taken from rib, has been described by Gillies (1920), Brown and McDowell (1951), and Millard (1957). Most commonly the periosteum at the osteochondral junction is left

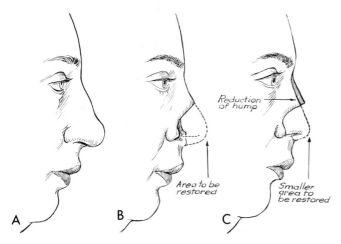

Figure 37–49. *A* to *C,* It is easier to reconstruct a small nose than a large one. The nasal stump is prepared before subtotal reconstruction by removing any hump or reducing a projecting dorsum.

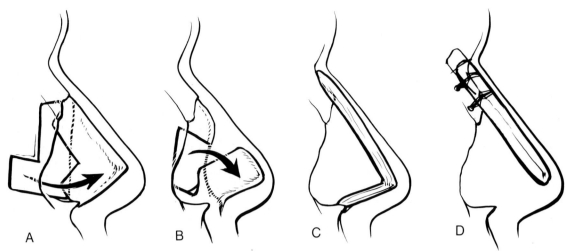

Figure 37–50. Methods of restoring midline skeletal support. *A*, A proximally based, L-shaped piece of septum rotated outward. *B*, A distally based septal hinge flap. *C*, An L-strut. *D*, A cantilever bone graft.

intact to serve as support for the septal angle. The L-strut helps to achieve nasal projection when an inadequate amount of septum remains to accomplish the reconstruction (Fig. 37–50*C*).

The disadvantage of the technique is that it offers no means of rigid stabilization. In nasal reconstruction the soft tissue tensions within the reconstructed wound not infrequently displace an L-strut from its midline position. The L-strut technique is therefore most applicable in saddle nose deformities, where the soft tissue sleeve is intact and balanced in tensions. An additional disadvantage of the L-strut is that the columellar portion necessary to achieve septal angle projection causes noticeable thickening in the columella.

Cantilever Bone Graft. In major reconstructions of the midline skeletal structure of the nose, the cantilever bone graft technique is the most reliable. Bone with a significant cortical component can be secured from rib, iliac crest, tibia, ulna, or cranial bone and anchored to the nasal bones with wire sutures (Fig. 37–50*D*).

Chait, Becker, and Cort (1980) recommend using an osteochondral rib graft as a cantilever, arguing that the bony portion of the graft in contact with the nasal bone solidifies while the distal cartilaginous portion keeps the nasal tip pliable.

Cortical bone placed as a cantilever graft shows less resorption than other onlay bone graft materials. Gerrie, Cloutier, and Woolhouse (1950), Wheeler, Kawamoto, and Zarem (1982), and Farina (Farina and Villano, 1971; Farina, 1984) reported long-term maintenance of the structural integrity of cortical bone grafts used for nasal cantilever support. After initial rarefaction during the first year, recalcification is shown to occur, and the grafts maintain their integrity for up to 21 years after insertion.

The great advantage of the cantilever method is that it is rigidly fixed to the remnant nasal bones and therefore does not easily displace. In addition, since it requires no columellar extension, no secondary distortion of the columella occurs. The remaining nasal bones often must be lowered to accommodate the bone graft, which is either imbedded into the frontal bone, wired to the nasal bones, or both.

Lateral Support

Support of the lateral nasal wall is usually achieved with autogenous cartilage in order to maintain the desired flexibility of the tissues.

Reconstruction of the arch of the *alar rim* is most commonly achieved with a strip of auricular (conchal) cartilage measuring 3 to 4 mm by 35 mm positioned between the dome of the medial crural remnant and the piriform aperture. Under normal anatomic conditions, the alar wing contains no cartilage, but rather the lateral crus of the alar cartilage defines the lateral boundary of the nasal tip. However, in reconstruction of the nasal ala it is necessary to implant the auricular cartilage in a position that follows the alar rim from the dome to the alar base.

The nasal wall in the location of the *upper lateral cartilage* is best replaced by the septal chondromucosal flap previously described (see Fig. 37–47). A portion of the vomer or perpendicular plate of the ethmoid can be included along with the septal quadrangular cartilage to replace the upper lateral cartilage or a portion of the frontal process of the maxilla. The septal chondromucosal flap will not support the lower nostril and alar rim, however, since a strut of cartilage in the midline must be maintained to ensure dorsal septal integrity.

TOTAL NASAL RECONSTRUCTION

As previously mentioned, a total nasal defect is defined as absence of the nasal bones, so that a cantilever bone graft has no base on which to be seated. The reconstruction must begin with provision of this platform.

A bone graft is placed across the root of the nose and secured to the frontal bone (Jackson, Smith, and Mixter, 1983). The graft is lined by turn-in flaps and temporarily covered by a midline forehead flap (Fig. 37–51A). After the platform has solidified, the reconstruction can be carried out by following the same

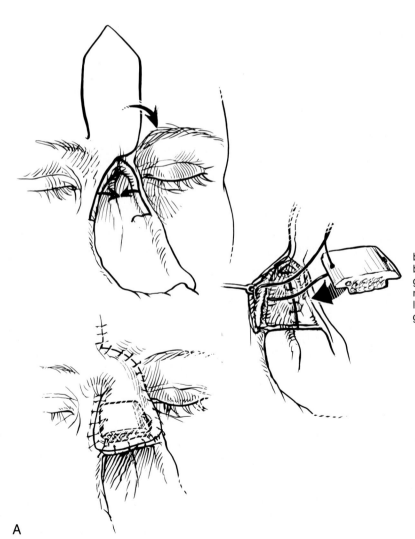

Figure 37–51. Preparing the bony platform at the nasal radix before seating a cantilever bone graft. *A,* Design and transfer of a median forehead flap and turn-in local flaps between which a bone graft is inserted.

A

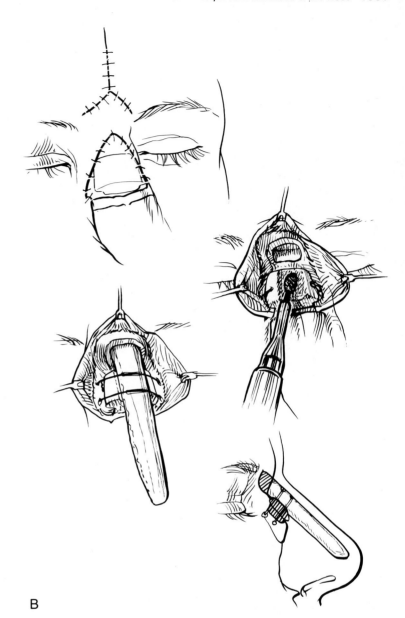

Figure 37–51 *Continued B,* At a later stage the healed bone graft serves as a bony platform for a cantilever graft.

B

sequence described for subtotal nasal reconstruction, i.e., using a cantilever bone graft for support (Fig. 37–51B) followed by lining and external nasal coverage.

RECONSTRUCTION OF COLUMELLA

The columella is probably one of the most difficult reconstructions in nasal restorative surgery, especially as an isolated defect. Many techniques have been described; Paletta and van Norman (1962) reviewed the literature and categorized the major historical approaches (Fig. 37–52). Joseph apparently published the earliest report of reconstruction in the modern literature in 1912; he utilized a composite graft from the ala.

Perhaps the best source of reconstruction of the columella is the midline forehead flap (Gillies, 1923, 1949; Ivy, 1925; Kazanjian, 1937; Shaw and Fell, 1948; Heanley, 1955; Malbec and Beaux, 1958; Cardoso, 1958; Paletta and van Norman, 1962; Millard, 1976). This is especially so when the columella is part of a larger defect that includes the nasal tip.

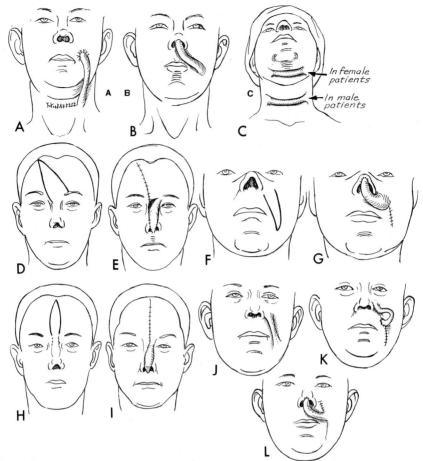

Figure 37–52. Various methods of reconstructing the columella. *A, B,* A horizontal cervical tube flap migrated to the nasolabial area and hence to the tip of the nose. *C,* Cervical tube flaps for columella reconstruction. *D, E,* Oblique median forehead flap. *F, G,* Nasolabial flap. *H, I,* Median forehead flap. *J to L,* Nasolabial tube flap.

The second most useful source of tissue for reconstruction of the columella is the nasolabial skin. Bilateral nasolabial flaps turned in on themselves were described by Gillies (1920) and later used by Millard (1976).

An excellent technique utilizing the nasolabial flap was described by da Silva in 1964, who tunneled a superiorly based nasolabial flap under the alar base to emerge in the nasal vestibule for columellar reconstruction (Fig. 37–53). At a second stage the flap is divided and the tunnel closed. This modification permits the use of a shorter and hence more reliable nasolabial flap.

Another refinement of columellar reconstruction with nasolabial tissue involves bilateral nasofacial island flaps based either inferiorly (Kaplan, 1972) or superiorly (Yanai, Nagata, and Tanaka, 1986) and elevated on subcutaneous vascular pedicles that are tunneled under the upper lip to the midline of the nose in one stage (Fig. 37–54).

Dieffenbach (1845) preferred the upper lip as a source of columellar tissue. Lexer (1931) formed a tube of mucosa and brought it through an opening in the upper lip, a procedure that has largely been abandoned be-

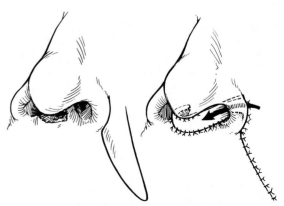

Figure 37–53. Columellar reconstruction with a nasolabial flap by a transnasal route.

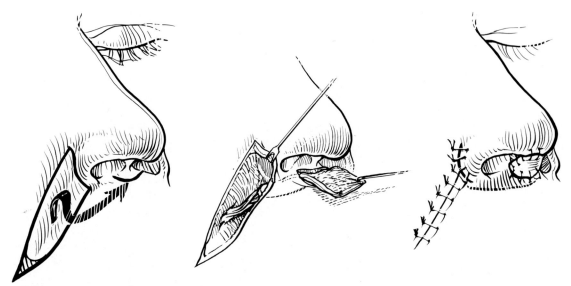

Figure 37–54. Nasolabial island flap raised on a subcutaneous pedicle and tunneled translabially for columellar reconstruction.

cause of the persistent reddish coloration of the labial mucosa. A modification of the technique suggested by Millard (1966) is the use of a horizontal labial flap as a vascular base on which a chondrocutaneous graft from the postauricular area can be seated. The technique provides adequate skin color for the anterior portion of the transplanted columella.

Composite grafts from the earlobe have also been used for columellar replacement. This procedure has been especially applied to children in whom there is minimal redundant nasolabial tissue to donate to the columella and in whom the donor scars would be unacceptable (Dupertuis, 1946; Gillies, 1950; Paletta and van Norman, 1962).

RHINOPHYMA

Although reportedly observed during the time of Hippocrates, rhinophyma was first named by Hebra in 1845 from the Greek *rhis*, meaning nose, and *phyma*, meaning growth (Matton and associates, 1962; Elliott, Ruf, and Hoehn, 1980). Rhinophyma has been referred to colloquially as "whisky nose," elephantiasis of the nose, and acne hyperplastica (Odou and Odou, 1961). These terms suggest an association with many different etiologies, particularly alcohol ingestion, yet no consistent causative factor has been identified to date. Most investigators agree that rhinophyma represents a severe stage of acne rosacea, as suspected by Virchow (1863–1867).

Rhinophyma is recognized clinically by bulbous enlargement of the nose with erythe-matous skin containing grossly hyperplastic sebaceous glands. Superficial infection of the foul-smelling sebaceous material is characteristic. Rhinophyma is 12 times more common in men than in women, the typical patient being a 60 year old male Caucasian.

PATHOLOGY

The histologic picture of rhinophyma is one of marked hypertrophy-hyperplasia of the sebaceous glands, fibrovascular proliferation in the dermis, and acanthosis of the epithelium (Fig. 37–55) (Acker and Helwig, 1967; Marks, 1968). The nasal cartilages are usually spared.

Malignant degeneration in rhinophyma is rare. Of the few reported malignancies, most

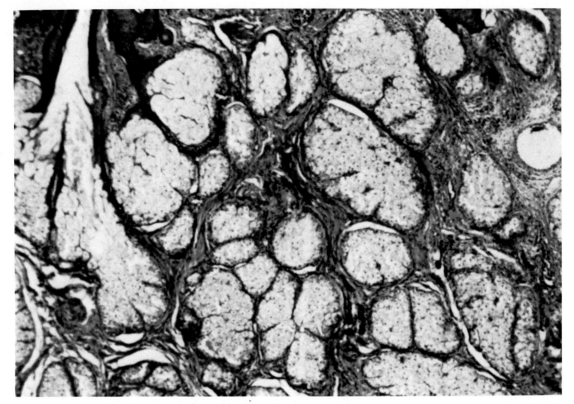

Figure 37–55. Histologic picture of rhinophyma.

are basal cell carcinomas (Novy, 1930; Eisenklam, 1931; Rees, 1955). Wende and Bentz (1904) suggested the presence of basal cell carcinoma in rhinophyma, but the first documented cases were those of Novy (1930) and Rees (1955). The definitive pathologic study was by Acker and Helwig (1967), who found basal cell carcinoma in five of 47 specimens of rhinophyma and reasoned that this ratio was significantly higher than would be expected from the natural occurrence of basal cell carcinoma on the nose. There have also been isolated reports of squamous carcinoma (Broadbent and Cort, 1977) and angiosarcoma (Traaholt and Eeg Larsen, 1978) in rhinophyma.

NONSURGICAL TREATMENT

In the 1920's irradiation was a popular form of treatment for a variety of skin maladies, acne rosacea included. Unfortunately the early benefit derived from shrinkage of the sebaceous glands was more than negated by the late occurrence of radiation-induced skin malignancies (MacKee and Cipollaro, 1946).

Today, conservative treatment of rhinophyma is similar to that of acne vulgaris: skin hygiene, meticulous cleansing, and avoidance of spicy foods, caffeine, and alcohol. Oral tetracycline may be helpful, especially if pustules are prominent (Roenigk, 1987). In the very early stages of the disease, isotretinoin may have a beneficial effect by shrinking the sebaceous glands (Goldstein and associates, 1982; Gomez, 1982; Strauss and Stranieri, 1982).

SURGICAL EXTIRPATION

For many decades the treatment of rhinophyma has been largely surgical. Extirpation can be either *partial* (tangential), maintaining the bases of the skin appendages, or *complete*, involving full-thickness removal of the affected skin.

Partial (Tangential) Excision. The most common approach to the treatment of rhinophyma is tangential excision of the skin and

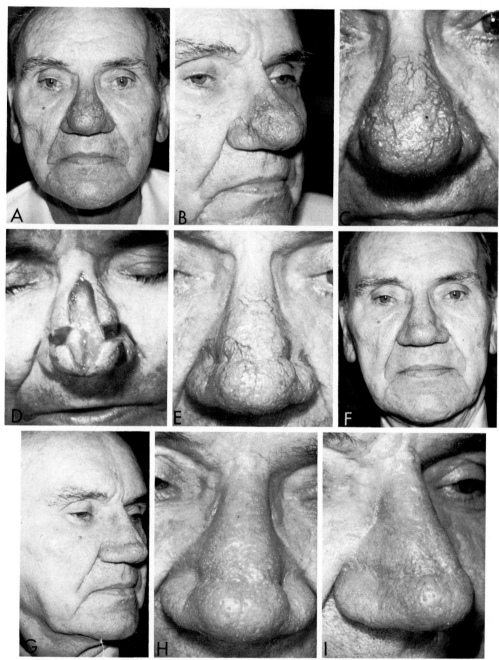

Figure 37–56. Full-thickness cruciate excision of rhinophyma in a 69 year old man. *A to C,* Preoperative views of the enlarged nose with increased vascularity and pitting. *D,* Full-thickness cruciate resection. *E,* Result six weeks after primary closure. *F to I,* Result six weeks after second-stage dermabrasion. Six months elapsed between stages. (From Elliott, R. A., Jr., Ruf, L. E., and Hoehn, J. G.: Rhinophyma and its treatment. Clin. Plast. Surg., 7:277, 1980.)

its hypertrophied appendages. The method is attributed to Stromeyer (1864), who suggested partial-thickness excision leaving the fundi of the sebaceous glands as a source of reepithelization. This technique was later termed "decortication" by Ollier (1875). It is crucial to spare the perichondrium and cartilages to avoid desiccation and distortion.

An almost limitless number of techniques for achieving tangential removal have been described. They include cryosurgery (Nolan, 1973), argon laser (Halsbergen Henning and van Gemert, 1983), CO_2 laser (Shapshay and associates, 1980; Wheeland, Bailin, and Ratz, 1987; Roenigk, 1987), electrocautery (Elliott, Ruf, and Hoehn, 1980), Shaw scalpel (Eisen and associates, 1986), dermabrasion (Elliott, Ruf, and Hoehn, 1980; Riefkohl and associates, 1983; Wiemer, 1987), and scalpel excision (Freeman, 1970; Riefkohl and associates, 1983).

Linehan, Goode, and Fajardo (1970) compared "cold knife" surgery with "electrosurgery" (electrocautery) in the treatment of rhinophyma. The authors noted that excision by electrocautery should not be as deep as that by scalpel, since an eschar layer of variable thickness is created by electrocautery. As would be expected, the destructive plane of the electrocautery is deeper than that of the initial dissection.

Nondesiccating dressings and topical bacteriostasis promote secondary epithelization after tangential excision.

Complete (Full-Thickness) Excision. Full-thickness excision of the entire dorsal nasal skin was initially suggested by von Langenbeck in 1851, and the method has enjoyed intermittent acceptance (Macomber, 1946; Freeman, 1970; Crikelair, 1972). Full-thickness excision necessitates resurfacing, usually by full-thickness skin graft. Crikelair (1972) reported the use of split-thickness skin grafts from the excised rhinophymatous skin to cover raw areas and exposed cartilage, but the possibility of replanting a nidus of basal cell carcinoma with the graft must be kept in mind.

Occasionally the pattern of enlargement in rhinophyma lends itself to cruciate full-thickness excision (Fig. 37–56) of portions of the dorsal nasal skin, followed by direct closure as described by Dieffenbach (1845). *Conservative* undermining of the flaps facilitates wound approximation, whereas *wide* undermining can lead to edge necrosis (Freeman, 1970). Rarely is this degree of excision necessary. Most authorities believe that the technique of tangential excision and spontaneous epithelization yields the best results.

THE FORESHORTENED NOSE

The short nose results from loss or lack of development of skeletal support, nasal lining, and cutaneous covering. Foreshortening as a result of full-thickness loss of nasal tissue has been previously described. This section deals with foreshortening secondary to congenital or traumatic causes as they relate to deficiencies of lining or skeletal support. (See also Chap. 29 under Nasomaxillary Hypoplasia).

DIAGNOSIS

The foreshortened nose is characterized by a broad and flattened nasal dorsum. The tip may be broad and underprojecting from a total lack of septal support, or it may be upturned (cephalic rotation) from contracture in the upper or middle third of the nose. Nasal foreshortening can be confirmed by measuring the distance from the root of the nose to the nasal tip. The root of the nose is taken at the level of the supratarsal fold of the upper eyelid. This length should be approximately 1.6 times the distance from the nasal tip to the level of the lip commissure (stomion), and equal to the distance from the stomion to the mentum (SM) (Fig. 37–57). Compared with the lower facial third, nasal length (RT) should be approximately 0.6 times the distance from the nasal tip to the mentum (TM).

Confusion can arise in association with a deep frontonasal angle when the dorsal incli-

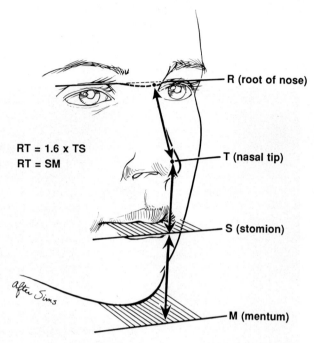

Figure 37–57. Ideal facial relationships between the nose and other facial structures (see text).

RT = 1.6 x TS
RT = SM

R (root of nose)

T (nasal tip)

S (stomion)

M (mentum)

nation begins at or below the level of the medial canthus (Fig. 37–58). The result is a nose that appears to be short even though the nasal tip may be a normal distance from the supratarsal fold.

ETIOLOGY

Congenital causes of short nose include nasoorbitoethmoid hypoplasia, nasomaxillary hypoplasia (Binder's syndrome), craniosynostosis, midline clefts, and other related developmental anomalies. Short noses, by Caucasian standards, may be found as a normal expression of development in several Oriental subgroups such as Filipinos and Koreans. With these diverse presentations, it is not surprising that many patients simply demonstrate noses that are disproportionately foreshortened relative to their facial skeleton (Fig. 37–59). All have in common an *unscarred* nasal framework, although deficiencies of lining, skeleton, and skin may be present to variable degrees.

Traumatic causes of short nose typically are malunited nasoethmoidoorbital fractures, impacting nasal fractures that telescope the framework, and complex septal fractures where buckling, collapse, and lining contracture are common. Because of the attachments

of the alar cartilages to the septum, cephalad rotation of the nasal tip is a frequent finding when shortening is secondary to septal injury (Fig. 37–60).

SURGICAL MANAGEMENT

Appropriate surgery begins with proper treatment planning that distinguishes between a nose that appears to be short and one that is truly disproportionate to the rest of the face. When the length is normal, correction usually involves dorsal augmentation to correct the vertical deficiency as well as to create a nasofrontal angle at the proper level and inclination to the face (Fig. 37–61). Bone, cartilage, and alloplasts have been successfully used for this purpose, although alloplastic implants are best reserved for nontraumatic deformities that are free of scar and have a nonconstricting soft tissue envelope.

When nasal shortening is confined to the cartilaginous septum, wide mobilization of the septal mucoperichondrium, upper lateral cartilages, and alar dome cartilages is generally required. Liberal resection of buckled, collapsed, and deformed septal cartilage is preferable to scoring and reshaping techniques. Structural support is provided in the form of cartilage grafts from the septum or

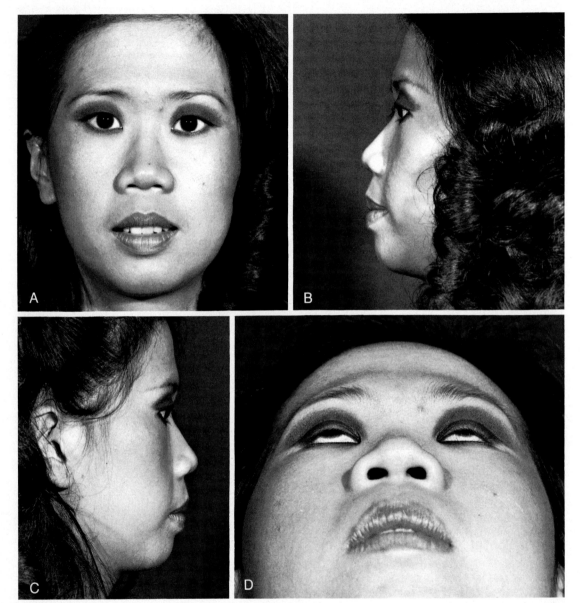

Figure 37–58. *A* to *D,* The nose appears to be foreshortened because the dorsal inclination begins below the level of the supratarsal folds.

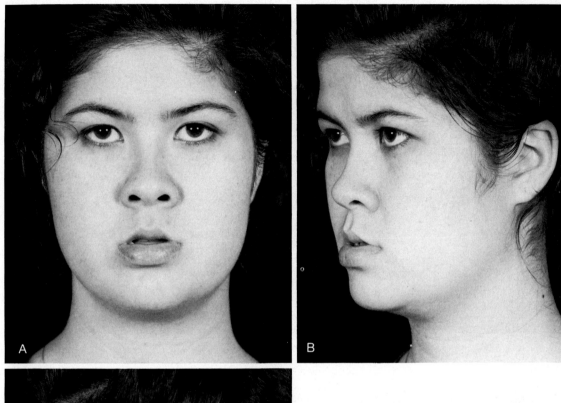

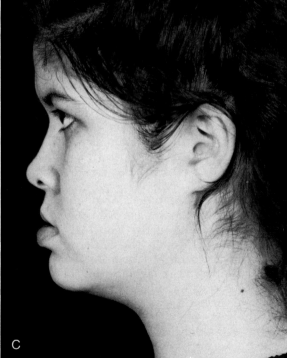

Figure 37–59. *A* to *C,* The nose appears foreshortened because of midfacial retrusion, but is actually of normal size and in proportion to other features in the lower face. There is also an anterior crossbite with Class III malocclusion.

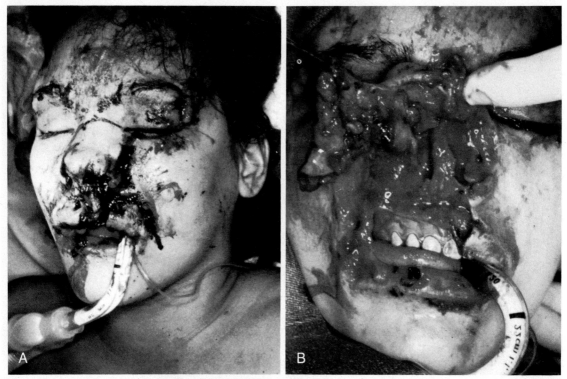

Figure 37–60. A, B, Traumatic foreshortening after septal injury.

rib. Lining deficiences can usually be augmented with mucosa mobilized and released from the undersurface of the nasal skeleton. Care should be taken to avoid rents and tears, in order to minimize exposure of supporting grafts.

External rhinoplasty approaches are preferable for severe septal deformities. Adequate visualization can be achieved with a transcolumellar skin incision connecting bilateral alar margin (rim) incisions (Fig. 37–62). The added exposure greatly facilitates septal dissection, lining release, and securing and positioning of the grafts. Linear and H-shaped dorsal transcutaneous incisions should be avoided because of attendant scarring.

Septal support is achieved by anchoring the osseous portion of an autogenous rib bone–cartilage graft to the bony nasal skeleton. Direct wiring and pinning with small Kirschner wires has been used to advantage (Figs. 37–63, 37–64). The cantilevering effect provides vertical support, and at the same time allows the upper lateral cartilages and alar cartilages to be fixed to the cartilaginous portion of the graft. Additional tip support

can be obtained by interposing a strut of septal cartilage between the medial crura, enhancing the tip so that an esthetic break occurs.

When foreshortening involves the entire osteocartilaginous skeleton (severe nasoethmoidoorbital fractures) or when there is major lining deficiency or contracture from extensive intranasal injury, *perinasal osteotomies* (see Chap. 29) mobilizing the nasal complex from the cranial base may be required (Fig. 37–65).

Exposure is obtained through bicoronal, intraoral, and intranasal incisions. Subperiosteal dissection of the nasofrontal junction is achieved through the bicoronal incision. The medial canthal tendon is identified and detached from the medial orbit, and the lacrimal sac is mobilized from the lacrimal groove. A transverse osteotomy is performed at the junction of the frontal bone and nasal bone. An extension is carried down into the medial orbit, where it passes behind and lateral to the lacrimal fossa.

Through the oral incision, subperiosteal dissection of the nasal floor and frontal proc-

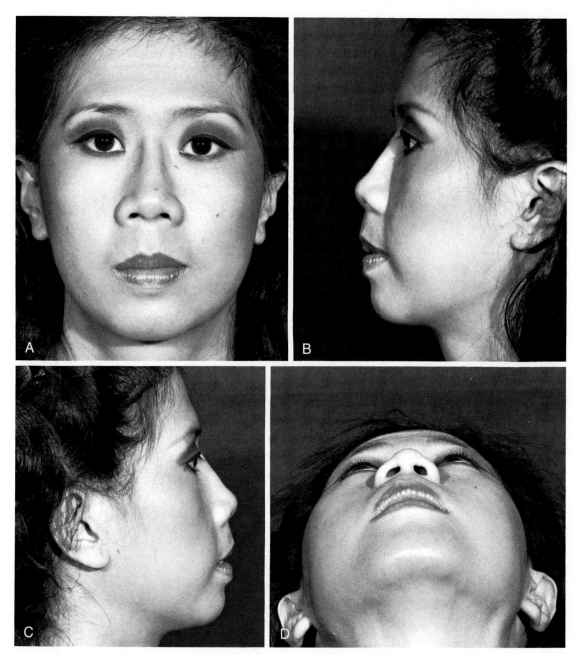

Figure 37–61. *A* to *D,* The same patient as in Figure 37–58 after augmentation of the nasal dorsum.

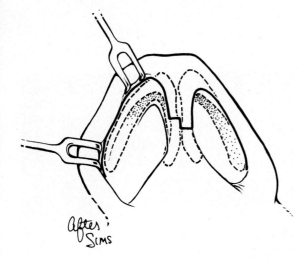

Figure 37–62. Transcolumellar skin incision combined with rim incisions.

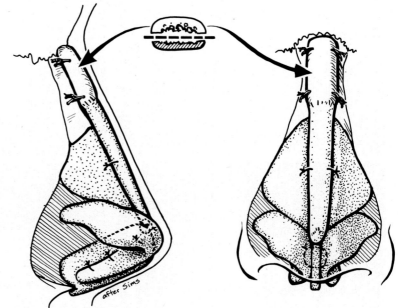

Figure 37–63. Septal graft support with direct wiring.

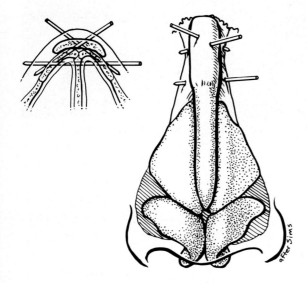

Figure 37–64. Costochondral graft to augment the nasal dorsum. Note the K-wire fixation.

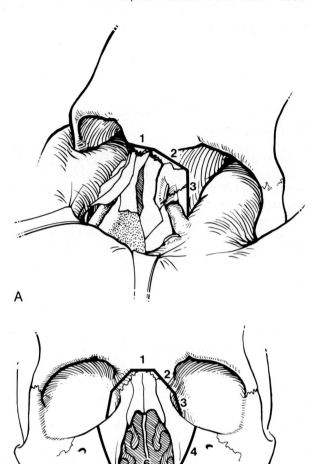

Figure 37–65. *A, B,* Lines of osteotomy of the perinasal osteotomy (Converse). A bicoronal incision is used to expose the nasofrontal junction; the medial canthal tendon is detached and the lacrimal sac mobilized. The frontal and nasal bones are separated, and subperiosteal degloving of the maxillary processes is possible through an intraoral incision. Various osteotomies: 1, 2, nasofrontal; 3, medial orbital; 4, 5, anterior wall of the maxilla; 6, septal.

ess of the maxilla is achieved. A maxillary osteotomy is performed through the anterior wall of the maxillary sinus immediately lateral to the frontal process of the maxilla. The osteotomy joins the orbital osteotomy through the infraorbital rim lateral to the lacrimal sac. A second maxillary osteotomy is made through the lateral wall of the nose (the medial wall of the maxillary sinus) below the opening of the nasolacrimal duct. A midline osteotomy severs the vomer and septal structures from the palate.

Attention is redirected to the frontonasal junction, where a small osteotome is driven through the midline septal structures toward the posterior nasal spine. Levering downward mobilizes the nasal complex from the cranial base and facial skeleton and opens a space at the root of the nose. The degree of downward displacement governs the amount of nasal lengthening.

A bone graft of appropriate width is wedged between the frontal bone and nasal bone to achieve the desired length. An osteocartilaginous rib graft may be incorporated in the fixation to redefine the nasal dorsum and provide additional support to the distal third of the nose. The canthal tendons are wired transnasally to the appropriate dimension.

Additional refinement is sometimes possible through intranasal incisions, allowing the nasal tip to be released and attached to supporting dorsal and columellar grafts. Septal obstructions can be removed and external skeletal irregularities may be recontoured if care is taken not to overdissect the skeletal constituents contained in the mobilized nasal pyramid. Overdissection may lead to relapse or collapse of the advanced parts if they are not secured to adjacent supporting grafts. When intranasal dissection is done prior to perinasal osteotomies, mobilization of the pyramid may be incomplete owing to the flail nature of the structures. The reader is also referred to Chapter 29.

POSTOPERATIVE NASAL SHORTENING

Nasal shortening after rhinoplasty is typically secondary to overzealous resection of lining and cartilage at the interface between the upper lateral and alar cartilages or along the caudal and membranous septum. Skin and mucosa grafts theoretically replace lining deficiencies, but in practice they invariably contract, contributing to a recurrence of the deformity. Accordingly, successful correction usually involves hard tissue (skeletal) backing to maintain length. These requirements can usually be satisfied by composite grafts taken from the septum or ear, or by intranasal mucosal advancements reinforced by thin grafts of septal cartilage. In the former, care should be taken to "step" the release so that an increased vascular interface with the graft is achieved and graft survival enhanced. In the latter, the advanced mucosa and distal nasal complex must be well secured to the interposed cartilage graft so that mucosal contraction across the release does not result in recurrence of the deformity (see Chap. 36).

CONGENITAL CHOANAL ATRESIA

Congenital choanal atresia is an obstruction between the nasal cavity and nasopharyngeal vault resulting in continuous nasal discharge, impaired sense of smell, and restricted nasal ventilation (Freng, 1978).

Choanal atresia was first described by Roederer in 1755 (Flake and Ferguson, 1984), and Ronaldson (1880–1881) is credited with the classic description of the syndrome.

EMBRYOLOGY

Five theories for the embryologic development of choanal atresia have been proposed: (1) persistence of the buccopharyngeal membrane from the foregut, (2) failure of the bucconasal membrane to rupture, (3) congenital adhesions, (4) medial overgrowth of the vertical and horizontal process of the palatal bone, and (5) misdirection of flow of the neural crest cells (Hengerer and Strome, 1982; Hall and associates, 1982).

Persistence of the buccopharyngeal membrane accounts for membranous atresias in the region of the nasopharyngeal passage posterior to the definitive nasal choana (Hengerer and Strome, 1982). Although the atresias are not truly of the nasal choana, they constitute approximately 10 per cent of the reported cases.

If persistent, the *bucconasal membrane* is located anterior to the hard palate edge. The differentiation of its cellular elements would allow such an obstructing septum to be entirely membranous, completely bony, or composed of membrane and bone (Theogaraj, Hoehn, and Hagan, 1983). The theory serves as a tenable explanation for patients who demonstrate a septate obstruction of the nasal choana.

Many patients have no clearly defined obstructing septum and demonstrate general *encroachment on the choanae from all sides*. This casts a doubt on the persisting membrane theory as an explanation in these cases.

Medial overgrowth of the horizontal and vertical processes of the palatal bone has been proposed as the cause of choanal atresia in cases that do not have an obstructing septum. A thickened, high-arched palate, medial displacement of the lateral nasal wall, and a decrease in the anteroposterior dimension of the nasopharynx serve as an anatomic basis for this theory (Theogaraj, Hoehn, and Hagan, 1983).

Misdirection of flow of neural crest cells has been proposed as an explanation for choanal atresia and the related structural anomalies of the cranial base and midface (Strome and

Hengerer, 1984). It is thought to occur between the fourth and 12th week of gestation. A failure in the precision with which normal cellular elements migrate to genetically predetermined positions in the facial processes results in significant structural alterations. The clinical import of the latter rests on the fact that choanal atresia is more than an isolated plate of bone, but rather is a component of a skull base anomaly.

Structural abnormalities are demonstrated on the undersurface of the body of the sphenoid bones superiorly, the medial pterygoid laminae laterally, the vomer medially, and the horizontal portion of the palatal bone inferiorly. These changes, together with other changes in the bone structure of the nasal vault, suggest a general developmental abnormality rather than the isolated persistence of the bucconasal membrane.

Normal nasal development begins with the migration of neural crest cells from their origin in the dorsal neural folds, laterally around the eye and across the frontonasal process. The migration begins at approximately the fourth week of embryonic life and has completed the nasal architecture by the 12th week. Once positioned, these pluripotential cells undergo rapid proliferation and differentiation into a matrix of mesenchymal tissue that will be further transformed into muscle, cartilage, and bone. This simple explanation assumes the accurate migration of the neural crest cells, both in terms of eventual location and of appropriate cell masses.

INCIDENCE

Choanal atresia is an uncommon malformation, occurring once in every 7000 to 8000 births. Its true incidence may be greater owing to missed diagnosis in stillbirths, unilateral presentations, and incomplete obstructions (choanal stenosis). Choanal atresia is twice as likely to be unilateral and right-sided. There is also a 2:1 greater incidence in females than in males.

Associated anomalies are a common occurrence and are reported to be as high as 40 to 50 per cent in most series (Theogaraj, Hoehn, and Hagan, 1983; Strome and Hengerer, 1984). The most commonly associated anomalies are craniofacial and cardiovascular malformations. Deafness and facial paralysis are also in frequent association.

ANATOMY

The obstruction may be complete or incomplete and may be membranous, cartilaginous, or bony (approximately 90 per cent). The location of the atretic plate is at the maxillopalatal junction and anterior to the posterior end of the vomer. It may vary in thickness from 1 to 12 mm (Hall and associates, 1982).

There is a medial compression of the lateral and superior walls, with greater thickness of bone in these regions. A narrowed nasopharyngeal vault is common. The palate may be elevated or high-arched, and structural abnormalities of the posterior septum are not unusual. The atresia is in a tangential plane and is bordered laterally by the medial pterygoid plate, superiorly by the sphenoid, inferiorly by the palatal bone, and medially by the vomer.

In osseous choanal atresia the posterior nasal cavity is obstructed by expanded medial pterygoid plates and a posterior vomer that is abnormally enlarged by endochondral bone formation. In membranous choanal atresia the nasal cavity is obstructed by a thin fibrous membrane, lined with respiratory epithelium, that links the posterior vomer to the medial pterygoid plate. The obstructing membrane thickens as it joins superiorly with the roof of the nasopharynx. Combined osseous and membranous atresia is characterized by a rim of bone surrounding a membranous septum, although osseous or chondroid islands within the membranous atretic plates have also been documented (Brown and associates, 1986).

DIAGNOSIS

Unilateral choanal atresia and bilateral stenosis may be asymptomatic in the neonatal period. In childhood a persistent mucous drainage or nasal airway obstruction with viral upper airway infections is characteristic.

Bilateral atresia becomes acutely symptomatic, since mouth breathing is not acquired owing to an obligatory nasorespiratory reflex that persists (in most neonates) for the first two to four weeks of life (Osguthorpe, Singleton, and Adkins, 1982). The classic presentation is cyclic cyanosis, in which the patient alternates between periods of apnea with progressive cyanosis and life-sustaining oral respiration during crying. Although most untreated infants survive, notwithstanding aspiration during feedings and failure to thrive, the cyclic pink-blue sequence left untreated may progress to exhaustion of the infant and respiratory death.

The diagnosis is strengthened when a small red rubber catheter or probe cannot be passed beyond 32 mm into the nose (Beinfield, 1956). If methylene blue placed in the nose fails to reach the oropharynx, atresia should be suspected.

Although choanograms and other specialized radiographs have been used to confirm the diagnosis of choanal atresia, the complete anatomic abnormality of the atresia and surrounding bony skeleton is best identified by computed tomography (Slovis and associates, 1985). A CT scan clearly distinguishes membranous atresias from the more complex and common bone atresias, and provides anatomic details about the surrounding skeleton (Fig. 37–66) that are essential to proper surgical planning (Brown and associates, 1986).

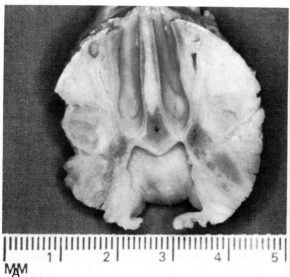

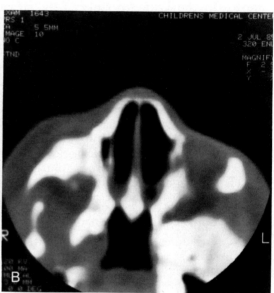

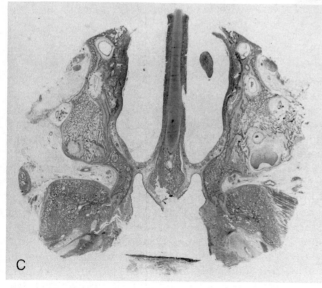

Figure 37–66. *A,* Axial section through the nasal cavity of a newborn with bilateral posterior choanal atresia (BPCA). The posterior vomer is thickened, thin atresia plates obstruct the nasal airway, and the nasal cavity is narrowed by medial protrusion of the pterygoid plates. A large vessel is seen in the abnormal posterior vomer. *B,* On axial CT scan, the nasal cavity is narrowed by abnormal medial pterygoid plates, the posterior vomer is thickened, and thin membranes obstruct the nasal airway. Small air-fluid levels are present bilaterally. *C,* Photomicrograph showing medial pterygoid plates and the posterior vomer enlarged by endochondral bone. A thin fibrous septum lined by respiratory epithelium joins the posterior vomer to the lateral nasal wall, obstructing the nasal airway.

TREATMENT

Opinion is divided regarding the optimal surgical approach for the correction of choanal atresia. There are also arguments about the proper timing for surgical intervention. Regardless of controversy, interval medical management of the airway is essential.

The airway may be established by the use of an orogastric tube, intraoral nipple, or oral airway (Theogaraj, Hoehn, and Hagan, 1983). Tracheostomy is entertained only when associated craniofacial anomalies preclude other management alternatives.

The insertion of a large orogastric feeding tube (No. 12 or 14 French) effectively breaks the obstructive seal between the tongue and the palate (Hough, 1955). The tube also serves as a feeding conduit and may be taped to a Logan's bow for security.

The top of a feeding nipple may be modified to serve as an efficient airway. The hole at the tip is enlarged and an additional hole is cut on either side of it (McGovern, 1961). When taped to the head, the nipple provides an efficient method of breaking the tongue-palate seal. A tiny feeding tube may be passed through one of the holes for feeding without interfering with respiration.

An oral airway may be placed in the mouth, providing the same benefit as the orogastric tube. Gavage feeding can be instituted by passing a feeding tube beside the airway into the stomach. Some advocates indicate that this method eliminates the palatal ulceration that can be problematic in the surgical approach (Strome and Hengerer, 1984).

Surgical Timing

Strome and Hengerer (1984) advocated surgical correction in the neonatal period after the child was cleared for general anesthesia in cases of bilateral atresia and in unilateral atresia with partial stenosis of the functioning side. Advances in neonatal anesthesia and microscopic surgical techniques allow for a definitive repair that minimizes the likelihood of prolonged hospitalization, intermittent aspiration, abnormal development in height and weight, and cardiac enlargement, all of which may accompany nasopharyngeal obstruction when left untreated. Others (Maniglia and Goodwin, 1981; Theogaraj, Hoehn, and Hagan, 1983; Harding, 1983) advocated deferring surgery until mouth breathing is learned or until the infant is 2 to 3 months of age. A semiemergent approach in the neonatal period is recommended by Samuel and Fernandes (1985), although a different surgical technique is employed.

Unilateral atresia with a normal contralateral side is repaired at 1 year of age or when symptoms lead to the diagnosis. There are arguments in favor of deferring surgery in these children until after the primary dentition has erupted, to minimize growth disturbance of the dentofacial skeleton.

Surgical Treatment

The four basic approaches to the correction of choanal atresia are the *transantral, transseptal, transnasal,* and *transpalatal.* The transantral and transseptal approaches have limited applicability and are best reserved for the adult patient. In the child the roots of the permanent teeth are situated high in the maxillary antrum and would likely sustain injury with the transantral approach. Similarly, the transseptal approach requires sacrifice of the septum, which contributes significantly to growth of the nose and midface. Accordingly, most of the controversy centers on the relative merits of the transnasal and transpalatal approaches.

Transnasal Approach. The transnasal approach has evolved from a blind puncture or curettage technique (Beinfield, 1959) to a puncture aided by endoscopic vision (Winther, 1978) to a microsurgical drill-out procedure under direct vision (Singleton and Hardcastle, 1968; Freng, 1978; Osguthorpe, Singleton, and Adkins, 1982; Samuel and Fernandes, 1985). The blind puncture procedures generally provided a limited correction, with recurrence of obstruction in 50 to 60 per cent of patients, and were associated with severe complications such as cerebrospinal fluid leaks, midbrain trauma, and injury to cranial nerves V and VI (Gradenigo's syndrome) (Herceg and Harding, 1971).

Advances with the microsurgical drill-out procedure in infants have resulted in a stable correction with minimal morbidity (Samuel and Fernandes, 1985). Children over 1 year of age must be approached individually depending on the nasopalatal dimensions, because the exposure afforded by the transnasal microsurgical route is progressively compro-

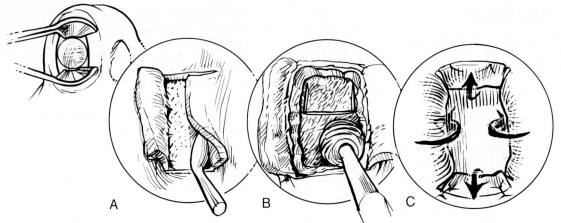

Figure 37–67. In the transnasal approach, the anterior mucosa is incised vertically, with medial and lateral flap elevation *(A)*. After the obstructing plate has been removed with a bur *(B)*, the posterior mucosa is incised horizontally to create superior and inferior flaps *(C)*.

mised as the depth of the nasal cavity increases.

Technique. With an aural speculum held firmly in the nares and the inferior turbinates fractured laterally, the entire atresia plate can be visualized in a 6 × field. In a neonate the inferior origin of an atresia plate is approximately 32 mm from the alar rim, and slopes posteriorly and superiorly to the sphenoid. The mucosa of the anterior face of the atresia plate is incised vertically, followed by medial and lateral flap elevation (Fig. 37–67). The inferomedial aspect of the bony plate is perforated with a 3 mm microsurgical cutting bur. Having penetrated the plate, the bur is brought backward to enlarge the perforation (Fig. 37–68). Repeated posterior to anterior cuts with the bur minimize the risk of injuring cranial structures.

Inferior and medial resection to include the posterior part of the vomer is crucial to achieving a permanent correction (Fearon and Dickson, 1968; Osguthorpe, Singleton, and Adkins, 1982; Samuel and Fernandes, 1985). After adequate bone resection, the posterior mucosa is split horizontally, followed by superior and inferior flap elevation (see Fig. 37–67*C*). These four interdigitating mu-

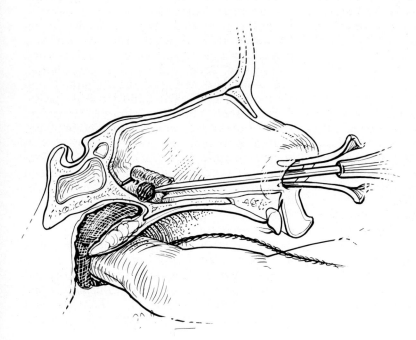

Figure 37–68. A 3 mm bur is introduced through the nares and the bony plate is drilled out. A gauze pack in the nasopharynx cushions the delicate structures in the area.

cosal flaps must be properly positioned and stabilized during obturator placement. A 3.5 to 4.0 mm soft endotracheal tube, cut almost in half, bent into a "U" shape, and fixed together by a suture through the membranous septum, is a satisfactory obturator. The tubes should remain in place for two to three months.

Transpalatal Approach. The transpalatal approach for the correction of choanal atresia is unequivocally endorsed by other authors (Freng, 1978; Theogaraj, Hoehn, and Hagan, 1983; Strome and Hengerer, 1984). Advantages cited include wide surgical exposure, larger fenestra, improved access to the posterior septum, ability to preserve mucosal flaps, decreased stenting time, fewer dilatations following stent removal, and decreased incidence of re-stenosis.

A number of incisions have been proposed (Fig. 37–69) (Brunk, 1909; Steinzeug, 1933; Ruddy, 1945; Wilson, 1957; Owens, 1965). The author prefers a modified Owens incision to gain access to the atretic plate. The exposure allows the superior lateral nasal wall to be approached with the microdrill, thereby effecting the maximal achievable choanal dimension.

Technique. The Dingman mouth gag is inserted for exposure and the palate is infiltrated with 0.5 per cent lidocaine with 1:200,000 epinephrine solution. The incision starts behind the maxillary tuberosity and is continued medially to the alveolar ridge, at which point it is carried cephalad to the canine region and angled back to the nasopalatine foramen (Owens incision). A similar incision is made on the other side (Fig. 37–70). The mucoperiosteal flaps are elevated in the standard manner posterior to the edge of the hard palate, preserving the greater palatine neurovascular pedicle. The nasal mucosa is elevated from the nasal surface of the hard palate with Cronin dissectors, and the posterior edge of the hard palate is removed with a Kerrison punch.

As the nasal cavity is entered, a definite web of bone may be encountered and should be removed to the roof of the nose. Hinged mucosal flaps from both sides of the obstruction are developed. The atretic area is enlarged by removing the posterior part of the palate, vomer, and septum. Additional enlargement is achieved by submucosal modeling of the epipharynx with the microdrill (Freng, 1978). The wall between the nasal cavity, maxillary sinus, and pterygopalatine fossa is made paper-thin to allow for the

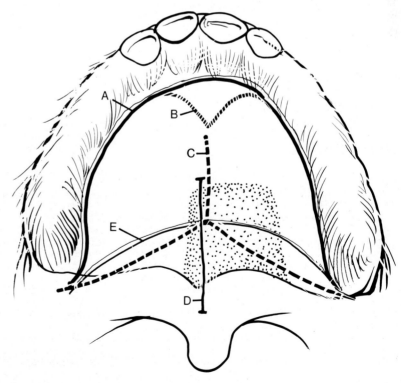

Figure 37–69. Incisions used in the transpalatal approach. *A,* Steinzeug. *B,* Owens. *C,* Wilson. *D,* Brunk. *E,* Ruddy. The dotted area represents the atresia.

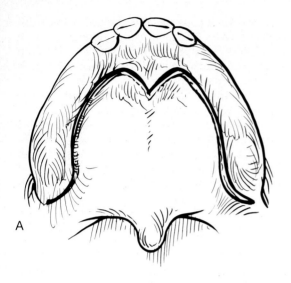

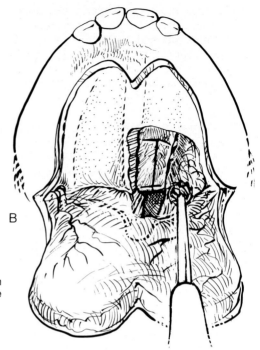

Figure 37–70. *A, B,* The author's preferred incision and flap in the transpalatal approach to the correction of choanal atresia. Note the burring of the bony atresia.

largest possible nasal diameter. The adequacy of removal is confirmed by the passage of a No. 14 French catheter through each nasal passage. The mucosal flaps are used to cover raw surfaces, and the nasal passages are stented with tubes equivalent to the No. 14 or 16 French size. Tubes are left in place for six to eight weeks or until complete epithelization is confirmed.

The development of maxillary hypoplasia and anterior crossbite following a transpalatal approach in infancy is well documented (Freng, 1978) and is attributed to removal of the midpalatal suture.

REFERENCES

Acker, D. W., and Helwig, E. B.: Rhinophyma with carcinoma. Arch. Dermatol., 95:250, 1967.

Antia, N. H.: The scope of plastic surgery in leprosy: a ten-year progress report. Clin. Plast. Surg., 1:69, 1974.

Antia, N. H., and Daver, B. M.: Reconstructive surgery for nasal defects. Clin. Plast. Surg., 8:535, 1981.

Argamaso, R. V.: An ideal donor site for the auricular composite graft. Br. J. Plast. Surg., 28:219, 1975.

Auvert, A.: Selecta praxis medico-chirurgicae quam Mosquae exercet. Tab. 31 and 32. Cancer nasi. 2nd Ed. Parisiis, V. Masson, 1856.

Ballantyne, D. L., and Converse, J. M.: Vascularization of composite auricular grafts transplanted to the chorioallantois of the chick embryo. Transplant. Bull., 5:373, 1958.

Ballantyne, D. L., Uhlschmid, G. K., and Converse, J. M.: Massive rabbit skin xenografts in rats. Transplantation, 7:274, 1969.

Barron, J. N., and Emmett, A. J. J.: Subcutaneous pedicle flaps. Br. J. Plast. Surg., 18:51, 1965.

Barton, F. E., Jr.: Aesthetic aspects of partial nasal reconstruction. Clin. Plast. Surg., 8:177, 1981.

Beare, R. L., and Bennett, J. P.: The naso-labial full thickness graft. Br. J. Plast. Surg., 25:315, 1972.

Beinfield, H. H.: Surgical management of the complete and incomplete bony atresia of the posterior nares. Trans. Am. Acad. Ophthalmol. Otolaryngol., 60:778, 1956.

Beinfield, H. H.: Surgery for bilateral bony atresia of the posterior nares in the newborn. Arch. Otolaryngol., 70:1, 1959.

Blair, V. P.: Reconstruction surgery of face. Surg. Gynecol. Obstet., 34:701, 1922.

Blair, V. P.: Total and subtotal restoration of the nose. J.A.M.A., 85:1931, 1925.

Bouisson, E. F.: De la réparation de l'aile du nez et du contour de la narine. Montpellier Med., 12:128, 1864.

Breach, N. M.: Pre-auricular full-thickness skin grafts. Br. J. Plast. Surg., 31:124, 1978.

Broadbent, N. R., and Cort, D. F.: Squamous carcinoma in longstanding rhinophyma. Br. J. Plast. Surg., 30:308, 1977.

Brown, J. B., and Cannon, B.: Composite free grafts of skin and cartilage from the ear. Surg. Gynecol. Obstet., 82:253, 1946.

Brown, J. B., and McDowell, F.: Plastic Surgery of the Nose. St. Louis, MO, C. V. Mosby Company, 1951.

Brown, O. E., Smith, T., Armstrong, E., and Grundfast, K.: The evaluation of choanal atresia by computed tomography. Int. J. Pediatr. Otorhinolaryngol., 12:85, 1986.

Brunk, A.: Ein neuer Fall von einseitigen knochernem Choanenverschluss. Operationsversuch von Gaumen aus Z. Ohrenheilk., 59:221, 1909.

Burget, G. C.: Aesthetic restoration of the nose. Clin. Plast. Surg., *12*:463, 1985.

Burget, G. C., and Menick, F. J.: The subunit principle in nasal reconstruction. Plast. Reconstr. Surg., *76*:239, 1985.

Burget, G. C., and Menick, F. J.: Nasal reconstruction: seeking a fourth dimension. Plast. Reconstr. Surg., *78*:145, 1986.

Cameron, R. R., Latham, W. D., and Dowling, J. A.: Reconstructions of the nose and upper lip with naso-labial flaps. Plast. Reconstr. Surg., *52*:145, 1973.

Cardoso, A. D.: Loss of columella after leishmaniasis; reconstruction with subcutaneous tissue pedicle flap. Plast. Reconstr. Surg., *21*:117, 1958.

Chait, L. A., Becker, H., and Cort, A.: The versatile costal osteochondral graft in nasal reconstruction. Br. J. Plast. Surg., *33*:179, 1980.

Chitrov, F. M.: Plastic Reconstruction of the Face and Neck Defects with Filatov's Tube Flap. Moscow, Medgiz, 1954.

Conley, J. J., and von Fraenkel, P. H.: The principle of cooling as applied to the composite graft in the nose. Plast. Reconstr. Surg., *17*:444, 1956.

Converse, J. M.: New forehead flap for nasal reconstruction. Proc. R. Soc. Med., *35*:811, 1942.

Converse, J. M.: Composite graft from the septum in nasal reconstruction. Trans. Lat. Am. Congr. Plast. Surg., *8*:281, 1956.

Converse, J. M.: Reconstruction of the nose by the scalping flap technique. Surg. Clin. North Am., *39*:335, 1959.

Converse, J. M.: Clinical applications of the scalping flap in reconstruction of the nose. Plast. Reconstr. Surg., *43*:247, 1969.

Converse, J. M. (Ed.): Reconstructive Plastic Surgery. 2nd Ed. Philadelphia, W. B. Saunders Company, 1977, Chap. 29, pp. 1040–1287.

Converse, J. M., and Wood-Smith, D.: Experiences with the forehead island flap with a subcutaneous pedicle. Plast. Reconstr. Surg., *31*:521, 1963.

Converse, J. M., Wood-Smith, D., and Shaw, W. W.: Congenital choanal atresia. *In* Converse, J. M. (Ed.): Reconstructive Plastic Surgery. 2nd Ed. Philadelphia, W. B. Saunders Company, 1977, pp. 1163–1169.

Crikelair, G. F.: Rhinophyma skin grafts. Plast. Reconstr. Surg., *49*:98, 1972.

Daniel, R. K., Terzis, J., and Schwarz, G.: Neurovascular free flaps—a preliminary report. Plast. Reconstr. Surg., *56*:13, 1975.

da Silva, G.: A new method of reconstructing the columella with a naso-labial flap. Plast. Reconstr. Surg., *34*:63, 1964.

Davis, J. S.: Plastic Surgery—Its Principle and Practice. Philadelphia, P. Blakiston & Son, 1919.

Davis, J. S.: The story of plastic surgery. Ann. Surg., *113*:641, 1941.

Delpech, J. M.: Observation d'opération de rhinoplastique. Rev. Med. Franc., *2*:182, 1824.

Denecke, H. J., and Meyer, R.: Plastic Surgery of Head and Neck. Vol. 1. Corrective and Reconstructive Rhinoplasty. New York, Springer-Verlag, 1967.

Denonvilliers, C. P.: Présentation de malades. Bull. Soc. Chir. Paris, Vol. 5, 1854.

de Quervain, F.: Ueber partielle seitliche Rhinoplastik. Zentralbl. Chir., *29*:297, 1902.

Dhawan, I. K., Aggarwal, S. B., and Hariharan, S.: Use of an off-midline forehead flap for the repair of small nasal defects. Plast. Reconstr. Surg., *53*:537, 1974.

Dieffenbach, J. F.: Die Nasenbehandlung in Operative Chirurgie. Leipzig, F. A. Brockhaus, 1845.

DiGeronimo, E. M.: Make a plan and a pattern for this plan: a useful material. Plast. Reconstr. Surg., *73*:310, 1984.

Dolmans, S., Guimberteau, J. C., and Baudet, J.: The upper-arm flap. J. Microsurg., *1*:162, 1979.

Dufourmentel, C., and Talaat, S. M.: The kite-flap. *In* Hueston, J. T. (Ed.): Transactions of the Fifth International Congress of Plastic and Reconstructive Surgery. Melbourne, Butterworths, 1971, p. 1223.

Dupertuis, S. M.: Free ear lobe grafts of skin and fat. Plast. Reconstr. Surg., *1*:135, 1946.

Eisen, R. F., Katz, A. E., Bohigian, R. K., and Grande, D. J.: Surgical treatment of rhinophyma with the Shaw scalpel. Arch. Dermatol., *122*:307, 1986.

Eisenklam, D.: Rhinophyma; case of carcinomatous degeneration with remarks on the treatment. Wien. Klin. Wochnschr., *44*:1407, 1931.

Elliott, R. A., Jr.: Rotation flaps of the nose. Plast. Reconstr. Surg., *44*:147, 1969.

Elliott, R. A., Jr., Ruf, L. E., and Hoehn, J. G.: Rhinophyma and its treatment. Clin. Plast. Surg., *7*:277, 1980.

Emmett, A. J.: The closure of defects by using adjacent triangular flaps with subcutaneous pedicles. Plast. Reconstr. Surg., *59*:45, 1977.

Esser, J. F.: Gestielte lokale Nasenplastik mit zweizipfligen Lappen, Deckung des sekundaren Defektes vom ersten Zipfel durch den Zweiten. Dtsch. Z. Chir., *143*:385, 1918.

Farina, R.: Deformity of nasal dorsum through loss of substance: correction by bone grafting. Ann. Plast. Surg., *12*:466, 1984.

Farina, R., and Villano, J. B.: Follow-up of bone grafts to the nose. Plast. Reconstr. Surg., *48*:251, 1971.

Farkas, L. G., Hreczko, T. A., and Deutsch, C. K.: Objective assessment of standard nostril types—a morphometric study. Ann. Plast. Surg., *11*:381, 1983.

Farkas, L. G., Kolar, J. C., and Munro, I. R.: Geography of the nose: a morphometric study. Aesth. Plast. Surg., *10*:191, 1986.

Fearon, B., and Dickson, J.: Bilateral choanal atresia in the newborn: plan of action. Laryngoscope, *78*:1487, 1968.

Flake, C. G., and Ferguson, C. F.: Congenital choanal atresia in infants and children. Ann. Otol. Rhinol. Laryngol., *73*:458, 1984.

Fomon, S.: The Surgery of Injury and Plastic Repair. Baltimore, Williams & Wilkins Company, 1939.

Freeman, B. S.: Reconstructive rhinoplasty for rhinophyma. Plast. Reconstr. Surg., *46*:265, 1970.

Freeman, B. S.: Rhinophyma. *In* Converse, J. M. (Ed.): Reconstructive Plastic Surgery. 2nd Ed. Philadelphia, W. B. Saunders Company, 1977, pp. 1185–1192.

Freng, A.: Surgical treatment of congenital choanal atresia. Ann. Otol. Rhinol. Laryngol., *87*:346, 1978.

Fujino, T., Harashina, T., and Nakajima, T.: Free skin flap from the retroauricular regions to the nose. Plast. Reconstr. Surg., *57*:338, 1976.

Galvao, M. S.: A postauricular flap based on the contralateral superficial temporal vessels. Plast. Reconstr. Surg., *68*:891, 1981.

Gan, K. B.: Inner arm flap for the reconstruction of nasal and facial defects. Ann. Plast. Surg., *6*:277, 1981.

Gerrie, J., Cloutier, G. E., and Woolhouse, F. M.: Carved cancellous bone grafts in rhinoplasty. Plast. Reconstr. Surg., *6*:196, 1950.

Gillies, H. D.: Plastic Surgery of the Face. London, Oxford Medical Publications, 1920.

Gillies, H. D.: Deformities of the syphilitic nose. Br. Med. J., *29*:977, 1923.

Gillies, H. D.: Experiences with the tubed pedicle flaps. Surg. Gynecol. Obstet., *60*:291, 1935a.

Gillies, H. D.: The development and scope of plastic surgery. Bull. Northwest. Univ. Med. Sch., *35*:1, 1935b.

Gillies, H. D.: A new free graft applied to the reconstruction of the nostril. Br. J. Surg., *30*:305, 1943.

Gillies, H. D.: The columella. Br. J. Plast. Surg., *2*:192, 1949–1950.

Gillies, H. D., and Millard, D. R., Jr.: The Principles and Art of Plastic Surgery. Boston, Little, Brown & Company, 1957, p. 576.

Goldstein, J. A., Comite, H., Mescon, H., and Pochi, P. E.: Isotretinoin in the treatment of acne: histologic changes, sebum production, and clinical observations. Arch. Dermatol., *118*:555, 1982.

Goldwyn, R. M., and Rueckert, F.: The value of healing by secondary intention for sizeable defects of the face. Arch. Surg., *112*:285, 1977.

Gomez, E. C.: Actions of isotretinoin and etretinate on the pilosebaceous unit. J. Am. Acad. Dermatol., *6*:746, 1982.

González-Ulloa, M.: Restoration of the face covering by means of selected skin in regional aesthetic units. Br. J. Plast. Surg., *9*:212, 1956.

Haberer, J. P. (1917): Quoted in Zoltan, J.: Ersatz der Nasenflugel. Zbl. Chir., *83*:545, 1958.

Hacker, V. von: Zur partiellen und totalen Rhinoplastik Bruns. Beitr. Klin. Chir., *18*:545, 1897.

Hagerty, R. F., and Smith, W. S.: The nasolabial cheek flap. Am. Surg., *24*:506, 1958.

Hall, W. J., Watanabe, T., Kenan, P. D., and Baylin, G.: Transseptal repair of unilateral choanal atresia. Arch. Otolaryngol., *108*:659, 1982.

Halsbergen Henning, J. P., and van Gemert, M. J.: Rhinophyma treated by argon laser. Lasers Surg. Med., *2*:211, 1983.

Hardin, J. C., Jr.: Alar rim reconstruction by a dorsal nasal flap. Plast. Reconstr. Surg., *66*:293, 1980.

Harding, R. L.: Discussion of "Practical management of congenital choanal atresia" by S. D. Theogaraj, J. G. Hoehn, and K. F. Hagan. Plast. Reconstr. Surg., *72*:641, 1983.

Heanley, C.: The subcutaneous tissue pedicle in columella and other nasal reconstruction. Br. J. Plast. Surg., *8*:60, 1955.

Hebra, F.: Versuch einer auf pathologische Anatomie gegrundeten Eintheilung der Hautkrankheiten. Z. der k. k. Gessellschaft der Aerzte zu Wien, Zweiter Jahrg., *B1*:148, 211, 1845.

Hebra, F., and Elfinger, A.: Atlas der Hautkrankheiten. Heft VIII, Taf 6. Wien, aus der k. k. Hof. und Staatsdruckerei, 1856–1876.

Hengerer, A. S., and Strome, M.: Choanal atresia: a new embryologic theory and its influence on surgical management. Laryngoscope, *92*:913, 1982.

Herbert, D. C., and Harrison, R. G.: Nasolabial subcutaneous pedicle flaps. I. Observations on their blood supply. Br. J. Plast. Surg., *28*:85, 1975.

Herceg, S. J., and Harding, R. L.: Gradenigo's syndrome following correction of a posterior choanal atresia. Case report. Plast. Reconstr. Surg., *48*:181, 1971.

Hough, J. V. D.: The mechanism of asphyxia in bilateral choanal atresia: the technic of its surgical correction in the newborn. South. Med. J., *48*:588, 1955.

Israel, J.: Zwei neue Methoden der Nasenplastik. Langenbecks Arch. Klin. Chir., *53*:255, 1896. (Reprinted in Plast. Reconstr. Surg., *46*:80, 1970.)

Ivy, R. H.: Repair of acquired defects of the face. J.A.M.A., *84*:181, 1925.

Jackson, I. T., Smith, J., and Mixter, R. C.: Nasal bone grafting using split skull grafts. Ann. Plast. Surg., *11*:533, 1983.

Jobert, A. J.: Traité de Chirurgie Plastique. Paris, J. B. Baillière & Fils, 1849.

Joseph, J.: Handbuch d. Spezielle Chirurgie. Kats, Preysing, Blumenfeld, 1912.

Joseph, J.: Nasenplastik und sonstige Gesichtsplastik. Leipzig, Kabitzsch, 1931.

Kaplan, E. N., and Pearl, R. M.: An arterial medial arm flap—vascular anatomy and clinical applications. Ann. Plast. Surg., *4*:205, 1980.

Kaplan, I.: Reconstruction of the columella. Br. J. Plast. Surg., *25*:37, 1972.

Kazanjian, V. H.: Plastic repair of deformities about the lower part of the nose resulting from loss of tissue. Trans. Am. Acad. Ophthalmol. Otolaryngol., *42*:338, 1937.

Kazanjian, V. H.: The repair of nasal defects with the median forehead flap. Primary closure of forehead wound. Surg. Gynecol. Obstet., *83*:37, 1946.

Kazanjian, V. H.: Nasal deformities of syphilitic origin. Plast. Reconstr. Surg., *3*:517, 1948.

Kazanjian, V. H., and Converse, J. M.: The Surgical Treatment of Facial Injuries. 2nd Ed. Baltimore, Williams & Wilkins Company, 1959.

Kilner, T. P.: Plastic surgery. In Maingot, R. (Ed.): Postgraduate Surgery. Vol. 3. New York, Appleton-Century-Crofts, 1937.

Koenig, F.: On filling defects of the nostril wall. Berl. Klin. Wochenschr., *39*:137, 1902.

Krauss, M.: Reconstruction of subtotal defects of the nose by abdominal tube flap. Br. J. Plast. Surg., *17*:70, 1964.

Labat, P. A.: De la rhinoplastie, art de restaurer ou de refaire complètement le nez. Thesis, Paris, 1834.

Langenbeck, B. von (1851): Quoted in Joseph, J.: Nasenplastik. Leipzig, Kabitzsch, 1931.

Lexer, E.: Die gesamte Wiederherstellungs-Chirurgie. Leipzig, Johann Ambrosius Barth, 1931.

Limberg, A. A. (1935): Quoted in Zoltan, J.: Ersatz der Nasenflugel. Zbl. Chir., *83*:545, 1958.

Limberg, A. A.: The Planning of Local Plastic Operations on the Body Surface: Theory and Practice. Leningrad, U.S.S.R., Government Publishing House for Medical Literature, 1963. (Translation by Wolfe, S. A., published in Lexington, MA by D. C. Heath, 1984.)

Linehan, J. W., Goode, R. L., and Fajardo, L. F.: Surgery vs electrosurgery for rhinophyma. Arch. Otolaryngol., *91*:444, 1970.

Lisfranc, J.: Rhinoplastie. Clin. Hôp. Paris, *2*:285, 1827.

Liston, S.: "How I do it"—head and neck. A targeted problem and its solution: stenting choanal atresia. Laryngoscope, *90*:1061, 1980.

Loeb, R.: Temporo-mastoid flap for reconstruction of the cheek. Rev. Lat. Am. Cir. Plast., *6*:185, 1962.

Lössen, H.: Über Rhinoplastik mit Einfügen einer Prosthesis. Munch. Med. Wochenschr., *45*:1527, 1898.

MacKee, G. M., and Cipollaro, A. C.: X-rays and Radium in the Treatment of Diseases of the Skin. 4th Ed. Philadelphia, Lea & Febiger, 1946.

Macomber, D. W.: Surgical cure of acne rosacea and rhinophyma. Rocky Mt. Med. J., *43*:466, 1946.

Maillard, G. F., and Montandon, D.: The Washio tempororetroauricular flap: its use in 20 patients. Plast. Reconstr. Surg., *70*:550, 1982.

Makara, L. (1908): Quoted in Zoltan, J.: Ersatz der Nasenflugel. Zbl. Chir., *83*:545, 1958.

Malbec, E. F., and Beaux, A. R.: Reconstruction of columella. Br. J. Plast. Surg., *11*:142, 1958.

Manders, E. K., Schenden, M. J., Furrey, J. A., Hetzler, P. T., Davis, T. S., and Graham, W. P., III: Soft-tissue expansion: concepts and complications. Plast. Reconstr. Surg., *74*:493, 1984.

Maniglia, A. J., and Goodwin, W. J., Jr.: Congenital choanal atresia. Otolaryngol. Clin. North Am., *14*:167, 1981.

Marchac, D., and Toth, B.: The axial frontonasal flap revisited. Plast. Reconstr. Surg., *76*:686, 1985.

Marks, B.: Pathogenesis of rosacea. Br. J. Dermatol., *80*:170, 1968.

Masson, J. K., and Mendelson, B. C.: The banner flap. Am. J. Surg., *134*:419, 1977.

Matton, G., Pickrell, K., Hugher, W., and Pound, E.: The surgical treatment of rhinophyma. An analysis of fifty-seven cases. Plast. Reconstr. Surg., *30*:403, 1962.

Mazzola, R. F., and Marcus, S.: History of total nasal reconstruction with particular emphasis on the folded forehead flap technique. Plast. Reconstr. Surg., *72*:408, 1983.

McCarthy, J. G., Lorenc, Z. P., Cutting, C., and Rachesky, M.: The median forehead flap revisited: the blood supply. Plast. Reconstr. Surg., *76*:866, 1985.

McDowell, F., Valone, J. A., and Brown, J. B.: Bibliography and historical note on plastic surgery of the nose. Plast. Reconstr. Surg., *10*:149, 1952.

McGovern, F. H.: Bilateral choanal atresia in the newborn. A new method of medical management. Laryngoscope, *71*:480, 1961.

McGregor, I. A.: Fundamental Techniques of Plastic Surgery and Their Surgical Applications. Edinburgh, Churchill Livingstone, 1960, p. 160.

McLaren, L. R.: Nasolabial flap repair for alar margin defects. Br. J. Plast. Surg., *16*:234, 1963.

McLaughlin, C. R.: Composite ear grafts and their blood supply. Br. J. Plast. Surg., 7:274, 1954.

Medawar, P. D.: Notes on problems of skin homografts. Bull. War Med., *4*:1, 1942.

Mendelson, B. C., Masson, J. K., Arnold, P. G., and Erich, J. B.: Flaps used for nasal reconstruction: a perspective based on 180 cases. Mayo Clin. Proc., *54*:91, 1979.

Millard, D. R., Jr.: Nasal fractures. *In* Gillies, H., and Millard, D. R., Jr.: The Principles and Art of Plastic Surgery. Boston, Little, Brown & Company, 1957, p. 575.

Millard, D. R., Jr.: Total reconstructive rhinoplasty and a missing link. Plast. Reconstr. Surg., *37*:167, 1966.

Millard, D. R., Jr.: Hemirhinoplasty. Plast. Reconstr. Surg., *40*:440, 1967.

Millard, D. R., Jr.: Reconstructive rhinoplasty for the lower half of a nose. Plast. Reconstr. Surg., *53*:133, 1974.

Millard, D. R., Jr.: Reconstructive rhinoplasty for the lower two-thirds of a nose. Plast. Reconstr. Surg., *57*:722, 1976.

Millard, D. R., Jr.: Aesthetic reconstructive rhinoplasty. Clin. Plast. Surg., *8*:169, 1981.

Miller, T. A.: The Tagliacozzi flap as a method of nasal and palatal reconstruction. Plast. Reconstr. Surg., *76*:870, 1985.

Morgan, R. F., Sargent, L. A., and Hoopes, J. E.: Midfacial and total nasal reconstruction with bilateral pectoralis major myocutaneous flaps. Plast. Reconstr. Surg., *73*:824, 1984.

Myer, C. M., III, and Cotton, R. T.: Nasal obstruction in the pediatric patient. Pediatrics, *72*:766, 1983.

Natvig, P., Sether, L. A., and Dingman, R. O.: Skin abuts skin at the alar margins of the nose. Ann. Plast. Surg., *2*:428, 1979.

Nélaton, C., and Ombrédanne, L.: La Rhinoplastie. Paris, G. Steinheil, 1904.

New, G. B.: Sickle flap for nasal reconstruction. Surg. Gynecol. Obstet., *80*:597, 1945.

Newsom, H. T.: Medial arm free flap. Plast. Reconstr. Surg., *67*:63, 1981.

Nichter, L. S., Morgan, R. F., and Nichter, M. A.: The impact of Indian methods for total nasal reconstruction. Clin. Plast. Surg., *10*:635, 1983.

Nolan, J. O.: Cryosurgical treatment of rhinophyma. Case report. Plast. Reconstr. Surg., *52*:437, 1973.

Novy, F. G., Jr.: Rhinophyma with carcinomatous degeneration; case. Arch. Dermatol. Syph., *22*:270, 1930.

Odou, B. L., and Odou, E. R.: Rhinophyma. Am. J. Surg., *102*:3, 1961.

Ohmori, K., Sekiguchi, J., and Ohmori, S.: Total rhinoplasty with a free osteocutaneous flap. Plast. Reconstr. Surg., *63*:387, 1979.

Ohtsuka, H., Shioya, N., and Asano, T.: Clinical experience with nasolabial flaps. Ann. Plast. Surg., *6*:207, 1981.

Ollier, L.: Application de l'ostéoplastie à la réstauration du nez; transplantation du périoste frontal. Bull. Gen. Therapeut., *61*:510, 1861.

Ollier, L.: Technique of rhinoplasty. Bull. Mem. Soc. Chir. Paris, *3*:184, 1875.

Orticochea, M.: A new method for total reconstruction of the nose: the ears as donor areas. Br. J. Plast. Surg., *24*:225, 1971.

Orticochea, M.: Refined technique for reconstructing the whole nose with the conchas of the ears. Br. J. Plast. Surg., *33*:68, 1980.

Ortiz-Monasterio, F.: Labat and the three-lobed forehead flap (letter to the editor). Plast. Reconstr. Surg., *73*:705, 1984.

Osguthorpe, J. D., Singleton, G. T., and Adkins, W. Y.: The surgical approach to bilateral choanal atresia. Analysis of 14 cases. Arch. Otolaryngol., *108*:366, 1982.

Owens, H.: Observations in treating twenty-five cases of choanal atresia by the transpalatine approach. Laryngoscope, *75*:84, 1965.

Paletta, F. X., and van Norman, R. T.: Total reconstruction of the columella. Plast. Reconstr. Surg., *30*:322, 1962.

Panje, W. R.: A new method for total nasal reconstruction. The trapezius myocutaneous island "paddle" flap. Arch. Otolaryngol., *108*:156, 1982.

Peet, E. W., and Patterson, T. J. S.: The Essentials of Plastic Surgery. Oxford, Blackwell Scientific Publications, 1964.

Pers, M.: Cheek flaps in partial rhinoplasty. Scand. J. Plast. Surg., *1*:37, 1967.

Preindelberger, J.: Zur partiellen Rhinoplastik. Wien Klin. Wochenschr., *11*:587, 1898.

Rawat, S. S., and Sharma, K.: One-stage repair of full-thickness alar defects. Br. J. Plast. Surg., *28*:317, 1975.

Rees, T. D.: Basal cell carcinoma in association with rhinophyma. Plast. Reconstr. Surg., *16*:282, 1955.

Rees, T. D., Wood-Smith, D., Converse, J. M., and Guy, C. L.: Composite grafts. *In* Transactions of the Third International Congress of Plastic and Reconstructive Surgery. Washington, DC, Excerpta Medica Foundation, 1963.

Reiner: Rhinoplastik. Munchen, 1817.

Riefkohl, R., Georgiade, G. S., Barwick, W. J., and Georgiade, N. G.: Rhinophyma: a thirty-five-year experience. Aesth. Plast. Surg., 7:131, 1983.

Rieger, R. A.: A local flap for repair of the nasal tip. Plast. Reconstr. Surg., 40:147, 1967.

Rigg, B. M.: The dorsal nasal flap. Plast. Reconstr. Surg., 52:361, 1973.

Roenigk, R. K.: CO_2 laser vaporization for treatment of rhinophyma. Mayo Clin. Proc., 62:676, 1987.

Ronaldson, T. R.: Note on a case of congenital closure of the posterior nares. Edinburgh Med. J., 26:1035, 1880–1881.

Ruddy, L. W.: A transpalatine operation for congenital atresia of the choanae in the small child or infant. Arch. Otolaryngol., 41:432, 1945.

Samuel, J., and Fernandes, C. M.: Surgery for correction of bilateral choanal atresia. Laryngoscope, 95:326, 1985.

Sawhney, C. P.: A longer angular midline forehead flap for the reconstruction of nasal defects. Plast. Reconstr. Surg., 58:721, 1976.

Schimmelbusch, C.: Rhinoplasty. Verhandl. Dtsch. Gesellsch. Chir., 24:57, 342, 1895.

Schmid, E.: Ueber neue Wege in der plastischen Chirurgie der Nase. Beitr. Klin. Chir., 184:385, 1952.

Schmid, E.: Über die Haut-Knorpel-Transplantationen aus der Ohrmuschel und ihre funktionelle und asthetische Bedeutung bei der Deckung von Gesichtsdefekten. Fortschr. Kiefer Gesichtschir., 7:48, 1961.

Shapshay, S. M., Strong, M. S., Anastasi, G. W., and Vaughan, C. W.: Removal of rhinophyma with the carbon dioxide laser: a preliminary report. Arch. Otolaryngol., 106:257, 1980.

Shaw, M. H., and Fell, S. R.: Columella reconstruction. Br. J. Plast. Surg., 1:111, 1948.

Shaw, W. W.: Microvascular reconstruction of the nose. Clin. Plast. Surg., 8:471, 1981.

Singleton, G. T., and Hardcastle, B.: Congenital choanal atresia. Arch. Otolaryngol., 87:74, 1968.

Slovis, T. L., Renfro, B., Watts, F. B., Kuhns, L. R., Belenky, W., and Spoylar, J.: Choanal atresia: precise CT evaluation. Radiology, 155:345, 1985.

Song, I. C., Wise, A. J., and Bromberg, B. E.: Total nasal reconstruction: a further application of the deltopectoral flap. Br. J. Plast. Surg., 26:414, 1973.

Song, R., Song, Y., Yu, Y., and Song, Y.: The upper arm free flap. Clin. Plast. Surg., 9:27, 1982.

Spear, S. L., Kroll, S. S., and Romm, S.: A new twist to the nasolabial flap for reconstruction of lateral alar defects. Plast. Reconstr. Surg., 79:915, 1987.

Steinzeug, A.: Ein neues Operationsverfaren zur Beseitigung der Choanenverwachsungen. Arch. Ohren Nasen Kehlkopfheilkd., 137:364, 1933.

Strauss, J. S., and Stranieri, A. M.: Changes in long-term sebum production from isotretinoin therapy. J. Am. Acad. Dermatol., 6:751, 1982.

Strome, M., and Hengerer, A. S.: Choanal atresia. Clinical considerations for management. J. Laryngol. Otol., 98:1207, 1984.

Stromeyer (1864): Quoted in Joseph, J.: Nasenplastik. Leipzig, Kabitzsch, 1931.

Tagliacozzi, G.: De Curtorum Chirurgia per Insitionem. Venezia, Bindoni, 1597.

Theogaraj, S. D., Hoehn, J. G., and Hagan, K. F.: Practical management of congenital choanal atresia. Plast. Reconstr. Surg., 72:634, 1983.

Thiersch, C.: Ueber eine rhinoplastiche Modifikation. Verh. Dtsch. Ges. Chir., 8:67, 1879.

Traaholt, L., and Eeg Larsen, T.: Rhinophyma and angiosarcoma of the nose. A case report. Scand. J. Plast. Reconstr. Surg., 12:81, 1978.

Twyman, E. D.: Nose defects, partial. A new modification of the "French" method of restoration with sliding flaps of adjoining tissue. West. J. Surg. Obstet. Gynecol., 48:106, 1940.

Verneuil, A.: Mémoires de Chirurgie. Paris, Masson, 1877–1888.

Virchow, R.: Die krankhaften Geschwültse. Berlin, A. Hirschwald, 1863–1867.

Volkmann, R.: Die frontale Rhinoplastik. Verh. Dtsch. Ges. Chir., 3:20, 1874.

von Graefe, C. F.: Rhinoplastik, oder die Kunst den verlust der Nase organisch zu ersetzen in ihren früheren Verhältnisse erforscht und durch neue Verfahrungsweisen zur höheren Vollkommenheit gefördert. Berlin, Realschulbuchhandlung, 1818.

von Mangoldt, F.: Correction of saddle nose by cartilage transplant. Verhandl. Dtsch. Gesellsch. Chir., 29:460, 1900.

Washio, H.: Retroauricular temporal flap. Plast. Reconstr. Surg., 43:162, 1969.

Washio, H.: Further experiences with the retroauricular temporal flap. Plast. Reconstr. Surg., 50:160, 1972.

Wende, G. W., and Bentz, C. A.: Rhinophyma: a pathological analysis and five separate tumors occurring in the same patient. Cutan. Dis., 22:447, 1904.

Wheeland, R. G., Bailin, P. L., and Ratz, J. L.: Combined carbon dioxide laser excision and vaporization in the treatment of rhinophyma. J. Dermatol. Surg. Oncol., 13:172, 1987.

Wheeler, E. S., Kawamoto, H. K., and Zarem, H. A.: Bone grafts for nasal reconstruction. Plast. Reconstr. Surg., 69:9, 1982.

Wiemer, D. R.: Rhinophyma. Clin. Plast. Surg., 14:357, 1987.

Wilson, C. P.: Treatment of choanal atresia. J. Laryngol. Otol., 71:616, 1957.

Winther, L. K.: Congenital choanal atresia. Anatomic, physiological, and therapeutic aspects, especially the endonasal approach under endoscopic vision. Arch. Otolaryngol., 104:72, 1978.

Yanai, A., Nagata, S., and Tanaka, H.: Reconstruction of the columella with bilateral nasolabial flaps. Plast. Reconstr. Surg., 77:129, 1986.

Young, F.: The repair of nasal losses. Surgery, 20:670, 1946.

Young, L., and Weeks, P. M.: Reconstruction of a large unilateral nasal defect. Ann. Plast. Surg., 1:485, 1978.

Zimany, A.: The bilobed flap. Plast. Reconstr. Surg., 11:424, 1953.

Zoltan, J.: Ersatz der Nasenflugel. Zbl. Chir., 83:545, 1958.

38

Barry M. Zide

Deformities of the Lips and Cheeks

LIPS

Anatomy

The main function of the lip (Fig. 38–1), i.e., oral competence, is controlled by the orbicularis oris muscle. Some fibers of this muscle are primarily oriented horizontally. The horizontal fibers start at the commissures, mingling with other muscle bundles in an area called the *modiolus*. They cross the lip from one commissure to the other, with insertions also into the opposite philtral columns and mucocutaneous junction. These muscle fibers compress the lips together. A more oblique component of orbicularis oris fibers, whose primary action is eversion of the lip, arise also from the commissure region. The oblique fibers travel more upward and medially to insert at the anterior nasal spine, septum, and anterior nasal floor.

The major elevators of the upper lip are the levator labii superioris (LLS), the zygomaticus major, and the levator anguli oris (Freilinger and associates, 1987). The levator originates from the inferior and medial orbital margin. Its fibers run superficially between the small elevator of the ala medially and the levator anguli oris, which arises just below the lateral edge of the LLS (Fig. 38–2). The LLS fibers curve around the alar base over the orbicularis oris to insert into the orbicularis oris fibers and lower philtral column on the ipsilateral side. The zygomaticus major muscle extends from the zygomatic surface at the zygomaticotemporal suture to insert into the modiolus. Three nasalis muscles arise from bone below the piriform apertures (Fig. 38–3). The most medial, the depressor septi, arises from the periosteum over the central and lateral incisors to insert cephalad into the footplates of the medial crura. Some fibers may actually arise superficial to the orbicularis oris fibers. Certain fibers may also bypass the usual insertions into the medial crura and proceed as far as the nasal tip. The function of this muscle relates primarily to depressing the tip of the

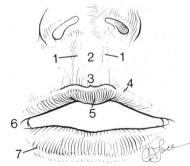

Figure 38–1. Topographic anatomy of the lips. *1,* Philtral columns. *2,* Philtral groove or dimple. *3,* Cupid's bow. *4,* White roll upper lip. *5,* Tubercle. *6,* Commissure. *7,* Vermilion.

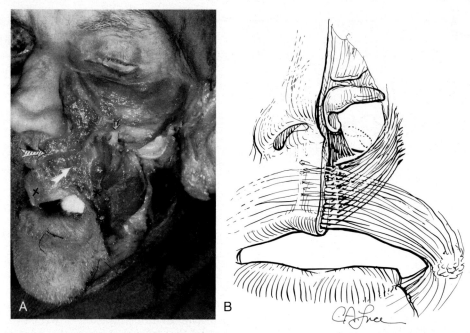

Figure 38–2. *A,* The skin of the left upper lip *(x)* has been reflected to expose the orbicularis oris muscle *(lowest arrow).* This muscle starts at the modiolus *(*)* just lateral to the commissure. The modiolus is the confluence of the cheek and lip muscles at the angle of the mouth. Note the levator labii superioris *(striped arrow),* which inserts into the lower philtral column and the peak of the Cupid's bow. The upper (small) arrow denotes the infraorbital nerve. Note the levator anguli oris muscle, which is medial to the nerve and also inserts into the modiolus. *B,* Lip: basic muscles. The orbicularis oris decussates in the midline. Some fibers continue while others insert into the contralateral philtral columns. The levator muscle helps to form the lower philtral columns and lies superficial to the orbicularis oris. The nasalis (depressor septi) arises from the periosteum over the central and lateral incisors and sometimes from the upper orbicularis fibers to insert into the medial footplates, and occasionally beyond into the nasal tip.

nose, and secondarily to lifting the upper central lip and forming the upper philtral columns. The more lateral nasalis muscles send fibers to the ala as well as to the nasal dorsum.

Elevation and protrusion of the central aspect of the lower lip is caused by the paired mentalis muscles. These muscles, which occasionally possess a firm septum between them, arise from the alveolar periosteum be-

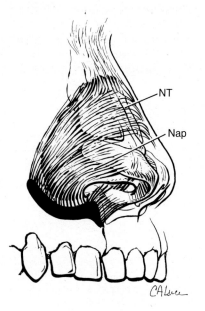

Figure 38–3. The nasalis muscle complex arises from the shaded area below the piriform aperture and over the incisor roots. The nasalis transversus (NT) and nasalis, alar part (Nap) arise from the lateral shaded area. From over the central and lateral incisors the depressor septi arises to insert into the medial footplates, and occasionally it goes between the footplates to insert into the tip. The depressor septi gives bulk to the upper philtral columns while functioning to pull down the tip of the nose.

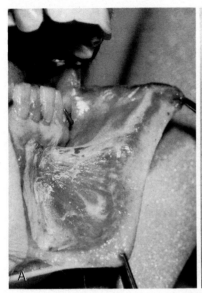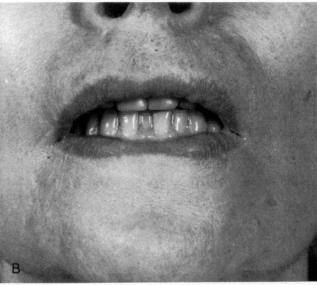

Figure 38–4. *A,* The mentalis muscle arises at the depth of the vestibule from the periosteum over the central and lateral incisor roots. It diverges horizontally and obliquely to insert into the skin of the chin prominence. It elevates the central portion of the lower lip. *B,* This patient had undergone multiple attempts at chin implantation, with subsequent infection. The mucosa is scarred and the mentalis muscle origin is lowered. The lips are incompetent.

low the vestibular sulcus. These muscles descend obliquely to insert into the skin of the chin (Fig. 38–4*A*). They often are hypertrophic in patients with lip incompetence who must voluntarily close their lips at rest (e.g., long face syndrome), causing the chin prominence to be heavily dimpled during use of these muscles. Loss of these muscles by tumor below the labiomental area, mucosal scarring, or inadequate muscle suture technique following degloving results in lip incompetence and lower incisor show (Fig. 38–4*B*).

The depressor labii inferioris (quadratus) arises from the lower border of the mandible between the symphysis and mental foramen. The fibers pass upward and medially, intermingling superiorly and more medially with the orbicularis oris (Fig. 38–5). This muscle displaces the lower lip inferiorly.

The depressor anguli oris (triangularis) arises inferior to the latter muscle and continues upward to the modiolus. At its origin the muscle mingles with the platysma fibers, which also help to draw the angle of the mouth downward and laterally. Functional loss of the latter two muscles, as is seen in marginal mandibular branch (VII) palsy, is manifest as an abnormally elevated lower lip on the affected side while the person is smiling.

The motor nerves to the lip muscles arise from the buccal and marginal mandibular rami of cranial nerve VII. The marginal branches supply the depressors from their inside, but the mentalis is supplied by the marginal branch from the outside (Freilinger and associates, 1987). The buccal branches alone innervate the orbicularis oris muscle. Sensory innervation to the upper lip (see Fig. 38–2) comes from branches of the infraorbital nerve (V^2), while the lower lip is innervated

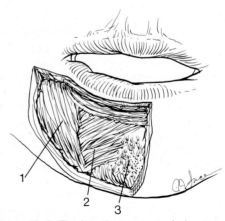

Figure 38–5. The key *depressors* and *elevators* of the lower lip: the depressor anguli oris (1) and depressor labii inferioris muscles (2); the mentalis muscle (3) *elevates* the central portion of the lower lip.

by the mental nerve (V^3), the end branch of the inferior alveolar nerve.

The blood supply to the lips is derived mainly from the facial arteries. On each side the superior and inferior labial arteries arise from the facial vessels to travel tangentially with the orbicularis oris muscles. This fact permits easy mobilization for sufficient muscle flap length without jeopardizing vascularity.

The lymphatic drainage from the lips occurs mainly via submental and submandibular nodes, which may be assessed easily by bimanual palpation. The upper lip drains primarily into the submandibular chain, as does the lateral lower lip. The central segment of the lower lip drains into the submental nodal area with easy crossover from one side to another.

LOWER LIP RECONSTRUCTION

Since the upper lip does not receive direct actinic radiation, only 5 per cent of lip tumors develop in the upper lip, while the lower lip is the site of the remainder (Lee and Wilson, 1970). Ninety per cent of patients with lower lip cancers are male (Wilson and Walker, 1981). It is fortunate that only 2 per cent of tumors involve the commissure, since this area is the most difficult to reconstruct. According to Backus and deFelice (1956) approximately 15.5 per cent show evidence of metastasis on admission to the hospital, and 4.8 per cent develop positive nodes subsequently. The incidence of positive lymph nodes with commissural involvement may be as high as 19 per cent (MacKay and Seller, 1964). Cruse and Radocha (1987) underscored the need for aggressive treatment of squamous cell carcinomas. They noted a decrease in survival from 90 to 50 per cent with positive cervical nodes. When prophylactic suprahyoid dissections were involved with tumor, later radical neck dissection showed positive cervical nodes in 83 per cent of cases. They advocated *wide* excision and 1 cm margins even for the smaller lesions, to minimize local recurrence. This means, of course, that the surgeon would have to employ more flap reconstructions than primary closures with the smaller lesions.

Although the above findings suggest that all lower lip reconstructions result from tumor ablation, they do not, of course. Lip defects may be due to acquired problems such as trauma (e.g., gunshot, auto accident), infectious disease (e.g., noma), vasculitis (e.g., lupus), or congenital nevi, hemangiomas, or clefts. The degree of substance loss may be skin, muscle, or mucosa or a combination of one or all layers.

The history of lip reconstructions for such defects is vast and the most recent relatively complete "who's who" list of lip reconstruction may be easily read (Mazzola and Lupo, 1984b). The following is an abridged version modified from the latter publication:

1000 B.C.	Sushruta	First mention of labial repair.
1597 A.D.	Tagliacozzi	Upper and lower lip repair by distant arm flap.
1768	Louis	First wedge excision and direct suture.
1834	Dieffenbach	Lower lip repair with two inferiorly based cheek flaps lined with mucosa.
1838	Sabbattini	Full-thickness switch flap from lower lip to upper lip.
1845	Dieffenbach	Nasolabial flap for upper lip repair.
1857	von Bruns	Nasolabial flaps for lower lip defect, curvilinear incisions for oral sphincter reconstruction (similar to Karapandzic).
1872	Estlander	Lateral triangular upper lip flap for lower lip reconstruction.
1909	Lexer	Tongue donor tissue for lip reconstruction.
1954	Schuchardt	Sliding inferiorly based cheek flap that pivots around the chin prominence.
1969	Bakamjian	Deltopectoral flap for lower lip defect.
1974	Karapandzic	Emphasis on oral sphincter reconstruction.

The neophyte embarking on lip reconstruction cannot help but be unsure of the ideal method of reconstruction owing to the myriad of proposed surgical methods. For that reason the following is a review of the questions and considerations that should go through the surgeon's mind in choosing a technique.

In an evaluation of the patient, the size of the tumor and thus the width of lip removal must be assessed. The reconstructive method may reduce the size of the oral aperture, and thus the surgeon must consider whether the patient will be able to pass his dentures in and out of the oral cavity. A microstomic result may require considerable postoperative lip stretching (Panje, 1982) or perhaps a denture especially constructed to collapse during insertion or removal. In addition, the dentulous patient must be able to open his mouth sufficiently to provide access for dental repair.

Although lip surgery has little long-term effect on speech (Stranc and Page, 1983), it may leave the lips with reduced sensation and elasticity (Stranc, Fogel, and Dische, 1987). Patients who have reduction of lip sensation in addition to poor sulcus depth have a tendency to lose liquid out of their mouths. This problem, which carries major social implications, is observed more often after lower lip reconstruction than after the repair of upper lip defects. Vestibuloplasty may be required as a secondary procedure.

Many lip repairs that utilize muscle from the adjacent cheek produce a muscle malalignment. The sphincteric action of the lip and thus its power are reduced. Movements of the lip with emotion are somewhat distorted. Reconstructive techniques that use full-thickness nasolabial tissue may also denervate the upper lip muscle to a great degree.

The surgeon must also carefully evaluate the vermilion along the remainder of the lip to determine whether total vermilionectomy is indicated in order to prevent tumor occurrence in the lateral margins. Many of the so-called "English" techniques suggest total vermilionectomy (Bretteville-Jensen, 1973; McGregor, 1983; Stranc and Robertson, 1983; Nakajima, Yoshimura, and Kami, 1984), which requires tongue flaps and thus division and later insetting. Tongue flaps for women should use the underside (ventral) surface so that lipstick can later be placed, whereas the dorsal, more papillated aspect may be adequate in males. Tongue color usually does not match the remaining vermilion and is noticeable at a conversational distance.

Elderly patients with more lax soft tissue may permit the use of transposition, advancement, or rotation flaps to greater advantage than those in the younger age groups (Gullane and Martin, 1983). The lower lip, which has no definitive central structure like the philtral columns of the upper lip, may sustain greater loss and in fact donate large amounts of tissue for upper lip reconstruction before obvious tightness or asymmetry occurs.

Finally, the nature of the tumor and its size play a role in overall therapy. The basal cell carcinomas of the upper lip do not require the same excisional margin as the lower lip tumors. The lower lip tumors present a spectrum of aggressiveness. The anaplastic tumors and commissural lesions often require wide margins and lymph node treatment. Thus, the nature of the cancer determines the reconstructive mode because of its effect on the size of the defect.

Vermilion

When a lesion needs to be excised from the vermilion alone, the surgeon should attempt to excise the mass with a vertical ellipse without crossing into the skin ("white lip"). If the lesion is oriented horizontally and vertical elliptic excision will require extension onto the skin, the transverse excision method should be used. The scar may be visible or tight when the patient stretches the lips, since it is actually in the direction opposite to the lines of relaxed skin tension. If the lesion extends onto the skin or requires extended excision that will include skin, the white roll must be marked with dye before the incision, since the white roll–vermilion junction will be paled by the epinephrine in the local anesthetic solution.

Anesthesia for the lower lip vermilion lesions that extend onto the skin should first include mental nerve block. In most individuals the lower lip sensory nerves can actually be seen before injection and the block need not be aimed at the foramen. By rolling the lower lip outward and stretching the mucosa, the mental nerves may be noted just below the mucosa at the canine root (Fig. 38–6A). If, as in some cases, the nerves are not readily apparent, submucosal infiltration at the apices of the canines into the lower lateral buccal sulcus may be performed. After this is done, blue dye is used to mark the white roll lateral to the incision, which *must cross the skin vermilion junction at 90 degrees* (Fig. 38–6C). Lateral to each line the blue dye is passed into dermis on a 25 gauge needle. The needle may be held in a straight clamp, but usually an applicator stick bud is forced into the needle hub (Fig. 38–6B). The other side of the applicator stick may be carved, dipped in dye, and used to outline the procedure. As stated previously, the marking of the white roll is critical since the direct infiltration of local anesthetic containing epinephrine will obliterate the white roll. A 1 mm discrepancy between skin and vermilion is noticeable at a conversational distance. Often an additional dot or two of blue dye is put into the dermis 1 to 2 mm lateral to the first dot just in case the first dot is inadvertently excised or becomes difficult to see, or frozen section

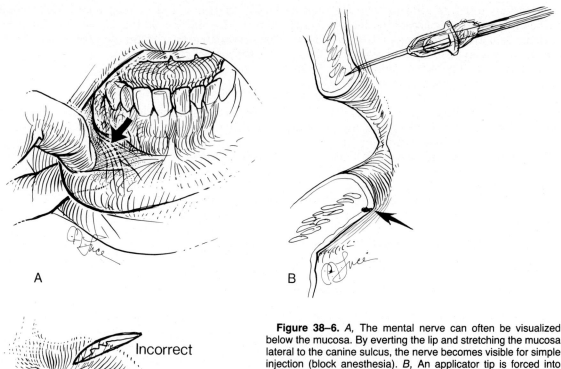

A

B

Incorrect

Correct

C

Figure 38–6. *A,* The mental nerve can often be visualized below the mucosa. By everting the lip and stretching the mucosa lateral to the canine sulcus, the nerve becomes visible for simple injection (block anesthesia). *B,* An applicator tip is forced into the hub of a 25 gauge needle. The needle, dipped in dye, is passed just into the dermis to mark the white roll. This is done after the nerve block but before direct local infiltration with epinephrine, which might obscure the vermilion-skin junction. *C,* Skin-vermilion incisions. Every effort should be made to cross the skin-vermilion border at a 90 degree angle. The white roll is marked with dye prior to local infiltration. Closure is better performed as noted in the lower figure.

findings dictate a wider excision. To block the chin point and region below the labiomental fold, it is necessary to anesthetize more than the mental nerve alone. Bilateral inferior alveolar nerve blocks along the medial border of the mandibular ramus provide sufficient anesthesia (DuBrul, 1980). Even bone surgery at the symphysis may be performed, if necessary.

The classical lip shave operation, or total vermilionectomy, is done for premalignant lesions or widespread carcinoma in situ. The lip vermilion from the mucocutaneous junction to the exposed contact area between upper and lower lips is usually removed. This represents the area directly targeted by the sun's rays (Esmarch and Kowalzig, 1982). In an earlier description of closure, the central lip mucosa was undermined and advanced for closure. Undermining was found to be unnecessary as it led to considerable swelling and ecchymosis. The criticisms of this type of

closure were that the new lower lip did not retain its fullness, that the tense free lip margin was pulled inward, and that the hairs on the lower lip margin were a source of irritation (Kurth, 1957). To prevent these complications, Wilson and Walker (1981) suggested making the advanced mucosa into a bipedicle flap with an incisional release at the depth of the labial sulcus to reduce tension (Fig. 38–7). This method has been taken a step further by including muscle in the advanced flap with a V-Y maneuver to augment the central portion (Kolhe and Leonard, 1988).

Many surgeons suggest vermilionectomy as part of tumor removal since the residual epithelium is unstable. The reconstructions, therefore, make use of tongue or adjacent buccal mucosa to reconstruct the vermilion (Bretteville-Jensen, 1973; Stranc and Robertson, 1983; Nakajima, Yoshimura, and Kami, 1984). Rayner and Arscott (1987) resurfaced

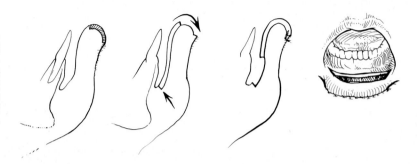

Figure 38–7. The usual vermilionectomy involved excision and primary closure without undermining. Wilson and Walker (1981) modified the procedure with an incisional release in the sulcus (bipedicle flap) to reduce some of the problems associated with simply approximating the wound.

the lower lip with adjacent sensate musculomucosal flaps. When tongue is used to resurface the lip, Wilson and Walker (1981) suggested suturing the tongue laterally to produce a uniform lip. The tongue flap is usually left attached for approximately two weeks, divided and inset a few days after division to allow for swelling to subside. Guerrosantos, Dicksheet, and Ruiz-Ruzura (1985) described a free tongue composite graft for a small lip vermilion defect.

When larger sections of lower vermilion must be excised, a bipedicle mucomuscular upper lip flap may be helpful if the upper lip has sufficient bulk (Converse, 1977).

Notch or whistle deformities of the lower lip that involve vermilion alone are best corrected by excision and Z-plasty, in the same way as clefts made in the lobules of ears (Converse, 1977). A Z-plasty at the edge may be required to reduce the tendency of the indentation to recur (Fig. 38–8).

The vermilion and muscle with its included axial labial artery may be released and used to resurface up to one-half of the lower lip (Goldstein, 1984). This technique may be use-

ful for certain localized lip defects (Fig. 38–9).

Wedge Excisions

Smaller lesions of the lower lip may be corrected by V-excision, but this technique is not optimal since the squamous tumors tend to spread laterally or infiltrate downward (Mazzola and Lupo, 1984a). The tumors should be treated more aggressively. In addition, any V-excision should not cross the labiomental fold since hypertrophic scars tend to occur there. The W-excision allows excision of a wider (approximately 2 cm) section of lower lip, but the inferior incision tends to cross the labiomental fold and result in an unsatisfactory scar. With larger lesions two options are more esthetic, namely, the flared W-plasty (Davidson, Bartlow, and Bone, 1980) or the barrel-shaped excision, which can also be tailored to accommodate more lateral midsized lesions (Fig. 38–10) (Wilson and Walker, 1981).

Larger Central and Paramedian Defects

When the defect involves approximately one-third to three-quarters of the lower lip, multiple techniques may be used. A critical decision that must be made before surgery is whether to remove all the remaining lower lip vermilion, since some techniques require a neovermilion for completion. In addition, certain techniques may be better suited for larger central defects than to the more lateral lip ablations. The surgeon should consider whether a denture can be inserted and removed. Described below are the lip repair techniques that tend to work best, with attendant benefits and disadvantages.

Schuchardt Flap(s) (1954). The so-called barrel-shaped excision may be extended around the labiomental fold to the submental region on each side. The original procedure

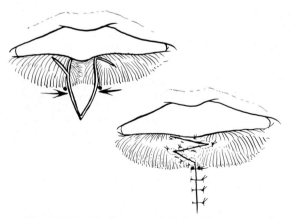

Figure 38–8. Significant notch deformities may require excision and Z-plasty to prevent further retraction. Other methods (Kapetansky, 1971; Spira and Stal, 1983) may also be applicable.

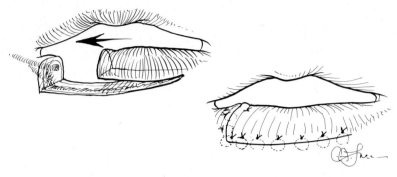

Figure 38–9. A mucomuscular advancement flap may be useful for localized vermilion defects. (Modified after Goldstein, 1984.)

involved the excision of triangles in the submental region to correct for the advancement. This triangular excision may not be necessary since a crescentic compensating excision, as noted, is sometimes possible (Fig. 38–11A). A 40 to 50 per cent lower lip excision may be closed with this method, but a larger defect makes the lip too tight. In some patients, however, this type of closure may not allow insertion of a denture, and the lip may appear tight. In such situations, the upper lip-switch flap (Abbé, 1898) may provide additional tissue (Fig. 38–11B, C, D).

Staircase or Stepladder Technique (Johanson and associates, 1974). This step technique allegedly allows closure of defects of up to two-thirds of the lower lip, although the lip will appear rather tight and the step scars are visible. This type of flap retains relatively good sensation, muscle continuity, and function and may be adjusted for lateral defects as well (Fig. 38–12). Usually two to four steps

are used. This technique, as well as the Schuchardt procedure, works well in conjunction with other methods (Fig. 38–13) (Pelly and Tan, 1981), but the incisions are more noticeable than those of the Schuchardt flap.

Abbé Flap (1898). When lower lip closure exceeds the 30+ per cent that can be closed by barrel-shaped excision or flared W-plasty, a flap from the upper lip may be helpful. Of course, the central portion of the upper lip should not be used for donor tissue, as the philtral columns and dimple are irreplaceable. A switch flap from the junction of the middle and lateral thirds of the upper lip is ideal. The flap can be square or tapered into the nasolabial fold, from which additional tissue can be extracted if required. Before the Abbé flap is incised, four blue dots must be placed on the white roll, one on each side of the incision. The dots on the inside of each incision line allow proper placement of the flap into the defect. The dots outside the Abbé

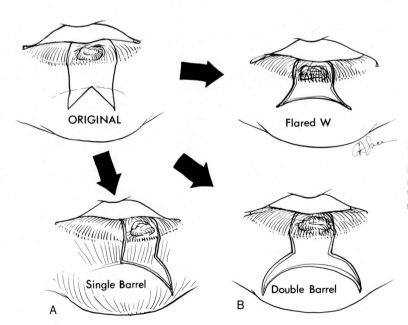

ORIGINAL

Flared W

Single Barrel

A

Double Barrel

B

Figure 38–10. The W-plasty results in a scar that crosses the labiomental fold, often providing a hypertrophic band. Modifications such as the flared W *upper right* or the barrel excisions *(A, B)* yield a more pleasing scar.

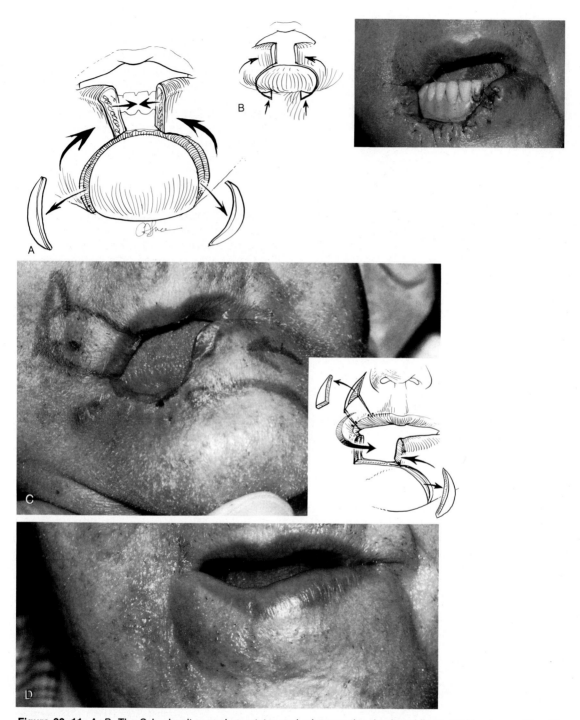

Figure 38–11. *A, B,* The Schuchardt procedure rotates and advances the cheek and lip to provide closure. The skin folds are removed as crescents *(A)* or submental triangles *(B). Inset:* Lip defect immediately after Mohs chemosurgery. *C,* An example of Abbé-type flap and unilateral Schuchardt procedure for reconstruction of the defect several months later. *D,* Final result after correction of minor notching.

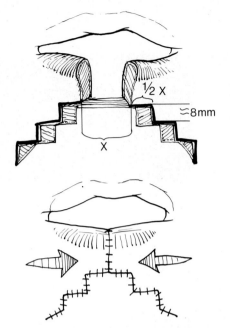

Figure 38–12. The staircase or stepladder method (Johanson and associates, 1974) may be used for both central and lateral defects. Although function and sensation may be preserved, the incisions are usually obvious.

incision lines provide for proper closure (Fig. 38–14). Either side of the flap may be used to carry the artery. The incision through the nonpedicle side should allow the surgeon to see where the labial artery lies within the muscle. The donor site for the Abbé flap should heal with minimal visible scar and rarely requires surgical revision. The flap inset, which is usually done at approximately two weeks, almost always requires secondary surgery owing to the mild discrepancies between the transferred flap vermilion and the vermilion in the area of inset. However, the flap becomes neurotized, as has been demonstrated by electromyographic (EMG) study (Smith, 1960). The flap tends to look biscuit-like or pin-cushioned in the earlier phases of healing after separation, but this tends to decrease in time. Juraha (1980) and Wexler and Dingman (1975) described the use of a double Abbé flap to reconstruct a 75 to 80 per cent central defect of the lower lip. Laterally based switch flaps were designed on each side of the philtral columns. The final results appeared satisfactory and the commissures were preserved. The flaps were left attached for three weeks since they were sutured to each other in the lower lip midline (Fig. 38–15).

Bernard Modification (1853). The original Bernard operation was reported as illustrated in Figure 38–16 (upper small figure). The tumor was removed as a wedge from the central lower lip. Incisions were extended outward from the commissures. Full-thickness triangles removed lateral to the upper lip provided relief space to advance bilateral lower cheek flaps medially. Multiple modifications of this original concept have yielded techniques that provide satisfactory results for larger lower lip defects.

Freeman Modification (1958). Freeman (1958) suggested excising only skin and subcutaneous tissue rather than full-thickness lateral triangles. He also moved the triangular excisions more laterally to conform to the graceful lines of the nasolabial fold. He sutured the muscles at the new labial angle and placed a removable nylon suture to stabilize the commissure.

Webster Modification (1960). See also Fries, 1973; Lentrodt, 1975; Platz and Wepner, 1977; and Wilson and Walker, 1981 (Fig.

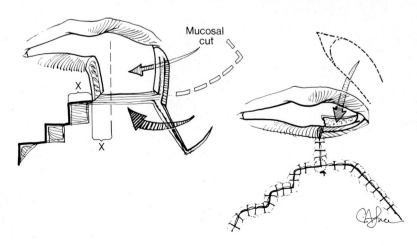

Figure 38–13. Techniques may be combined as noted in Figure 38–11. The stepladder method is illustrated with the method of Pelly and Tan (1981). The vermilion may also be reconstructed with a tongue flap.

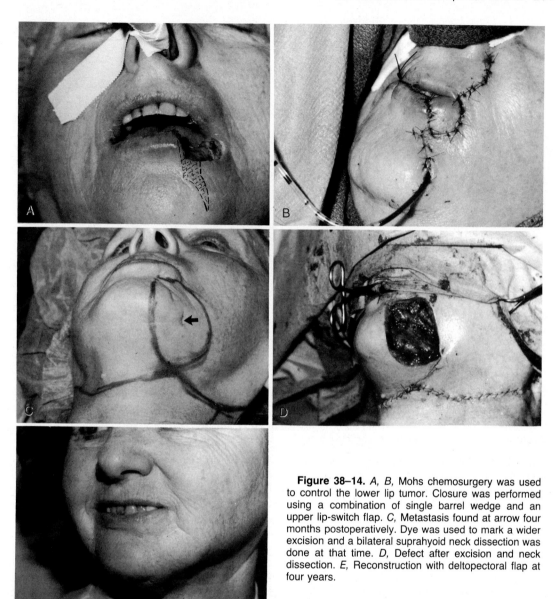

Figure 38–14. *A, B,* Mohs chemosurgery was used to control the lower lip tumor. Closure was performed using a combination of single barrel wedge and an upper lip-switch flap. *C,* Metastasis found at arrow four months postoperatively. Dye was used to mark a wider excision and a bilateral suprahyoid neck dissection was done at that time. *D,* Defect after excision and neck dissection. *E,* Reconstruction with deltopectoral flap at four years.

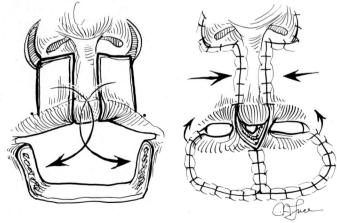

Figure 38–15. The double Abbé flap (Wexler and Dingman, 1975) may be used to close 75 per cent central defects of the lower lip.

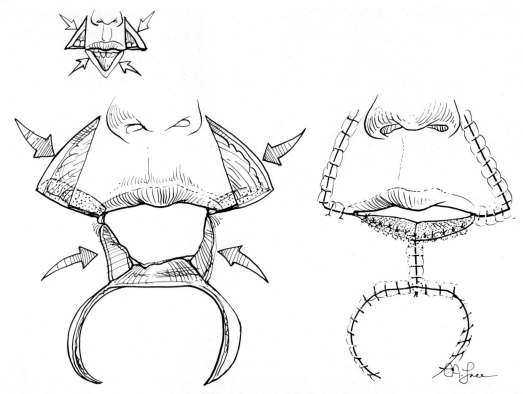

Figure 38–16. *Small figure:* The original Bernard operation used for full-thickness triangular excisions. *Large figures:* The Webster modification (1960) provided major technical advances. Mucosal flaps (stippled) were used for vermilion reconstruction. The nasolabial excisions became partial thickness. Schuchardt flaps facilitated cheek advancement.

38–16). Webster (1960) applied many of the above suggested Freeman (1958) modifications and added additional refinements to provide what he termed the "physiologic" repair. The principles of his reconstructive technique also hold for complete upper lip repairs. The tumor is excised as a quadrilateral segment. Flaps of buccal mucous membrane are left to provide the new vermilion for the lip. The vertical suture lines may be interrupted by Z-plasty. Lapped joint or offset closure methods are applied to prevent notching of the lip. The lower cheek flap incisions are extended inferiorly according to the Schuchardt principle (1954). In this way, innervated muscle is brought into the new lip to provide a sensate, cosmetically superior, watertight, and functioning lip.

The Meyer–Abul-Failat technique (1982) marks the most recent modification of the Bernard procedure and may be applied to 80 per cent defects of the central portion of the lower lip (Fig. 38–17). An upper lip Abbé flap followed by perialar crescents and lateral advancement for upper lip closure may be required for total lower lip reconstruction. In this technique the tumor is excised as a full-thickness trapezium. The mucosal lining for vermilion reconstruction is raised inferior to Stensen's duct, and advanced by excising triangles anterior or posterior to the duct for tension relief. The mucosal incisions are horizontal but not through muscle. The lower skin incisions are made similar to the Schuchardt technique but may be reduced in length for reconstruction of smaller defects. The orbicularis oris muscles at the commissures are not divided, but "pulled out and laterally displaced." Skin resection is performed as triangles at the vermilion border. If the Schuchardt incisions are extended completely around the prominence of the chin, a vertical extension inferiorly may be made to provide access to the submental suprahyoid region for lymph node dissection (Lentrodt, 1975) (see Fig. 38–22). *Any of the above procedures for larger defects may be applied unilaterally for the more laterally positioned lower lip lesions* (Fries, 1973; Platz and Wepner, 1977; Wilson and Walker, 1981).

Estlander --→ Gillies --→ Karapandzic. The Estlander flap (1872) employs a full-

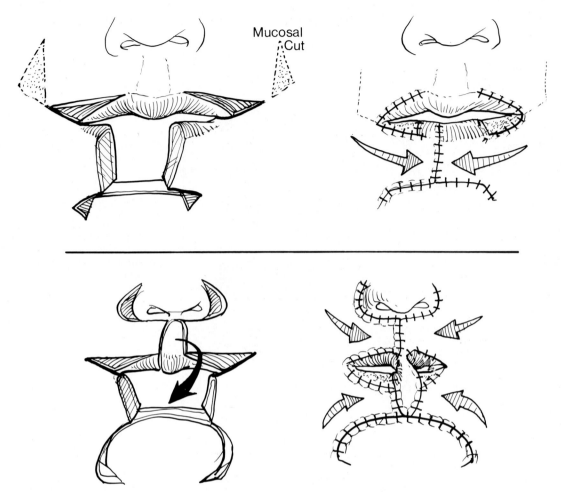

Mucosal Cut

Figure 38–17. Meyer and Abul-Failat (1982). A modification of the Bernard-Webster method involves supravermilion excisions and mucosal back cuts while the muscle is left intact. As noted in the text, a central Abbé flap is used in conjunction with this technique when a defect approaches 80 to 90 per cent of the lower lip width. The author avoids the central Abbé flap whenever possible.

thickness, medially based, triangular *upper* lip flap, which is transferred to reconstruct the lower lateral lip and commissure. Although the oral sphincter is maintained, the shape of the "neocommissure" may require a secondary revision (Fig. 38–18). The Estlander technique works well for reconstruction of lower lip (lateral) defects with minor commissural involvement. Of course, a combined procedure that brings the contralateral lower lip into proper position, e.g., Schuchardt or stepladder technique, could be employed to reduce the size of the defect in preparation for the Estlander flap.

The Gillies fan flap (Gillies and Millard, 1957) and its modifications actually represent an extended version of the Estlander flap (Fig. 38–19). It carries the commissure and lower lateral lip inward for the more medially

located lower lip defects. The commissure is somewhat distorted and the lower lip is shortened.

Karapandzic (1974) and later Jabaley, Clement, and Orcutt (1977) modified the Gillies fan flap to reconstruct 3.5 to 7 cm central lower lip defects. By leaving the neurovascular supply intact, these authors rotated myocutaneous flaps inward to provide a functional lower lip. They provided the proper muscular direction and thus restored the lip sphincter to prevent drooling, with a totally adequate labial sulcus. The scars, however, remain noticeable and the larger reconstructions may leave the patient with a microstomia (Fig. 38–20). The latter may require later prosthetic stretching (Panje, 1982).

McGregor (1983) criticized the classic fan flap as well as its neurovascular modification,

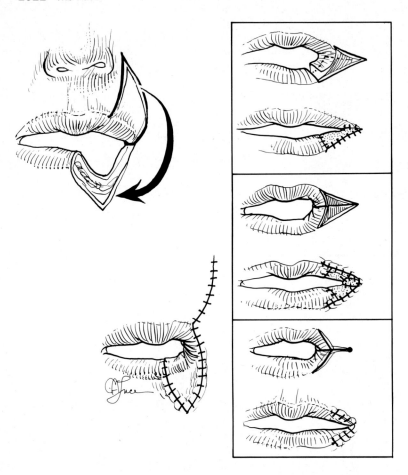

Figure 38–18. The Estlander flap produces a rounded commissure that may require secondary revision. Three methods of commissuroplasty *(insets)* have been proposed, each of which provides only fair results.

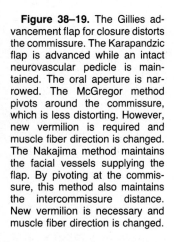

Figure 38–19. The Gillies advancement flap for closure distorts the commissure. The Karapandzic flap is advanced while an intact neurovascular pedicle is maintained. The oral aperture is narrowed. The McGregor method pivots around the commissure, which is less distorting. However, new vermilion is required and muscle fiber direction is changed. The Nakajima method maintains the facial vessels supplying the flap. By pivoting at the commissure, this method also maintains the intercommissure distance. New vermilion is necessary and muscle fiber direction is changed.

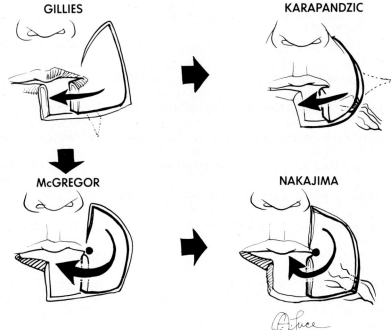

GILLIES

KARAPANDZIC

McGREGOR

NAKAJIMA

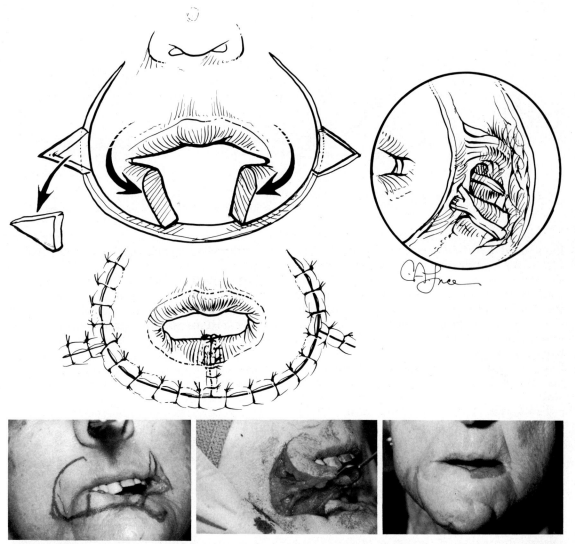

Figure 38–20. The Karapandzic technique (1974) produces a functioning sphincter and may be used bilaterally as noted. Central defects of up to 80 per cent may be reconstructed. *Left,* An 80 year old woman had a verrucous carcinoma that resulted in loss of 75 per cent of the vermilion as well as lip height. The area had been treated by Mohs chemosurgery and allowed to heal partially. *Center,* A right-sided Karapandzic flap and left-sided Pelly-Tan flap were used. Note the preserved vessels. The tongue resurfaces on the left side. *Right,* There is a vast color difference between normal lip and tongue.

because they do not rid the patient of the malignant potential of the remaining lower lip vermilion. Adequate prophylactic treatment should include vermilion lip shave and reconstruction at the time of carcinoma resection. Thus, McGregor modified the fan flap to cope with the problem of damaged vermilion. Both the Gillies fan flap and the McGregor modification contain the superior labial vessels; however, the flap transfer differs. The Gillies fan rotates into position with the resected lip margin sutured to residual medial lip. The advancement of the flap rotates the angle of the mouth along with the flap. The rectangular McGregor modification in contrast pivots around the commissure point, transposing the cut edge upward (Fig. 38–21). Thus, the angle or commissure remains in position, but the transfer leaves the lip devoid of vermilion along the free border of the flap. The preferable method of lip vermilion reconstruction is the tongue flap, used to resurface not only the free flap edge but also the remaining lower lip (McGregor, 1966). The classic fan flaps, their associated neurovascular modifications, and the McGregor

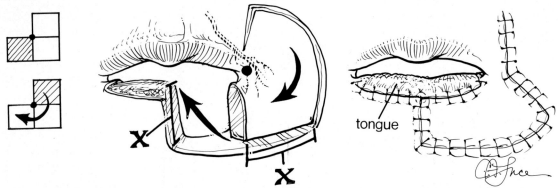

Figure 38–21. The McGregor flap requires an intact labial artery. It pivots around the commissure, thus reducing the microstomia. The tongue may be used to reform the vermilion, which is often removed from the remaining lip as well.

flaps used nasolabial skin for closure. The McGregor modification, of course, changes the direction of the muscle fibers, and thus sphincteric action is not as strong as following the Karapandzic (1974) technique. In addition, since this method denervates the motor and sensory supply of the flap, one might expect more drooling. According to McGregor, however, the sensory loss was not commented on by patients and recovery did "occur slowly."

Nakajima, Yoshimura, and Kami (1984) further modified the McGregor flap by leaving it supplied by the facial artery as opposed to the superior labial vessels (see Fig. 38–19). This allowed the back cut toward the vermilion in the upper lip to be extended. The flap could be made larger and rotated more easily. Stranc and Robertson (1983) designed a similar flap as an island based on the facial vessels and called it the "steeple flap." This flap, in essence a medial nasolabial island, was then "tumbled" into position. Although microstomia was prevented and there was some motor recovery, marked sensory loss occurred in most patients. The published pictures made the flap look like biscuits below the lips, especially during function; the muscle units were obviously misdirected.

Total Lower Lip Reconstruction

Some of the subtotal lip reconstruction techniques may be adapted to total lower lip reconstruction. The Karapandzic procedure may reconstruct 80 per cent central defects. The bilateral McGregor-Nakajima procedures may be used for 90+ per cent defects while pivoting around the remnants of the commissures. The Webster-Bernard technique may

be modified to reconstruct even 100 per cent defects.

Webster-Bernard. As noted above, the original Bernard operation advanced full-thickness local flaps with concomitant triangular excisions to allow proper mobilization. Webster, Coffey, and Kelleher (1960) reported modifications of this technique, which, although applicable for partial lower lip losses, may be extended to full-thickness reconstruction.

The basic technique consisted of the following:

1. Quadrilateral or rectangular resection.
2. Medial advancement of one or two cheek-lip flaps.
3. Excision of skin and subcutaneous tissue only for removal of tissue excesses.
4. Minimal incisions through the muscle laterally.
5. Buccal mucosa flaps for vermilion replacement.
6. Z-plasties on all vertical suture lines.
7. Offset closure to prevent lip notching.

The Webster flap method may be extended to the neck for suprahyoid and submental neck dissection as required (Fig. 38–22) (Lentrodt, 1975).

Nasolabial Variations. Nasolabial flaps and their modifications (Bretteville-Jensen, 1973; Walker and Schewe, 1967; Fujimori, 1980; Wilson and Walker, 1981; Meyer and Abul-Failat, 1982; Stranc and Page, 1983) may be used for total lip reconstruction. Unfortunately, full-thickness nasolabial flap elevation destroys the innervation to the upper lip (Bradley and Leake, 1984). Bipedicled tongue flaps are usually provided for vermilion reconstruction. As noted by Fujimori (1980), who designed arterialized nasolabial

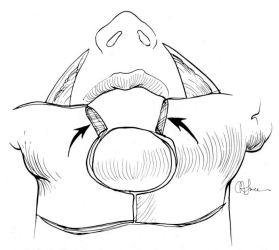

Figure 38–22. Commissural and large lower lip tumors often extend to the submental nodes. The incision for the Webster reconstruction may be carried around the chin prominence to provide access to the neck for lymph node dissection (Lentrodt, 1975).

The final result, although adequate for closure, appeared cosmetically inferior to the Bernard technique. In this case, however, more normal tissue would have been sacrificed to provide room for the usual Bernard technique. When the lower lip lesion is extensive, neck visor flaps or distant flaps, such as the deltopectoral flap, may be required.

Commissure Reconstruction

The commissure has received relatively little literary attention, probably because the area is difficult to reconstruct. Three methods have been proposed for small defects (approximately 2 cm) at the commissure. The Converse "over and out" flap (1977) involves taking a pedicled upper lip switch flap and moving it laterally instead of into the lower lip. Of course, the neocommissure obtained by this technique is round and must be revised.

The techniques of Zisser (1975) (Fig. 38–24) and Platz and Wepner (1977) (Fig. 38–25) produce a commissure with better definition at the angle. Zisser (1975) excised the tumor as a crescent. The tumor and a safe margin were removed in full-thickness fashion but only partial-thickness triangles were excised superiorly and inferiorly. A horizontal incision through all layers was made lateral to the tumor excision along the lip line for the same length as the excised lip portion. The two triangles were deepithelized and covered with buccal mucosa.

Platz and Wepner (1977) turned the Bernard operation on its side for commissural lesions. Triangular excisions were removed in the submental region and the nasolabial area as well, after advancing inferior and superior cheek flaps to close the defect. More

"gate flaps" (Fig. 38–23), final retouch operations involving Z-plasty and defatting are often necessary when the tissues have become soft and supple. Wilson and Walker (1981) presented a case report of a total lower lip reconstruction by inferiorly based nasolabial flaps that "developed a good functioning lower lip," since these were actually myocutaneous flaps. Although most authors tend to abut the end of one nasolabial flap against the other in either a straight line (Wilson and Walker, 1981) or a staggered line closure (Fujimori, 1980), Meyer and Abul-Failat (1982) developed full-thickness arterialized island flaps that were tunneled subcutaneously and placed sidewise one atop the other (1982). This technique was used for the total lower lip defect that did not extend far inferiorly.

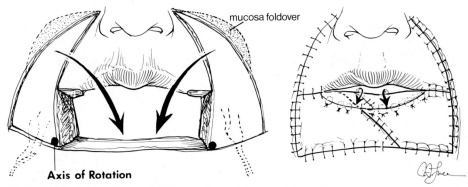

Axis of Rotation

mucosa foldover

Figure 38–23. Fujimori "gate flaps" (1980) may be used for total lower lip reconstruction. Mucosal flaps provide vermilion coverage. The facial vessels are left intact. Revisional operations are usually necessary.

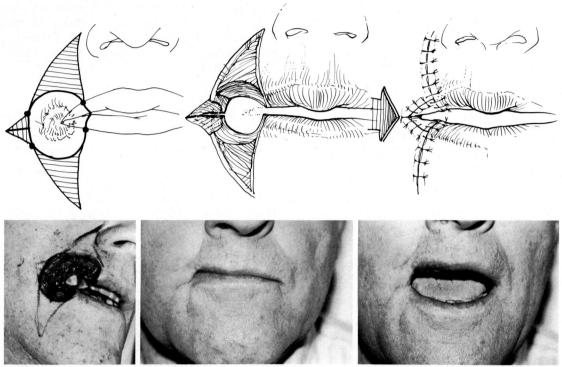

Figure 38–24. *Upper panel,* Commissure reconstruction: Zisser method (1975). The tumor is excised as a vertical crescent. The lateral lip is reformed from cheek tissue located lateral to the defect. *Lower panel,* Mohs chemosurgery defect. *Center* and *right,* Final result.

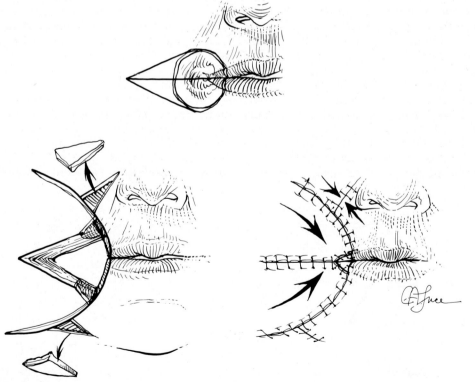

Figure 38–25. Platz and Wepner commissure reconstruction (1977). The tumor is excised as a wedge. Superior and inferior flaps are mobilized for closure. Tissue excess is removed along the upper nasolabial fold and in the submental region.

recently Jackson (1985) reported the use of double rhomboid flaps for commissure reconstruction.

UPPER LIP RECONSTRUCTION

Anesthesia

Although some patients may choose general anesthesia for extirpative or reconstructive lip procedures, local anesthesia is also effective. The entire upper lip may be anesthetized easily by bilateral infraorbital nerve blocks (Fig. 38–26). A 25 or 27 gauge 1 to 1½ inch needle may be passed transcutaneously or transmucosally for block anesthesia. For skin entrance the needle is placed lateral to the alar base and medial to the nasolabial fold. For intraoral injection the needle is passed transmucosally above the canine eminence. The infraorbital foramen, which faces downward and medial, lies about 4 to 7 mm from the inferior orbital rim. The needle need not pass into the foramen to desensitize the lip. Following block anesthesia, a 25 gauge

needle should be dipped in blue dye to mark the white roll exactly on each side of the tumor. This allows proper approximation of the vermilion-cutaneous border after injection and tumor removal.

Vermilion

The vermilion of the upper lip tends to camouflage scars even in the male, who cannot use lipstick. The usual contour of the upper lip is thicker in the central portion owing to the tubercle, but great variation in tubercle size occurs. Whenever possible, excisions should be kept within the vermilion, since incisions into the skin of the lip tend to be more noticeable. In cases of small lesions a vertical ellipse and occasionally a horizontal ellipse, which is the "wrong" direction, may be preferred to extending an incision onto skin ("white lip"), as long as symmetric contour is maintained. If the required excision extends through the white roll, the surgeon should mark the white roll and make elective incisions perpendicular to the ver-

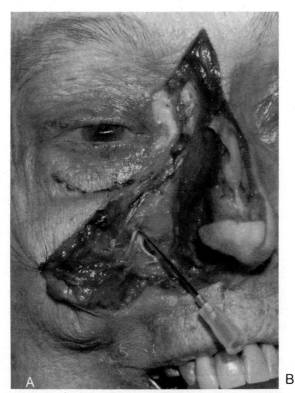 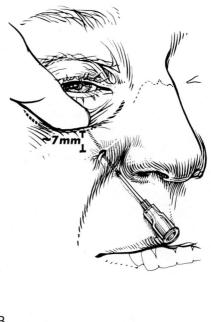

Figure 38–26. *A, B,* Local anesthesia works well for upper lip procedures. The infraorbital nerve block should be performed. The needle is passed into the skin between the upper nasolabial fold and alar base. With the eye looking forward, the needle is directed upward and laterally in a line with the medial limbus. (*A* from Zide, B. M.: Nasal anatomy: the muscles and tip sensation. Aesthetic Plast. Surg., 9:193, 1985.)

milion skin junction as previously discussed. This is especially true for emergency room debridements as well as for removal of any lip lesions.

Whenever a laceration passes through muscle, closure of that layer is required. Such lacerations through vermilion and muscle tend to be firm and look symmetric at first, but the scar droops in time owing to the pull of gravity. *Patients with upper lip incisions, therefore, should always be told that minor vermilion revisions are common.* Placement of sutures exactly into the white roll in both upper and lower lips should be avoided since the subsequent redness tends to blend with the vermilion, making the mucocutaneous junction indistinct.

When deficits of vermilion and muscle are present, the use of local tissue is always preferred. Slight whistle or notching defects, or defects wherein more tubercle might be required, may be helped by double flaps (Kapetansky, 1971), mucomuscular advancement flaps, or simple V-Y advancement of the upper buccal mucosa (Fig. 38–27). When larger areas of vermilion and muscle are required, bipedicle or unipedicle flaps (Kawamoto, 1979) from the lower lip work nicely, as do tongue flaps (Rees, Tabbal, and Aston, 1983) and modified Abbé flaps (Holmstrom, 1987). Of course the lower lip, when used, must be of sufficient size to tolerate the loss. The lip flaps should be left attached for 10 to 14 days before division. In most cases in which exactness of tissue bulk is crucial, the author has used block or general anesthesia via a nasal route without injecting the lip per se. In this way, minimal distortion of the lip occurs from anesthetic solution injection, but the procedure is more time consuming and associated with more blood loss.

Kawamoto (1979) presented a flap for vermilion muscle deficiency, as is frequently seen in hemifacial atrophy. The flap consists of lower lip mucous membrane and muscle, is based centrally, and is tapered beyond one commissure. It is turned upward 180 degrees and sutured into the pre-made defect in the upper lip. The lips are later separated and the inset is performed (Fig. 38–28). The identical defect may also be treated with a tongue flap (Rees, Tabbal, and Aston 1983), although in women the papillated dorsum of the tongue does not match the lip well nor does it accept lipstick in a satisfactory manner. Ortiz-Monasterio and Factor (1980) used tongue flaps for electrical burn reconstruction at the commissure, and Zarem and Greer (1974) reported their use for lower lip electrical injuries.

When the bulk of the white roll is missing, Vecchione (1980) suggested splitting the proposed mucocutaneous junction and placing a free dermis graft subcutaneously.

Smaller Skin and Vermilion Defects

Up to one-quarter of the upper lip may be resected and closed primarily, and in older patients up to one-third of the upper lip could be so handled. Defects that remove the philtrum may leave the lip without a Cupid's bow. This defect may be covered with the mustache in males (Fig. 38–29). In females this defect gives the lip a flattened appearance (see Fig. 38–37).

Low-lying lesions between the philtral columns and more than 0.5 cm medial to the commissure may be treated by many techniques (Fig. 38–30). If the lesion extends across the mucocutaneous border, partial- or full-thickness wedge excision and primary closure may be performed with excellent results. As noted by Spira and Stal (1983), double V-Y advancements may transfer both skin and vermilion into proper alignment

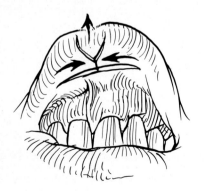
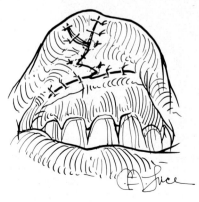

Figure 38–27. For midline whistle deformity or deficiency of the tubercle, a V-Y mucomuscular flap may be advanced. Closure with interdigitating flaps is accomplished with the buccal mucosa behind the advanced flap.

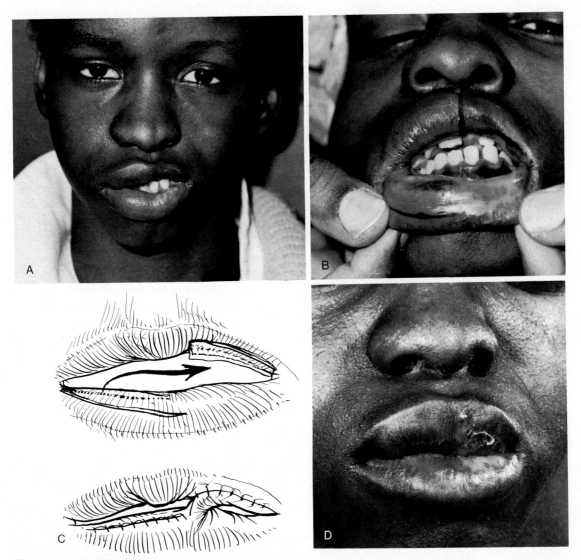

Figure 38–28. *A–D,* Vermilion lip switch (Kawamoto, 1979). Unilateral lip deficiencies may often be treated with a transversely oriented flap as noted. The flap is left attached for 10 to 14 days. The patient demonstrates the procedure for correction of the lip deformity associated with hemifacial atrophy.

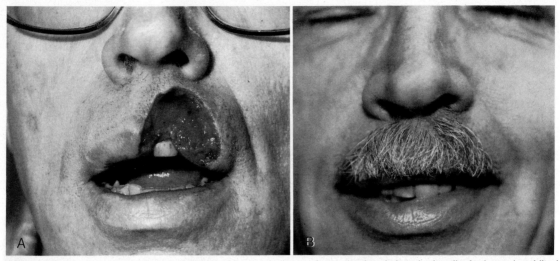

Figure 38–29. *A, B,* One-quarter to one-third of the upper lip may be excised and closed primarily. In the male, philtral distortion is easily concealed with a mustache.

with minimal sacrifice of tissue. Finally a combination of transposition flap and muco-muscular advancement may be performed (Converse, 1977). When the lesion is situated in a lateral position, a lower lip wedge can be used to assist in closure (Zisser, 1975; Madden and associates, 1980) even when 40 per cent or more of the lateral lip requires

reconstruction (Fig. 38–31). This technique is actually a unilateral Webster-Bernard procedure for the upper lip.

Larger Skin Defects/Full Lip Reconstruction

When larger amounts of upper lip skin must be excised, the inferiorly based nasola-

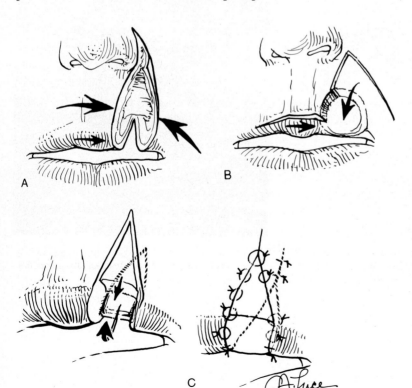

Figure 38–30. Lesions of the skin and vermilion. *A,* Transformation of the lesion into a wedge excision. *B,* Transposition flap closure of the skin defect; muco-muscular flap advancement for vermilion reconstruction. *C,* Inside and outside V-Y advancement flaps.

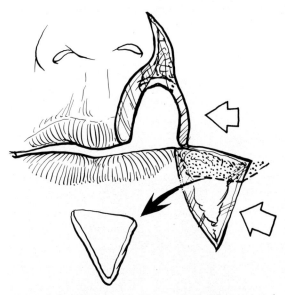

Figure 38–31. Zisser-Madden method. When approximately 40 per cent of the upper lip is excised laterally, a partial-thickness wedge may be excised inferiorly, leaving mucosa for "neovermilion." This, in reality, is an upside-down version of the Webster-Bernard procedure.

bial transposition flap provides excellent donor tissue. The flap brings hairless cheek skin into the lip. In the male, however, this may be noticeable as the beard grows adjacent to the glabrous flap later in the day. However, hairy skin may be brought in by a nasolabial flap when based superiorly (Jackson, 1985). The hair direction will not be proper and a second stage is required to eradicate the dog-ear. Allowing the wound to heal secondarily with subsequent excision often provides the best results in these cases. The hair direction is proper and the scar is minimally visible. The same defect should therefore be handled differently for each sex (Fig. 38–32). When total upper lip skin requires resurfacing, bilateral nasolabial flaps provide an excellent cosmetic result (Fig. 38–33). Burget (in Millard, 1986) championed a tailored nasolabial flap to fill the upper lateral lip esthetic unit even if a less than total unit was removed for the original problem.

The male upper lip requires hair, and multiple techniques for reconstruction may be used. In 1974, Harii, Ohmori, and Ohmori transferred a microvascular scalp flap containing hair to reconstruct half of the upper lip. Walton and Bunkis (1983) transferred by microsurgical techniques sufficient occipital hair to reconstruct total upper lip skin. Tzur, Shafir, and Orenstein (1983) devised a uni-

pedicle or bipedicle neck flap that can be used for reconstruction of the mustache as well as the mucosal lining if required (Fig. 38–34A). Although this technique involves one or more delays, they may all be performed under local anesthesia on an outpatient basis. Hair-bearing scalp flaps may be used in similar fashion. Wilson, Falvao, and Brough (1980) presented many variations of these flaps. The glabrous forehead skin may be used for lining while the scalp provides cover (Fig. 38–34B). The hair may not grow in the right direction, however, and the donor site defect is visible. The bipedicle tongue flap may then be developed to reconstruct the vermilion. The central portion of the upper lip may later be the recipient for an Abbé flap, even in males, as the mustache is usually less full centrally.

The technique of the lip-switch flap from the lower lip to the upper lip should be available to reconstruct full-thickness central defects (Fig. 38–35) as well as lateral defects of approximately half of the lip. Burget and Menick (1986) carried the Abbé lip-switch principle to the maximum by using it to reconstruct one-half of the upper lip. This method (Fig. 38–36) relies on the surgical formation of an esthetic unit for the defect. This topographic unit is then exactly replaced with a replica from the lower lip. Excision of perialar crescents may allow the surgeon to decrease the defect size considerably to accommodate the lip-switch flap. Perialar crescentic excisions and cheek advancement may facilitate closure in defects of 50 to 60 per cent (Fig. 38–37). The lip-switch flaps may be double, quadrilateral, forked, or winged as required to provide sufficient tissue to the upper lip. The lower lip can easily sacrifice 25 to 35 per cent of itself for these reconstructions without a residual functional or cosmetic disability.

Full-thickness nasolabial flaps combined with a lower lip-switch flap have been used for total upper lip reconstruction (Panje, 1982), but the lip appeared tight and required secondary stretching with a prosthesis. The Bernard operation may be easily modified for large full-thickness lateral defects. Large lateral defects of the upper lip may also be closed with lip-switch flaps, or lower triangle excision and sulcal release similar to that illustrated in Figure 38–31 (Zisser, 1975; Madden and associates, 1980). The Bernard operation may be adapted for the *full* upper lip as modified by Fries (1973). Bilateral flaps reconstruct approximately a three-quarters

Text continued on page 2037

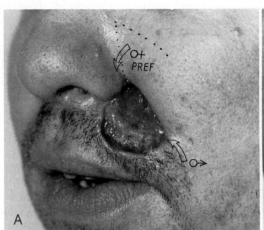
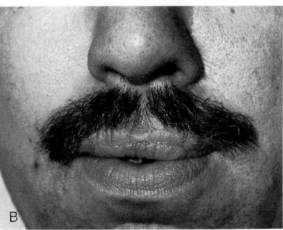

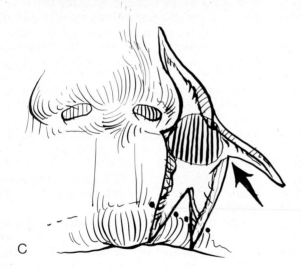

Figure 38–32. *A* to *C,* Males (○→) and females (○+) have different requirements in reconstruction of the upper lip. The nasolabial flap should be avoided in men, or an abnormal hair growth pattern will be obvious later in the day. Advancement from the adjacent lip and cheek brings hair into its proper position (*C*). Additional skin and vermilion should be excised in men below the defect.

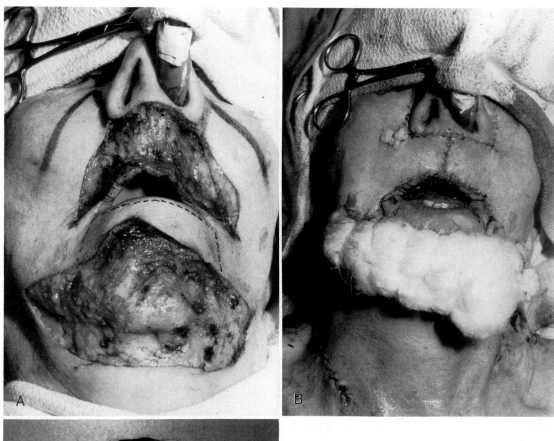

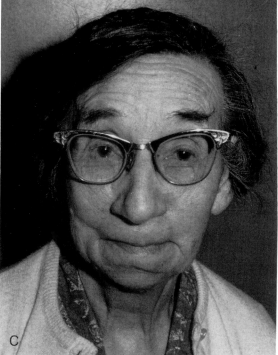

Figure 38–33. *A* to *C,* A woman who suffered radiation injury as an adolescent. The entire upper lip skin was excised and replaced by bilateral nasolabial flaps. The chin would have been better dealt with by total excision along the dotted line, i.e., as an esthetic unit with skin graft coverage (performed with Peter Calamel, M.D.).

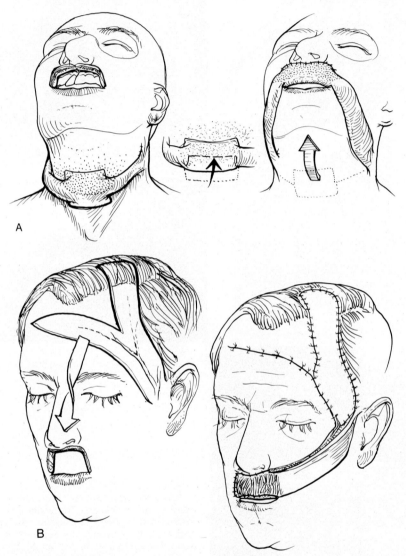

Figure 38–34. *A,* Tzur and associates (1983). When the skin of the upper lip is removed in the male, a delayed neck flap may provide hairy skin. In addition, an inferior extension of glabrous skin may be used for lining (as drawn). The donor defect may be skin grafted and/or closed primarily. *B,* Wilson and associates (1980). The forehead and scalp may be used to provide lining and cover.

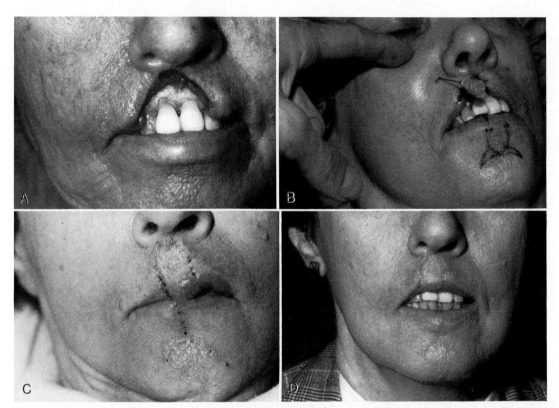

Figure 38–35. Lower to upper lip-switch flap. *A,* Defect after excision; the mucosa was sutured to the skin while all margins were studied. *B,* Flap drawn on the lower lip. Note the *four* white roll dots on the lower lip donor site. Infraorbital nerve block is given bilaterally. Crescents used to adjust the labiomental fold reduce the hypertrophic scar that forms if the fold is crossed. *C,* Switch flap in position at 10 days; separation done at 15 days. *D,* Result at six months.

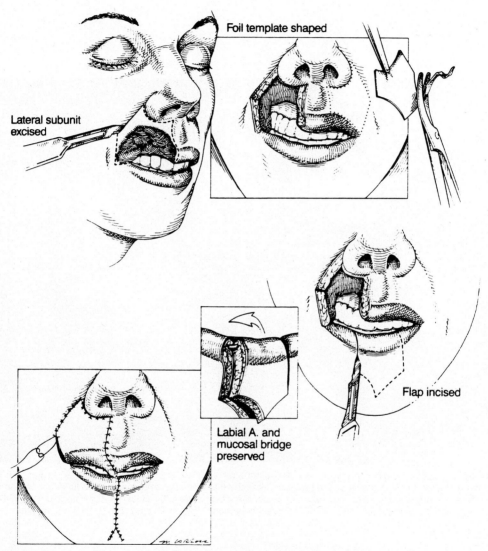

Labels within the figure: Foil template shaped; Lateral subunit excised; Labial A. and mucosal bridge preserved; Flap incised

Figure 38–36. A full-thickness defect occupied half the lateral topographic subunit of the upper lip. The remaining tissues of the lateral topographic subunit were excised. A foil template was cut as an exact replica of the opposite normal lateral subunit. The lip-switch flap was based on a 1 cm bridge of posterior vermilion and mucosa and the marginal labial vessels on the side of the defect. At three months a vermilion excision was performed to achieve symmetry. (From Burget, G. C., and Menick, F. J.: Aesthetic restoration of one-half the upper lip. Plast. Reconstr. Surg., 78:583, 1986.)

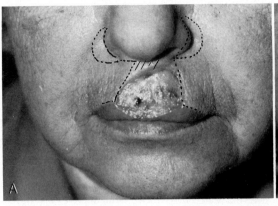
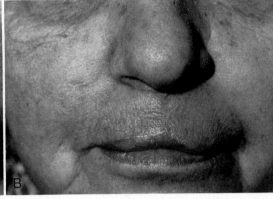

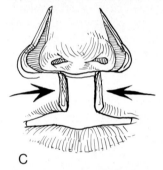
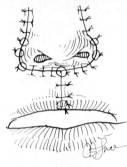

Figure 38–37. *A* to *C,* Perialar crescentic excisions may facilitate closure in both full-thickness and partial-thickness defects of the central upper lip. The Cupid's bow is lost.

C

central defect. In the male, however, non–hair-bearing skin may be transferred from the cheek by means of this method. The patient should be forewarned.

Many methods may be used to reconstruct the philtral dimple, and when available the lower lip-switch flap may provide a satisfactory first choice. However, as noted by Feldman (1984), in burn cases an auricular composite graft removed from between the crura of the antihelix provides the best dimple for philtral reconstruction. An overview of methods of lip reconstruction is presented in Figure 38–38.

CHEEK RECONSTRUCTION

Just as the lips may be subdivided into central, lateral, and commissural reconstruction, so also the cheek may be zoned arbitrarily. Ideally, the best-looking reconstructions for the larger defects involve total esthetic unit replacement (Gonzalez-Ulloa and associates, 1954) (see Chap. 41), but this may not be feasible or desirable for smaller or medium-sized lesions. For the sake of simplicity, the cheek can be divided into three zones (Fig. 38–39): (1) suborbital, (2) preauricular, and (3) buccomandibular. Of course,

Figure 38–38. Overview of methods of repairing upper lip defects. *A,* Lip-switch flap (Abbé). *B,* Advancement cheek flap with perialar crescentic excisions. *C,* Modified Zisser-Madden-Bernard. *D,* Karapandzic method. *E,* Perialar crescent excision combined with a lower lip-switch flap to provide a philtral dimple. *F,* Combination of Karapandzic and lip-switch flap.

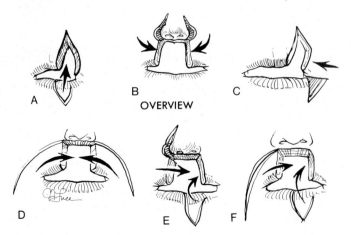

OVERVIEW

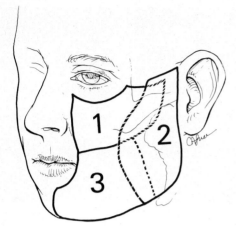

Figure 38–39. Cheek zones. The cheek is arbitrarily divided into three zones: Zone 1 (suborbital), Zone 2 (preauricular), and Zone 3 (buccomandibular). In reality, the zones may overlap considerably. Zone 3 may require lining as well as cover.

these areas overlap somewhat. Certain Zone 3 defects require lining as well as cutaneous cover, and options are provided for that eventuality. The replacement of subcutaneous bulk is also discussed in this chapter.

Zone 1 Defects (Suborbital)

The border of Zone 1 extends along the lateral border of the nose to the nasolabial fold, across the cheek below the gingival sulcus toward the sideburn, up the anterior sideburn to the lateral crow's foot line, and then along the lower eyelid cheek junction. Deep lesions in this area do not require lining as the soft tissue excision will extend to bone or the mucosal excision usually allows primary closure in the upper buccal vestibule.

ANATOMY

As the skin of the lower eyelid extends onto the cheek, it begins to thicken. Subjacent to the cheek skin superiorly are the lower orbital fibers of the orbicularis oculi muscle. Below the lower edge of this muscle are the origins of the quadratus muscle complex, which elevates or pulls the upper lip laterally. More laterally the tendinous origin of the masseter muscle arises from the outer surface of the maxillary buttress. The facial nerve branches lie on the masseter but on the underside of the orbicularis oculi and quadratus muscles (Fig. 38–40).

Skin Grafts

Split-thickness skin grafts do *not* usually work satisfactorily since the contraction involved in wound healing tends to pull down the lower lid. Full-thickness skin grafts, although superior in this respect, may be hidden with make-up or glasses but can be noticeable when applied to defects that are greater than 5 mm in depth. Such full-thickness skin grafts may be harvested from the postauricular, preauricular, or supraclavicular region. Although the texture, color match, and resilience of this skin are excellent, the use of local flap skin produces even better results. Full-thickness skin grafts usually look patchlike on an otherwise ungrafted face. Unless the edges are hidden along natural lines, this is their greatest disadvantage.

The Smaller Flaps

Modified Limberg. For defects of the cheek skin that might result in ectropion

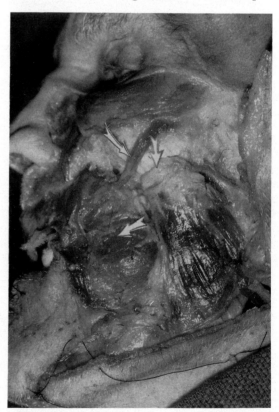

Figure 38–40. Cheek anatomy. The tail of the upper arrow rests on the lower fibers of the orbicularis oculi muscle. The upper arrow points to the zygomaticus major, which overlies the tendinous origin of the masseter muscle. The middle arrow points to the parotid duct below which a large buccal nerve branch (VII) is noted. The lower arrow denotes the buccinator muscle.

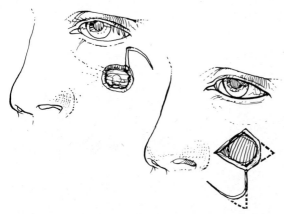

Figure 38–41. When primary closure along relaxed skin tension lines will produce ectropion, local flap closure is indicated. *Left,* Local transposition flap. *Right,* Limberg-type flap. This flap works well when the defect lies over the midcheek or malar prominence, because donor site closure will not pull down the lower eyelid. (Quaba and Sommerlad, 1987.)

after primary closure, a Limberg flap, or some modification, may be used (Quaba and Sommerlad, 1987) (Fig. 38–41). Schrudde and Petrovici (1981) presented a case of a large nevus of the cheek resurfaced with a "swing-slide plasty" (Fig. 38–42), which produced a satisfactory result.

Skin defects over the malar prominence may be dealt with by multiple techniques that use adjacent inferior and posterior cheek skin for resurfacing. A local transposition flap

(Mustardé, 1980) may be sufficient for smaller areas, but this depends on the amount of preauricular skin remaining for the flap. In addition, a preauricular skin graft may be required for the donor site—an obvious drawback of the method.

Ohtsuka, Shioya, and Asano (1981) described the use of an island-type nasolabial flap, medially based, for both medial and lateral Zone 1 reconstructions. Although such subcutaneous pedicle flaps provide reliability and a satisfactory rotational arc (Herbert and DeGeus, 1975; Herbert and Harrison, 1975), the final result always looks bulky. Secondary defatting, peripheral Z-plasties, or steroid injections are required in most cases.

When Zone 1 cheek defects approach 4 × 6 cm in area, the smaller flaps must yield to the cervicofacial flaps. Juri and Juri (1979) described a reconstructive method that required extensive cervical cheek, retroauricular, and chin undermining for flap advancement. The facial portion *was rotated* and *advanced* upward (Fig. 38–43). The Mustardé method used for eyelid repairs in a slightly higher area is primarily a rotation flap (1980). The flap incision can actually be extended onto the chest by extending the incision behind the anterior border of the trapezius, or constructing a bilobed flap by using soft tissue inferoposterior to the ear (Weisberger and Hanke, 1983).

A similar flap may be elevated but based

Figure 38–42. Schrudde and Petrovici (1981). The "swing-slide plasty" takes advantage of the mobility of local tissue to reduce the defect size. The flap may be considerably smaller than the defect.

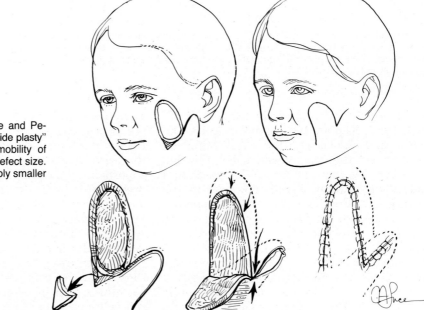

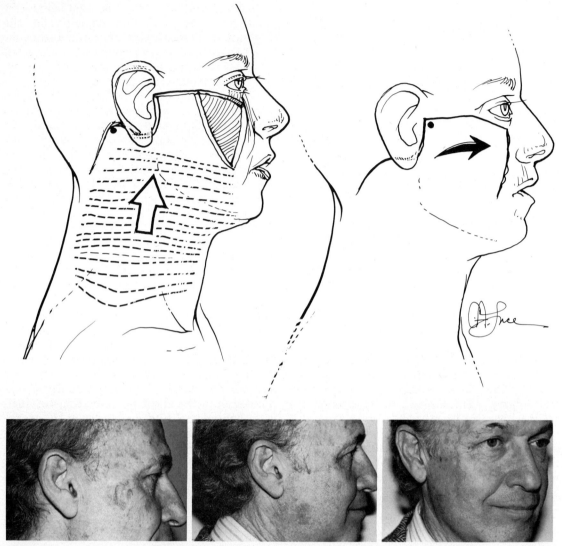

Figure 38–43. Juri and Juri (1979). *Upper panel,* An anteriorly and inferiorly based cervicofacial flap may be widely undermined for rotation and advancement to close the lateral aspect of the suborbital region. *Lower panel, Left,* A 60 year old male with melanoma in situ of the zygomatic area. *Center and right,* Postoperative appearance after resection and closure with a Juri flap.

posteriorly or inferolaterally (Bray and Eichel, 1977; Kaplan and Goldwyn, 1978; Domarus and associates, 1985). Depending on the extent of the upper cheek defect, this flap is formed by incising along the nasolabial fold in an inferior direction lateral to the commissure (Fig. 38–44) across the mandibular border approximately 2 cm anterior to the facial artery notch. From here, if required, the incision curves posteriorly across the submandibular triangle, ending over the sternocleidomastoid muscle approximately 3 fingerbreadths below the mandibular angle (Fig. 38–45). The flap moves superomedially

along the nasolabial fold. The incision across the chin is *cosmetically inferior* to the posterior or inferomedial preauricular incision of the cervicofacial flap. The dissection is kept superficial to the platysma (Kaplan and Goldwyn, 1978), and the incision may extend posterior to the mastoid or earlobe to allow for sufficient flap movement. Ectropion caused by the weight of a flap sutured to the lower eyelid should be avoided by deep anchoring sutures placed around the bony orbit. Closure of the neck defect may require undermining and incision toward the opposite side. Closure should proceed from the poste-

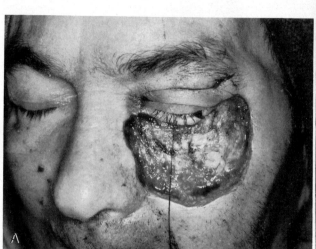
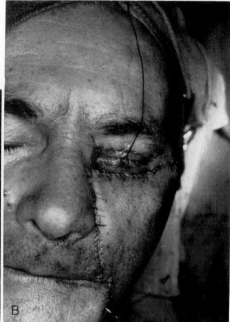
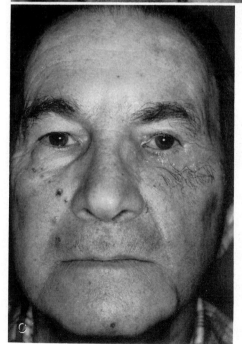

Figure 38–44. Upper suborbital lesions. The lower eyelid skin was replaced with an upper eyelid banner flap. The defect below was covered with an advancement flap. The incision extended along the nasolabial fold and into the submental region. (Courtesy of Dr. Glenn Jelks.)

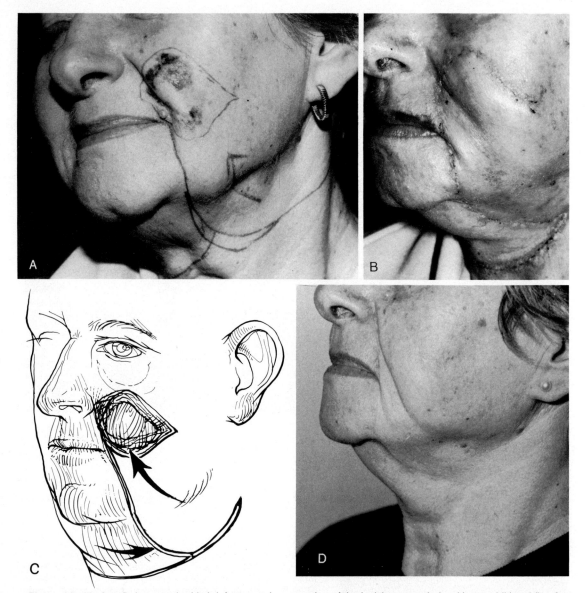

Figure 38–45. *A* to *D*, Lower suborbital defects require extension of the incision posteriorly with an additional flap from the opposite side of the neck to close the resultant defect.

riormost point toward the chin, using the anterior skin flap to achieve closure. Males should be warned that the position of the beard line must be altered. Postoperative positioning of the head in a flexed position reduces the pull on the flap.

Medial reconstructions in Zone 1, an especially difficult area, may also be performed with tissue expansion techniques (see Chap. 13). When there are no time constraints for the reconstruction (e.g., in the case of large nevi or old skin grafts), a large tissue expander may be placed subcutaneously in the cheek via a face lift approach. The reservoir should be placed behind the ear or under the scalp for ease in access and inflation over a two to three month interval to provide sufficient flap tissue for mobilization. The flap must be anchored along the orbital rim to prevent subsequent ectropion (Fig. 38–46).

Zone 2 Defects (Preauricular)

The preauricular region extends from the junction of the helix and the cheek across the

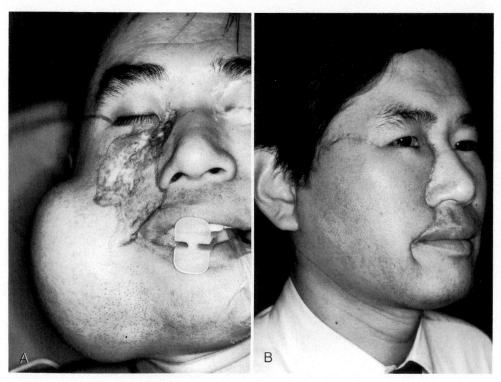

Figure 38–46. *A, B,* Skin expansion. A chronic postirradiation lesion. Expansion and advancement were used to reconstruct the defect resulting from excision. (Courtesy of Dr. Glenn Jelks.)

sideburn to overlap with Zone 1 at the malar prominence. It includes the tissues over the parotid-masseteric fascia and extends inferiorly to the mandibular angle and lower border of the mandible.

Smaller Flaps

Although skin grafts may certainly be used for reconstruction in this area, the laxity of adjacent neck skin, especially in older patients, makes flap closure relatively simple. Advancement flaps, perhaps using a preauricular incision with extension onto the neck, as well as local transposition flaps, provide well-vascularized tissue in sufficient amounts (Fig. 38–47).

Larger Defects

When the cheek defect is much larger in the preauricular area, resurfacing may require a large neck flap. Upper Zone 2 reconstructions may utilize an anteriorly based neck flap (Crow and Crow, 1976), taking advantage of the elastic neck tissue. The distal end of the flap may, if necessary, approach the posterolateral hairline (Fig. 38–48). The flap's design may allow a sufficient amount of tissue to be sutured on a plane between the helical attachment and the lateral brow. This suture level is chosen since placement of the flap at a lower level produces ectropion. As the flap is transposed, a dog-ear may form that can be resected later. The lower level of the flap incision should be just above the clavicle. The donor site may often require skin grafting. A preliminary delay will provide greater reliability. When the defect is in the temporozygomatic area, the flap may be rotated for closure, as opposed to the transposition noted above (Patterson and associates, 1984). This maneuver takes full advantage of the lax neck skin without producing a donor defect.

When the cheek defect in this zone is very large, the medially based cervicopectoral flap (Becker, 1978) offers many advantages (Fig. 38–49). This flap is vascularized by anterior thoracic perforators of the internal mammary artery. As emphasized by Feldman (1984), when this flap is delayed (at least three to four times), the entire cheek may be replaced as an esthetic unit. Becker (1978) noted that the upper border of the flap is determined by the lower border of the excision. From the

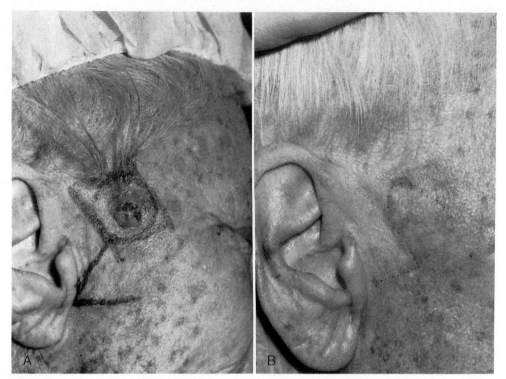

Figure 38–47. *A, B,* Small preauricular defects may be reconstructed by upward cheek advancement or local flap transposition.

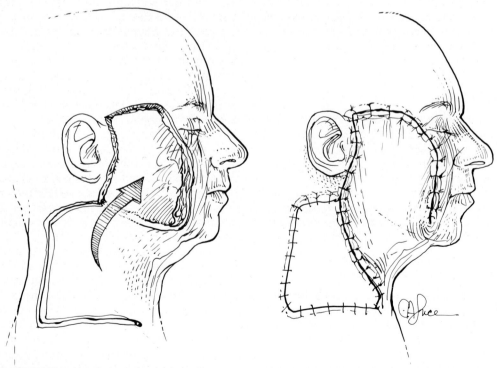

Figure 38–48. If neck and cheek advancement flaps are insufficient to achieve closure, an anteriorly based neck flap can be employed. Preliminary delay reduces the likelihood of partial necrosis of the distal end of the flap. A graft is required to cover the donor site.

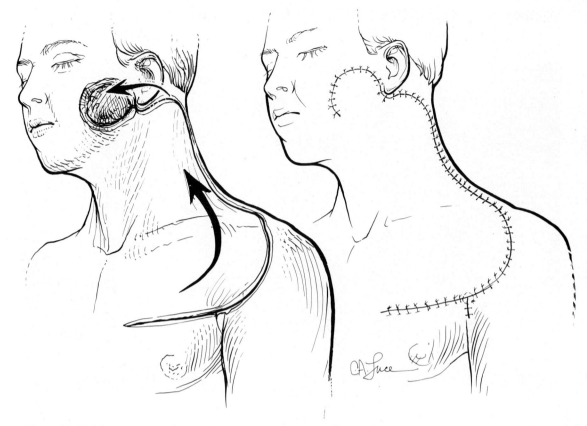

Figure 38–49. The cervicopectoral flap (Becker, 1978) transposes the neck and chest skin in a superior direction for closure of larger lower cheek defects. When possible, delay may help to ensure the viability of the flap, but this is not usually necessary.

posterior limit of the excision, the surgeon marks around the earlobe to the hairline behind the ear. The incision continues along the cervical hairline and passes down a line 2 cm *behind* the anterior trapezius border. The line crosses the acromioclavicular region of the shoulder and along the lateral pectoralis border. The flap edge then passes medially and parallel to the clavicle approximately 3 cm above the male nipple or the third intercostal space. The flap is elevated deep to the platysma muscle and anterior pectoral fascia to provide access for a neck dissection if necessary. The flap is checked for fluorescence after rotation; the dog-ears are trimmed, and suction drainage is placed through the posterior neck skin. A skin graft was not required for donor site closure in either young or older patients.

Multiple regional flaps have been used to resurface this zone and beyond. Examples include (1) a deltopectoral flap, (2) a cervicohumeral flap, (3) a trapezius flap, (4) a pec-

toralis major flap, and (5) a latissimus dorsi flap.

The medially based *deltopectoral flap* (Bakamjian, 1965) provides reliable cover from the shoulder and upper arm region. This flap may need defatting and usually does not require delay. The working end of the flap may be widened considerably by previous expansion (Fig. 38–50), thus allowing primary donor site closure. This flap may thus be used to resurface almost the entire cheek. When staging is not feasible, the deltopectoral flap may be transferred by microvascular anastomoses.

The *cervicohumeral flap* may also be applied to Zone 2 defects, but can also be extended for nasal, Zone 1, and lip defects (Mathes and Vasconez, 1978). This flap, based on the supraclavicular region, extends inferiorly on the lateral aspect of the upper arm. The flap, elevated subfascially and centered over the acromioclavicular joint, rotates around an arc centered where the transverse

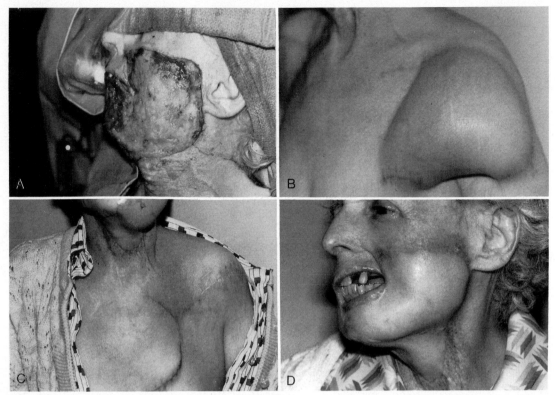

Figure 38–50. Expanded deltopectoral flap. As a delayed cervicopectoral flap may be used for partial cheek resurfacing, an expanded deltopectoral flap may be similarly employed for total cheek resurfacing. *A,* Cheek and chin defect after resection of radiated skin. *B,* 700 ml expander at the distal end of the deltopectoral flap. The flap was delayed also by ligation of the thoracoacromial perforator vessels. The device was expanded eventually to 1000 ml. *C,* Donor site closed primarily. *D,* Flap in place. The right facial nerve paralysis is due to an excision of an anaplastic cancer of the right preauricular area with tumor invading the right parotid gland.

cervical artery and vein enter the trapezius muscle. The poorer color match and less reliable nature of the flap, when not delayed, have not made it part of the usual head and neck reconstructive armamentarium.

The *trapezius muscle flap* may be used to provide bulk or cover with or without scapular bone for head and neck reconstruction (Panje and Cutting, 1980). The most important blood supply for the trapezius muscle is derived from the transverse cervical artery, which usually (in 80 per cent of cases) arises from the thyrocervical trunk. This artery, which passes over the phrenic nerve, the brachial plexus, and the scalenus anterior muscle, divides finally into a superficial and deep branch. The superficial branch runs beneath the fascia on the deep surface of the lateral portion of the trapezius muscle. The deep branch nourishes the posterior trapezius and rhomboid muscles. When not arising from the thyrocervical trunk, the transverse cervical artery usually comes off the subcla-

vian and may pass through the brachial plexus before branching. The venous system that accompanies the artery varies in its drainage and may restrict placement of the flap (Goodwin and Rosenberg, 1982).

The lower trapezius flap may be elevated as an island based on the above blood supply. It can reach the chin (Zone 3), cover exposed mandibular prostheses (Zones 2 and 3), and provide subcutaneous padding (Baek and associates, 1980) after deepithelization. With the patient in the lateral decubitus position, the arm is internally rotated to widen the space between the scapula and the vertebrae. The island is outlined with skin dissection to separate the muscle from the overlying tissue for several centimeters. The flap is elevated (Fig. 38–51), leaving the rhomboid muscles intact. These are adherent to the underside of the trapezius. When the trapezius requires considerable mobilization anteriorly, the eleventh nerve must be sacrificed. For Zone 2 defects, however, the upper trapezius at

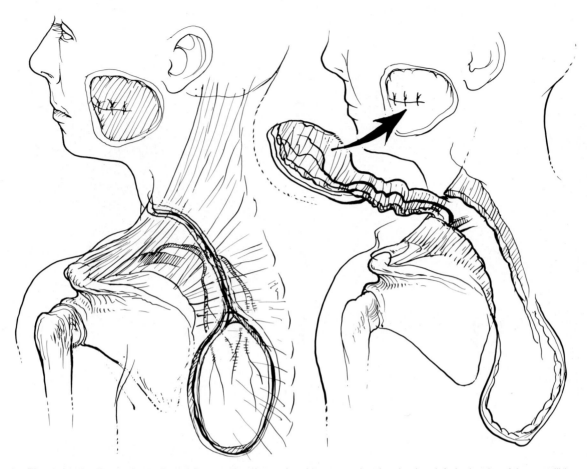

Figure 38–51. The trapezius island flap may be elevated and transposed to the cheek or inferior border of the mandible. The pedicle may require skin grafting or tunneling (Baek and associates, 1980; Panje and Cutting, 1980).

least may be left intact with the reconstruction.

The *pectoralis major myocutaneous flap* provides good quality chest skin for cover and/or cheek lining with minimal morbidity and an acceptable donor site (Ariyan, 1979). The random portion of this flap may actually extend beyond the edge of the muscle to the sternum and opposite perforating vessels. Thus, thin, pliable skin and fascia may be transferred in a cephalad direction to the upper face. In elevating the thinner distal skin beyond the muscle, Baek, Lawson, and Biller (1982) suggested beveling beyond the skin island to include as much subcutaneous tissue as possible under the island. The width of the muscle used to carry the skin may vary from an area just sufficient to carry the major vessel to the entire sternocostal portion. By increasing the amount of muscle, distal skin necrosis may be decreased and there is the more valuable benefit of covering the major

neck vessels. Loss of the pectoralis major muscle is of minimal functional consequence, although some elderly patients may have difficulty in lifting themselves in bed. Baek, Lawson, and Biller (1982) and Sharzer and associates (1981) have reconstructed full-thickness cheek defects with the double-island technique. The proximal island, which rests on muscle, is used for lining, while the distal random extension is folded for the cutaneous portion. The double-paddle technique provides excellent primary reconstruction for through and through cheek defects (Fig. 38–52).

The *latissimus dorsi myocutaneous flap* is technically simple to raise and shows great reliability as both a myocutaneous and free flap. Based on the subscapular thoracodorsal pedicle, which measures 8 to 12 cm in length from the axillary vessel to muscle penetration, this muscle has a sufficient rotational arc to be used for facial reconstruction. The

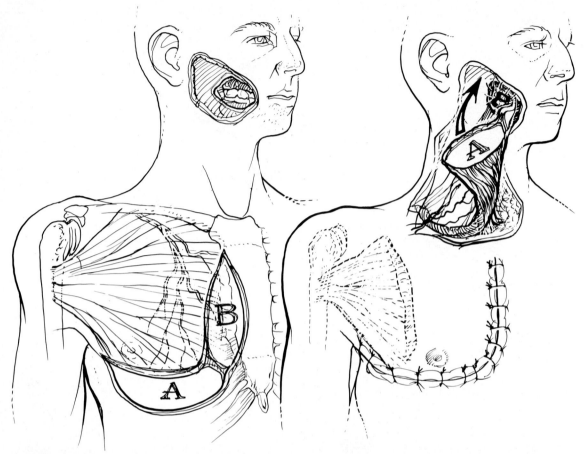

Figure 38–52. The parasternal paddles of the pectoralis major myocutaneous flap may be used to provide both lining *(B)* and cutaneous cover *(A)* (Sharzer and associates, 1981; Baek and associates, 1982).

subscapular trunk arises approximately 0.5 cm below the pectoral humeral junction. The flap may be transferred into the neck by passing the flap via a tunnel over or through the pectoralis major muscle (Quillen, 1979). The exact route should be the shortest and depends on the patient's anatomy. The muscle may require judicious thinning to prevent a bulge in the neck. The island pedicle flap may be used for reconstructions of the cheek, neck, temple, ear, and floor of the mouth, especially following composite resection. Its free flap potential is limitless. This flap may provide unradiated bulk in large quantity from a distant inconspicuous donor site without significant functional loss.

Zone 3 Defects and Variations (Buccomandibular)

Many of the myocutaneous and cutaneous flaps used for surface reconstruction for Zone 2 defects may also be applied to Zone 3 problems. The deltopectoral flap provides excellent thin cheek skin for the lower cheek and neck region; it may, however, require defatting. The cervicohumeral flap does so less reliably. The pectoralis major myocutaneous flap, or even the latissimus dorsi or trapezius myocutaneous flaps, may reach the lower Zone 3 defects. When the surface defects are smaller, simple transposition flaps from the neck, e.g., either the posteriorly or the anteriorly based cervicofacial flap, may provide sufficient cover.

The surgeon must adapt to local requirements in this area, since (1) lining may be required for full-thickness cheek reconstruction, (2) very large areas adjacent to Zone 3 may also need resurfacing, or (3) subcutaneous bulk alone may be required.

LINING

Although the forehead flap may be effectively used for lining (McGregor and Reid,

1970) and for cutaneous cover (Kavarana, 1975; Grewal, Pusalkar, and Hiranandani, 1982), its donor defect is visible and unsightly. It should be reserved as a last possibility, because better, less conspicuous options exist. The other possibilities for lining are (1) tongue, (2) local, hinged turnover flaps, (3) flaps for lining or cover, which may be split or combined (two flaps), or (4) free flaps used for lining or cover, folded or double paddled.

TONGUE

Tongue flaps have been used primarily for cleft palate fistulas or floor of mouth resurfacing. For substantial defects of the cheek, the dorsal flap (Bracka, 1981) rarely provides sufficient tissue or rotational arc for cheek lining. The anatomy of the tongue is such, however, that a hemitongue flap based on one-third or one-half of the tongue may be used (see Chap. 71). This is because the lingual arteries are axial on each side with the anastomoses occurring primarily anteriorly.

As noted by Ganguli (1968), the tongue may be split longitudinally at the two-thirds–one-third junction, back cut, and rotated anteriorly after incising the base. The raw muscular surface of the tongue may be prepared by longitudinal incisions along the long axis. If there is time for two stages, the tongue may be split first and skin grafted. At a second stage it is transposed more easily and directly for providing oral lining.

TURNOVER FLAPS

The use of a subcutaneous pedicle flap (Chongchet, 1977) or hinge flaps, as often employed for nasal reconstruction, may be an alternative to full-thickness cheek defects when the angle of the mouth is involved (Grewal, Pusalkar, and Hiranandani, 1982). For the heavily bearded male, this method may bring hirsute tissue intraorally and thus preclude its use. Coverage of this neolining may be made with a deltopectoral flap, cervicofacial flap, or forehead flap, among others (see Chap. 71).

SKIN FLAPS

Just as the forehead flap may have its end folded on itself for lining and cover, so too may other skin flaps be folded. The deltopectoral flap, long a workhorse for head and neck reconstruction, may be folded primarily or during a preliminary delay stage at the shoulder (Bakamjian, Long, and Rigg, 1971). The pectoralis major myocutaneous flap (Ariyan, 1979) may accomplish the dual task of lining and cover by using a double skin paddle (Sharzer and associates, 1981) (Fig. 38–52) or by vertically splitting its end along the long axis of the flap (Morain and Geurkink, 1980). Either of these flaps may be used to provide lining or cover (McGregor, 1980), although the deltopectoral flap usually has the superior external skin quality (Bunkis and associates, 1982).

McGregor (1981) outlined his "defensive" approach to elevating the pectoralis major flap (Fig. 38–53) to save the deltopectoral for either simultaneous or later back-up use.

Skow (1983) solved the problem of full-thickness cheek defect reconstruction by using the pectoralis major flap for lining while transposing the cervicopectoral flap (Becker, 1978) for cutaneous cover. The outline of the cervicopectoral flap may also be adapted defensively to save the deltopectoral flap for later use (Fig. 38–54).

The lateral trapezius musculocutaneous flap may also be transposed and folded on itself (Guillamondegui and Larson, 1981) for cheek reconstruction. The skin over the shoulder is always pliable. The potential eleventh nerve loss poses a problem, but the excellent blood supply of the flap makes it a good choice for reconstruction of an irradiated bed. Moreover, the additional capability of including an osseous flap component for undelayed reliable mandible reconstruction is obvious (Panje and Cutting, 1980).

The sternocleidomastoid (SCM) flap may be transposed for oral lining, but its reliability is less than ideal. Parkash, Ramakrishnan, and Ananthakrishnan (1980) reported 19 cases of use of the SCM island flap for intraoral lining. Although eight (42 per cent) resulted in orocutaneous fistulas, six were associated with primary closure. As noted by Ariyan and Krizek (1977), the SCM is a *nonaxial* muscle with three separate blood supplies, the occipital artery (superior), the superior thyroid artery (middle), and the thyrocervical trunk (inferior). Jabaley and associates (1979) noted that the number of musculocutaneous branches from the lower "working" third are few and the skin carried on this end is unreliable. In spite of this, Ariyan (1980) suggested using the SCM flap for inner lining while employing a pectoralis

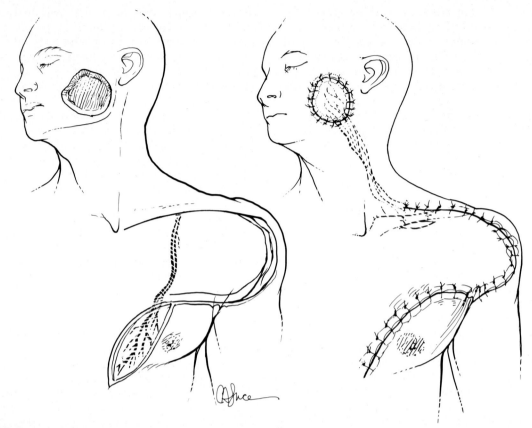

Figure 38–53. The "defensive" method of elevating the pectoralis myocutaneous flap reserves the deltopectoral flap for later use. The deltopectoral flap may also be used for cutaneous cover when the pectoralis is transposed for lining (McGregor, 1981).

major flap tunneled under the skin of the chest and neck for cutaneous cover.

Hurwitz, Rabson, and Futrell (1983) and Coleman, Nahai, and Mathes (1983) presented the anatomic rationale and clinical experience for using the platysma for cheek lining. This flap may be arced on branches of the submental artery as well as on the cutaneous branch of the superior thyroid artery. Platysma flap dissection is tedious but it may also be used to provide mild bulk. According to Hurwitz, Robson, and Futrell (1983), the flap also has motor and sensory capabilities.

FREE FLAPS

Flaps may be split, folded, or double paddled, and microvascular free flaps may also be so treated. Harashina, Imai, and Wada (1979) presented a case in which the omentum was sandwiched between two skin grafts for a full-thickness cheek defect. Harii, Ono, and Ebihara (1982) demonstrated two cases of cheek closure using a double myocutaneous

free flap. The double flap consisted of the latissimus dorsi and serratus anterior based on the common thoracodorsal nutrient pedicle. The serratus anterior was turned into the buccal mucosal defect, while the latissimus dorsi was used to cover the cutaneous defect. The functional deficit was minimal. This same concept of double free flap may be applied using the parascapular and latissimus dorsi territories to surface extra large cheek defects, or when the defect extends far out of the cheek region (Fig. 38–55).

Lining may also be required for the sinus. Fujino, Maruyama, and Inuyama (1981) have folded and doubled the latissimus dorsi for a total cheek defect after radical maxillectomy with orbital exenteration. In addition, a neural anastomosis was performed between the thoracodorsal nerve and a local buccal facial nerve branch in an attempt to maintain bulk and restore the motion of some of the missing muscle.

The use of free flaps for surface defects of the cheek is covered in Chapter 70. Depend-

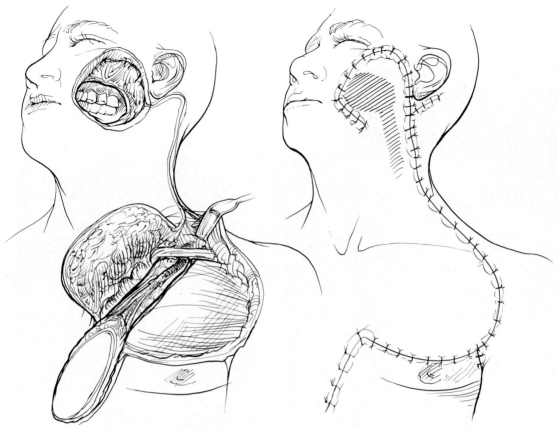

Figure 38–54. Another method of achieving both lining and cutaneous cover of the cheek employs the cervicopectoral flap (Becker, 1978) for cover, again using the pectoralis major flap for lining.

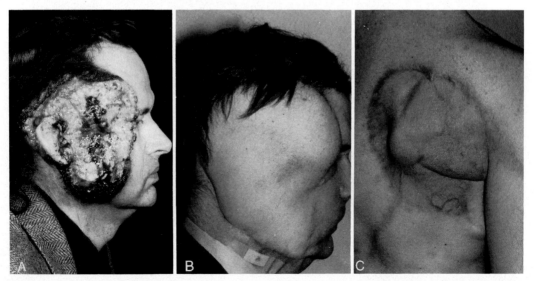

Figure 38–55. *A, B,* Long neglected basal cell carcinoma treated by excision of the right globe and lateral orbit, partial maxillomandibulectomy, total auriculectomy, partial mastoidectomy, and temporal bone excision. The defect was reconstructed by a parascapular-latissimus free flap. The donor site *(C)* required skin grafting. Recurrence was noted at 14 months for which additional radiation was provided. (Case performed with Dr. David Hidalgo.)

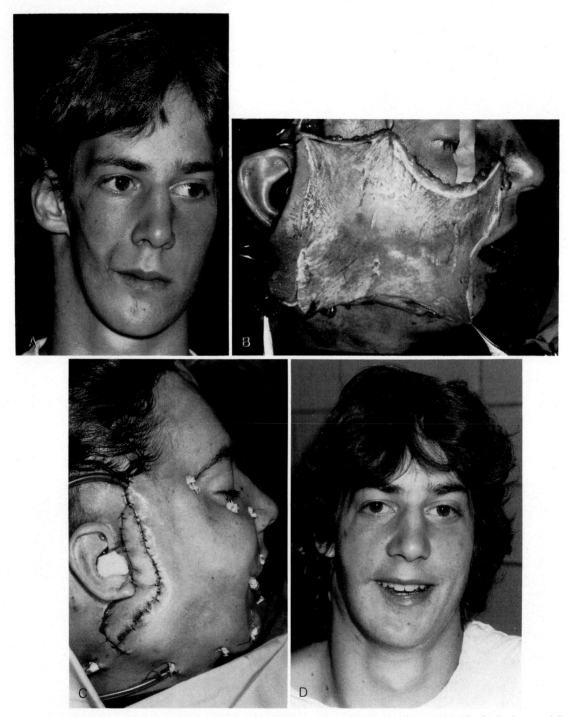

Figure 38–56. *A,* College-aged male with inactive Romberg's disease (hemifacial atrophy). *B,* Groin flap partially deepithelized. *C,* Groin flap in position with monitoring shin paddle in front of the ear. *D,* Final result at two years. The skin paddle was excised subsequently.

ing on the requirements, there are many possibilities, including groin flaps, tensor fascia lata flaps, parascapular flaps, and latissimus dorsi flaps.

Restoration of Cheek Bulk

Hemifacial atrophy (Romberg's disease), scleroderma, lipodystrophic conditions, and the first and second branchial arch syndromes may present with varying degrees of subcutaneous atrophy. Depending on the degree of deformity and the time of onset, the process may affect the cartilaginous or bony substructures of the face. In some situations, bone or cartilage grafts may be successful. The maxillary teeth on the side of involvement often do not erupt, and the alveolar process may be hypoplastic.

The use of silicone liquid to augment small areas remains illegal but somewhat effective. Dermis fat grafts resorb to a large degree, yielding a graft of mainly dermis and little adipose. This technique frequently necessitates a second operation to correct insufficient contour.

Deepithelized free flaps are superior in reconstructing bulk defects of the cheek. The groin flap, superficial inferior epigastric flap, parascapular flap, or deltopectoral flap (Fujino, Tanino, Sugimoto, 1975) may be deepithelized and sutured dermis side down (Shintomi and associates, 1981) or up (Fig. 38–56). The flap must be anchored at the orbital rim as it tends to droop at that area. Fascial strips may also be helpful. Some flap skin must be left exposed in the preauricular area to monitor the postoperative flap vascularity, as well as to provide room for the inevitable edema that occurs in these skin flaps. Deepithelized skin flaps provide a more reliable amount of tissue than free muscle flaps (e.g., rectus, serratus, latissimus, and gracilis) owing to the expected postoperative denervation atrophy that often accompanies such procedures.

Wallace and associates (1979) and Upton and associates (1980) suggested using omentum (see Chap. 63, Fig. 63–30) for subcutaneous deficiency to avoid the "bulky" groin flap that "could not be fashioned." The problem of the short pedicle of the groin flap may be overcome with the parascapular or epigastric flap. The omental transfer seemed better to these authors because of the long pedicle and easy contouring. Upton and associates

divided the cheek into pockets to prevent gravitational droop. The results seemed satisfactory in three patients, although another major problem exists with the omentum. If the patient becomes pregnant or gains weight for any reason, there is increased bulk in the flap in the face. This does not occur with the deepithelized flaps to any great degree. Postoperative sag is much greater with omentum than with deepithelized flaps. Also, laparotomy is required to obtain the omental flap, which results in a midline abdominal scar. Spear and Oldham (1986) showed that the omentum can actually be left pedicled and tunneled to restore bulk to the cheek in a moderate-sized defect.

When the area of subcutaneous loss is primarily preauricular, as may occur after subtotal parotidectomy, a deepithelized pectoralis myocutaneous flap, deltopectoral flap, or trapezius flap may all be successfully used for reconstruction.

REFERENCES

Abbé, R. A.: A new plastic operation for the relief of deformity due to double harelip. Med. Rec., *53*:477, 1898.

Ariyan, S.: The pectoralis major myocutaneous flap, a versatile flap for reconstruction in the head and neck. Plast. Reconstr. Surg., *63*:73, 1979.

Ariyan, S.: Pectoralis major, sternomastoid, and other musculocutaneous flaps for head and neck reconstruction. Clin. Plast. Surg., *7*:89, 1980.

Ariyan, S., and Krizek, T. J.: Reconstruction after resection of head and neck cancer. Cine Clinics. Clinical Congress of the American College of Surgeons, Dallas, TX, October 19, 1977.

Backus, L. H., and deFelice, C. A.: Five year end results in epidermoid carcinoma of the lip with indications for neck dissection. Plast. Reconstr. Surg., *17*:58, 1956.

Baek, S. M., Biller, H. F., Krespi, Y. P., and Lawson, W.: The lower trapezius island myocutaneous flap. Ann. Plast. Surg., *5*:108, 1980.

Baek, S., Lawson, W., and Biller, H. F.: An analysis of 133 pectoralis major myocutaneous flaps. Plast. Reconstr. Surg., *69*:460, 1982.

Bakamjian, V. Y.: A two-stage method of pharyngoesophageal reconstruction with a primary pectoral skin flap. Plast. Reconstr. Surg., *36*:173, 1965.

Bakamjian, V. Y.: Total reconstruction of the pharynx with a medially based deltopectoral skin flap. N.Y. State J. Med., *68*:2771, 1968.

Bakamjian, V. Y., Culf, N. K., and Bales, H. W.: Versatility of the deltopectoral flap in reconstruction following head and neck cancer surgery. *In* Sanvenero-Roselli, G., and Boggio-Robutti, G. (Eds.): Trans. Fourth Int. Congr. Plast. Surg., Rome, 1967. Amsterdam, Excerpta Medica Foundation, 1969, p. 808.

Bakamjian, V. Y., Long, M., and Rigg, B.: Experience with the medially based deltopectoral flap in reconstructive surgery of the head and neck. Br. J. Plast. Surg., *24*:174, 1971.

Becker, D. W.: A cervicopectoral rotation flap for cheek coverage. Plast. Reconstr. Surg., *61*:868, 1978.

Bernard, C.: Cancer de la lèvre inférieure opéré par un procédé nouveau. Bull. Soc. Chir. Paris, *3*:357, 1853.

Bracka, A.: The blood supply of dorsal tongue flaps. Br. J. Plast. Surg., *34*:379, 1981.

Bradley, C., and Leake, J. E.: Compensatory reconstruction of the lips and mouth after major tissue loss. Clin. Plast. Surg., *11*:637, 1984.

Bray, D. A., and Eichel, B. S.: Closure of large nose-cheek groove defects. Arch. Otolaryngol., *103*:29, 1977.

Bretteville-Jensen, G.: Reconstruction of the lower lip after central excisions. Br. J. Plast. Surg., *26*:247, 1973.

Bruns, V. von: Chirugischer Atlas. Bildliche Darstellung der chirurgischen Krankheiten und der zu inrer Heilung erforderlichen Instrumente, Bandagen und Operationen. II. Abt.: Kau- und Geschmaks-Organ. Tables XIII, XIV, XV. Tübingen, Laupp, 1857/1860.

Bunkis, J., Mulliken, J. B., Upton, J., and Murray, J. E.: The evolution of techniques for reconstruction of full-thickness cheek defects. Plast. Reconstr. Surg., *70*:319, 1982.

Burget, G. C., and Menick, F. J.: Aesthetic restoration of one-half of the upper lip. Plast. Reconstr. Surg., *78*:583, 1986.

Caffee, H. H., and Asokan, R.: Tensor fascia lata myocutaneous free flaps. Plast. Reconstr. Surg., *68*:195, 1981.

Chan, S. T. S.: A technique of undermining a V-Y subcutaneous island flap to maximise advancement. Br. J. Plast. Surg., *41*:62, 1988.

Chongchet, V.: Subcutaneous pedicle flaps for reconstruction of the lining of the lip and cheek. Br. J. Plast. Surg., *30*:38, 1977.

Coleman, J. J., III, Nahai, F., and Mathes, S. J.: The platysma musculocutaneous flap: experience with 24 cases. Plast. Reconstr. Surg., *72*:315, 1983.

Converse, J. M.: The "over and out" flap for restoration of the corner of the mouth. Plast. Reconstr. Surg., *56*:575, 1975.

Converse, J. M.: Plastic and Reconstructive Surgery. 2nd Ed. Vol. 3. Philadelphia, W. B. Saunders Company, 1977.

Crow, M. L., and Crow, F. J.: Resurfacing large cheek defects with rotation flaps from the neck. Plast. Reconstr. Surg., *58*:196, 1976.

Cruse, C. W., and Radocha, R. F.: Squamous cell carcinoma of the lip. Plast. Reconstr. Surg., *80*:787, 1987.

Davidson, T. M., Bartlow, G. A., and Bone, R. C.: Surgical excisions from and reconstructions of the oral lips. J. Dermatol. Surg. Oncol., *6*:133, 1980.

Dieffenbach, J. F.: Chirurgische Erfahrungen, besonders über die Wiederherstellung Zerstörter Theile des menschlichen Körpers. Abt. 3, 4. Berlin, Enslin, 1834, p. 101.

Dieffenbach, J. F.: Die Operative Chirurgie. Leipzig, Brockhaus, 1845.

Domarus, H. von, Johanisson, R., and Schmauz, R.: Merkel cell carcinoma of the face. Case report and review of the literature; J. Maxillofac. Surg., *13*:39, 1985.

DuBrul, E.: Sicher's Oral Anatomy. St. Louis, C. V. Mosby Company, 1980.

Eriksson, E., and Johanson, B.: Reconstruction of the oral commissure with Z-plasty. Scand. J. Plast. Reconstr. Surg., *16*:305, 1982.

Esmarch, F. von, and Kowalzig, E.: Chirurgische Technik. Kiel, Lipsius and Tischer, 1982.

Estlander, J. A.: Eine Methode aus der einen Lippe Substanzverluste der anderen zu ersetzen. Arch. Klin. Chir., *14*:622, 1872.

Feldman, J. J.: Reconstruction of the burned face in children. *In* Serafin, D., and Georgiade, N. G. (Eds.): Pediatric Plastic Surgery. Vol. 1. St. Louis, C. V. Mosby Company, 1984.

Franklin, J. D., Newton, E. D., Madden, J. J., and Lynch, J. B.: The deltoid free flap: a refinement in head and neck reconstruction. Plast. Surg. Forum, *4*:95, 1981.

Freeman, B. S.: Myoplastic modification of the Bernard cheiloplasty. Plast. Reconstr. Surg., *21*:453, 1958.

Freilinger, G., Gruber, H., Happak, W., and Pechmann, U.: Surgical anatomy of the mimic muscle system and the facial nerve: importance for reconstructive and aesthetic surgery. Plast. Reconstr. Surg., *80*:686, 1987.

Fries, R.: Advantages of a basic concept in lip reconstruction after tumor resection. J. Maxillofac. Surg., *1*:13, 1973.

Fujimori, R.: "Gate flap" for the total reconstruction of the lower lip. Br. J. Plast. Surg., *33*:340, 1980.

Fujino, T., Maruyama, Y., and Inuyama, I.: Double-folded free myocutaneous flap to cover a total cheek defect. J. Maxillofac. Surg., *9*:96, 1981.

Fujino, T., Maruyama, Y., and Yoshimura, Y.: Primary functional cheek reconstruction: a case report. Br. J. Plast. Surg., *34*:136, 1981.

Fujino, T., Tanino, R., and Sugimoto, C.: Microvascular transfer of free deltopectoral dermal-fat flap. Plast. Reconstr. Surg., *55*:428, 1975.

Ganguli, A.: Use of tongue flap to line cheek defects in surgery for cancer. Plast. Reconstr. Surg., *41*:390, 1968.

Gillies, H., and Millard, R.: The Principles and Art of Plastic Surgery. London, Butterworth, 1957.

Goldstein, M. H.: A tissue-expanding vermilion myocutaneous flap for lip repair. Plast. Reconstr. Surg., *73*:768, 1984.

Gonzalez-Ulloa, M., Castillo, A., Stevens, E., Alvarez Fuertes, G., Leonelli, F., et al.: Preliminary study of the total restoration of the facial skin. Plast. Reconstr. Surg., *13*:151, 1954.

Goodwin, W. J., Jr., and Rosenberg, G. J.: Venous drainage of the lateral trapezius musculocutaneous island flap. Arch. Otolaryngol., *108*:411, 1982.

Grewal, D. S., Pusalkar, A. G., and Hiranandani, N. L.: A surgical technique for reconstruction of full-thickness defects of the cheek and lips after cancer surgery. J. Laryngol. Otol., *96*:1033, 1982.

Guerrosantos, J., Dicksheet, S., and Ruiz-Ruzura, A.: Free tongue composite graft for correction of a vermilion defect. Plast. Reconstr. Surg., *76*:451, 1985.

Guillamondegui, O. M., and Larson, D. L.: The lateral trapezius musculocutaneous flap: its use in head and neck reconstruction. Plast. Reconstr. Surg., *67*:143, 1981.

Gullane, P. J., and Martin, G. F.: Minor and major lip reconstruction. J. Otolaryngol., *12*:75, 1983.

Harashina, T., Imai, T., and Wada, M.: The omental sandwich reconstruction for a full-thickness cheek defect. Plast. Reconstr. Surg., *64*:411, 1979.

Harii, K., Ohmori, K., and Ohmori, S.: Successful clinical transfer of 10 free flaps by microvascular anastomosis. Plast. Reconstr. Surg., *53*:259, 1974.

Harii, K., Ono, I., and Ebihara, S.: Closure of total cheek defects with two combined myocutaneous free flaps. Arch. Otolaryngol., *108*:303, 1982.

Herbert, D. C., and DeGeus, J.: Nasolabial subcutaneous pedicle flaps. Br. J. Plast. Surg., *28*:90, 1975.

Herbert, D. C., and Harrison, R. G.: Nasolabial subcutaneous pedicle flaps. Br. J. Plast. Surg., 28:85, 1975.

Holmstrom, H.: The Abbé island flap for the correction of whistle deformity. Br. J. Plast. Surg., 40:176, 1987.

Hurwitz, D. J., Rabson, J. A., and Futrell, J. W.: The anatomic basis for the platysma skin flap. Plast. Reconstr. Surg., 72:302, 1983.

Jabaley, M. E., Clement, R. L., and Orcutt, T. W.: Myocutaneous flaps in lip reconstruction. Applications of the Karapandzic principle. Plast. Reconstr. Surg., 59:680, 1977.

Jabaley, M. E., Heckler, F. R., Wallace, W. H., and Knott, L. H.: Sternocleidomastoid regional flaps: a new look at an old concept. Br. J. Plast. Surg., 32:106, 1979.

Jackson, I. T.: Local Flaps in Head and Neck Reconstruction. St. Louis, C. V. Mosby Company, 1985.

Johanson, B., Aspelund, E., Breine, U., and Holmstrom, H.: Surgical treatment of non-traumatic lower lip lesions with special reference to the step technique. Scand. J. Plast. Reconstr. Surg., 8:232, 1974.

Juraha, Z. L. G.: Reconstruction of the lower lip with two flaps from the upper lip hinged on the superior labial vessels. Br. J. Plast. Surg., 38:87, 1980.

Juri, J., and Juri, C.: Advancement and rotation of a large cervicofacial flap for cheek repairs. Plast. Reconstr. Surg., 64:692, 1979.

Juri, J., and Juri, C.: Cheek reconstruction with advancement-rotation flaps. Clin. Plast. Surg., 8:223, 1981.

Kapetansky, D. I.: Double pendulum flaps for whistling deformities in bilateral cleft lip. Plast. Reconstr. Surg., 47:321, 1971.

Kaplan, I., and Goldwyn, R. M.: The versatility of the laterally based cervicofacial flap for cheek repairs. Plast. Reconstr. Surg., 61:390, 1978.

Karapandzic, M.: Reconstruction of lip defects by local arterial flaps. Br. J. Plast. Surg., 27:93, 1974.

Kavarana, N. M.: Use of a folded forehead flap for reconstruction after a large excision of the full-thickness of the cheek. Plast. Reconstr. Surg., 56:629, 1975.

Kawamoto, H. K.: Correction of major defects of the vermilion with a cross-lip vermilion flap. Plast. Reconstr. Surg., 64:315, 1979.

Kolhe, P. S., and Leonard, A. G.: Reconstruction of the vermilion after "lip shave." Br. J. Plast. Surg., 41:68, 1988.

Kurth, M. E.: "Lipshave" or vermilionectomy: indications and technique. Br. J. Plast. Surg., 10:156, 1957.

Langdon, J. D., and Ord, R. A.: The surgical management of lip cancer. J. Craniomaxillofac. Surg., 15:281, 1987.

Lee, E. S., and Wilson, J. S. P.: Cancer of the lip. Proc. R. Soc. Med., 63:685, 1970.

Lentrodt, J.: Contribution to the reconstruction of the lower lip after tumour resection combined with neck dissection. J. Maxillofac. Surg., 3:139, 1975.

Lexer, E.: Wangenplastik. Dtsch. Z. Chir., 100:206, 1909.

Louis, A.: Mémoire sur l'opération du bec de lièvre, ou l'on établi le premier principe de l'art de réunir les plaies. Mem. Acad. Roy. Chir., 4:385, 1768.

MacKay, E. N., and Seller, A. H.: A statistical review of carcinoma of the lip. Can. Med. Assoc. J., 90:670, 1964.

Madden, J. J., Jr., Erhardt, W. L., Jr., Franklin, J. D., Withers, E.H., and Lynch, J.B.: Reconstruction of the upper and lower lip using a modified Bernard-Burow technique. Ann. Plast. Surg., 5:100, 1980.

Maruyama, Y., Nakajima, H., Fossati, E., and Fujino, T.: Free latissimus dorsi myocutaneous flaps in the dynamic reconstruction of cheek defects: a preliminary report. J. Microsurg., 1:231, 1979.

Mathes, S. J., and Vasconez, L. O.: The cervicohumeral flap. Plast. Reconstr. Surg., 61:7, 1978.

Mazzola, R. F., and Lupo, G.: Evolving concepts in lip reconstruction. Clin. Plast. Surg., 11:583, 1984a.

Mazzola, R. F., and Lupo, G.: Our experience with lip reconstruction: a lesson from history. Clin. Plast. Surg., 11:619, 1984b.

McGregor, I. A.: The tongue flaps in lip surgery. Br. J. Plast. Surg., 19:253, 1966.

McGregor, I. A.: Fundamental Techniques of Plastic Surgery And Their Surgical Applications. 7th Ed. Edinburgh, Churchill Livingstone, 1980.

McGregor, I. A.: A "defensive" approach to the island pectoralis major myocutaneous flap. Br. J. Plast. Surg., 34:435, 1981.

McGregor, I. A.: Reconstruction of the lower lip. Br. J. Plast. Surg., 36:40, 1983.

McGregor, I. A., and Reid, W. H.: Simultaneous temporal and deltopectoral flaps for full-thickness defects of the cheek. Plast. Reconstr. Surg., 45:326, 1970.

Meyer, R., and Abul-Failat, A. S.: New concepts in lower lip reconstruction. Head Neck Surg., 4:240, 1982.

Millard, D. R., Jr.: Principlization of Plastic Surgery. Boston, Little, Brown & Company, 1986, p. 266.

Morain, W. D., and Geurkink, N. A.: Split pectoralis major myocutaneous flap. Ann. Plast. Surg., 5:358, 1980.

Mustardé, J. C. (Ed.): Plastic Surgery in Infancy and Childhood. 2nd Ed. New York, Churchill Livingstone, 1979.

Mustardé, J. C.: Repair and Reconstruction in the Orbital Region. Edinburgh, Churchill Livingstone, 1980.

Nakajima, T., Nagamine, T., Masumura, N., and Asai, Y.: Primary reconstruction of cheek defect following excision of a large malignant melanoma: report of a case. Int. J. Oral Surg., 10:140, 1981.

Nakajima, T., Yoshimura, Y., and Kami, T.: Reconstruction of the lower lip with a fan-shaped flap based on the facial artery. Br. J. Plast. Surg., 37:52, 1984.

Ohtsuka, H., Shioya, N., and Asano, T.: Clinical experience with nasolabial flaps. Ann. Plast. Surg., 6:207, 1981.

Ortiz-Monasterio, F., and Factor, R.: Early definitive treatment of electric burns of the mouth. Plast. Reconstr. Surg., 65:169, 1980.

Panje, W., and Cutting, C.: Trapezius osteomyocutaneous island flap for reconstruction of the anterior floor of the mouth and mandible. Head Neck Surg., 3:66, 1980.

Panje, W. R.: Lip reconstruction. Otolaryngol. Clin. North Am., 15:169, 1982.

Parkash, S., and Ramakrishnan, K.: Tongue-flaps—turntable and a two-stage forked flap in primary reconstruction after excision of oral carcinomas. Plast. Reconstr. Surg., 65:580, 1980.

Parkash, S., Ramakrishnan, K., and Ananthakrishnan, N.: Sternomastoid based island flap for lining after resection of oral carcinoma. Br. J. Plast. Surg., 33:115, 1980.

Patterson, H. C., Anonsen, C., Weymuller, E. A., and Webster, R. C.: The cheek-neck rotation flap for closure of temporozygomatic cheek wounds. Arch. Otolaryngol., 110:388, 1984.

Pelly, A. D., and Tan, E. P.: Lower lip reconstruction. Br. J. Plast. Surg., 34:83, 1981.

Platz, H., and Wepner, F.: Results of standardized lip repair after tumour resection. J. Maxillofac. Surg., 5:108, 1977.

Psillakis, J. M., Kamakura, L., and Spina, V.: Reconstruction of the labial philtrum with auricular composite grafts. Rev. Assoc. Med. Brasil, 20:297, 1974.

Quaba, A., and Sommerlad, B.: "A square peg into a round hole": a modified rhomboid flap and its clinical application. Br. J. Plast. Surg., 40:163, 1987.

Quillen, C. G.: Latissimus dorsi myocutaneous flaps in head and neck reconstruction. Plast. Reconstr. Surg., 63:664, 1979.

Rayner, C. R., and Arscott, G. D.: A new method of resurfacing the lip. Br. J. Plast. Surg., 40:454, 1987.

Rea, J. L., Davis, W. E., and Rittenhouse, L. K.: Reinnervation of an Abbé-Estlander and a Gillies fan flap of the lower lip: electromyographic comparison. Arch. Otolaryngol., 104:294, 1978.

Rees, T. D., Tabbal, N., and Aston, S. J.: Tongue flap reconstruction of the lip vermilion in hemifacial atrophy. Plast. Reconstr. Surg., 72:643, 1983.

Sabattini, P.: Cenno storico dell'origine e progressi della rinoplastica e cheiloplastica. Bologna, Belle Arti, 1838.

Schrudde, J., and Petrovici, V.: The use of slide-swing plasty in closing skin defects: a clinical study based on 1,308 cases. Plast. Reconstr. Surg., 67:467, 1981.

Schuchardt, K.: Operationen im Gesicht und im Kieferbereich. Operationen an den Lippen. In Bier, Braun, and Kümmel (Eds.): Chirurgische Operationslehre. Leipzig, J. A. Barth, 1954.

Shah, J. P.: Folded forehead flap for reconstruction of full-thickness defects of the cheek. Head Neck Surg., 2:248, 1980.

Sharzer, L. A., Kalisman, M., Silver, C. E., and Strauch, B.: The parasternal paddle: a modification of the pectoralis major myocutaneous flap. Plast. Reconstr. Surg., 67:753, 1981.

Shintomi, Y., Ohura, T., Honda, K., and Iida, K.: The reconstruction of progressive facial hemi-atrophy by free vascularized dermis fat grafts. Br. J. Plast. Surg., 34:398, 1981.

Skow, J.: One-stage reconstruction of full-thickness cheek defects. Plast. Reconstr. Surg., 71:855, 1983.

Smith, J. W.: The anatomical and physiologic acclimatization of tissue transplanted by the lip-switch technique. Plast. Reconstr. Surg., 26:40, 1960.

Spear, S. L., and Oldham, R. J.: A lengthened omental pedicle in facial reconstruction. Plast. Reconstr. Surg., 77:828, 1986.

Spira, M., and Stal, S.: V-Y advancement of a subcutaneous pedicle in vermilion lip reconstruction. Plast. Reconstr. Surg., 72:562, 1983.

Stein, S. A. W.: Laebedannelse (Cheiloplastik) udfört paa en ny methode. Hospitalsmeddelelser (Copenhagen), 1:212, 1848.

Stranc, M. F., Fogel, M., and Dische, S.: Comparison of lip function: surgery vs. radiotherapy. Br. J. Plast. Surg., 40:598, 1987.

Stranc, M. F., and Page, R. E.: Functional aspects of the reconstructed lip. Ann. Plast. Surg., 10:103, 1983.

Stranc, M. F., and Robertson, G. A.: Steeple flap reconstruction of the lower lip. Ann. Plast. Surg., 10:4, 1983.

Tripier, L.: Cited in Imbert, G.: Étude sur la Restauration de la Lèvre Inférieure suivie de la Description d'un Nouveau Procédé pour Refaire le Bord Libre au Moyen d'un Lambeau Mugueux en Forme de Pont. Lyon, 1883.

Tzur, H., Shafir, R., and Orenstein, A.: Hair-bearing neck flap for upper lip reconstruction in the male. Plast. Reconstr. Surg., 71:262, 1983.

Upton, J., Mulliken, J. B., Hicks, P. D., and Murray, J. E.: Restoration of facial contour using free vascularized omental transfer. Plast. Reconstr. Surg., 66:560, 1980.

Vatanasapt, V., Chadbunchachai, W., Taksaphan, P., and Komthong, R.: Bilateral neurovascular cheek flaps for one-stage lower lip reconstruction. Br. J. Plast. Surg., 40:173, 1987.

Vecchione, T. R.: Reconstruction of the oral mucocutaneous junction. Plast. Reconstr. Surg., 63:430, 1980.

Walker, A. W., and Schewe, J. E., Jr.: Nasolabial flap reconstruction for carcinoma of the lower lip. Am. J. Surg., 113:783, 1967.

Wallace, J. G., Schneider, W. J., Brown, R. G., and Nahai, F. M.: Reconstruction of hemifacial atrophy with a free flap of omentum. Br. J. Plast. Surg., 32:15, 1979.

Walton, R. L., and Bunkis, J.: A free occipital hair-bearing flap for reconstruction of the upper lip. Br. J. Plast. Surg., 36:168, 1983.

Webster, J. P.: Crescentic peri-alar cheek excision for upper lip flaps advancement with a short history of upper lip repair. Plast. Reconstr. Surg., 16:434, 1955.

Webster, R. C., Coffey, R. J., and Kelleher, R. E.: Total and partial reconstruction of the lower lip with innervated muscle bearing flaps. Plast. Reconstr. Surg., 25:360, 1960.

Weisberger, E. C., and Hanke, W.: Reconstruction of full-thickness defects of the cheek. Arch. Otolaryngol., 109:190, 1983.

Wexler, M. R., and Dingman, R. O.: Reconstruction of the lower lip. Chir. Plast. (Berlin), 3:23, 1975.

Wilson, J. S. P., Falvao, M. S. L., and Brough, M. D.: The application of hair-bearing flaps in head and neck surgery. Head Neck Surg., 2:386, 1980.

Wilson, J. S. P., and Walker, E. P.: Reconstruction of the lower lip. Head Neck Surg., 4:29, 1981.

Zarem, H., and Greer, D. M.: Tongue flap for reconstruction of the lips after electrical burns. Plast. Reconstr. Surg., 53:310, 1974.

Zisser, G.: Ein Beitrag zur Deckung malignumbedingter Oberlippen und Mundwinkeldefekten. Acta Chir. (Austria), 4:36, 1972.

Zisser, G.: A contribution to the primary reconstruction of the upper lip and labial commissure. J. Maxillofac. Surg., 3:211, 1975.

Zook, E. G., Van Beek, A. L.. Russell, R. C., and Moore, J. B.: V-Y advancement flap for facial defects. Plast. Reconstr. Surg., 65:786, 1980.

39

Thomas D. Cronin
Alfonso Barrera

Deformities of the Cervical Region

COMPLETE CERVICAL CONTRACTURES

Scars of the anterior cervical region are prone to be unusually severe because the area from the chin to the sternum is a concave flexor surface. The skin is rather thin and thus easily destroyed. Vertical incisions in the skin of the anterior cervical area, whether accidental or surgical, are likely to result in contracted scar bands.

Most scar contractures of the neck result from thermal burns. Less frequently, neck contractures are caused by electrical, radiation, or chemical burns. Severe infection with gangrene of the skin may also cause scar contractures; surgical or accidental vertical incisions may produce linear scars.

The proper treatment of severe contractures of the anterior neck has always been a most difficult problem. Many authorities (Dowd, 1927; Mixter, 1933; MacCollum, 1938a; Couglin, 1939; Aufricht, 1944; McIndoe, 1949; Smith, 1950; Ho, Sykes, and Bailey, 1975; Shchipacheva, 1975; Thomas, 1980) advocated skin flaps despite the number of operations entailed. Others (Babcock, 1932; Padgett, 1932; Brown, Byars, and Blair, 1935; Kazanjian, 1936; Blocker, 1941) recommended full-thickness skin grafts as a means of avoiding postoperative contracture. Spina (1955) and Pitanguy (1957) advised coverage with a thick, split-thickness skin graft in the region from the chin to the mandibulocervical angle and with a flap to the front of the neck below the mandibulocervical angle.

Split-thickness skin grafts have been advocated by Greeley (1944), Padgett and Stephenson (1948), Frackelton (1957), and Brown and McDowell (1958). As ordinarily used, they have been disappointing in these cases because of the high incidence of postoperative contracture and wrinkling of the graft. Preventive measures to avoid contracture were described by the author (Cronin, 1957, 1961, 1964, 1973, 1977) and they make possible the use of split-thickness skin grafts as the treatment of choice. In fact, whereas the anterior neck was one of the most unsatisfactory sites for split-thickness skin grafts, successful, wrinkle-free grafts can be reliably obtained with the splinting-pressure technique. Dingman (1961), Mendoza and associates (1961), Gottlieb (1963), Cramer (1964), Tanzer (1964), Gibbons (1965), Pitanguy and Bisaggio (1967), Converse (1967), Fujimori, Hiramoto, and Ofuji (1968), Ousterhout and associates (1969), Moore (1970), and Evans and associates (1970) have confirmed this principle, although several have suggested modification of the splint. Other writers making use of split-thickness skin grafts with splinting include Willis (1970), Dey (1972), Noordhoff (1974), Larson and associates (1974), Bunchman and Huang (1975), and Parks (1977).

Burn contractures of the neck may involve only limited areas, and when these areas lie more or less vertical, some type of scar band usually forms. Actually, a complete anterior neck contracture may be simpler to correct than one involving only one-half or one-third of the neck. In the former situation all the scar is excised and replaced with a thick, split-thickness skin graft, and a uniform result is obtained. However, relief of incomplete contractures with only a split-thickness skin graft may not be ideal, because one part of the neck is covered by normal elastic skin, while the relatively inelastic skin-grafted area stands in marked contrast. Therefore, repair with local flaps or Z-plasties is often preferable, augmented when necessary with split-thickness skin grafts.

Scar contractures of the neck should be prevented rather than surgically corrected at a later date. Following a thermal burn the neck should be kept extended and the use of a pillow avoided. Willis (1970) used isoprene splints molded to the neck early in the healing phase to prevent contracture. To be successful, however, a definitive thick, split-thickness skin graft must be applied and splinted within four to six weeks (Fig. 39–1). If (1) the burn wound cannot be prepared for definitive grafting within this time, (2) the extent of the surrounding burn is so great as to interfere with the proper use of a splint, or (3) the general condition is such that a definitive graft is not possible, it is preferable to use a thin graft and accept a contracture until conditions are favorable for scar excision and application of a thick, split-thickness skin graft with prolonged splinting, according to the authors' technique.

Anesthesia

The accomplishment of safe anesthesia is perhaps the most important problem to be solved when there is a severe anterior neck contracture. Induction with thiopental (Pentothal) or any of the inhalation agents is likely to result in sudden respiratory obstruction. Introduction of an endotracheal tube under these circumstances is extremely difficult, if not impossible. The use of a paralyzing agent for intubation only compounds the problem and is, therefore, contraindicated.

According to Wilson and associates (1970), ketamine is the safest anesthetic agent for children with severe neck contractures. While producing anesthesia, it also stimulates rather than depresses respiration, and the protective pharyngeal and laryngeal reflexes persist during anesthesia. The authors recommend two alternatives, both involving the use of ketamine. In one method, ketamine is used alone. Premedication consists of 0.1 mg scopolamine one hour preoperatively; ketamine, 8 mg per kg of body weight, is given intramuscularly in the patient's room. The authors would use a smaller dosage of ketamine, 0.5 to 1.5 mg per kg I.V., or 4 to 6 mg per kg I.M. No obstruction occurred with this regimen in the five cases so treated, and the only objection was the accumulation of carbon dioxide if the surgical drapes were placed over the airway. Consequently, minimal draping was used in these cases. Wilson (1974) stated that he prefers ketamine alone and that the following method of endotracheal intubation with halothane is used, especially when it is necessary to remove the anesthesiologist from the surgical field:

1. Premedication with 0.1 mg scopolamine one hour before surgery.

2. Ketamine, 8 mg/kg, is administered intramuscularly in the patient's room. (Again, the authors would use a smaller dosage of ketamine.)

3. In the operating room, brief administration of halothane is followed by spraying the larynx with 2 to 4 per cent lidocaine; after additional inhalation of halothane, nasotracheal intubation is accomplished under direct vision.

Jacobacci and Towey (1978) also reported the use of ketamine to anesthetize a child with a severely contracted neck.

Tanzer (1964) and Pitanguy and Bisaggio (1967), suggested initial incision of the scar contracture under local anesthesia, followed in turn by general anesthesia and endotracheal intubation. This is a sound method that probably should be used if there is any question as to the experience of the anesthesiologist with ketamine, or if there is a difficult problem with endotracheal intubation.

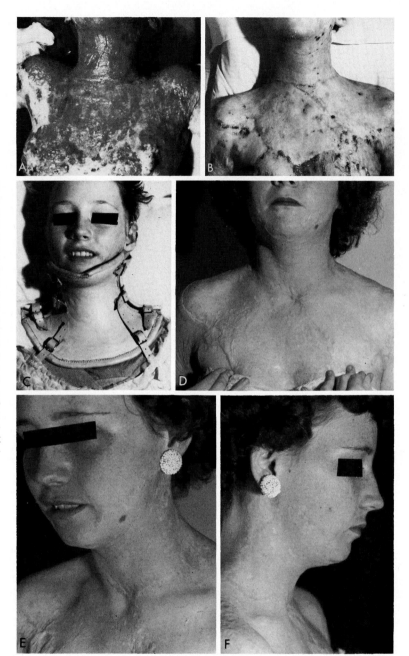

Figure 39–1. Patient with thermal burn. *A,* Clean granulating wounds 27 days following thermal burn. *B,* Appearance approximately three weeks after the application of a split-thickness skin graft (0.20 inch) to the neck, shoulders, and upper chest. *C,* Molded splint was worn day and night for six months, and for an additional three weeks only at night. *D,* Appearance two years later. The circular linear scar on the right side of the chin outlines a small skin graft that was necessary to cover an area of pressure necrosis four months after the original grafting. *E, F,* Appearance 3½ years after skin grafting. (From Cronin, T. D.: The use of a molded splint to prevent contracture after split skin grafting on the neck. Plast. Reconstr. Surg., 27:9, 1961. Copyright 1961, The Williams & Wilkins Company, Baltimore.)

For a severe contracture of the neck, the use of a fiberoptic bronchoscope or a fiberoptic laryngoscope (Fig. 39–2) might be the safest approach. There is prior application of topical anesthetic agents to the nose, oropharynx, and hypopharynx (5 per cent cocaine for the nose and 4 per cent lidocaine spray for the oropharynx and hypopharynx). If doubt exists as to the reach of the lidocaine spray to the larynx, a superior laryngeal nerve block should be done bilaterally. The block is easily done by injecting 2 to 3 ml of 1 or 2 per cent lidocaine, with or without epinephrine, on each side of the neck halfway between the greater horns of the hyoid bone and the upper border of the thyroid laminae; and 1 ml is also instilled into the upper tracheal lumen. Anesthesia of these areas prevents laryngospasm. With the patient breathing spontaneously, a flexible fiberoptic bronchoscope or

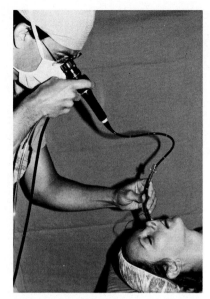

Figure 39–2. A fiberoptic laryngoscope has been passed through a No. 7 endotracheal tube in preparation for intubation. For insertions of smaller tubes, a fiberoptic pediatric bronchoscope is recommended. (From Cronin, T. D.: Burn scar contractures of the neck. *In* Stark, R. B. (Ed.): Plastic Surgery of the Head and Neck. New York, Churchill Livingstone, 1987.)

laryngoscope is passed completely through an endotracheal tube. It is then inserted through the anesthetized and decongested nasal passage, or transorally if the former route is not possible. When the hypopharynx is reached, the epiglottis is passed and the glottis visualized. At this point the tip of the fiberoptic instrument is advanced between the vocal cords into the trachea, followed by the endotracheal tube, and the fiberoptic instrument is withdrawn.

Other useful methods include the blind technique of nasotracheal intubation. After prior topical anesthesia, as described above, an endotracheal tube may be gradually advanced along the floor of the nose and into the oropharynx and hypopharynx; as long as breath sounds are well heard, one may continue advancing the tube. If the breath sounds cease, the vallecula or one of the piriform sinuses has been entered. At this point the tube is withdrawn slowly until the breath sounds are again audible. The tube is maneuvered and gently advanced again. It is important to hold the larynx against the vertebral column during this maneuver. Intubation is verified by adequate air exchange through the tube and the inability to phonate. The cuff may then be inflated and general

anesthesia instituted (Gaskill, 1967; Mulder and Wallace, 1975; Applebaum, 1979; Brown and Sataloff, 1981).

Excision of Scar

Complete excision of the scar is indicated to minimize postoperative contracture (Fig. 39–3). If the scar extends over the chin or lower border of the mandible, it is usually advisable to excise this area, because the splint can be made with an extension to apply pressure against the grafts (Fig. 39–4). The excision should extend inferiorly to a level slightly below the clavicles. If a heavy scar is continuous with scarring over the upper chest, it is advisable to excise as much scar as possible and to apply split-thickness skin grafts, with plans to repeat the procedure at a later date. When this is not done, the author has seen continued contraction of the scar pull the newly applied skin graft of the neck toward the chest (Fig. 39–5), thereby impairing its efficiency in relieving the neck contracture.

On each side of the neck, the vertical margins of the wound are interrupted by making one arm of a Z-plasty and transposing it, the other arm to be formed from the skin graft when it is later applied (see Fig. 39–3). If the chin-neck angle remains obtuse, it may be accentuated by performing a Z-plasty of the platysma muscle and its overlying subcutaneous tissue.

If the neck fails to extend completely after excision of the scar, overhead traction with a weight, cord, and pulley to a hook (made from a Kirschner wire) in the symphysis can be applied for as long as necessary before application of the skin graft (Fig. 39–6).

It is not wise to apply the skin grafts at the time of excision, because a 100 per cent take of the graft is extremely important. Despite the greatest care, small to large hematomas are prone to occur with loss of the skin graft if it has been applied at the time of the scar excision.

The wound may be dressed with fine mesh nitrofurazone (Furacin) gauze or an antibiotic ointment and fluffed Kerlex or cotton waste secured by an elastic bandage (Fig. 39–6). This dressing, plus the padding behind the shoulders, keeps the neck extended; it is *not* changed until the skin graft is applied at about five days. If available, porcine xenografts may be applied to the fresh wound.

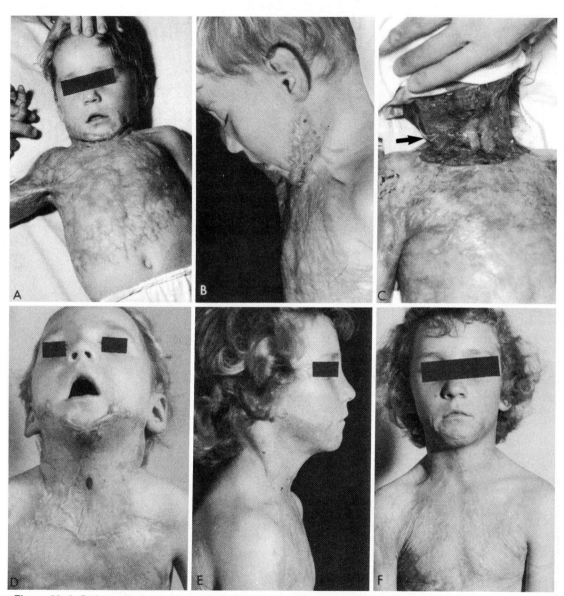

Figure 39–3. Patient with thermal burn. *A, B,* Complete contracture of the neck despite skin grafting (applied without splinting). *C,* The neck extended on the operating table after excision of the scar. Arrow shows arm of the Z-plasty. *D,* Loss of skin over the larynx caused by swallowing movements. To avoid this complication, dressings are removed from the neck after the first 24 hours. *E, F,* Appearance almost four years after a single operation to release the scar and apply split-thickness skin grafts. A splint was worn continuously for 6½ months. (From Cronin, T. D.: The use of a molded splint to prevent contracture after split skin grafting on the neck. Plast. Reconstr. Surg., 27:13, 1961. Copyright 1961, The Williams & Wilkins Company, Baltimore.)

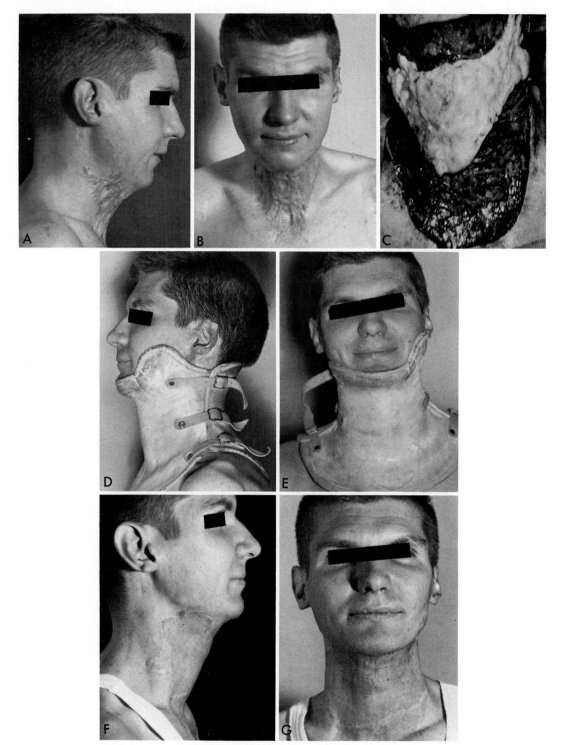

Figure 39–4. Patient with neck contracture. *A, B,* Moderate contracture involving most of the anterior aspect of the neck. *C,* After excision, the scar has been laid in the center of the wound to show the extent of expansion. Contracted parts of the platysma were also excised. A split-thickness skin graft was applied one week later. *D,E,* Splint with extension on one cheek to apply pressure to a graft of this area. The splint was worn continuously for eight months. *F, G,* Appearance eight months after application of the skin graft. Note the Z-plasty on the side of the neck at the junction of the graft with the neck skin. (From Cronin, T. D.: The use of a molded splint to prevent contracture after split skin grafting on the neck. Plast. Reconstr. Surg., *27*:11, 1961. Copyright 1961, The Williams & Wilkins Company, Baltimore.)

Figure 39–5. *A,* Scar contractures following 50 per cent third degree burn. *B,* Appearance nine months after release of scar contracure and split-thickness skin grafting. A poorly designed splint failed to prevent contracture. *C,* Appearance five months after complete excision of the skin graft and application of a thick (0.02 inch) split-thickness skin graft. The patient wore the splint for five months. *D,* Appearance 20 months after grafting. It was noticed that the heavy scarring of the chest was tending to pull the neck skin down. A large area of the scar of the upper chest was excised and covered with a split-thickness skin graft. (From Cronin, T. D.: The use of a molded splint to prevent contracture after split skin grafting on the neck. Plast. Reconstr. Surg., *27:*7, 1961. Copyright 1961, The Williams & Wilkins Company, Baltimore.)

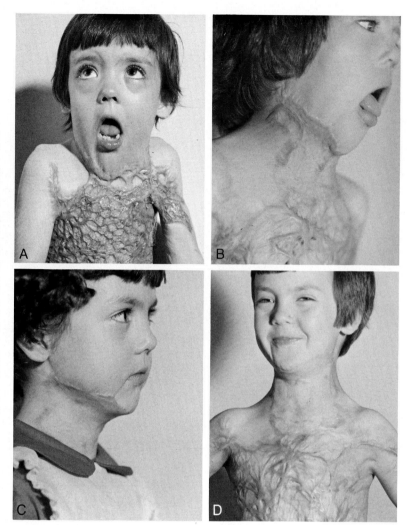

Split-Thickness Skin Grafting

An interval of five days between scar excision and skin grafting seems to be the optimum. By this time, a fine layer of granulation tissue has begun to form. Any areas of fat necrosis can be curetted. With shorter periods, bleeding upon removal of the dressing may still be troublesome. After a lapse of five days, epithelium begins to grow in from the wound margins and may need to be trimmed, with the possibility of additional bleeding.

The skin graft should be removed in one large piece if possible. The Padgett-Hood or Reese dermatomes are preferred, since a graft of 4 × 8 inches (10 × 20 cm) can be obtained, a size usually adequate for a young child. These dermatomes are preferred also because a thick graft (0.020 inch) is desired and can

be more accurately obtained than with other dermatomes or knives. If more than one piece is required, the line of junction should be transverse. The grafts should be carefully sutured in a slightly stretched state, completing the second arm of a Z-plasty wherever a first arm has previously been made on the lateral margin of the wound. Scattered interrupted sutures may be left long to tie over a large bolster dressing of fluffed gauze or mechanic's waste. The latter is piled on a layer of gauze impregnated with Furacin or an antibiotic ointment. A pressure dressing is preferred initially to ensure that the graft is in contact with the surface depressions and irregularities.

Postoperative Care. On the first postoperative day, the bolster dressing is removed and the graft is carefully inspected for evi-

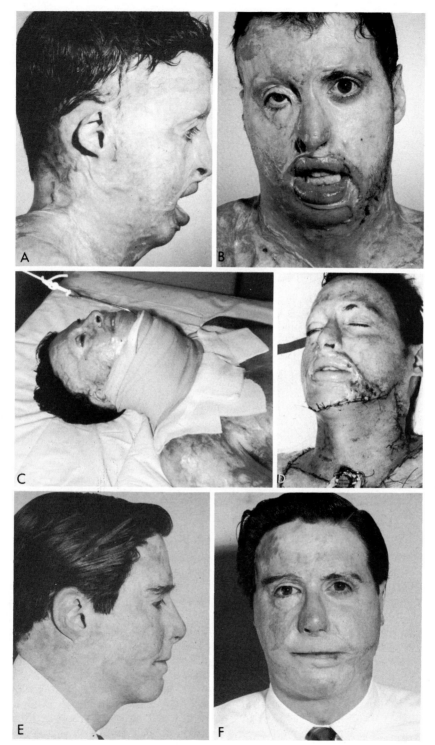

Figure 39–6. Patient with thermal burns of the face, neck, and trunk. *A, B,* Proper splint was not possible after an early skin graft, and a contracture resulted. *C,* Complete extension of the neck was not obtained immediately following scar excision; overhead traction was applied to the symphysis for several days. *D,* Two days after application of a split-thickness skin graft. *E, F,* Appearance two years following thick, split-thickness skin grafting and prolonged use of a molded splint. (From Cronin, T. D.: Burn scar contractures of the neck. *In* Lynch, J. B., and Lewis, S. R. (Eds.): Symposium on the Treatment of Burns. Vol. 5. St. Louis, MO, C. V. Mosby Company, 1973, p. 191.)

dence of hematoma and serum collections. Hematomas should be removed with power suction through a small transverse incision in the skin graft. Serum and liquid blood collections may be aspirated with syringe and needle. Daily inspection and care are essential.

The bulky dressing is not reapplied because of the danger of loss of skin over the larynx. The graft tends to stick to the dressing and is therefore prevented from adhering to the underlying moving tissues over the larynx during deglutition (see Fig. 39–3D). The extended position of the neck is, of course, maintained.

If as much as 1 sq cm of skin is lost, it is advisable to resurface it promptly with a skin graft. Refrigerated skin autograft can be used if available, otherwise a fresh piece of skin can be procured under local anesthesia. If areas of skin loss are permitted to heal without regrafting, the scars contract and are unsightly, even though a splint is used as prescribed below.

Daily observation is essential until it is certain that the splint fits well (see below) and any pressure points have been detected and corrected by the splint maker. If pressure necrosis of the skin graft develops, the area must be promptly regrafted and the splint modified. The splint should be worn even if there are small unhealed areas, which must be covered with a thin dressing.

Infection is rarely a problem in the clean wound after scar excision, but is more likely to occur in primary grafting of granulating burn wounds. It is best, therefore, not to attempt a definitive graft unless the local condition of the wound is ideal.

The Splint. The use of a splint is absolutely essential for about six months if a split-thickness skin graft has been used to relieve the contracture of the neck. The splint is designed to accomplish three goals: (1) to keep the neck extended; (2) to mold the chin-neck angle; and (3) to apply even pressure to the grafted area.

The successful use of the splint presupposes complete surgical correction of the scar contracture and restoration of the cutaneous contour of the neck.

The need for keeping the neck extended is obvious, but the advisability of applying pressure to the graft and molding the chin-neck line is often overlooked, as it was by Gibbons (1965) and Koepke (1970), who reported the use of four-post adjustable cervical braces. The four-poster cervical splint fails to achieve two of the three essential goals. Although it may keep the chin elevated, it does not mold the chin-neck angle and it does not apply pressure to all of the graft. The pressure is important in preventing the development of a hypertrophic scar and in producing a soft, smooth graft.

Making the Neck Mold. In the construction of the splint, it is best to make a plaster mold of the neck with the splint maker present, so that he will understand the problem (Fig. 39–7). The mold is made during the first two or three days after the graft is applied. The graft is covered with strips of Furacin or petrolatum gauze one or two layers thick. The patient is then allowed to sit up in a comfortable position with the neck extended slightly. The position must be carefully chosen because the splint is molded to this exact position and shape, and it determines the contour of the neck when the graft contracts against it. The entire success of this method depends on the accuracy of the mold and the resultant splint. A strip of malleable metal or cardboard is laid along each side of the neck and shoulders. When the cast is removed the line of section through the cast is extended over these strips, which protect the patient's skin from injury. A complete circular cast is applied directly to the neck, the

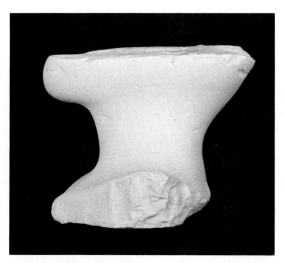

Figure 39–7. A complete circular cast is made of the neck. The cast is divided on each side and removed. A positive model, on which the splint will be constructed, is then made. (From Cronin, T. D.: Burn scar contractures of the neck. *In* Stark, R. B. (Ed.): Plastic Surgery of the Head and Neck. New York, Churchill Livingstone, 1987.)

adjacent parts of the shoulders, and the clavicular area. It extends superiorly to the chin, and if the graft reaches the cheeks, the cast should also cover that area. As the plaster begins to warm, it is divided on one side and removed. If the plaster is already set, both sides are divided and the two halves of the cast can be separated.

The patient is returned to bed and to the previous hyperextended position. As mentioned before, the graft is left exposed, or it may be covered with a single layer of Furacin or other medicated gauze.

In the construction of the splint, a positive model is made from the negative cast by pouring plaster around a heavy wooden post, which is inserted in the center and is used as a handle. The negative mold must be kept rigid, with no expansion from front to back. After the plaster has set, the negative mold is removed, the rough positive model is smoothed with a coarse file, and a piece of ordinary screen wire (approximately 7 × 35 cm) is used in the manner of a shoeshine cloth. The angle between the chin and neck is deepened, as are the depressions above and below the clavicles and the manubrium sterni. It is necessary, however, to avoid excessive smoothing of the bony prominences (the clavicles and the inferior border of the mandible), as this could cause undue pressure at these points by the splint.

The collar or splint is made from ½-inch Plastizote (a polyurethane) or 3/16 inch Vicrathene. The Plastizote is not quite as strong and needs a brace riveted to it for strength. The Vicrathene is stiffer and requires no additional bracing. Whichever material is selected, it is first heated to 300°F and is molded to the positive plastic model, covering all grafted areas on neck, chin, and cheeks. Another piece of the material is molded to the back of the model. After trimming as needed, a Velcro hook with pressure sensitive back and Velfoam straps are added (Fig. 39–8).

A splint in which a plaster impression is taken only of the front of the neck can also be constructed (Fig. 39–9). A positive model was made from this, and as the model did not have an occiput, the back of the splint was made from the back half of a Philadelphia collar.

The splint is usually applied about five to seven days after grafting. It should be worn continuously day and night until approximately six months have elapsed, or until the grafted site is soft and pliable and there is no tendency for wrinkling of the graft. This may be determined after five or six months by removing the splint for a few hours or a day at a time, and in turn for longer intervals if there is no wrinkling.

Any splint that will efficiently fulfill the three requirements mentioned above may be used. Gottlieb (1963), Gibbons (1965), and Converse (1967) have used a ready-made collar sometimes constructed with the addition of foam rubber. Tanzer (1964) employed a 4 inch block of foam rubber trimmed to fit the neck and secured with an elastic bandage. Frackelton (1957) recommended a cervical wrap collar dressing of the Sayre type. All these methods may produce satisfactory pressure on the skin of the neck, but they are

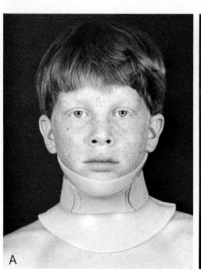 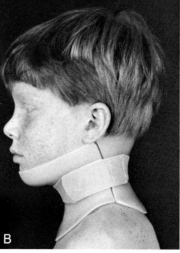

Figure 39–8. *A,* A 3/16-inch Vicrathene splint (single layer). The Vicrathene is stiffer and requires no additional bracing. It is first heated to 300°F and is then molded to the positive model. *B,* Another piece of the material is molded to the back of the model. After trimming as needed, a Velcro hook with a pressure sensitive back and Velfoam straps are added. (From Cronin, T. D.: Burn scar contractures of the neck. *In* Stark, R. B. (Ed.): Plastic Surgery of the Head and Neck. New York, Churchill Livingstone, 1987.)

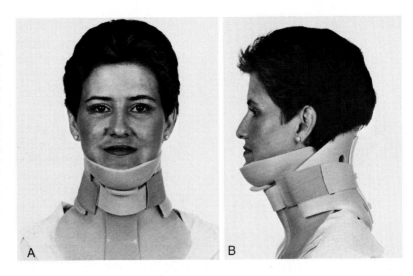

Figure 39–9. *A,* A splint made from Plastizote (polyurethane). An impression with plaster was taken of only the anterior aspect of the neck and chin. *B,* A positive model was made from this, upon which the Plastizote could be molded after heating at 300°F. The back half of a Philadelphia collar was used to complete the splint. (From Cronin, T. D.: Burn scar contractures of the neck. *In* Stark, R. B. (Ed.): Plastic Surgery of the Head and Neck. New York, Churchill Livingstone, 1987.)

somewhat deficient in extending the neck, and also are not able to produce pressure on adjacent skin over the jaws, on the cheeks and chin, or in the clavicular area.

Willis (1970) described in detail a splint made of Orthoplast isoprene,* a thermoplastic material. Another similar material, Polyform, has excellent conforming properties superior to those of the Orthoplast, yet it is stiffer afterward.

Malick and Carr (1980) described the use of Dow Corning Elastomere† to line Polyform or Orthoplast splints for better conformation to the surface (Fig. 39–10):

Materials
  Splint Perforated Polyform, a low temperature thermoplastic
  Mold 382 Medical Grade Elastomere Dow Corning
    Dow Corning Catalyst M
  Straps Two 1 inch D-ring straps
    Velcro hook with pressure sensitive back
    Velfoam straps
  Edging Moleskin 1 cm wide
Time of Application. Five days post graft

The patient is positioned during fabrication of the splint in a sitting position, head at midline, erect and neutral. Two measurements are made: one from the chin to about 1 inch below the sternoclavicular joint, and another from just below the ear around the

*Johnson & Johnson, 501 George St., New Brunswick, NJ 08903.
†Rolyan Medical Products.

jaw line to the same point on the other side of the neck. A elliptic pattern is cut out using these dimensions. The Polyform is placed in a pan of hot water (160°F); 16 oz of Elastomere is mixed with approximately 2 oz of catalyst until the substance becomes tacky. The Polyform is then taken out of the hot water, wiped off, and laid on a flat surface. The Elastomere is applied with tongue depressors over the entire surface to a thickness of perhaps 1 cm. The Polyform is lifted and applied to the front of the neck, molding it carefully around the neck and cupping over the chin. If the skin graft extends on the cheek, the splint is constructed to cover it. It extends inferiorly over the sternoclavicular area and flares slightly over the shoulders. It is kept in this position until it cools and solidifies, attempts being made to avoid any undue pressure points from the fingertips. A second piece of Polyform is fabricated to fit directly on the posterior neck from ear to ear and from T_2 level to the external occipital protuberance. The purpose of this splint is to provide a stable base for the anterior splint. The two splints are fastened by two 1 inch D-rings secured by Velcro to the anterior splint on either side of the area covering the neck. Two Velfoam straps are attached to the lateral borders of the posterior splint, passed through the D-rings, and secured by Velcro to the posterior splint. Two 17 cm long pieces of Velfoam are used to strap together the distal ends of the two splints. They are placed just medial to the acromion on both sides. This maneuver stabilizes the total neck splint. The edges around both splints are

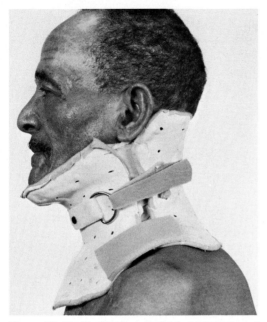

Figure 39–10. The Polyform splint is fabricated as described in the text. It is simple and inexpensive to make and may be easily replaced, if necessary. After several months it is possible that the elastomers may be dispensed with if care is taken to conform the Polyform carefully to the contour and surface. (From Cronin, T. D.: Burn scar contractures of the neck. *In* Stark, R. B. (Ed.): Plastic Surgery of the Head and Neck. New York, Churchill Livingstone, 1987.)

covered with 1 cm wide moleskin that is folded over (Fig. 39–10).

The splint is worn continuously for approximately six months. It may be removed for cleaning.

Skin Flaps

In the past, skin flaps have been widely used because they undergo little contraction, and if the donor site is carefully selected and the flap is of adequate size, excellent results can be obtained. However, since postoperative scar contracture can be prevented after application of thick, split-thickness skin grafts on the anterior neck, the need for skin flaps should be greatly reduced. Their use should be limited to repair of severe radiation burns and extremely deep thermal burns with resultant loss of contour, such as that of the chin prominence. Even in such instances, it may be possible to combine a thick, split-thickness skin graft applied to most of the neck with a supplementary flap to augment the chin (Fig. 39–11).

Converse (1967) restored the chin prominence by advancement of the anteroinferior border of the mandible after a horizontal osteotomy through an intraoral approach (Fig. 39–12).

When all or most of the anterior neck skin has been lost, an extremely large flap is required. In an adult this requires a rectangle of at least 35 × 18 cm, entailing the mutilation of some other part of the body, several major operations, and secondary debulking procedures. Aside from the general risk to the patient of repeated anesthesia, the technique also causes a great economic burden. In the mobilization of large flaps, there is also the risk of partial loss from circulatory embarrassment. Unless expert thinning of the flap is accomplished (Aufricht, 1944), the cervicomental angle can be obscured by the bulky flap.

Sources of Skin Flaps. If adjacent skin is available, its use is generally preferable for convenience and simplicity, although this may result in scarring of an exposed area. When the use of local skin is not possible or desirable, skin flaps should be obtained from parts of the body that are not exposed. Many sources have been used, including the acromiocervical (Figs. 39–13, 39–14), acromiopectoral (Fig. 39–15), thoracoepigastric (axilloabdominal), shoulder-back, transabdominal via the forearm, and oblique abdominal via the forearm. Many of these techniques are of only historical interest.

As tube flaps must, of necessity, be prepared in advance, it is important that an accurate estimate be made of the amount of skin that will be needed when the scar is excised and the neck extended. The decision concerning the choice of donor site may be simple, because in many cases it is determined by finding a sufficiently large skin donor site that is free of burn scar.

The Epaulette or Charreterra Flap (Acromiocervical). Arufe, Cabrera, and Sica (1978) attributed the first such flap to Thomas D. Mutter (1843, United States). They also credited Iturraspe and Fernandez (1951) with the precise description of the anatomic zone. Arufe, Cabrera, and Sica (1978), with experience of 286 cases since 1953, described their technique with the epaulette or Charreterra flap. This flap is indicated for the relief of neck contractures only; skin grafts are required if the chin or sternal areas are also involved. It may be used from one or both sides, depending on the extent of the burn.

Text continued on page 2073

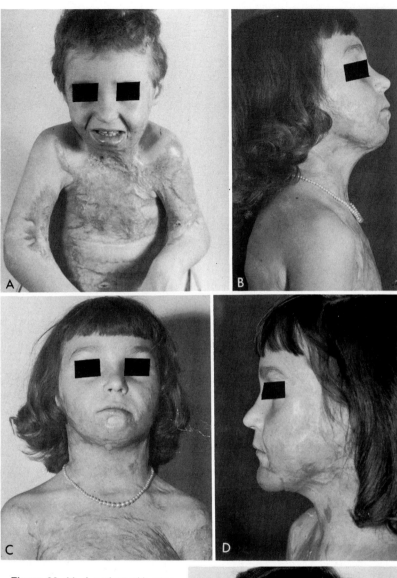

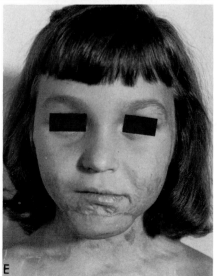

Figure 39–11. A patient with scar contracture corrected by skin grafting and skin flap. *A*, Severe contracture of the neck. *B, C*, Appearance 19 months after a single operative procedure in which the scar was released and a thick, split-thickness skin graft was applied. The splint was worn for seven months. Note the flatness of the chin caused by the depth of the burn. *D, E*, Appearance six weeks after transfer of an oblique abdominal tube flap via the wrist. (From Cronin, T. D.: The use of a molded splint to prevent contracture after split skin grafting on the neck. Plast. Reconstr. Surg., *27*:1, 7, 1961. Copyright 1961, The Williams & Wilkins Company, Baltimore.)

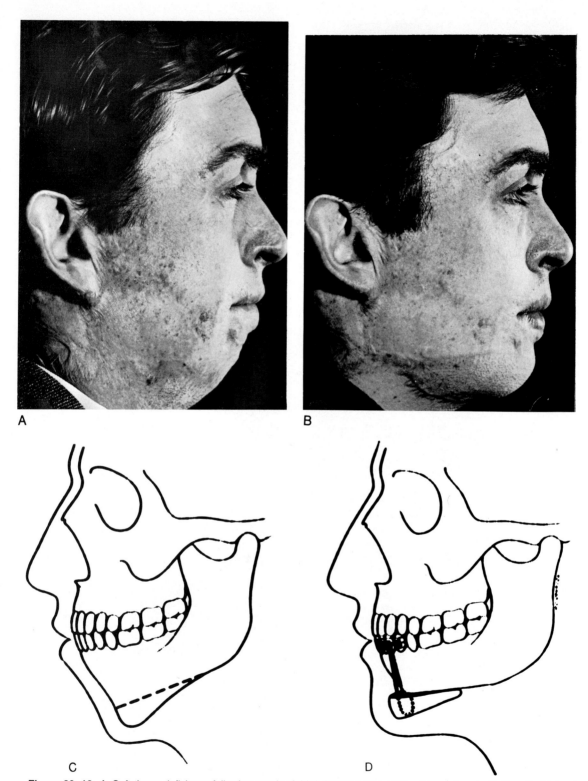

A

B

C

D

Figure 39–12. *A*, Soft tissue deficiency following repair of third degree burns of the chin and neck. *B*, Result obtained by use of a horizontal advancement osteotomy of the mandible. *C*, Horizontal advancement osteotomy of the mandible. *D*, The mandibular segment has been advanced and is maintained in position by a stainless steel wire attached to a dental appliance. This wire fixation is maintained for six weeks postoperatively (see Chap. 29 for alternative fixation techniques). (From Converse, J. M.: Burn deformities of the face and neck. Reconstructive surgery and rehabilitation. Surg. Clin. North Am., *47*:323, 1967.)

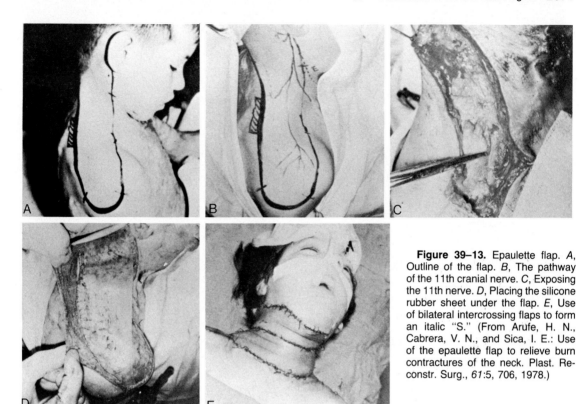

Figure 39–13. Epaulette flap. *A*, Outline of the flap. *B*, The pathway of the 11th cranial nerve. *C*, Exposing the 11th nerve. *D*, Placing the silicone rubber sheet under the flap. *E*, Use of bilateral intercrossing flaps to form an italic "S." (From Arufe, H. N., Cabrera, V. N., and Sica, I. E.: Use of the epaulette flap to relieve burn contractures of the neck. Plast. Reconstr. Surg., *61*:5, 706, 1978.)

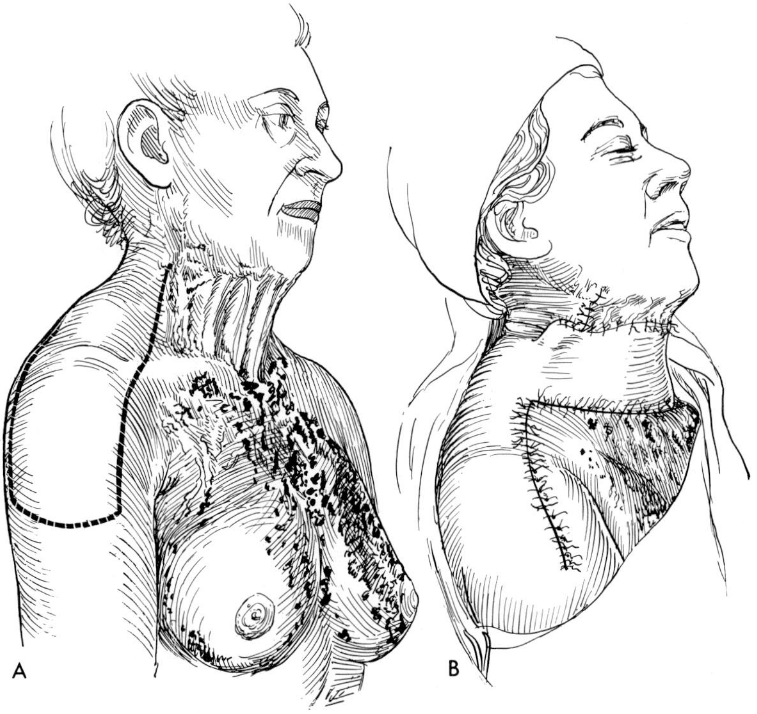

Figure 39–14. Acromiocervical flap. *A*, A burn scar contracture of the neck. Proposed flap incisions. *B*, Relief of contracture by transposition of a "Charreterra" (acromiocervical) flap in one stage. (Drawings after photographs from Kirschbaum, 1958.)

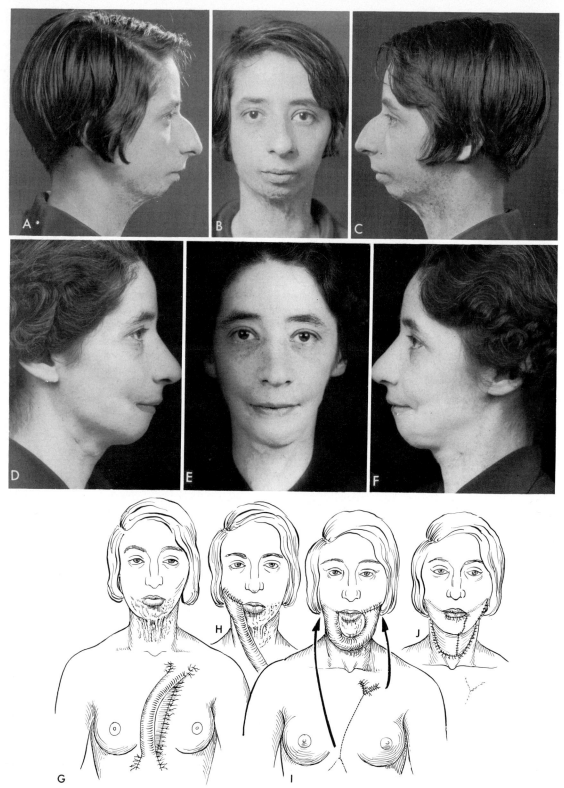

Figure 39–15. Correction of a cervical contracture with an acromiopectoral flap. *A, B, C,* Preoperative photographs of a patient following thermal burn. Hypertrophic scars had been treated with irradiation. Several years later, radiation dermatitis and ulceration appeared on the chin despite previous skin grafting procedures. *D, E, F,* Postoperative photographs after reconstruction of the chin and neck with an acromiopectoral tube flap. The patient had also had a corrective rhinoplasty. *G, H, I, J,* Diagrams of the surgical technique. (From Aufricht, G.: Evaluation of pedicle flaps versus skin grafts in reconstruction of surface defects and scar contractures of the chin, cheeks, and neck. Surgery, *15*:75, 1944.)

First Stage. Two parallel incisions are marked 5 to 9 cm apart (see Fig. 39–13). The anterior line starts at the ear lobule and runs toward the shoulder. The posterior one begins at the hair-bearing line toward the back of the scalp. The length of the flap depends on the length of the defect across the neck. The distal end can reach the deltoid region. The lines are incised in their full length and the flap is completely undermined. The 11th cranial nerve, which lies beneath the flap, should be visualized and preserved during the dissection. A thin sheet of silicone rubber is placed beneath the flap to isolate the nerve and prevent early revascularization of the flap.

Second Stage. Fourteen days later the distal end of the flap is incised under local anesthesia. This incision should enter the space previously dissected.

Third Stage. After one more week the flap is completely elevated, and if the circulation is satisfactory, the contracted scar is excised from the front of the neck and the flap is transposed. When two flaps are used, both should cross the midline and form a large "S." The donor site is usually closed.

Kirschbaum (1958), after treating 31 patients, advocated the use of the Charreterra flap for severe contractures, but unlike Arufe, Cabrera, and Sica (1978), he raised and transferred the flap in one stage (see Fig. 39–14).

Aufricht (1944) employed a transabdominal flap with transfer via the hand and forearm. He also used the axilloabdominal and acromiopectoral flaps for chin and neck reconstruction. In regard to securing good cosmetic results with tube flaps, Aufricht (1944) observed:

1. The size of the defect should be carefully considered. There is always the danger of lacking sufficient tissue in the flap.

2. Large flaps provide a better cosmetic result than small ones.

3. No scar should be spared between the transplanted and healthy skin.

4. In extensive reconstruction of the chin, the flap should extend to the vermilion border, even if uninvolved skin has to be sacrificed. Small islands of healthy skin spoil the esthetic effect and do not provide functional aid.

5. The flap can be thinned and modeled after transfer has been completed.

Rather than defatting the flap after it has been transferred, Thomas (1980) advocated defatting at the subdermal level before transfer. He described a groin flap that was raised and, after defatting to the subdermal level, was attached to the wrist. The flap was delayed at three weeks; at four weeks it was carried to the neck, and approximately one-half of the flap was inset. At seven weeks the flap was detached and spread out without evidence of necrosis. Pitanguy and Bisaggio (1967) attached both ends of the transabdominal flap to the forearm, leaving the middle attached to the abdomen. Along with Spina (1955), they applied a split-thickness skin graft from the chin to the mandibulocervical angle and transferred a flap to the anterior aspect of the neck. Harii, Torii, and Sekiguchi (1978) reported the use of the lateral thoracic flap for reconstruction of various defects, including the neck.

Microvascular Transfers

For surgeons trained and experienced in microvascular anastomosis, another method of resurfacing the neck is available. Harii, Ohmori, and Ohmori (1975) transferred groin flaps, ranging in size from 7 × 14 cm to 18 × 28 cm, supplied by either the superficial circumflex iliac artery or the superficial epigastric artery and subcutaneous vein. End to end anastomosis was made with the facial artery and vein. The donor sites were closed either by direct approximation or by split-thickness skin grafting.

Eleven patients were treated by this technique, with an excellent result in nine. There was partial necrosis of one flap and complete necrosis of another. Although the flap is transferred in one stage, two or more additional stages may be required to debulk and shape the flap. The groin microvascular free flap for resurfacing burn contractures of the neck has also been reported by Visse and associates (1976), who used the facial artery and external jugular vein as recipient vessels. Figure 39–16 demonstrates a case report by Ohmori (1978). Mühlbauer, Herndl, and Stock (1982), on a visit to the People's Republic of China in 1980, saw several patients who had had severe burn contractures of the neck and other sites repaired with forearm microvascular free flaps (Song, 1982). They reported a case in which the contracture of the neck was released by a transverse section

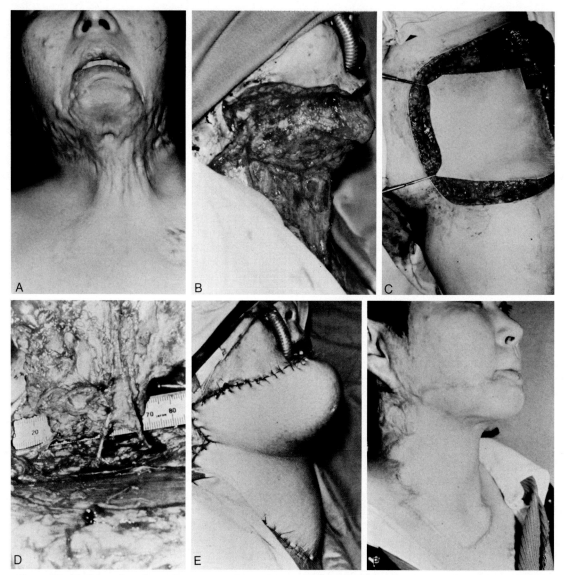

Figure 39–16. Correction of a neck contracture by a microvascular free groin flap. *A*, A 33 year old female with a burn contracture of the anterior neck. *B*, The anterior neck scar was excised, preserving the left facial artery and vein as recipient vessels. *C*, A free flap measuring 23 × 24 cm was designed in the groin area. *D*, Vascular pedicle in the groin island flap. *From left to right*: cutaneous veins, venae comitantes, common trunk of circumflex iliac artery, and epigastric artery. *E*, The free flap has been transferred, revascularized, and sutured in place. *F*, The final result after defatting the flap in three stages. (From Ohmori, K.: Application of microvascular free flaps to burn deformities. World J. Surg., 2:193, 1978.)

and a large flap consisting of most of the skin of the flexor aspect of the forearm (Fig. 39–17). The proximal end of the radial artery (3 mm) was anastomosed end to end to the facial artery (1 mm) at the level of the submandibular gland. The cephalic vein (3 mm) was easily anastomosed to the right external jugular vein (3.5 mm). The medial cutaneous nerve of the forearm was sutured to a branch of the cervical plexus. The donor area in the left forearm was covered with a split-thickness skin graft.

Badran, El-Helaly, and Safe (1984) described a lateral intercostal flap and showed that this large flap could be used to correct severe neck contractures.

Full-Thickness Skin Grafts

A "take" or vascularization is less certain when full-thickness skin grafts are used because of the thickness of the grafts. Coverage

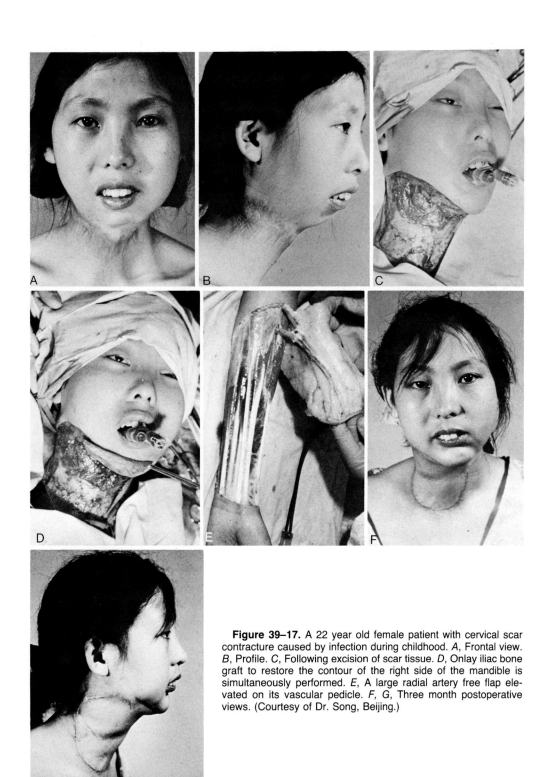

Figure 39–17. A 22 year old female patient with cervical scar contracture caused by infection during childhood. *A*, Frontal view. *B*, Profile. *C*, Following excision of scar tissue. *D*, Onlay iliac bone graft to restore the contour of the right side of the mandible is simultaneously performed. *E*, A large radial artery free flap elevated on its vascular pedicle. *F*, *G*, Three month postoperative views. (Courtesy of Dr. Song, Beijing.)

of the donor sites with split-thickness skin grafts may be required. Full-thickness grafts are not recommended for resurfacing large areas of the neck, but may profitably be used in small ones, as there is little postoperative contracture. Brown and McDowell (1958) used full-thickness grafts to restore a chin-neck line after contracture of previously applied split-thickness skin grafts.

LIMITED CONTRACTURES

In limited contractures, Z-plasties, local flaps, or a combination of local flaps and split-thickness skin grafts may be successfully used.

In using the Z-plasty, the surgeon should remember that one large Z-plasty provides greater length than several small ones in the same area. Mukhin and Mamonov (1970) described a four-flap, 90 degree Z-plasty of the Limberg type with the flaps divided in half (Fig. 39–18).

The use of local transposition flaps combined with split-thickness skin grafts and subsequent prolonged splinting is illustrated in Figure 39–19.

CONGENITAL WEBBING OF THE NECK (PTERYGIUM COLLI)

Turner's Syndrome

Turner (1938) reported a syndrome in females consisting of webbed neck, infantilism, and cubitus valgus. Webbing of the neck was already well known, having been reported by Kobylinski (1882) and named pterygium colli by Funke (1902). Turner (1938) considered these patients to have pituitary insufficiency, but Wilkins and Fleischmann (1944) reported absence of the ovaries, there being only a streak of rudimentary tissue, and termed the syndrome "ovarian agenesis and dwarfism." Barr, Bertram, and Lindsay (1950) discovered that certain cells of the female contained a peripheral nuclear chromatin mass not present in males. Polani, Hunter, and Lennox (1954) and Wilkins, Grumbach, and Van Wyk (1954) found that the cells of girls with the syndrome described by Turner, for the most part, were chromatin negative or lacked the typical chromatin mass. In most series, about 80 per cent of patients were found to be chromatin negative. This finding led investigators to postulate that dysgenesis of the fetal gonad had occurred, resulting in the invariable development of the müllerian structures. Jost (1947) had previously shown that gonadectomy of the fetus in experimental animals resulted in 100 per cent of the offspring being females. In abnormal individuals, however, chromatin negativity or positivity ("nuclear sexing") may not necessarily indicate true chromosomal sex (Polani, Lessof, and Bishop, 1956). Ford and associates (1959) suggested "the findings in gonadal dysgenesis might be abnormal sex differentiation following anomalous sex determination in the zygote."

Tjio and Levan (1956) and Ford and Hamerton (1956) discovered that humans have 46 chromosomes. Ford and associates (1959) subsequently found that girls with Turner's syndrome had only 45 chromosomes, having 44 autosomes and only one sex chromosome—the XO. These females are typically dwarfed, and this may be the only finding, or they may also have webbed neck with low and wide hairline, webbed elbows and knees, epicanthal folds, malformation of the mandible, anomalies of the nails, coarctation of the aorta, hypertension of unknown cause, lymphedema of the hands and feet, and mental retardation.

The diagnosis is made by obtaining a buccal smear and examining the cells for the periph-

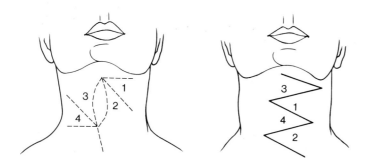

Figure 39–18. Z-plasties are helpful when a scar band is present and in most cases the single 60 degree Z-plasty is satisfactory. Occasionally with a long scar, as illustrated, a right angle or double Z-plasty is indicated. (From Mukhin, M. V., and Mamonov, A. F.: Classification of scarred neck contractures and their surgical therapy by methods of local plastic operation. Acta Chir. Plast. (Praha), *12*:48, 1970.)

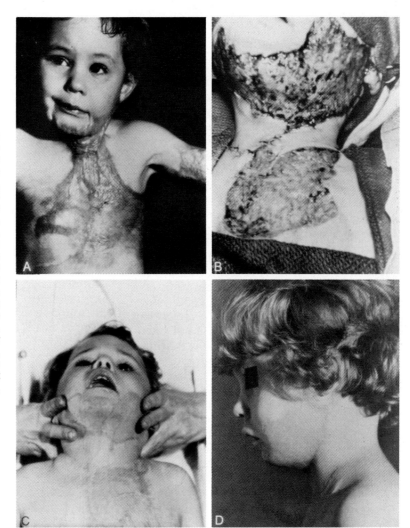

Figure 39–19. Correction of a cervical contracture by transposition flaps combined with skin grafts. *A,* Heavy scar contracture of the left side of the neck, face, and chest. *B,* Excision of scar and transposition of local flaps across the anterior aspect of the neck. *C,* Appearance six months later, showing that the flaps have spread out over the neck. The split-thickness skin grafts above and below the flaps are smooth and soft after the patient has worn a molded splint. *D,* Profile six months after surgery. Note the well defined chin-neck angle. (From Cronin, T. D.: Burn scar contractures of the neck. *In* Lynch, J. B., and Lewis, S. R. (Eds.): Symposium on the Treatment of Burns. Vol. 5. St. Louis, MO, C. V. Mosby Company, 1973.)

eral chromatin mass. In postpubertal patients the urinary gonadotropins are elevated.

Medical treatment consists of administration of estrogen at the age of puberty. Consultation with the endocrinologist or interested gynecologist or pediatrician is indicated in the diagnosis and systemic treatment of these patients.

Sybert (1984) reported that androgen therapy in adult individuals with Turner's syndrome does not seem to alter the height significantly in comparison with their untreated counterparts.

Ullrich-Noonan Syndrome (Turner Phenotype)

Other terms for the Ullrich-Noonan syndrome are Bonnevie-Ullrich syndrome and chromatin positive Turner's syndrome. This is one of the most common syndromes transmitted by a mendelian mode. Nora and Sinha (1970) and Levy, Pashayan, and Fraser (1970) demonstrated an autosomal dominant mode of inheritance. Nora, Nora, and Sinha (1974) stated:

General findings are that the patient with the Ullrich-Noonan syndrome may be male (eliminating XO Turner syndrome) or female and will have normal chromatin and chromosomes for their phenotype sex. Thus, a buccal smear that is chromatin positive with Barr bodies that are normal in size (to differentiate from isochromosome X) and normal in number (to distinguish from XX/XO mosaicism) will represent strong evidence that a female patient with Ullrich-Noonan and Turner stigmata has Ullrich-Noonan syndrome rather than Turner syndrome. The stature is usually, but not invariably, small.

Surgical Correction of Cervical Webs

The usual low hairline and its anterior extension on the neck increase the difficulties of designing flaps that will not transpose hair-bearing skin to the lateral or anterior aspect of the neck. In the typical case of Turner's syndrome, the hair extends so far forward on the web and so low on the neck that it is impossible to design a classical Z-plasty with flaps of equal size (Fig. 39–20). If the skin of the web is pulled backward, a normal contour is obtained. Some cases may be relieved by excision of a half-moon or ellipse of hair-bearing skin on each side (Fig. 39–21). Foucar (1948) excised an ellipse from the midline of the back of the neck. A combination of excision of hair-bearing skin plus rotation of a flap was described by Schröder (1958). However, his flap, being based below and posteriorly, would in most cases contain hair-bearing skin and would therefore be unsuitable. La Ruffa (1970) described a technique of excision of hair-bearing skin from the upper neck with a Z-plasty below, the posterior arm being based below and the anterior arm above. In this design the posterior flap would ordinarily be hair bearing and thus unsuitable. Cronin (1964, 1977) used one arm of a Z from the anterior non–hair-bearing part of the web to transpose skin medially on the lower neck. A large piece of the hair-bearing skin was excised, providing a satisfactory correction (see Fig. 39–20).

Mennig (1956) described an operation in which a posterior flap was advanced and concomitantly the excess hair-bearing skin was excised to improve the hairline.

One male patient, in addition to having club feet and the Robin sequence with cleft palate and bilateral inguinal hernia, had a short neck. There was generalized vertical shortening of the skin of the anterior aspect of the neck in addition to lateral webbing (Fig. 39–22). A large Z-plasty on each side of the neck relieved the webbing, but the anterior shortness remained, with resultant limitation of extension. The condition therefore had to be managed as if it were an extensive cicatricial contracture. A transverse incision was made and the skin of the neck retracted widely. A thick, split-thickness skin graft was inserted and a molded splint applied, which was worn for six months.

There have been two proponents of a posterior midline approach for the correction of the webbed neck deformity. Shearin and De Franzo (1980) suggested the butterfly technique, a posterior approach similar to that described by Foucar (1948). A large butterfly pattern of hair-bearing skin was excised, and lateral, superior, and inferior flaps were elevated and mobilized to close the defect in a double Y fashion (Fig. 39–23). However, there were problems with the spread of the vertical scar owing to the tightness of the closure and with partial recurrence of the webbing, so that secondary surgery was required.

Another posterior midline approach described by Agris, Dingman, and Varon (1983) was designed to camouflage the scars in the scalp and provide a smooth hairline and an acceptable neck contour (Fig. 39–24).

Menick, Furnas, and Achauer (1984) proposed a lateral advancement flap technique. The scars lie along the hairline or on the posterior neck, and neck contour is restored (Fig. 39–25).

CONGENITAL MIDLINE CERVICAL CLEFT AND WEB

A congenital midline cervical cleft with webbing is uncommon. Although patients with associated median cleft of the lower lip have been reported, there have been few in whom cervical webbing existed. Davis (1950) reported such a case, and Wynn-Williams (1952) cited two examples. In the first, a 7 year old child had a midline cleft in the anterior cervical region that extended to the symphysis menti. The base of the cleft appeared fibrotic but was not attached to the deeper structures. The floor of the cleft was slightly depressed below the normal skin at its cranial end and gradually increased in depth to end in a blind pit at the suprasternal notch. The cleft was excised and a large Z-plasty done to relieve the web.

The second patient was a 12 year old girl. There was a projecting tag of skin with a small depression in the skin caudal to it in the midline of the neck just below the symphysis menti. A subcutaneous fibrous band extended inferiorly from the caudal end of the cleft to the suprasternal notch. The soft tissues of the neck were tight and the normal cervicomental angle was obliterated. The mandible was underdeveloped. Roentgenograms of the mandible showed a congenital

Text continued on page 2085

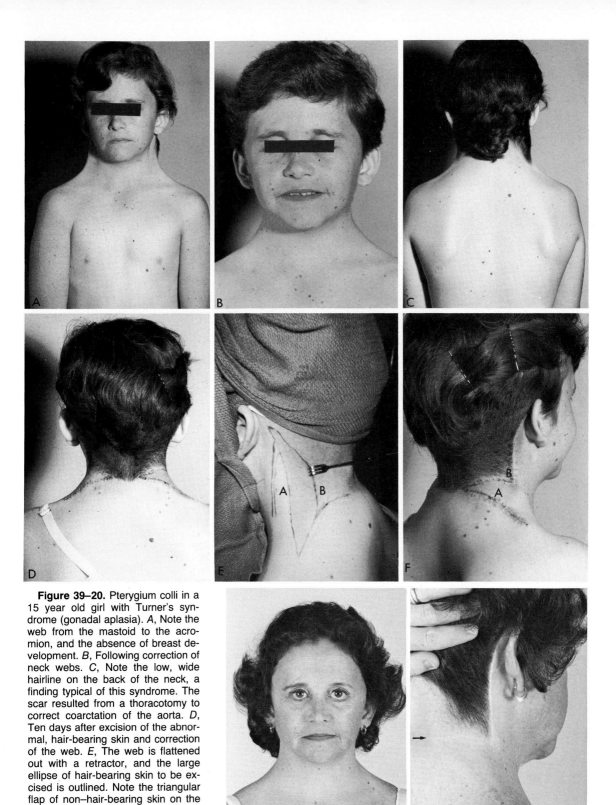

Figure 39–20. Pterygium colli in a 15 year old girl with Turner's syndrome (gonadal aplasia). *A,* Note the web from the mastoid to the acromion, and the absence of breast development. *B,* Following correction of neck webs. *C,* Note the low, wide hairline on the back of the neck, a finding typical of this syndrome. The scar resulted from a thoracotomy to correct coarctation of the aorta. *D,* Ten days after excision of the abnormal, hair-bearing skin and correction of the web. *E,* The web is flattened out with a retractor, and the large ellipse of hair-bearing skin to be excised is outlined. Note the triangular flap of non–hair-bearing skin on the anterior aspect of the web, which will be transposed 90 degree to fill the space created when the horizontal incision is made across the lower part of the neck. *F,* Ten days after excision of the excess hair-bearing skin and transposition of the flaps. *G, H,* Long-term follow-up: 22 years after a single operation to correct the web neck. Note the inconspicuous scar.

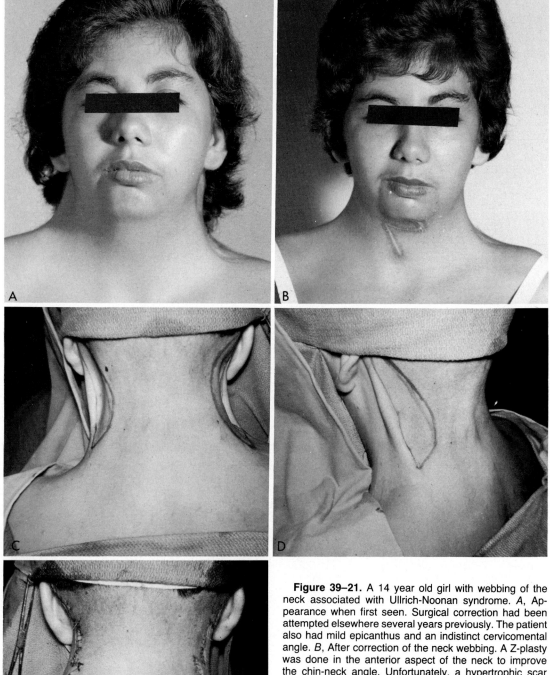

Figure 39–21. A 14 year old girl with webbing of the neck associated with Ullrich-Noonan syndrome. *A,* Appearance when first seen. Surgical correction had been attempted elsewhere several years previously. The patient also had mild epicanthus and an indistinct cervicomental angle. *B,* After correction of the neck webbing. A Z-plasty was done in the anterior aspect of the neck to improve the chin-neck angle. Unfortunately, a hypertrophic scar developed. *C,* Appearance of the webs at the time of surgery. The large ellipses of hair-bearing skin to be excised are outlined. *D,* Ellipse of hair-bearing skin to be excised. *E,* After excision of the ellipse of hair-bearing skin on each side, several small Z-plasties were done to combat the tendency for a hypertrophic, contracted scar to form.

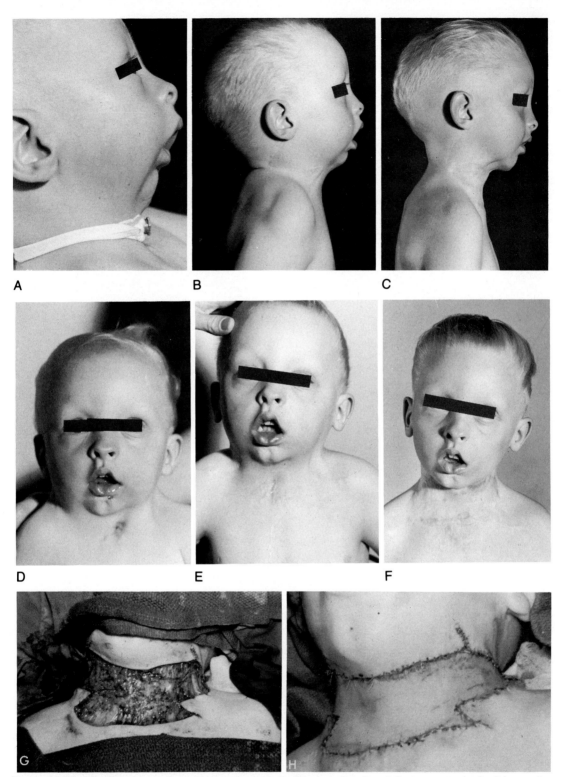

Figure 39–22. The Robin anomalad with short neck. *A*, Profile view. Suturing of the tongue to the lip did not relieve respiratory obstruction, and a tracheotomy had been performed. *B*, Appearance after large Z-plasty correction of the lateral webs. *C*, After addition of skin to the neck by the split-thickness skin graft technique. *D*, Frontal view showing generalized vertical shortness of the skin of the neck with lateral webbing. Note the tracheostomy. *E*, Appearance after large Z-plasty on each side of the neck. *F*, Appearance after split-thickness skin grafting of the anterior neck. *G*, Size of the wound after transverse releasing incision of the anterior neck. *H*, Thick (0.17 inch) split-thickness skin graft immediately after application. A special molded collar splint, as shown in Figure 39–8, was worn continuously for five months.

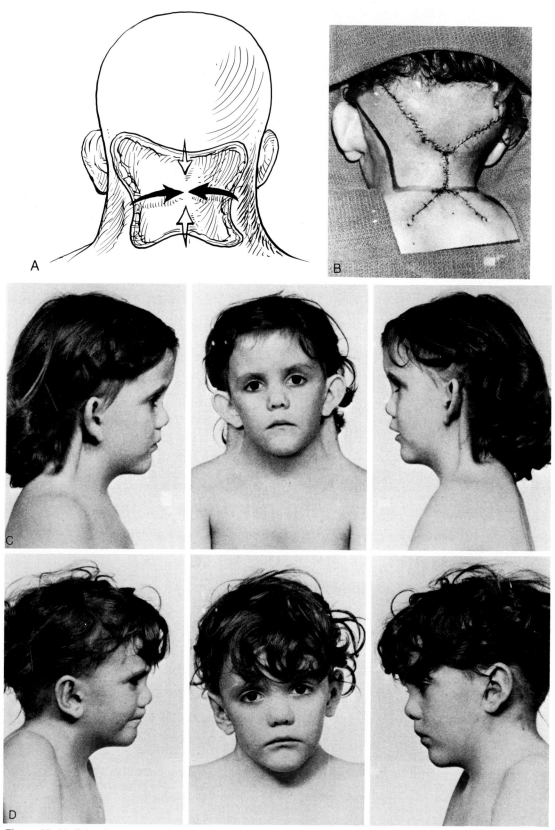

Figure 39–23. Butterfly correction of webbed neck in Turner's syndrome. *A*, Redundant skin excised. *B*, Flaps sutured together at the midline. *C*, Webbed neck deformity of Turner's syndrome, preoperative appearance. *D*, Postoperative appearance. (From Shearin, J. C., and DeFranzo, A.: Butterfly correction of webbed-neck deformity in Turner's syndrome. Plast. Reconstr. Surg., *66*:129, 1980.)

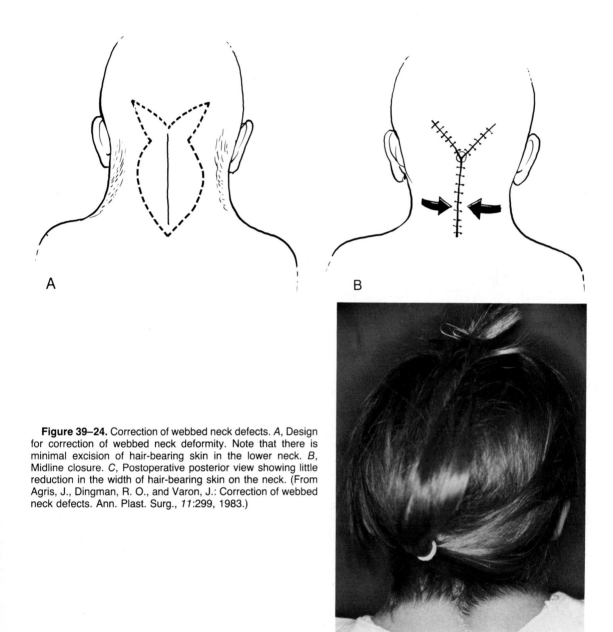

Figure 39–24. Correction of webbed neck defects. *A*, Design for correction of webbed neck deformity. Note that there is minimal excision of hair-bearing skin in the lower neck. *B*, Midline closure. *C*, Postoperative posterior view showing little reduction in the width of hair-bearing skin on the neck. (From Agris, J., Dingman, R. O., and Varon, J.: Correction of webbed neck defects. Ann. Plast. Surg., *11*:299, 1983.)

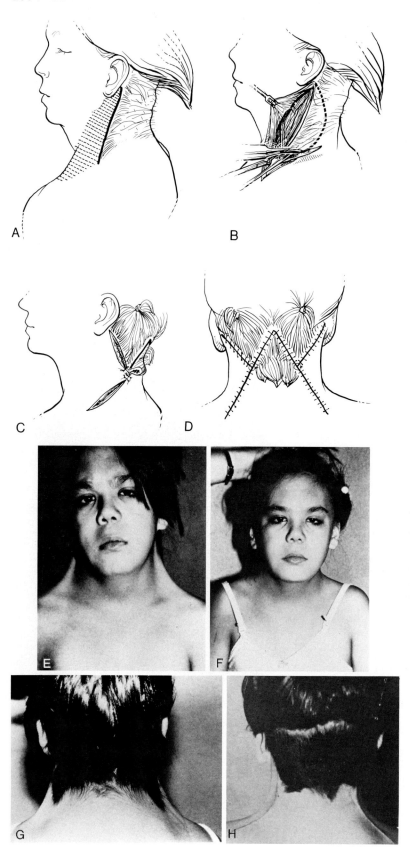

Figure 39–25. Lateral cervical advancement flaps for the correction of webbed neck deformity. *A,* Incision marked along or within abnormal hairline from mastoid onto the posterolateral neck. Area of required anterior undermining is outlined by fine dashed lines. *B,* Glabrous anterior aspect of web elevated with platysma muscle exposing external jugular vein. The proposed hairline is marked and excised on the posterior hair-bearing aspect of the web. *C,* Lateral cervical advancement flap positioned to recontour neck and establish the new hairline. Triangle of scalp excised to equalize wound margins. *D,* Incisional closure at completion of bilateral correction. *E,* Preoperative view of 12 year old girl with Turner's syndrome. *F,* Postoperative view. *G,* Preoperative view. *H,* Postoperative view one year after advancement of lateral cervical flaps. (From Menick, F. J., Furnas, D. W., and Achauer, B. M.: Lateral cervical advancement flaps for the correction of webbed neck deformity. Plast. Reconstr. Surg., *73*:222, 1984.)

midline cyst. The skin tag, cleft, and the fibrous band were excised as far as the suprasternal notch, and a double Z-plasty was done. A similar case is illustrated in Figure 39–26.

CONGENITAL MUSCULAR TORTICOLLIS

Torticollis (literally "twisted neck") is the term used for both congenital and acquired deformities of both organic and psychogenic origin. The deformity is frequently known as wryneck. Other terms are collum distortum and caput obstipum (Hough, 1934). Scoliosis capitis is descriptive of the skeletal deformity of the head (Middleton, 1930).

The condition results from a shortening of the sternocleidomastoid muscle and is characterized by a tilting of the head to the affected side, while the chin points up and to the opposite side. The shoulder is higher on the affected side, and the external ear may sometimes be more prominent on that side. Either the sternal or the clavicular head of the muscle may predominate (Figs. 39–27, 39–28), or both heads may participate equally. Attempts to turn the head in the opposite direction are limited by the tightness of the shortened sternocleidomastoid muscle. Bilateral torticollis has been reported by von Muralt (1946).

When the condition persists beyond a few weeks in infancy, an asymmetry develops in which the face and skull on the affected side appear smaller.

The skeletal deformity is reversible if the contracture is released during the period of growth. However, in adults and older teenagers few, if any, changes in skeletal contour can be expected.

History. Torticollis has been recognized and reported for centuries, and treatment is

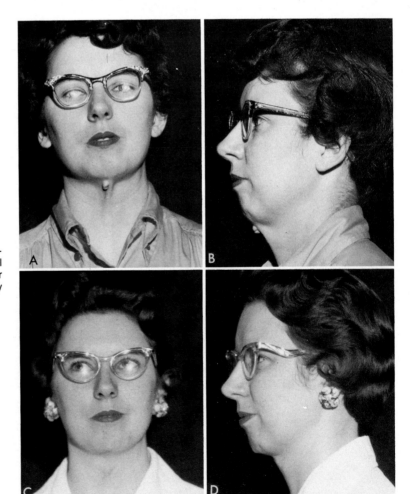

Figure 39–26. Congenital midline web of the neck. *A,* Frontal view. *B,* Profile view. *C, D,* After excision of the skin tag and Z-plasty correction of the web.

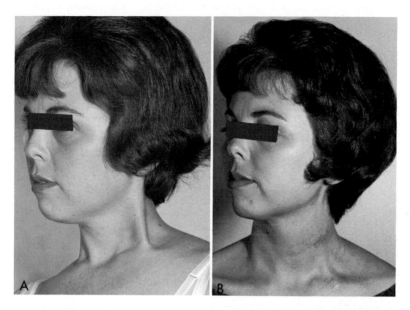

Figure 39–27. A 30 year old woman without history of tumor of the sternocleidomastoid muscle. Torticollis was first noted when she was 10 years of age. *A,* Shortness is predominant in the clavicular head of the muscle. Note the elevation of the shoulder and the head tilt. *B,* Appearance following excision of the upper 3.7 cm of the sternocleidomastoid muscle and all of the clavicular head; the sternal head was left intact. The incisions were made below the tip of the mastoid and over the middle of the neck. A small stab incision was made over the clavicle, through which a bony exostosis was removed.

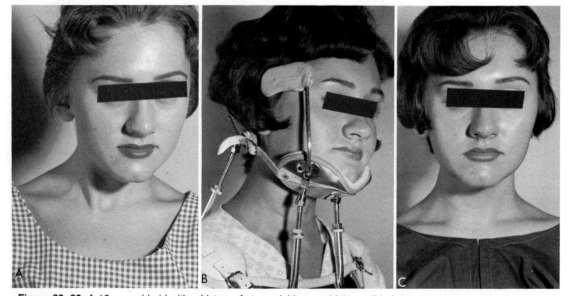

Figure 39–28. A 16 year old girl with a history of sternocleidomastoid "tumor" in infancy. Attempts to correct the head tilt by positioning were not successful. *A,* Frontal view. The sternal head predominates. *B,* Adjustable brace worn for two months following surgery according to the technique of the author. Note extension on the temple to secure additional positive overcorrection of the head tilt. *C,* Appearance two months after surgical correction.

known to have been attempted long ago. Lidge, Bechtol, and Lambert (1957) stated that Girolama Fabrizio d'Aguapendente (1537–1619) devised an apparatus to correct torticollis. They also credited a Dutch surgeon, Isacius Minnius, with performance of the first tenotomy. Hulbert (1950), however, stated that tenotomy probably dates at least from the second century. Taylor (1875) was the first to describe the pathology of the sternocleidomastoid muscle.

Classification. Many classifications of the different forms of torticollis have been suggested, including the following simple one:

1. Congenital
   a. Muscular
   b. Vertebral maldevelopment
2. Acquired
   a. Secondary or acute (infection or trauma)
   b. Ocular (hypertropia or hypotropia)
   c. Spasmodic or neurogenic
   d. Psychogenic

Etiology. The cause of congenital torticollis is unknown. Many explanations have been suggested but none has been fully substantiated.

Stromeyer (1838) suggested that rupture of the sternomastoid and hematoma formation during labor could cause the condition, but the presence of a hematoma within the muscle has never been demonstrated.

Middleton (1930) offered experimental evidence to support his theory of venous occlusion, and this is perhaps the most reasonable explanation of the pathogenesis yet offered.

Lidge, Bechtol, and Lambert (1957) cited 87 references to the high incidence of breech and other abnormal obstetric presentations, but torticollis has been reported in infants delivered by cesarean section (Roemer, 1954). Chandler (1948) believed that intrauterine malposition causes pressure and ischemia of the muscle, predisposing it to damage by a traumatic or even normal delivery that would not injure a normal muscle. Kiesewetter and associates (1955) thought that intrauterine malposition resulting in ischemia and fibrosis of the muscle might be the cause of the abnormal delivery.

Hellstadius (1927) proposed a genetic factor, although a positive family history is rarely obtained. Reye (1951) suggested the possibility of a congenital defect in the development of the muscle anlage.

Incidence. Coventry and Harris (1959) reported an incidence of 0.4 per cent (35 out of 7835). The "tumor" was first discovered by the physician in half the cases and by the mother in the other half. This could easily explain the lack of a history of "tumor" in some children who subsequently develop torticollis. Hough (1934) cited the following incidence figures: Tubby reported 0.3 per cent of the children in a surgical hospital (eight of 2324 admissions), 0.3 per cent of orthopedic cases (15 of 5079 at Royal National Orthopedic Hospital), and less than 0.2 per cent of other patients (nine of 5190); Colonna reported 0.5 per cent (269 of 55,000 at the Hospital for the Ruptured and Crippled); and Grieve (1946) found only two cases of muscular torticollis among 4500 recruits, as opposed to 16 cases of ocular torticollis in the same group.

No significant differences according to sex or to the side of the neck involved have been noted.

Clinical Course. In the typical case, a firm, cartilaginous-like "tumor" involving the sternocleidomastoid muscle is discovered about 10 to 14 days after birth, or sooner. The muscle feels short and inelastic. The head may be tilted to the affected side to a variable degree, while the chin points to the opposite side. The cervical vertebrae are normal. The swelling may increase for two to four weeks and remain stationary for two or three months, gradually regressing and disappearing in four to eight months. In a few cases, residual shortness of the sternocleidomastoid may remain, producing torticollis and asymmetry. In another small group, torticollis may not be apparent until three or four years later, when the neck elongates.

Coventry and Harris (1959) suggested that whether or not torticollis occurs and when it occurs are dependent on the ratio of normal muscle to fibrous tissue that remains after disappearance of the sternocleidomastoid muscle "tumor" of infancy.

Differential Diagnosis. The diagnosis is established by a history of a sternocleidomastoid "tumor," a short sternocleidomastoid muscle in early life, and normal cervical vertebrae.

Severe maldevelopment of the cervical vertebrae may rarely be confused with torticollis, but a roentgenogram will clarify the nature of the deformity.

Ocular torticollis is distinguished by a

milder degree of head tilt and the absence of contracture of the sternocleidomastoid muscle. The face looks toward the side of tilt and down, whereas in the muscular form the face looks up and away from the side of tilt. Conjugate ocular movements are abnormal, and hypertropia or hypotropia are present.

Secondary torticollis is usually a temporary, acutely painful condition ascribed to exposure to drafts of cold air, pharyngeal or cervical spine infection, or trauma.

Spasmodic torticollis occurs most frequently in adult life and is characterized by recurring attacks of irregular clonic or tonic contractions of neck muscles, which cause intermittent rotation and lateral flexion or extension of the head. Grimacing and blepharospasm may also be present. No single etiologic factor has been established.

Hanukoglu, Somekh, and Fried (1984) described benign paroxysmal torticollis, which is a self-limited disorder. It usually starts in early infancy and is characterized by attacks of torticollis associated with vomiting, ataxia, and drowsiness. The episodes may last from 30 minutes to several days, and occur every few weeks to every few months, eventually disappearing by age 1 to 5 years. It is seen most commonly in females. The cause is unknown but peripheral vestibular dysfunction has been suggested.

Sandyk (1984) reported the successful use of sodium valproate combined with baclofen in the treatment of one case of idiopathic spasmodic torticollis.

Pathology. Middleton (1930) described a cut section of the sternocleidomastoid "tumor" as having the appearance of glistening fibrous tissue. On microscopic examination, immature cellular fibrous tissue is seen containing dispersed remnants of muscle fibers. Many of the muscle fibers show absence of nuclei and vacuolation and evidence of continued degeneration.

Middleton (1930) believed that the microscopic picture in a fully developed case of torticollis could be interpreted only as representing the terminal stage of a sternocleidomastoid tumor. No degenerating muscle or immature fibrous tissue was observed; instead, swathes of adult noncellular fibrous tissue were seen. Scattered throughout were collections of muscle fibers that, although smaller than normal and varying in size and outline, were living, healthy fibers and bore no stigmata of degeneration.

No cases of fibrosarcoma of the sternocleidomastoid muscle have been reported (Gruhn and Hurwitt, 1951).

Treatment. Lee (1984), speaking only about spasmodic torticollis (which usually begins after the age of 40), reported that multiple drugs have been used alone and in combination (anticholinergics, benzodiazepines, dopaminergics, neuroleptics, carbamazepine, adrenergic blocking agents, and amantadine), but to date none has proved effective on a consistent basis.

In view of the observed tendency for "tumors" of the sternocleidomastoid muscle in infants to disappear spontaneously with no residual shortening, most writers (Hulbert, 1950; Gruhn and Hurwitt, 1951; Horsley, Pitman, and Schuler, 1954; and Coventry and Harris, 1959) advised against surgery on the sternocleidomastoid "tumor." They advocated surgery only for those cases in which torticollis persisted after a year. The authors also recommend this program.

Chandler and Altenberg (1944), Brown and McDowell (1950), and Clader, Sawyer, and McCurdy (1958) advised early total excision of the fibrous sternocleidomastoid muscle in well-developed cases. Brown performed the resection through a 5 cm collar incision, ligating the external jugular vein but preserving the 11th cranial nerve, phrenic nerve, internal jugular vein, and carotid artery. If necessary, the deep fascia or scalene muscles or the anterior border of the trapezius are divided. No postoperative splinting is necessary in these infants.

Those who do not operate on the "tumor" usually suggest massage, stretching, or the like, but Coventry and Harris (1959) believe that no treatment is as effective as the surgical one.

Treatment of a well-established muscular torticollis has included subcutaneous and open tenotomy of the inferior end of the sternocleidomastoid muscle. Lange (Steindler, 1940) divided the muscle at the upper end, and this approach has been combined with an inferior tenotomy. In Foelderl's procedure (Steindler, 1940), the clavicular head is divided near its middle third. The clavicular head is transposed to the distal sternal head and sutured, thereby lengthening the muscle. LaFerte (1947) felt that a 4 cm vertical incision between the clavicular and sternal heads, being in the line of traction when the deformity is corrected, might show less tendency to hypertrophy. He also pointed out that the platysma might be shortened, and if so should also be divided, otherwise failure might result and prolonged overcorrection becomes necessary.

In choosing the proper surgical procedure, consideration should be given to both the functional and the cosmetic result. Although complete excision of the sternocleidomastoid muscle in infancy does not seem to leave an objectionable hollow in the neck as the child grows, it does so in the teenager or adult. Penn and Kark (1954) performed a dermis-fat graft to correct the unsightly hollow two years after removal of the muscle in a 13 year old girl. Tenotomy at the clavicular end of the muscle may also tend to eliminate the normal prominence of the sternal head.

Ferkel and associates (1983) reported their experience in 12 patients with the use of bipolar release of the sternocleidomastoid muscle and lengthening of the sternal attachment, as illustrated in Figure 39–29. They

also released the contracted bands of fascia or muscle and postoperatively used a head halter traction for two to four weeks, followed by a Plastizote cervical collar in an overcorrected position associated with muscle stretching exercises for three to four months.

They selected the patients only after conservative treatment had failed, or from older children who had had previous operations. With this technique they reported 92 per cent good to excellent results, using for their assessment of results the following variables: facial asymmetry, neck movement, head tilt, scar formation, loss of the sternocleidomastoid column, and recurrence of the torticollis. Their results compared favorably with those of other procedures, such as simple division of the sternal and clavicular heads of the sternocleidomastoid muscle.

Ling (1976) studied the influence of age on the results of open sternocleidomastoid tenotomy in muscular torticollis. In his long-term study of 103 patients over the period from

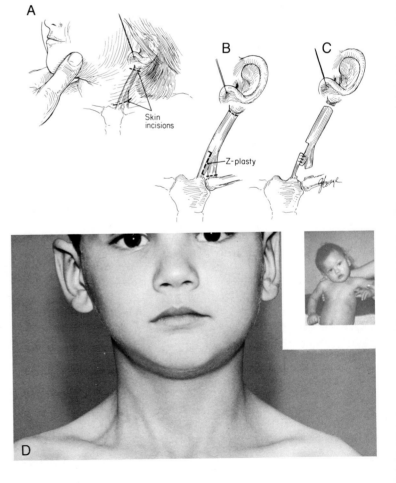

Figure 39–29. Ferkel's torticollis operation. *A,* The ear lobule has been retracted. Location of skin incisions. *B,* The clavicular and mastoid attachments are divided and the sternal attachment is lengthened. *C,* Operation completed. *D,* Pre- and postoperative photographs. The patient had the above-described operation with lengthening of the sternal head, and in this way the sternomastoid column is preserved. (From Ferkel, R. D., Westin, G. W., Dawson, E. G., and Oppenheim, W. L.: Muscular torticollis. A modified surgical approach. J. Bone Joint Surg., 65A:894, 1983.)

1962 to 1972, Ling concluded that the best results were obtained when surgery was performed between the ages of 1 and 4 years.

The preferred technique of the authors is an oblique incision made about 2.0 cm below the tip of the mastoid down to the muscle. The upper 4 cm of the sternocleidomastoid muscle is exposed, avoiding injury to the greater auricular nerve. The muscle is divided at its bony insertion, care being taken to identify and preserve the spinal accessory nerve that descends through the muscle. Approximately 2.5 to 4 cm of the muscle is excised. The head is tilted to the opposite side with the chin down and to the affected side, and any other restricting fascial or muscle (platysma, anterior scalene, and trapezius) bands are severed. When this has been completed, some tightness usually remains in the lower part of the sternocleidomastoid muscle. A short, transverse incision is made over the muscle approximately 4 cm above the clavicle. The muscle is completely divided, again with care taken to preserve the spinal accessory nerve. The procedure usually provides freedom of motion of the neck, but the short sternoclavicular heads that remain present an unsightly depression. If the clavicular head predominates, as in Figure 39–27, it is completely excised, leaving the sternal head undisturbed.

In all patients who have had torticollis for over one year, it is absolutely essential to hold the head in an overcorrected position for six to eight weeks or longer after the operation. If this is not done, the tendency of the patient to hold the head in the preoperative position and the development of scar contracture deep in the wound will result in recurrence of the torticollis.

Soeur (1940) applied a plaster cast that extended from the iliac crest to the top of the head. A ready-made brace (see Fig. 39–28), which rests on the shoulders and can be adjusted to hold the head in any position, is efficient if properly adjusted. The plaster cast or brace should generally be applied a day or two after the operation when the patient has recovered from the effects of the anesthesia.

In severe cases of long-standing torticollis, diplopia may be noted postoperatively, and Soeur (1940) reported that the patient's equilibrium might also be disturbed for a few days.

REFERENCES

Agris, J., Dingman, R. O., and Varon, J.: Correction of webbed neck defects. Ann. Plast. Surg., *11*:299, 1983.

Applebaum, E. L.: Laryngeal and tracheal problems in patients with central nervous system and spinal disorders. Otolaryngol. Clin. North Am., *12*:4, 829, 1979.

Arufe, H. N., Cabrera, V. N., and Sica, I. E.: Use of the epaulette flap to relieve burn contractures of the neck. Plast. Reconstr. Surg., *61*:707, 1978.

Aufricht, G.: Evaluation of pedicle flaps versus skin grafts in reconstruction of surface defects and scar contractures of the chin, cheeks and neck. Surgery, *15*:75, 1944.

Babcock, W. W.: Contracted dense scar of the neck despite the use of many Thiersch grafts. Surg. Clin. North Am., *12*:1405, 1932.

Badran, H. A.: The use of free groin flap in the treatment of post-burn contracted neck. Egypt. J. Plast. Reconstr. Surg., *1*:161, 1977.

Badran, H. A., El-Helaly, M. S., and Safe, I.: The lateral intercostal neurovascular free flap. Plast. Reconstr. Surg., *73*:17, 1984.

Barr, M. L., Bertram, L. F., and Lindsay, H. A.: The morphology of the nerve cell nucleus, according to sex. Anat. Rec., *107*:283, 1950.

Bizzarro, A. H.: Brevicollis. Lancet, *2*:828, 1938.

Blocker, T. G., Jr.: Free full thickness skin graft for the relief of burn contractures of the neck. South. Surg., *10*:849, 1941.

Brown, A. C. D., and Sataloff, R. T.: Special anesthetic techniques in head and neck surgery. Otolaryngol. Clin. North Am., *14*:3, 587, 1981.

Brown, J. B., Byars, L. T., and Blair, V. P.: The repair of surface defects from burns and other causes with thick split skin grafts. South. Med. J., *28*:408, 1935.

Brown, J. B., and McDowell, F.: Wry-neck facial distortion prevented by resection of fibrous stenomastoid muscle in infancy and childhood. Ann. Surg., *131*:721, 1950.

Brown, J. B., and McDowell, F.: Skin Grafting. Philadelphia, J. B. Lippincott Company, 1958, p. 234.

Bunchman, H. H., and Huang, T. T.: Prevention and management of contractures in patients with burns of the neck. Am. J. Surg., *130*:700, 1975.

Chandler, F. A.: Webbed neck (pterygium colli). Am. J. Dis. Child., *53*:798, 1937.

Chandler, F. A.: Muscular torticollis. J. Bone Joint Surg., *30A*:566, 1948.

Chandler, F. A., and Altenberg, A.: "Congenital" muscular torticollis. J.A.M.A., *125*:476, 1944.

Clader, D. N., Sawyer, K. C., and McCurdy, R. E.: Surgical treatment of congenital torticollis. Am. Surg., *24*:132, 1958.

Converse, J. M.: Burn deformities of the face and neck. Reconstructive surgery and rehabilitation. Surg. Clin. North Am., *47*:323, 1967.

Couglin, W. T.: Contractures due to burns. Surg. Gynecol. Obstet., *68*:352, 1939.

Coventry, M. B., and Harris, L. E.: Congenital muscular torticollis in infancy. J. Bone Joint Surg., *41A*:815, 1959.

Cramer, L. M.: Cervical splinting for burn contractures. Plast. Reconstr. Surg., *34*:293, 1964.

Cronin, T. D.: Successful correction of extensive scar

contractures of the neck using split skin grafts. *In* Skoog, T., and Ivy, R. H. (Eds.): Transactions of the International Society of Plastic Surgeons (First Congress, 1955). Baltimore, Williams & Wilkins Company, 1957, p. 123.

Cronin, T. D.: The use of a molded splint to prevent contracture after split skin grafting on the neck. Plast. Reconstr. Surg., 27:7, 1961.

Cronin, T. D.: Deformities of the cervical region. *In* Converse, J. M. (Ed.): Reconstructive Plastic Surgery. 1st Ed. Philadelphia, W. B. Saunders Company, 1964, p. 1175.

Cronin, T. D.: Burn scar contractures of the neck. *In* Lynch, J. D., and Lewis, S. R. (Eds.): Symposium on the Treatment of Burns. Vol. 5. St. Louis, MO, C. V. Mosby Company, 1973, p. 191.

Cronin, T. D.: Deformities of the cervical region. *In* Converse, J. M. (Ed.): Reconstructive Plastic Surgery. 2nd Ed. Philadelphia, W. B. Saunders Company, 1977, p. 1643.

Cronin, T. D.: Burn scar contractures of the neck. *In* Stark, R. B. (Ed.): Plastic Surgery of the Head and Neck. New York, Churchill Livingstone, 1987.

Cunningham, G. C., and Harley, J. F.: A case of Turner's syndrome. J. Pediatr., 38:738, 1951.

Davis, A. D.: Medial cleft of the lower lip and mandible. Plast. Reconstr. Surg., 6:62, 1950.

Davis, A. D.: Congenital webbing of the neck (pterygium colli). Am. J. Surg., 92:115, 1956.

Davis, J. S., and Kitlowski, E. A.: The theory and practical use of the Z-incision for the relief of scar contractures. Ann. Surg., 109:1001, 1939.

Dey, D. L.: Burn contractures in the child. Med. J. Aust., 2:604, 1972.

Dingman, R. O.: Some applications of Z-plasty procedure. Plast. Reconstr. Surg., 16:246, 1955.

Dingman, R. O.: The surgical correction of burn scar contractures of the neck. Surg. Clin. North Am., 41:1169, 1961.

Dowd, C. N.: Some details in the repair of cicatricial contractures of the neck. Surg. Gynecol. Obstet., 44:396, 1927.

Durham, R. H.: Encyclopedia of Medical Syndromes. New York, Paul B. Hoeber, 1960.

Evans, E. B., Larson, D. L., Abston, S., and Willis, B.: Prevention and correction of deformity after severe burns. Surg. Clin. North Am., 50:1361, 1970.

Ferkel, R. D., Westin, G. W., Dawson, E. G., and Oppenheim, W. L.: Muscular torticollis. A modified surgical approach. J. Bone Joint Surg., 65:894, 1983.

Flavell, G.: Webbing of neck, with Turner syndrome in the male. Br. J. Surg., 31:150, 1943.

Ford, C. E., and Hamerton, J. L.: The chromosomes of man. Nature, 178:1020, 1956.

Ford, C. E., Jones, K. W., Polani, P. E., de Almeida, J. C., and Briggs, J. H.: A sex-chromosome anomaly in a case of gonadal dysgenesis (Turner's syndrome). Lancet, 1:711, 1959.

Foucar, H. O.: Pterygium colli and allied conditions. Can. Med. Assoc. J., 59:251, 1948.

Frackelton, W. H.: Neck burns—early and late treatment. *In* Skoog, T., and Ivy, R. H. (Eds.): Transactions of the International Society of Plastic Surgeons (First Congress, 1955). Baltimore, Williams & Wilkins Company, 1957, p. 130.

Fujimori, A., Hiramoto, M., and Ofuji, S.: Sponge fixation method of early scars. Plast. Reconstr. Surg., 42:322, 1968.

Funke: Pterygium colli. Dtsch. Z. Chir., 3:162, 1902.

Furnas, D., and Fischer, G. W.: The Z-plasty: biomechanics and mathematics. Br. J. Plast. Surg., 24:144, 1971.

Gaskill, J. R.: Nasotracheal intubation in head and neck surgery. "Blind technique in the conscious patient." Arch. Otolaryngol., 86:697, 1967.

Gibbons, W. P.: Innovations of skin grafting as applied to chin-chest contractures. Plast. Reconstr. Surg., 35:322, 1965.

Gillies, H.: Experience with tubed pedicle flaps. Surg. Gynecol. Obstet., 60:291, 1935.

Gilmour, J. R.: The essential identity of the Klippel-Feil syndrome and iniencephaly. J. Pathol. Bacteriol., 53:117, 1941.

Ginestet, G., Merville, L., and Dupuis, A.: Le traitement des sequelles de brulures de la face et du cou par lambeaux cylindriques. Ann. Chir. Plast., 4:81, 1959.

Gottlieb, E.: Prolonged postoperative cervical pressure as an adjunct to plastic surgery of the neck. Plast. Reconstr. Surg., 32:600, 1963.

Greeley, P. W.: The plastic repair of scar contractures. Surgery, 15:224, 1944.

Grieve, J.: The relative incidence of sternomastoid and ocular torticollis in aircrew recruits. Br. J. Surg., 33:285, 1946.

Gruhn, J., and Hurwitt, E. S.: Fibrous sternomastoid tumor of infancy. Pediatrics, 8:522, 1951.

Hanukoglu, A., Somekh, E., and Fried, D.: Benign paroxysmal torticollis in infancy. Clin. Pediatr., 23:272, 1984.

Harii, K., Ohmori, K., and Ohmori, S.: Utilization of free composite tissue transfer by microvascular anastomoses for the repair of burn deformities. Burns, 1:237, 1975.

Harii, K., Torii, S., and Sekiguchi, J.: The free lateral thoracic flap. Plast. Reconstr. Surg., 62:212, 1978.

Hellstadius, A.: Torticollis congenita. Acta Chir. Scand., 62:586, 1927.

Ho, L. C. Y., Sykes, P. J., and Bailey, B. N.: Extensive deep neck burns. Burns, 1:149, 1975.

Horsley, G. E., Pitman, N., and Schuler, J. D.: Fibrous sternocleidomastoid tumor of infancy. J. Tenn. Med. Assoc., 47:20, 1954.

Hough, G. de N., Jr.,: Congenital torticollis. Surg. Gynecol. Obstet., 58:972, 1934.

Hulbert, K. F.: Congenital torticollis. J. Bone Joint Surg., 32B:50, 1950.

Jackson, W. P. U., and Sougin-Mibashan, R.: Turner's syndrome in the female. Br. Med. J., 2:368, 1953.

Jacobacci, S., and Towey, R. M.: Anesthesia for severe burn contractures of the neck: a case report. East Afr. Med. J., 55:11, 543, 1978.

Jones, P. G.: Torticollis in infancy and childhood: sternomastoid fibrosis and sternomastoid "tumor." Springfield, IL, Charles C Thomas, 1968.

Jost, A.: Sur les effets de la castration précoce de fembryon mâle de Lapin. C. R. Soc. Biol., 141:126, 1947.

Kazanjian, F. H.: The repair of contractures resulting from burns. N. Engl. J. Med., 215:1104, 1936.

Kiesewetter, W. B., Nelson, P. K., Palladino, V. S., and Koop, C. E.: Neonatal torticollis. J.A.M.A., 157:1281, 1955.

Kirschbaum, S.: Mentosternal contracture, treatment by acromial flap. Plast. Reconstr. Surg., 21:131, 1958.

Klippel, M., and Feil, A.: Anomalie de la colonne vertébrale par absence des vertebres cervicales—cage thoracique remontant jusqu'à la base du crane. Bull. Soc. Anat. (Paris), 87:185, 1912.

Kobylinski, O.: Ueber eine flughautahnliche Austreitung am Halse. Arch. Anthropol., *14*:343, 1882.

Koepke, G. H.: The role of physical medicine in the treatment of burns. Surg. Clin. North Am., *50*:1385, 1970.

Koepke, G. H., and Feller, I.: Physical measures for the prevention and treatment of deformities following burns. J.A.M.A., *199*:791, 1971.

LaFerte, A. D.: The role of the platysma muscle in torticollis deformity. Plast. Reconstr. Surg., *2*:72, 1947.

Larson, D. L., Abston, S., Willis, B., et al: Contracture and scar formation in the burn patient. Clin. Plast. Surg., *1*:653, 1974.

La Ruffa, H.: Cirugia de las membranas cervicales alares (pterygium colli). Bol. y Trab. Soc. Argentina de Cir., *31*:572, 1970.

Lee, M. C.: Spasmodic torticollis and other idiopathic torsion dystonias. Medical management. Postgrad. Med., *75*:139, 1984.

Levy, E. P., Pashayan, H., and Fraser, F. C.: XX and XY Turner phenotypes in a family. Am. J. Dis. Child, *120*:36, 1970.

Lidge, R. T., Bechtol, R. C., and Lambert, C. N.: Congenital muscular torticollis. J. Bone Joint Surg., *39A*:1165, 1957.

Ling, C. M.: The influence of age on the results of open sternomastoid tenotomy in muscular torticollis. Clin. Orthop., *116*:142, 1976.

MacCollum, D. W.: The early and later treatment of burns in children. Am. J. Surg., *39*:275, 1938a.

MacCollum, D. W.: Congenital webbing of the neck. N. Engl. J. Med., *219*:251, 1938b.

Malick, M. H., and Carr, J. A.: Flexible elastomer mold in burn scar control. Am. J. Occup. Ther., *34*:603, 1980.

Martins, A. G.: Burn contractures. Br. J. Plast. Surg., *13*:152, 1960.

May, H.: The correction of cicatricial deformities. Surg. Clin. North Am., *29*:611, 1949.

May, H.: Reconstructive and Reparative Surgery. 2nd Ed. Philadelphia, F. A. Davis Company, 1958.

McIndoe, A. H.: Total facial reconstruction following burns. Postgrad. Med., *6*:187, 1949.

Mendoza, C. A., Benzecry, A., Hernandez, M., et al.: Prevention of contractures following burns. Bol. Soc. Venez. Cirurg., *15*:381, 1961.

Menick, F. J., Furnas, D. W., and Achauer, B. M.: Lateral cervical advancement flaps for the correction of webbed neck deformity. Plast. Reconstr. Surg., *73*:223, 1984.

Mennig, H.: Die plastiche Operation des Pterygium colli. Z. Laryngol. Rhinol. Otol., *35*:153, 1956.

Middleton, D. S.: The pathology of congenital torticollis. Br. J. Surg., *18*:188, 1930.

Mixter, C. G.: Contractions of the neck following burns. N. Engl. J. Med., *208*:190, 1933.

Moore, D. J.: The role of the maxillofacial prosthetist in support of the burn patient. J. Prosthet. Dent., *24*:58, 1970.

Mukhin, M. V., and Mamonov, A. F.: Classification of scarred neck contractures and their surgical therapy by methods of local plastic operation. Acta Chir. Plast. (Praha), *12*:48, 1970.

Mühlbauer, W., Herndl, E., and Stock, W.: The forearm flap. Plast. Reconstr. Surg., *70*:336, 1982.

Mulder, D. S., and Wallace, D. H.: The use of the fiberoptic bronchoscope to facilitate endotracheal intubation following head and neck trauma. J. Trauma, *15*:638, 1975.

Mutter, T. D.: Cases of Deformity From Burns Relieved by Plastic Surgery. Philadelphia, Merrihew & Thompson Company, 1843.

Noordhoff, M. S.: Control and prevention of hypertrophic scarring and contracture. Clin. Plast. Surg., *1*:49, 1974.

Nora, J. J., Nora, A. H., and Sinha, A. K.: The Ullrich-Noonan syndrome (Turner phenotype). Am. J. Dis. Child, *127*:48, 1974.

Nora, J. J., and Sinha, A. K.: Direct male-to-male transmission of the XY Turner phenotype. Lancet, *1*:250, 1970.

Ohmori, K.: Application of microvascular free flaps to burn deformities. World J. Surg., *2*:193, 1978.

Ousterhout, D. K., Yeakel, M. H., Lau, B. M., and Tumbusch, W. T.: Inflatable splint: an adjunct to prevention and treatment of cervical scar contractures. Br. J. Plast. Surg., *22*:185, 1969.

Padgett, E. C.: The full thickness skin graft in the correction of soft tissue deformities. J.A.M.A., *98*:18, 1932.

Padgett, E. C., and Stephenson, K. L.: Plastic and Reconstructive Surgery. Springfield, IL, Charles C Thomas, 1948, p. 627.

Parks, D. H.: Late problems in burns. Clin. Plast. Surg., *4*:547, 1977.

Penn, J., and Kark, W.: Surgical treatment of a case of wry-neck. S. Afr. Med. J., *28*:929, 1954.

Pitanguy, I.: Cervical contractures. *In* Skoog, T., and Ivy, R. H. (Eds.): Transactions of the International Society of Plastic Surgeons (First Congress, 1955). Baltimore, Williams & Wilkins Company, 1957, p. 147.

Pitanguy, I., and Bisaggio, S.: Retracoes, cicatriciais do pescoco. Rev. Bras. Cirurg., *53*:469, 1967.

Polani, P. E., Hunter, W. F., and Lennox, B.: Chromosomal sex in Turner's syndrome with coarctation of the aorta. Lancet, *2*:120, 1954.

Polani, P. E., Lessof, M. H., and Bishop, P. M. F.: Colour blindness in "ovarian agenesis" (gonadal dysplasia). Lancet, *2*:118, 1956.

Reye, R. D. K.: Sterno-mastoid tumour and congenital muscular torticollis. Med. J. Aust., *1*:867, 1951.

Roemer, F. J.: Relation of torticollis to breech delivery. Am. J. Obstet. Gynecol., *68*:1146, 1954.

Sandyk, R.: Beneficial effect of sodium valproate and baclofen in spasmodic torticollis: a case report. S. Afr. Med. J., *65*:62, 1984.

Schmid, E., and Romacher, W.: Chirurgie reparation du cou et du menton après brulures. Ann. Chir. Plast., *4*:51, 1959.

Schneider, K. W., and McCullagh, E. P.: Infantilism congenital webbed neck and cubitus valgus (Turner syndrome). Cleve. Clin. Q., *10*:112, 1943.

Schröder, R.: Die operative Korrektur des Pterygium colli. Arch. Klin. Chir., *289*:643, 1958.

Shchipacheva, V. I.: Plastic treatment of scar contractures of neck with Filatov pedicle flap in children. Acta Chir. Plast., *17*:49, 1975.

Shearin, J. D., and De Franzo, A. J.: Butterfly correction of webbed neck deformity in Turner's syndrome. Plast. Reconstr. Surg., *66*:129, 1980.

Smith, F.: Plastic and Reconstructive Surgery. Philadelphia, W. B. Saunders Company, 1950, p. 666.

Soeur, R.: Treatment of congenital torticollis. J. Bone Joint Surg., *22*:459, 1940.

Song, R.: Discussion of the forearm flap by Mühlbauer, W., Herndl, E., and Stock, W. Plast. Reconstr. Surg., *70*:343, 1982.

Sougin-Mibashan, R., and Jackson, W. P. U.: Turner's syndrome in the male. Br. Med. J., 2:371, 1953.

Spina, V.: Tratamento Cirurgico das Cicatrizes do Pescoco Pos-Queimadura. Sao Paulo, Brazil, V. Spina, 1955.

Steiker, D. D., Mellman, W. J., Bongiovanni, A. M., Eberlein, W. K., and Leboeuf, G.: Turner's syndrome in the male. J. Pediatr., 58:321, 1961.

Steindler, A.: Orthopedic operations. Springfield, IL, Charles C Thomas, 1940.

Stromeyer, G. F. L.: Beitrage zur operativen Orthopädik. Hannover, Helwing, 1838, cited by Gruhn and Hurwitt (1951).

Sybert, V. P.: Adult height in Turner syndrome with and without androgen therapy. J. Pediatr., 104:365, 1984.

Tanzer, R. C.: Burn contracture of the neck. Plast. Reconstr. Surg., 33:207, 1964.

Taylor, F.: Induration of the sternomastoid muscle. Trans. Pathol. Soc. (Lond.), 26:224, 1875.

Thomas, C. V.: Thin flaps. Plast. Reconstr. Surg., 65:747, 1980.

Tjio, J. H., and Levan, A.: The chromosome number of man. Hereditas, 42:1, 1956.

Turner, H. H.: A syndrome of infantilism congenital webbed neck and cubitus valgus. Endocrinology, 23:566, 1938.

Visse, J. H., Adendorff, D. J., Malherbe, W. D., et al.: Free flap transfer with microvascular anastomosis. S. Afr. Med. J., 50:2026, 1976.

von Muralt, R. H.: Bilateral occurrence of congenital muscular torticollis. Helv. Paediatr. Acta, 1:349, 1946.

Wilkins, L., and Fleischmann, W.: Ovarian agenesis: pathology, associated clinical symptoms and the bearing on the theories of sex differentiation. J. Clin. Endocrinol., 4:357, 1944.

Wilkins, L., Grumbach, M. M., and Van Wyk, J. J.: Chromosomal sex in "ovarian agenesis." J. Clin. Endocrinol., 14:1270, 1954.

Willis, B.: A follow-up. The use of orthoplast isoprene splints in the treatment of the acutely burned child. Am. J. Occup. Ther., 24:187, 1970.

Wilson, R. D.: Personal communication, 1974.

Wilson, R. D., Knapp, C., Traber, D. L., and Evans, B.: Safe management of the child with a contracted neck: a new method. South Med. J., 63:1420, 1970.

Wynn-Williams, D.: Congenital midline cervical cleft and web. Br. J. Plast. Surg., 5:87, 1952.

Reconstruction of the Auricle

CONGENITAL DEFORMITIES

Total auricular reconstruction with autogenous tissues is one of the greatest technical feats that a reconstructive surgeon may encounter. An inherent understanding of sculpture and design influences the success of surgery, but strict adherence to basic principles of plastic surgery and tissue transfer is of equal importance.

During the years, ear reconstruction has stimulated the imagination of many surgeons who have provided innumerable contribu-

tions. This chapter is meant to document various techniques that have stood the test of time and to provide the reader with guidelines for managing a variety of ear deformities.

History

Ear reconstruction was first referred to in the *Susruta Samhita* (Bhishagratna, 1907), in which the use of a cheek flap was suggested for repairing the earlobe. As early as 1597, Tagliacozzi described repair of both upper and lower ear deformities with retroauricular flaps. In 1845 Dieffenbach reported the repair of the middle third of the ear with an advancement flap (see Fig. 40–45). This technique may occasionally have application today.

Early surgical attention focused mainly on traumatic deformities. However, by the end of the nineteenth century surgeons began to address congenital defects, in particular prominent ears (Ely, 1881).

The concept of microtia repair had its beginnings in 1920, when Gillies buried carved costal cartilage under mastoid skin and subsequently separated it from the head with a cervical flap. Pierce (1930) modified this method by lining the new sulcus with a skin graft and building the helix with a tubed flap. Gillies (1937) repaired more than 30 microtic ears using maternal ear cartilage; these were found to have progressively resorbed (Converse, 1977).

Peer (1948) turned to autogenous rib cartilage, which he ingeniously diced and placed in a Vitallium ear mold beneath the abdominal skin. After five months he retrieved the banked mold, opened it, and harvested the framework of cartilage chips, which had united by scar tissue that had grown through the fenestrations of the mold. Although the framework's matricial scar contracted and the shape withered, this technique led to a wave of enthusiasm for ear surgery, which again turned to allograft cartilage. Experiencing the same frustration as others (Kirkham, 1940; Brown and associates, 1947; Pierce, Klabunde, and Brobst, 1952; Dupertuis and Musgrave, 1959), Steffensen (1952) used preserved rib cartilage to produce excellent results, but later reported progressive resorption of the same cartilage frameworks (Steffensen, 1955).

A major breakthrough came in 1959, when Tanzer rekindled the use of autogenous rib cartilage, which he carved in a solid block. His excellent results have persisted during the years.

In an effort to circumvent extensive surgical procedures, Cronin (1966) introduced silicone ear frameworks, but found that, like other inorganic implants (e.g., polyethylene, nylon mesh, Marlex, polyester net, and Teflon), they suffered a high incidence of extrusion (Curtin and Bader, 1969; Lynch and associates, 1972). Initially, Cronin (1974) minimized this problem by providing fascia lata or galeal and fascial flaps for extra autogenous rim coverage, but later, when he found that the alloplastic frameworks still extruded, he discontinued this practice.

To this date, autogenous cartilage remains the most reliable material that produces results with the least complications (Tanzer, 1959, 1963, 1971; Fukuda, 1974; Brent, 1980a,b, 1987). Furthermore, rib cartilage provides the most substantial source for fabricating a total ear framework. Although contralateral conchal cartilage has been used for this purpose (Gorney, Murphy, and Falces, 1971; Davis, 1972), it seems best to reserve auricular cartilage for repairing partial ear defects, for which considerably less tissue bulk is needed.

Anatomy

The ear is difficult to reproduce surgically because it is made up of a complexly convoluted frame of delicate elastic cartilage surrounded by a thin skin envelope (Fig. 40–1). The denuded cartilage framework conforms almost exactly to the ear's surface contours except for its absence in the earlobe, which consists of fibrofatty tissue rather than cartilage. In most microtic vestiges, the presence of the lobular tissue is a valuable asset in the repair (see Fig. 40–14). When the lobule is lost in total ear avulsions, it is best recreated by shaping the bottom of the carved ear framework to resemble the lobe.

The ear's rich vascular supply comes from the superficial temporal and posterior auricular vessels, which can nourish a nearly avulsed ear even on surprisingly narrow tissue pedicles (see Fig. 40–30).

The sensory supply is chiefly derived from the inferiorly coursing great auricular nerve. The upper portions of the ear are supplied by the lesser occipital and auriculotemporal

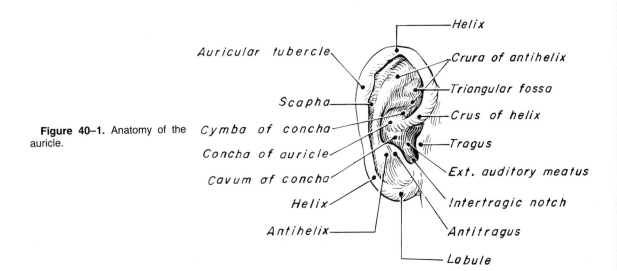

Figure 40–1. Anatomy of the auricle.

nerves, whereas the conchal region is supplied by a vagal nerve branch.

An understanding of the anatomy facilitates nerve blocking of the ear with local anesthetic solution (Fig. 40–2). First, the great auricular nerve is blocked by injecting a wheal underneath the lobule. After awaiting its effect, one continues injecting upward along the auriculocephalic sulcus, around the top of the ear and down to the tragus. Finally, the vagal branch can be anesthetized without discomfort by traversing the conchal cartilage with a needle placed through the already anesthetized auriculocephalic sulcus to raise a skin wheal just behind the canal.

Embryology and the Middle Ear Problem

At consultation the parents of a microtic infant are usually most concerned with the hearing problem. They think either that the child is completely deaf on the affected side or that hearing can be restored by merely opening a hole in the skin. The physician can do much to alleviate their anxieties and to correct these misconceptions by an explanation of fundamental ear embryology.

As the human ear's receptive (inner) portion is derived from embryologic tissue different from that of the conductive (external and middle) portion (Fig. 40–3), the inner ear is rarely involved in microtia and these patients have at least some hearing in the affected ear.

The problem is conduction, which is blocked by the malformed middle and external ear complex. Typically, these patients have approximately 40 per cent hearing on the affected side.

Tissues of both the middle and external ear are derived chiefly from the first (mandibular) and second (hyoid) branchial arches. The auricle itself is formed from six "hillocks" of tissue that lie along these arches and are first seen in the five week embryo (Figs. 40–4, 40–5) (His, 1899; Streeter, 1922; Arey, 1974).

On the other hand, the inner ear first appears at three weeks and is derived from tissues of distinctly separate ectodermal origin. Perhaps this explains why it is usually spared the developmental mishap that almost invariably involves the middle ear of microtic patients. Refinements in polytomography have occasionally demonstrated dysplasia and hypoplasia of the inner ear (Nauton and Valvassori, 1968; Reisner, 1969). However, in evaluating approximately 1000 microtic cases over a 15 year period, the author has seen only three patients who were totally deaf. These were patients with unilateral

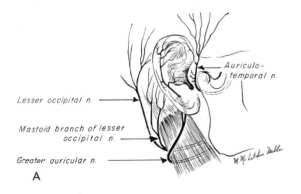

A

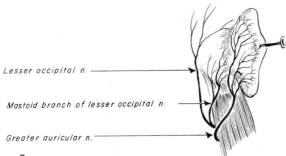

B

Figure 40–2. Sensory nerve supply of the auricle.

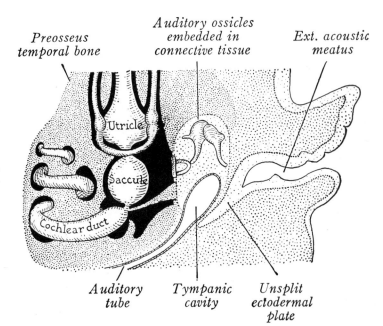

Figure 40–3. Partly schematic section of the ear in a three month embryo. (From Arey, L. B.: Developmental Anatomy. 6th Ed. Philadelphia, W. B. Saunders Company, 1954.)

microtia who had no family history of microtia. Because of their normal inner ear, patients with bilateral microtia usually have serviceable hearing, and use bone conductive hearing aids to overcome the transmission block. They usually develop normal speech.

However, surgical correction of the conductive problem is difficult because the middle ear lying beneath the closed skin is not normal. Exploration involves cautiously avoiding the facial nerve while drilling a canal through solid bone. One must usually create the tympanum with tissue grafts; the distorted or fused ossicles may be irreparable. As skin grafts are not readily vascularized on the drilled bony canal, chronic drainage is a frequent complication and meatal stenosis

is common. Finally, unless the surgeon can close the functional difference between the repaired and normal ear to within 15 to 20 decibels (an elusive feat in most surgeons' hands), binaural hearing will not be achieved.

As children do well without middle ear surgery (eight out of nine microtic cases are unilateral and the infants are "born adjusted" to the monaural condition), most surgeons presently consider that potential gains from middle ear surgery in unilateral microtia are outweighed by the potential risks and complications of the surgery itself.

The author believes that middle ear surgery should be reserved for cases of bilateral microtia, for which a team approach must be planned with an experienced, competent otologist. In these cases, the auricular construction should precede the middle ear surgery, since once an attempt is made to "open the ear," the virgin skin is scarred, a condition that compromises a satisfactory auricular construction. On the horizon lie implantable acoustic devices, which may offer a solution for these patients.

An otologist's viewpoint is presented later in the chapter.

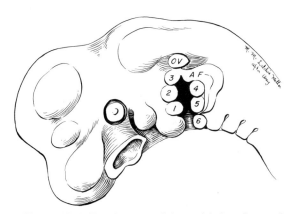

Figure 40–4. Development of the auricle in a five week human embryo: *1* to *6,* elevations (hillocks) on the mandibular and hyoid arches. ov = otic vesicle. (After Arey.)

Etiology

INCIDENCE

According to an extensive study conducted by Grabb (1965), microtia occurs once in

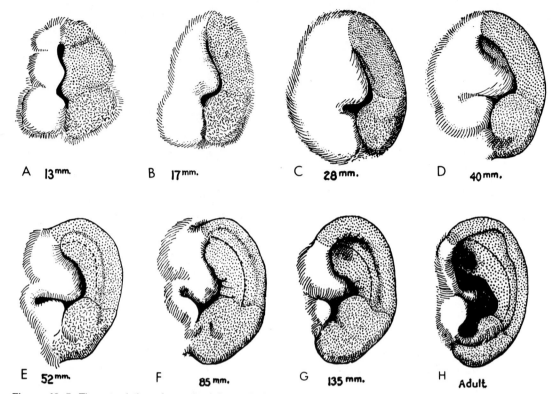

A 13mm.   B 17mm.   C 28mm.   D 40mm.

E 52mm.   F 85mm.   G 135mm.   H Adult

Figure 40–5. The retardation of growth of the auricular component of the mandibular arch and the expansion and forward rotation of the component of the hyoid arch. (After Streeter; from Patten, M.: Human Embryology. 3rd Ed. New York, McGraw-Hill Book Company, 1968.)

every 6000 births. The occurrence is estimated at one in 4000 in the Japanese and as high as one in 900 to 1200 births in Navajo Indians (Aase and Tegtmeier, 1977).

HEREDITARY FACTORS

In a study conducted by Rogers (1968), morphologic, anatomic, and genetic interrelationships were shown to exist among microtic, constricted, and protruding ears. In this thorough investigation, it was demonstrated that these deformities not only are interrelated but can also be hereditary.

Preauricular pits and sinuses and a combination of pits, preauricular appendages, cupping deformity, and deafness are hereditarily dominant (Wildervanck, 1962; Minkowitz and Minkowitz, 1964). Both dominant and recessive characteristics have been revealed in deafness associated with several auricular abnormalities (Königsmark, 1969). Ear deformities frequently recur in families of patients with mandibulofacial dysostosis (Treacher Collins syndrome) (Rogers, 1964). In the author's experience, these are frequently constricted ear deformities, an ab-

normality that is known to be hereditary (Potter, 1937; Hanhart, 1949; Erich and Abu-Jamra, 1965; Kessler, 1967). Hanhart (1949) reported a severe form of microtia associated with a cleft or high palate in 10 per cent of family members studied, and Tanzer (1971) found that approximately 25 per cent of his series of 43 patients with microtia had relatives with evidence of the first and second branchial arch syndrome (craniofacial microsomia); microtia was present in four instances.

In a thorough, intensive survey of 96 families of their 171 microtic patients, Takahashi and Maeda (1982) ruled out chromosomal aberrations, concluding that inheritance must be multifactorial and that there is a 5.7 per cent risk of recurrence. In previous studies, others found between 3 and 8 per cent multifactorial inheritance in first degree relatives.

SPECIFIC FACTORS

McKenzie and Craig (1955) theorized that tissue ischemia resulting from an obliterated stapedial artery is the cause of developmental auricular abnormalities (see also Chap. 62). The occurrence of deafness and occasional microtia resulting from rubella during the first trimester of pregnancy is well known. Also, certain drugs during this critical period may be causative; the author has seen at least three cases of microtia that resulted from the mother's ingestion of the tranquilizer thalidomide.

Diagnosis

CLASSIFICATION

Rogers (1968) noted that one could classify most types of auricular hypoplasia in a descending scale of severity. This corresponds to Streeter's (1922) depiction of embryologic patterns of auricular development. Rogers divided developmental ear defects into four groups: (1) microtia; (2) lop ear, i.e., folding or deficiency of the superior helix and scapha; (3) "cup" or constricted ear, with a deep concha and deficiency of the superior helix and anthelical crura; and (4) the common prominent or protruding ear.

Using a system that correlates with embryologic development, Tanzer (1975) classified congenital ear defects according to the approach necessary for their surgical correction (Table 40–1).

Associated Deformities

As discussed previously, embryologic development dictates that the microtic ear is usually accompanied by middle ear abnormalities. In full-blown, classic microtia, it is usual to find canal atresia and ossicular abnormalities. The middle ear deformity may range from diminished canal caliber and minor ossicular abnormalities to fused, hypoplastic ossicles and failure of mastoid pneumatization.

Table 40–1. Clinical Classification of Auricular Defects (Tanzer)

I. Anotia
II. Complete hypoplasia (microtia)
   A. With atresia of external auditory canal
   B. Without atresia of external auditory canal
III. Hypoplasia of middle third of auricle
IV. Hypoplasia of superior third of auricle
   A. Constricted (cup and lop) ear
   B. Cryptotia
   C. Hypoplasia of entire superior third
V. Prominent ear

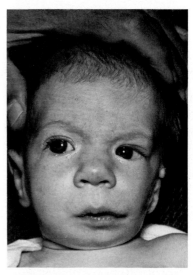

Figure 40–6. Patient with unilateral craniofacial microsomia (first and second branchial arch syndrome) displaying microtia; macrostomia; hypoplasia of the zygoma, maxilla, and mandible; and soft tissue hypoplasia.

Because the auricle develops from tissues of the mandibular and hyoid branchial arches, it is not surprising that a significant percentage of microtic patients exhibit deficient facial components that originate from these embryologic building blocks. These deformities are defined as unilateral craniofacial microsomia (first and second branchial arch syndrome) (Fig. 40–6). The most complete genetic expression of this condition includes defects of the external and middle ear; hypoplasia of the mandibular, maxillary, zygomatic, and temporal bones; macrostomia and lateral facial clefts; paresis of the facial nerve; and atrophy of the facial muscles and parotid gland (May, 1962; Longacre, de Stefano, and Holmstrand, 1963; Grabb, 1965). Dellon, Claybaugh, and Hoopes (1983) showed that the palatal muscles are rarely spared in this syndrome (see Chap. 62).

Urogenital tract abnormalities are increased in the presence of microtia (Longenecker, Ryan, and Vincent, 1965), particularly when the patient is afflicted with other manifestations of unilateral craniofacial microsomia (Taylor, 1965).

Complete Microtia (Hypoplasia)

CLINICAL CHARACTERISTICS

Microtia varies from the complete absence of auricular tissues (anotia) to a somewhat normal but small ear with an atretic canal.

Between these extremes there is an endless variety of vestiges, the most common being a vertically oriented, sausagelike remnant (see Fig. 40–14A). Microtia is nearly twice as frequent in males as in females, and the right-to-left-to-bilateral ratio is roughly 5:3:1 (Dupertuis and Musgrave, 1959; Ogino and Yoshikawa, 1963).

The microtic lobule is usually displaced superiorly to the level of the opposite, normal side, although incomplete ear migration occasionally leaves it in an inferior location. Approximately half the patients exhibit gross characteristics of unilateral craniofacial microsomia, although Converse and associates (1973, 1974) demonstrated tomographically that skeletal deficiencies exist in all cases. Whatever the deformity, the author has been impressed with its potential for causing psychologic havoc among the entire family, varying from the patient's emotional insecurity to the parents' deep-seated guilt.

GENERAL CONSIDERATIONS

During the initial consultation, it is imperative to describe to the patient and/or the family the technical limitations involved in surgically correcting microtia, and to outline alternative methods of managing each individual's particular deformity. The author strongly favors autogenous rib cartilage for auricular construction. Although its use necessitates an operation that carries a significant morbidity rate, it must be noted that, unlike a reconstruction with alloplastic materials, a successful construction with autogenous tissue is less susceptible to trauma; it therefore eliminates the problem of patients who may be excessively cautious about the performance of normal, everyday activities.

The age at which an auricular construction should begin is governed by both psychologic and physical considerations. Since the body image concept usually begins to form around the age of 4 or 5 years (Knorr, Edgerton, and Barbarie, 1974), it would be ideal to begin construction before the child enters school and becomes psychologically traumatized by the ridicule of peers. However, surgery should be postponed until rib growth provides substantial cartilage to permit a quality framework fabrication.

In the author's experience with over 400 patients with microtia whose ages range from 1 month to 62 years, the patients or families consistently stated that the psychologic disturbances rarely began before age 7 years but usually became overt from ages 7 to 10. Hence, in general, the author prefers to delay the initial cartilage graft until the patient is 6 years old, when there is usually sufficient rib cartilage for the repair. At age 6, the normal ear has grown to within 6 or 7 mm of its full vertical height (Farkas, 1974), which permits the construction of an ear that has reasonably constant symmetry with the opposite normal ear. Tanzer (1974a) demonstrated comparable increases in vertical height in both normal and reconstructed ears over periods of 10 to 16 years, but the roles played in this growth by soft tissues and by cartilage have not been determined.

If the patient is small for his or her age, or if the opposite (normal) ear is large, the author finds it prudent to postpone surgery for several years.

CORRELATION WITH CORRECTION OF OTHER FACIAL DEFICIENCIES

Before repairing the microtic ear, it is necessary to correlate timing with any other facial surgery that may be necessary, e.g., surgical correction of mandibular or maxillary hypoplasia or soft tissue atrophy.

In the author's experience, the patient and family are usually more concerned about the ear defect initially; thus, auricular surgery is usually under way before other corrections begin. By careful planning of the auricular location with reference to the opposite, normal side, it should be possible to meet this psychologic urgency without compromising other facial repairs. If mandibular or soft tissue repairs are begun before that of the ear, every effort must be made to preserve the auricular site free of scar.

Author's Method of Microtia Repair

The cartilage graft is the "foundation" of an auricular construction and, as in the construction of a house, it should be built and well established under ideal conditions before further stages or refinements are undertaken. By implanting the cartilage graft as the first surgical stage, one takes advantage of the optimal elasticity and circulation of an unviolated, scar-free skin "pocket." For these reasons, the author prefers to avoid initial lobule transposition or vestige division, since the resulting scars cannot help but inhibit the circulation and restrict the skin's elasticity, factors that in turn diminish its ability to accommodate a three-dimensional cartilage graft safely. In the author's experience, it seems easier both to judge the placement of the lobule and to "splice" it correctly into position with reference to a well-established, underlying framework. Although Tanzer (1978) transposed the lobule simultaneously with implantation of the cartilage graft during the last three cases of his clinical practice, the author finds it safer and far more accurate to transpose the lobule as a secondary procedure (see Fig. 40–11) (Brent, 1980a, 1987).

The third stage generally combines tragus construction, conchal excavation, and contralateral otoplasty, if indicated. By combining these procedures, tissues that are normally discarded from an otoplasty can be employed advantageously as free grafts in the tragus construction.

During a fourth stage, the ear is separated from the head and surfaced on its underside with a skin graft to create an auriculocephalic sulcus.

Preoperative Consultation

During the initial consultation, surgical expectations and psychologic considerations should be discussed with the patient and family, emphasizing the goals of reconstruction.

Although costal cartilage can be carved to form a delicate framework, it must be remembered that the volume and projection of the furnished three-dimensional framework are limited by the two-dimensional skin flap under which it is placed. Furthermore, because the retroauricular-mastoid skin that covers the framework is somewhat thicker than the normal, delicate anterolateral auricular skin, it blunts the details of a carved framework.

Hence, the plastic surgeon's aim is to achieve accurate representation, i.e., to create an acceptable facsimile of an ear of the proper size, position, and orientation to other facial features.

During the consultation, the discomforts and inconveniences of the surgery should be described, including the expected chest pain, the length of time that dressings must be worn, and the need for limited activities for four to six weeks. Finally, the risks and possible complications of the surgery are thoroughly discussed. The latter include pneumothorax, cartilage graft loss secondary to infection, skin flap necrosis, and hematoma. It should be stressed that, with proper precautions, these risks are less severe than the emotional trauma created by an absent ear.

Planning and Preparation

The result of a total ear reconstruction depends not only on meticulous surgical technique, but also on careful preoperative planning. It is essential to practice carving techniques on a number of human cadaver cartilages before applying them to a live patient. An acrylic or plaster replica of a normal ear serves as an excellent model for practice carvings.

During the patient's second office consultation, preoperative study photographs are obtained and an x-ray film pattern is traced from the opposite, normal ear. This pattern is reversed, and a framework pattern is designed for the new ear. After sterilization, these patterns serve as guidelines for framework fabrication at the time of surgery.

The location of the reconstructed ear is predetermined by first noting the topographic relationship of the opposite, normal ear with facial features, and then duplicating its position at the proposed reconstruction site. First, the height of the vestige from the front view is compared with that of the opposite, normal ear (Fig. 40–7). From the side, it should be noted that the ear's axis is roughly parallel to the nasal profile (Broadbent and Mathews, 1957; Gorney, Murphy, and Falces, 1971). Finally, the distance between the lateral canthus and the normal ear's helical root is noted and recorded.

FIRST STAGE OF RECONSTRUCTION

Almost invariably, the author's first-stage "foundation" in correcting microtia is fabricating and inserting the cartilaginous ear framework. As discussed previously, because resulting scars can be a significant handicap, the author rarely employs a preliminary procedure.

Obtaining the Rib Cartilage

Rib cartilages are obtained en bloc from the side contralateral to the ear being constructed, so as to utilize natural rib configu-

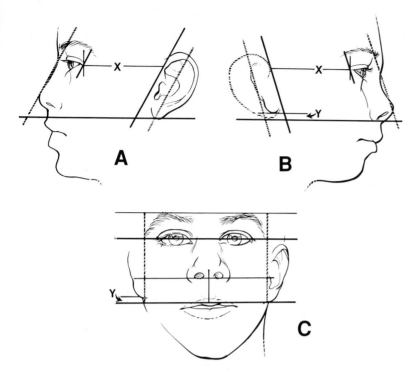

Figure 40–7. *A* to *C,* Preoperative determination of auricular location. The ear's axis is positioned to match the opposite side, roughly parallel to the nasal profile; the helical root is positioned equidistant from the lateral canthus. The reversed auricular pattern is traced 6 mm below the lobule, as determined by frontal measurement.

ration (Fig. 40–8). The rib cartilages are removed through a horizontal or slightly oblique incision, which is made just above the costal margin. After division of the external oblique and rectus muscles, the film pattern is placed on the exposed cartilages to determine the necessary extent of rib resection.

The helical rim is fashioned separately with cartilage from the first free-floating rib (Fig. 40–8). Excision of this cartilage facilitates access to the synchondrotic region of the sixth and seventh ribs, which supplies a sufficient block to carve the framework body. Extraperichondrial dissection is preferable in order to obtain an unmarred specimen.

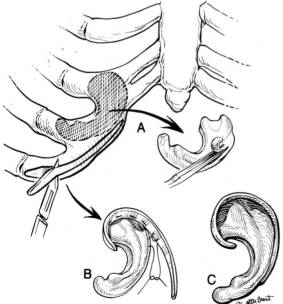

Figure 40–8. Sculpting an ear framework from costal cartilage. Obtaining the cartilage specimens from the contralateral chest utilizes natural cartilage configuration. *A,* Sculpting the base framework and thinning the helix. *B,* Suturing the helix to the base framework. *C,* The completed framework. See also Figure 40–9.

In cases in which the pleura is entered during the dissection, there is no reason for concern, since a leak in the lung has not been produced. However, when a pleural tear is discovered, a rubber catheter is inserted into the chest through the pleural opening; the chest wound is closed in layers by the assistant, while the surgeon fabricates the framework, thus conserving operative time. When skin closure is complete, the catheter is attached to suction, the lung is expanded, and the catheter is rapidly withdrawn. As a final precaution, a portable upright chest radiograph is taken in the operating room.

Framework Fabrication

In fabricating an ear framework, the surgeon's aim is to exaggerate the helical rim and the details of the anthelical complex (Fig. 40–9). This is achieved with scalpel blades and a rounded, wood-carving chisel. To minimize possible chondrocytic damage, the use

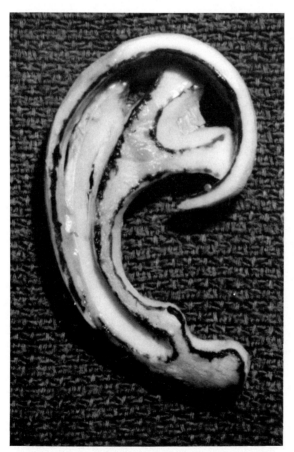

Figure 40–9. A right ear framework, sculpted from autogenous rib cartilage as illustrated in Figure 40–8.

of power tools for sculpting is strictly avoided; one should keep in mind that cartilage sculpting differs from basic wood carving in that a satisfactory long-term result ultimately depends on living tissue.

The basic ear silhouette is carved from the previously obtained cartilage block (see Fig. 40–8B). It is necessary to thin little, if any, of the basic form for a small child's framework, but it is essential for framework fabrication in most older patients. When thinning is necessary, care should be taken to preserve the perichondrium on the lateral, outer aspect of the framework to facilitate its adherence, "take," and subsequent nourishment from surrounding tissues. Because warping must be taken into consideration (Gibson and Davis, 1958), the cartilage is sculpted and thinned to cause a deliberate warping in a favorable direction. This allows one to produce the acute flexion necessary to create a helix, which is fastened to the framework body with horizontal mattress sutures; the knots are buried on the frame's undersurface.

Framework Implantation

A cutaneous pocket is created with meticulous technique so as to provide an adequate recipient vascular covering for the framework. Because several hours elapse during the rib removal and framework fabrication, the auricular region is prepared and scrubbed just before the cutaneous pocket is created. If two surgeons well versed in ear reconstruction work together, one can develop the cutaneous pocket while the other finishes the cartilage sculpture.

Through a small incision anterior to the auricular vestige (Fig. 40–10A), a thin flap is raised by sharp dissection, care being taken to preserve the subdermal vascular plexus. In order to evaluate the vascular status of the flap and to ensure accurate hemostasis, epinephrine-containing solutions are avoided. With great care, the skin is dissected from the gnarled, native cartilage remnant, which is excised and discarded (Fig. 40–10B). Finally, the pocket is completed by dissecting 1 or 2 cm peripherally to the projected framework markings (Fig. 40–10D).

Insertion of the framework into the cutaneous pocket takes up the valuable skin slack that was created when the native cartilage remnant was removed (Fig. 40–10D). The

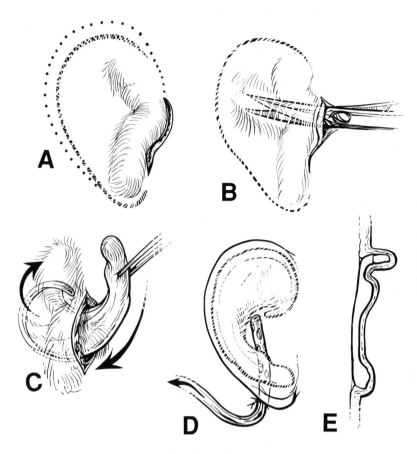

Figure 40–10. Total ear construction, Stage 1: implanting the cartilage framework. *A,* Preauricular incision. Dotted lines indicate the extent of the undermining. *B,* Dissecting the covering skin "pocket." *C,* Inserting the cartilage framework. *D,* Completion of the procedure. The skin is coapted to the framework by a suction drain. *E,* The auricular convolutions can be filled with Vaseline gauze.

framework displaces this skin centrifugally in an advantageous posterosuperior direction so as to displace the hairline behind the helical rim. The principle of anterior incision and centrifugal skin relaxation, introduced by Tanzer (1959), not only permits advantageous use of the hairless skin cover, but also preserves circulation by avoiding incisions and scars along the helical border.

Although Tanzer (1959, 1971) initially suggested the use of bolster sutures to coapt the skin flap to the underlying framework, the author finds it much safer to do this with suction, which simultaneously prevents fluid collection and minimizes the risk of flap necrosis along the helical margin.

To attain skin coaptation via suction, the surgeon uses a silicone catheter or fashions a perforated drain from an infusion catheter with the needle inserted into a rubber-topped vacuum tube (Fig. 40–10*D*), the tubes being retained on a rack so that changes in quantity and quality of drainage may be observed. Although a dressing is applied that accurately conforms to the convolutions of the

newly created auricle (Fig. 40–10*E*), firm pressure is dangerous and unnecessary and must be avoided. Hemostasis and skin coaptation are provided by the suction drain (Cronin, 1966; Brent, 1980a,b, 1987).

Postoperative Care

Attentive postoperative management is imperative for a successful ear reconstruction that is to remain unhampered by disastrous complications. The newly constructed auricle is scrutinized frequently and carefully for signs of infection or vascular compromise.

Early infection manifests itself neither by auricular pain nor by fever, but through local erythema, edema, subtle fluctuance, drainage, or a combination of the above. Hence, frequent observations and the immediate institution of aggressive therapy can deter an overwhelming infection.

Immediately an infection is suspected, an irrigation drain is introduced below the flap and continuous antibiotic drip irrigation is begun. Appropriate adjustments are made in the antibiotic drip irrigation and in the systemic therapy when sensitivities are available from the initial culture. Cronin (1966) salvaged Silastic framework reconstructions impressively by this technique, and the author has had success in managing the occasional infection in cartilage graft reconstructions (an incidence of less than 1 per cent).

Skin flap necrosis results from excessive tension in a pocket of inadequate size, tight bolster sutures, or damage to the subdermal vasculature during the flap dissection. This complication is best avoided by meticulous technique; however, once skin necrosis becomes evident, appropriate steps must be taken without delay.

Although at times a small local flap may be required to cover exposed cartilage, *small* localized ulcerations may heal with proper local wound care. This consists of keeping the wound continuously covered with antibiotic ointment to prevent cartilage desiccation, and using restraints to prevent the patient from lying on the ear during sleep.

However, major skin flap necrosis merits a more aggressive approach if the framework is to be salvaged. The necrotic skin is excised early, and the framework is covered by transposing a local skin flap or by using a small fascial flap and skin graft.

Postoperative Activities and Care

Once healing has taken place, no specific care is necessary for an ear constructed with autogenous tissues. To avoid flattening of the helical rim, the patient is instructed to sleep on the opposite side. A soft pillow ensures protection if the patient turns during sleep.

The patient may return to school two and one-half to three weeks postoperatively. However, running and sports are discouraged for an additional three weeks while the chest wound heals.

The ear itself withstands trauma well, since, like the normal ear, it houses a framework of autogenous cartilage. To date, the author has witnessed numerous traumatic incidents on reconstructed ears, e.g., baseball and soccer blows, a bee sting, and a dog bite. They have all healed well. For these reasons, the author does not recommend protective headgear, except in certain sports in which such equipment is used routinely.

OTHER STAGES OF AURICULAR CONSTRUCTION

The major stages of auricular construction subsequent to the initial framework implantation are lobule rotation, separation of the ear with a skin graft, deepening of the concha, and formation of a tragus. These stages can be planned independently or in various combinations, depending on which best achieves the desired end result.

Rotation of the Lobule

The author prefers to perform earlobe transposition as a secondary procedure, as it seems easier both to judge placement of the earlobe and to "splice" the lobule correctly into position with reference to a well-established underlying framework. The "rotation" or repositioning of this normal but displaced structure is accomplished essentially by Z-plasty transposition of a narrow, inferiorly based triangular flap (Fig. 40–11).

Tragal Construction and Conchal Definition

It is possible to form the tragus, excavate the concha, and mimic a canal in a single operation. This is accomplished by placing a thin, elliptic, chondrocutaneous composite graft beneath a J-shaped incision in the conchal region (Fig. 40–12) (Brent, 1980a,b, 1987). The main limb of the J is placed at the proposed posterior tragal margin; the crook of the J represents the intertragal notch (Fig. 40–12*B*). Extraneous soft tissues are excised beneath the tragal flap to deepen the

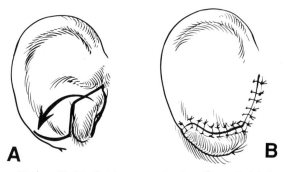

A   **B**

Figure 40–11. Total ear construction, Stage 2: lobule transposition. *A,* Healed Stage one repair and proposed lobule transposition. The appropriate lobule position will be deepithelized to receive the transposed earlobe. *B,* Completed procedure. The lobule has been transposed as an inferiorly based flap.

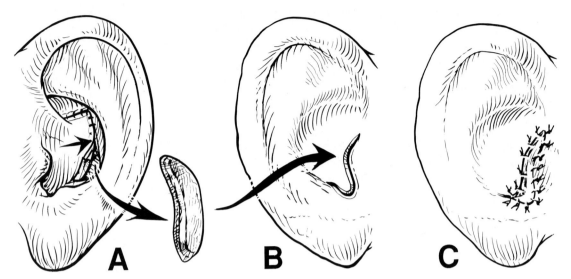

Figure 40–12. Total ear construction, Stage 3: tragus construction. *A,* Harvesting a chondrocutaneous composite graft from the contralateral concha. The donor ear is repaired. *B,* Composite graft at the site of the proposed tragus construction, marked by a J-shaped incision. The J's main limb is at the posterior tragal margin, and the crook of the J represents the intertragal notch. *C,* Composite graft placed under the J-shaped skin flap and sutured into place.

concha; the excavated region looks like a meatus when the newly constructed tragus casts a shadow on it (Fig. 40–14C).

It is advantageous to harvest the composite graft from the normal ear's anterolateral conchal surface, because of its ideal shape and the paucity of subcutaneous tissue between the delicate anterolateral skin and adjacent cartilage. This technique is particularly ideal when a prominent concha exists in the normal donor ear, since closure of the donor site facilitates an otoplasty, which often is needed to gain frontal symmetry.

Detaching the Posterior Auricular Region

Auricular separation with skin grafting is done solely to eliminate the cryptotic appearance by defining the ear through creation of a sulcus. This procedure will not project a framework that has been carved with insufficient depth.

The posterior auricular margin is defined by separating the ear from the head and covering its undersurface with a thick split-thickness skin graft. This should not be attempted until the edema has subsided and the auricular details have become well defined. When this occurs, an incision is made several millimeters behind the rim, taking care to preserve a protective connective tissue layer on the cartilage framework (Fig. 40–13). The retroauricular skin is then advanced

into the newly created sulcus so that the only graft requirement is on the ear's undersurface. To secure the graft, the sutures are left long and tied over a gauze bolster (Fig. 40–13D). Patients who underwent ear reconstruction are illustrated in Figures 40–14 and 40–15.

Managing the Hairline

A persistent problem, scalp hair on the reconstructed rim has largely been eliminated in microtia by the anterior incision–centrifugal relaxation principle (Tanzer, 1959), but the hairline remains a perplexing problem in major acquired auricular deformities.

Although the "scalp roll" and free graft provide a hairless skin cover (Letterman and Harding, 1956), this new cover lacks the elasticity of virgin skin. Instead, the author prefers first to implant the framework and later eradicate any undesirable hair. This can be done with electrolysis or by replacing the follicular skin with a graft. In trying to avoid hairy skin over the superior helix, the surgeon may be tempted to place the ear too low. Another complication arises when the framework is displaced anteriorly by the hairline, which acts as a constricting band at the juncture between the thin, hairless retroauricular skin and the thick scalp skin. This can be avoided by limiting the anterior dis-

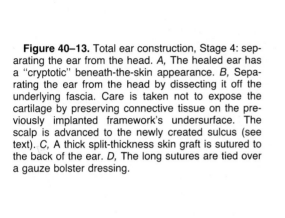
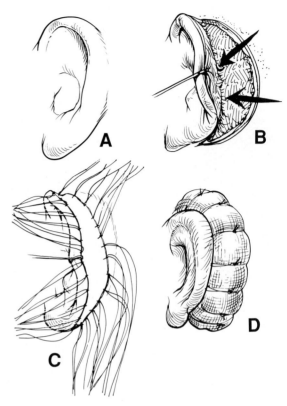

Figure 40–13. Total ear construction, Stage 4: separating the ear from the head. *A,* The healed ear has a "cryptotic" beneath-the-skin appearance. *B,* Separating the ear from the head by dissecting it off the underlying fascia. Care is taken not to expose the cartilage by preserving connective tissue on the previously implanted framework's undersurface. The scalp is advanced to the newly created sulcus (see text). *C,* A thick split-thickness skin graft is sutured to the back of the ear. *D,* The long sutures are tied over a gauze bolster dressing.

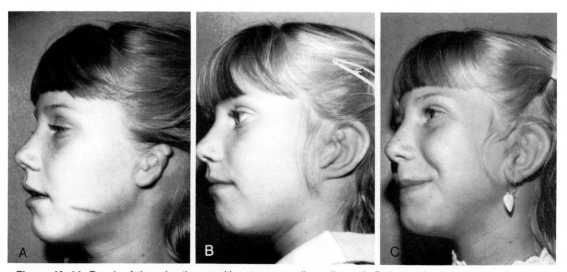

Figure 40–14. Repair of the microtic ear with autogenous rib cartilage. *A,* Patient with a microtic ear, preoperative view. *B,* Appearance several months after the sculpted rib cartilage framework has been implanted. The lobule is still in its original displaced position. *C,* Final appearance after lobule transposition, tragus construction, and separation of the reconstructed ear from the head with a skin graft.

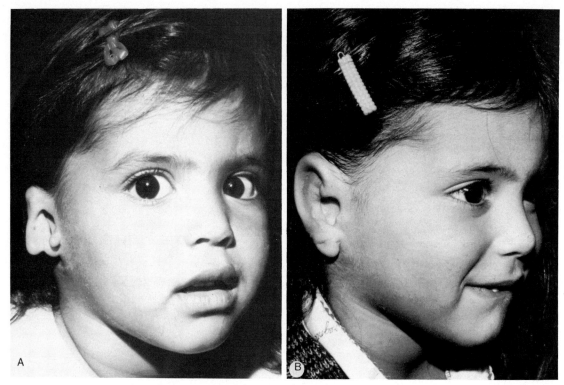

Figure 40–15. Repair of microtia with a sculpted rib cartilage graft. (From Brent, B.: The versatile cartilage autograft: current trends in clinical transplantation. Clin. Plast. Surg., 6:163, 1979.)

section of the cutaneous pocket and by checking the framework's position before closing the incision.

If a tight pocket and a hairline that will cover half the new ear are anticipated, the surgeon may consider creating a primary temporal fascial flap to cover an ear framework (Brent and Byrd, 1983).

SECONDARY RECONSTRUCTION

The difficulties in constructing an ear surgically are substantiated by the often disheartening result that emerges despite the surgeon's efforts. Discouragingly, at times the end result bears no resemblance to an auricle, apart from its location. Furthermore, the scars that result from multiple procedures may extend the defect well beyond the original deformity (see Fig. 40–17A). The impact of such failures is emotionally devastating to the patient and proportionately frustrating for the surgeon.

Tanzer (1974b) managed secondary reconstruction by first excising the scar and skin grafting the defect, and then waiting for the graft to mature before implanting a new cartilage framework. However, this approach often is beset with compromises, in that skin grafted tissues have limited elasticity as a cutaneous pocket, and a detailed framework with depth cannot be introduced without significant tension. Furthermore, deeply scarred tissue beds may be so severely damaged that this approach is not even possible, and the patient is apparently left with no solution to the problem.

In an effort to resolve this skin coverage impasse, Brent and Byrd (1983) implemented a more optimal method for treating secondary ear reconstruction: excising the entire auricular scar area, immediately placing a sculpted autogenous rib cartilage graft, and covering the latter with a temporoparietal fascial flap and skin graft (Figs. 40–16, 40–17).

Bilateral Microtia

Although it is relatively rare, bilateral microtia frequently afflicts patients with such conditions as Treacher Collins syndrome, bilateral craniofacial microsomia, and other

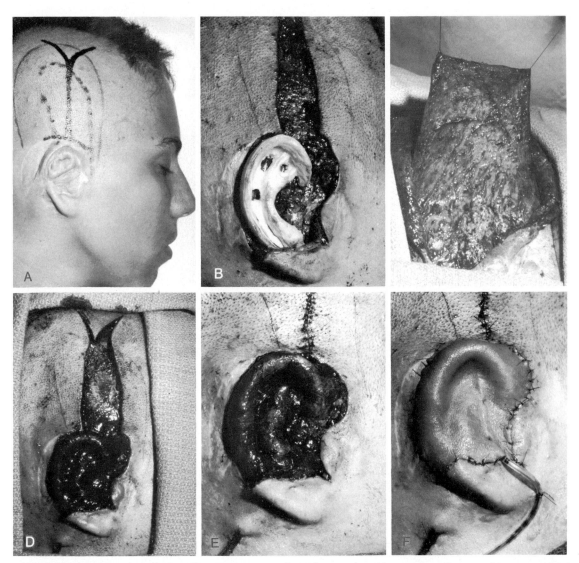

Figure 40–16. Ear reconstruction with an autogenous rib cartilage surfaced by a skin graft–covered temporoparietal fascial flap. *A,* A patient with a scarred auricular region. Doppler vessels, the flap extent, and the Y-shaped incision are indicated. *B,* Scar excision, framework fabrication and scalp dissection are begun. *C,* Raising a fascial flap that contains the superficial temporal vessels. *D,* Fascial flap draped over the ear framework. *E,* Scalp wound sutured. *F,* Skin graft applied over the fascia-covered ear framework. (From Brent, B., and Byrd, H. S.: Secondary ear reconstruction with cartilage grafts covered by axial, random, and free flaps of temporoparietal fascia. Plast. Reconstr. Surg., 72:141, 1983.)

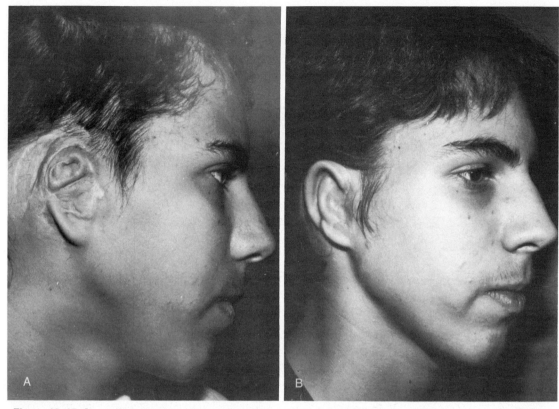

Figure 40–17. Secondary ear reconstruction with a rib cartilage graft surfaced with a superficial temporoparietal fascial flap and skin graft. *A,* A patient with a scarred auricular region after multiple failed procedures. *B,* Result achieved in one surgical stage with rib cartilage graft and fascial flap by the techniques outlined in Figure 40–16.

uncommon craniofacial malformations (see Chaps. 62, 63). The reconstructive principles for managing bilateral microtia are the same as for the unilateral deformity.

As mentioned previously, when middle ear surgery is contemplated, a team approach must be planned with an experienced otologist. In these instances, the auricular reconstruction must precede the middle ear surgery so that the reconstructive surgeon has the advantage of virgin skin to cover the cartilage framework. In bilateral microtia, the author first constructs one ear with a rib cartilage graft, and then after several months constructs the other side. After several more months of healing, both earlobes are transposed at a single surgical procedure.

With construction of the two auricles now well under way, the middle ear surgery can begin. With the plastic surgeon and otologist working as a team, the former preserves connective tissue on the undersurface of the framework as he elevates it from the side of the head to provide exposure for the otologist, who drills out the bony canal and performs

the tympano-ossiculoplasty. After this is accomplished, the canal is exteriorized in the conchal region by excising soft tissues, and the auricle is sutured back to its original bed. Finally, the new canal is skin grafted and packed.

Once the operative site is well healed, the auricle can be lifted and skin grafted, or the middle ear surgery itself can proceed.

The Constricted Ear

Tanzer (1975) applied the term "constricted ear" to a group of ear anomalies in which the encircling helix seems tight, as if constricted by a pursestring (Fig. 40–18). Once loosely termed "cup" or "lop" ears, these deformities collectively have helical and scaphal hooding and varying degrees of flattening of the anthelical complexes.

Although Tanzer (1975) gave these ears a numerical classification that corresponds to the severity of each deformity, in practical terms the surgeon needs to determine whether he can repair the ear by reshaping the existing tissues, or whether he must supplement skin coverage and/or the supporting cartilage.

It is necessary to individualize constricted ear repairs for each specific ear deformity. If helical lidding is the main defect and the height discrepancy is minimal, the surgeon can merely excise the overhanging tissue. At times, the cartilage lid can be used as a "banner flap" to increase ear height (Fig. 40–19). Moderate height discrepancies necessitate augmentation of the cartilage height by modification of the ipsilateral ear cartilage (Cosman, 1974, 1987) or the use of contralateral conchal cartilage grafts (Brent, 1980b). The key to repairing these moderate deformities is to visualize the defective cartilage armature, which is possible only after the skin envelope is "degloved" (Figs. 40–20, 40–21).

When constriction is sufficiently severe to produce a height difference of 1.5 cm, it is necessary to add both skin and cartilage and essentially to correct the deformity as if it were a formal microtia repair (Fig. 40–22).

Cryptotia

Cryptotia is an unusual congenital deformity in which the upper pole of the ear cartilage is buried beneath the scalp (Fig. 40–23). The superior auriculocephalic sulcus is absent but can be demonstrated by gentle finger pressure. This has stimulated Japanese physicians (Kageyama, 1928; Matsumoto, 1977) to correct this deformity nonsurgically, since it occurs in Japan as commonly as in one in 400 births (Ohmori and Matsumoto, 1972). The nonoperative procedure is accomplished by applying an external conforming splint. If this is done before the infant is 6 months of age, it may successfully mold a permanent retroauricular sulcus (Torikai, 1982).

Surgical repairs entail the addition of skin to the deficient retroauricular sulcus, by means of either skin grafts and Z-plasties (Gosserez and Piers, 1959), V-Y advancement flaps (Fukuda, 1968), or rotational flaps (Torikai, 1982). When a cartilage deformity accompanies the skin deficiency, various remodeling techniques are needed to facilitate the repair (Ohmori and Matsumoto, 1972; Washio, 1973).

The Prominent Ear

PATHOLOGY

During the third month of gestation, the protrusion of the auricle increases; by the end of the sixth month the helical margin curls, the anthelix forms its fold, and the anthelical crura appear. Anything that interferes with this process results in prominent ears.

The most common deformity arises from failure of the anthelix to fold. This widens the conchoscaphal angle as much as 150 degrees or more (Fig. 40–24) flattening the superior crus and, in severe forms, the anthelical body and inferior crus. In extreme cases the helical roll may be absent, producing a flat, shell-like ear without convolutions.

Text continued on page 2116

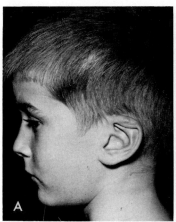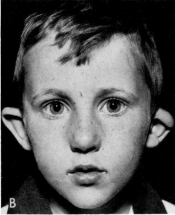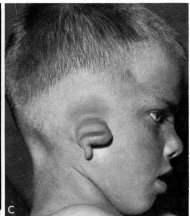

Figure 40–18. Varying types of constricted ear. *A,* Involvement of the helix only. *B,* Involvement of the helix and scapha (left auricle). *C,* Severe cupping deformity coupled with incomplete migration of the auricle.

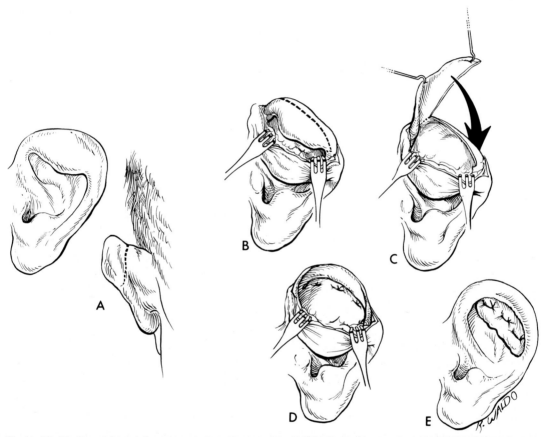

Figure 40–19. Correction of Group I ear constriction. *A,* The incision for exposure of the skeletal deformity. *B,* The deformed cartilage has been filleted from its soft tissue cover. The line of detachment of the angulated segment is marked. *C,* The deformed cartilage is lifted on a medially based pedicle and rotated into an upright position. *D,* The repositioned cartilage is sutured to the scapha. *E,* The skin is redraped and the helical sulcus is maintained by through and through sutures tied over gauze pledgets. (From Tanzer, R. C. *In* Tanzer, R. C., and Edgerton, M. T. (Eds.): Symposium on Reconstruction of the Auricle. St. Louis, MO, C.V. Mosby Company, 1974, p. 141.)

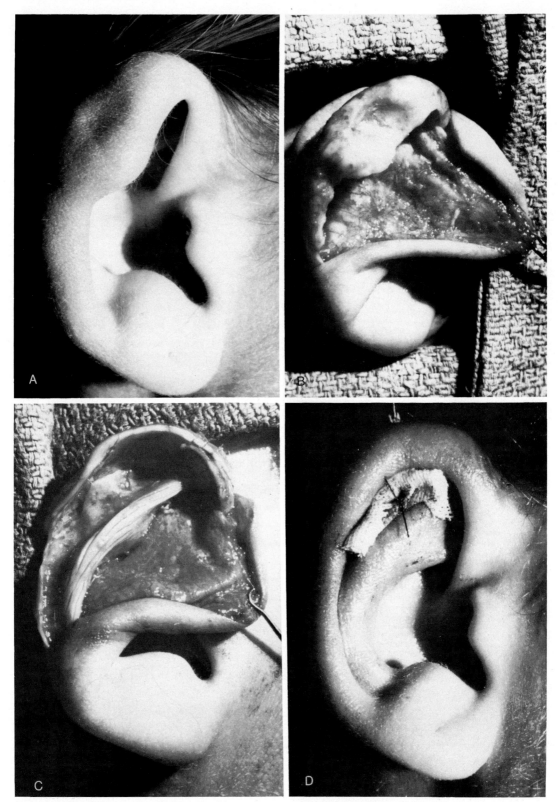

Figure 40–20. Repair of a moderately constricted ear. *A,* Preoperative appearance. *B,* "Degloving" the ear to expose the distorted cartilage. *C,* The cartilage is expanded, the antihelix is formed, and a contralateral conchal cartilage graft repairs the deficient upper third. *D,* Skin redraped to complete the repair. See Figure 40-21*B*. (From Brent, B.: The correction of microtia with autogenous cartilage grafts. II. Atypical and complex deformities. Plast. Reconstr. Surg., *66*:13, 1980.)

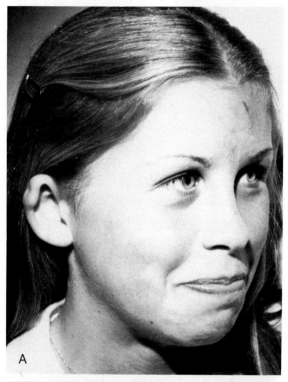

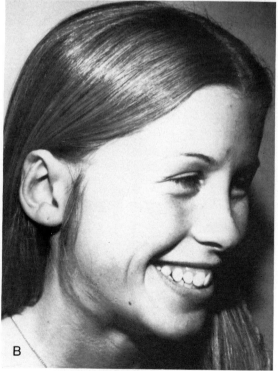

Figure 40–21. Repair of a moderately constricted ear by the technique shown in Figure 40–20. (From Brent, B.: The correction of microtia with autogenous cartilage grafts. II. Atypical and complex deformities. Plast. Reconstr. Surg., *66*:13, 1980.)

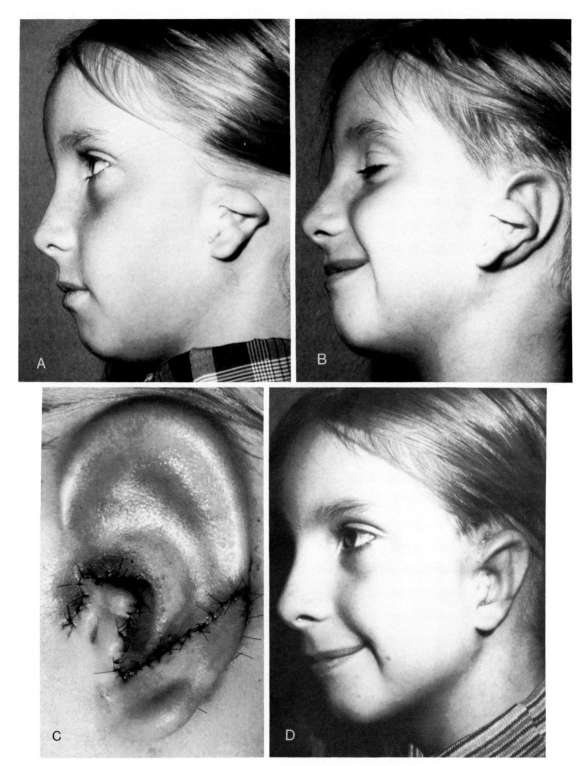

Figure 40–22. Repair of severe ear constriction by the classic microtia technique. *A,* A patient with a severely constricted ear. *B,* Appearance after insertion of total ear framework of rib cartilage. *C,* Utilizing the vestige to form the earlobe and tragus. *D,* Final result after separation from the head with a skin graft. (From Brent, B.: The correction of microtia with autogenous cartilage grafts. II. Atypical and complex deformities. Plast. Reconstr. Surg., *66*:13, 1980.)

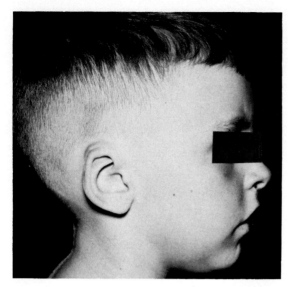

Figure 40–23. Cryptotia.

Conchal widening may also occur as an isolated deformity or may occur in conjunction with the anthelical deformities described above. This abnormality is usually bilateral and is frequently noted in siblings and parents.

TREATMENT

In repairing prominent ears, symmetry is most important and, paradoxically, may be more difficult to achieve in unilateral than in bilateral cases. The repaired ear convolutions should appear smooth and betray no

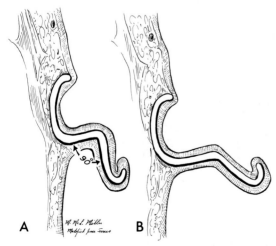

Figure 40–24. *A*, Cross section of a normal ear. *B*, Prominent ear resulting from an increased conchoscaphal angle.

signs of surgery. The most lateral point of the completed repair should be between 1.7 and 2.0 cm from the head, and the helix should be visible behind the anthelical body when the ears are viewed from the front (McDowell, 1968).

To attain these goals a number of techniques have been described, many of which produce acceptable results. However, the author recommends that the surgeon should direct his efforts toward correcting the specific problem areas of each individual ear rather than following a routine "cookbook recipe."

If the upper third of the ear protrudes because of an absent or weak anthelix, an exaggerated anthelix must be formed. If the middle third is too prominent, the concha must be recessed either by cartilage excision or by suture fixation (Furnas, 1968). Finally, if the lobule protrudes, the surgeon should either resect or reposition the cartilaginous tail (cauda helicis) (Webster, 1969) and/or excise retrolobular skin.

Conchal Alteration

Dieffenbach (1845) is credited with the first otoplastic attempt, which consisted of excising skin from the auriculocephalic sulcus and suturing the conchal cartilage to the mastoid periosteum.

In addition to narrowing the auriculocephalic sulcus, Ely (1881) and others excised a strip of conchal wall, a procedure attributed to Morestin (1903). This old method of tacking back the concha to mastoid periosteum (Fig. 40–25) has been revived throughout the past several decades (Owens and Delgado, 1955; Stark and Saunders, 1962; Paletta, Ship, and Van Norman, 1963; Furnas, 1968; Spira and associates, 1969).

One can also correct the wide concha by excising a cartilaginous ellipse beneath the anthelical body. This may create a redundant skin fold, which then may require excision.

Restoration of the Anthelical Fold

Luckett (1910) first conceptualized that prominent ears result from failure of the anthelix to fold. He restored the fold by excising a crescent of medial skin and cartilage (Fig. 40–26). Most subsequent otoplasty procedures have focused on creating a smoother anthelix than that produced by employing

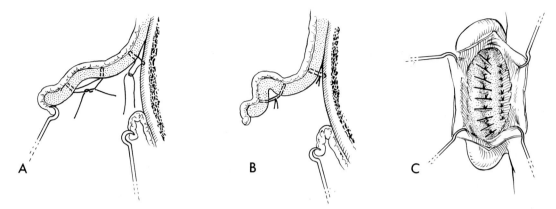

Figure 40–25. Technique of reducing prominence by conchomastoid sutures. *A,* Cross section of the auricle, showing placement of the sutures to reduce the conchomastoid angle and to restore the anthelical fold. *B,* Correction of the prominence. *C,* View of the medial surface of the auricular cartilage after correction of the prominence. (From Spira, M., McCrea, P., Gerow, F., and Hardy, B.: Analysis and treatment of the protruding ear. Trans. 4th Internatl. Congr. Plast. Surg. Amsterdam, Excerpta Medica, 1969.)

Luckett's sharp, cartilage-breaking technique (Erich, 1958; Straith, 1959; Cloutier, 1961; McDowell, 1968).

Alteration of the Medial Cartilage Surface

In order to permit its smooth molding, the scaphal cartilage can be recontoured by a number of techniques. McEvitt (1947) and Paletta, Ship, and Van Norman (1963) weakened the scapha with multiple parallel cuts, while Converse and associates (1955) used bur abrasion. Becker (1949, 1952), Converse and associates (1955), and Tanzer (1962) used parallel cuts and permanent sutures to form a smooth, cornucopia-like anthelix. The cartilage tube encases substantial scar to lock the cartilage into position and prevent the recurrence of deformity (Figs. 40–27, 40–28).

Reviving a long-forgotten suggestion of Morestin (1903), Mustardé (1963, 1967) created the anthelix by inserting permanent mattress sutures through the cartilage without using any actual cartilage incisions. The author finds this technique particularly useful in the pliable ear cartilage of children.

Alteration of the Lateral Cartilage Surface

Exploiting the tendency of cartilage to warp when one surface is cut (Gibson and Davis, 1958), Chongchet (1963) scored the anterior scaphal cartilage with multiple cartilage cuts to roll it back and form an anthelix. Chongchet did this under direct vision using a scalpel, but Stenström (1963) produced the same effect by using a short-tined rasp instrument to "blindly" score the ant-

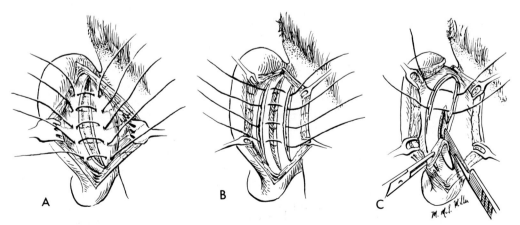

Figure 40–26. Evolution of the tubing principle for correction of prominent ears. *A,* Luckett; *B,* Barsky; *C,* Becker.

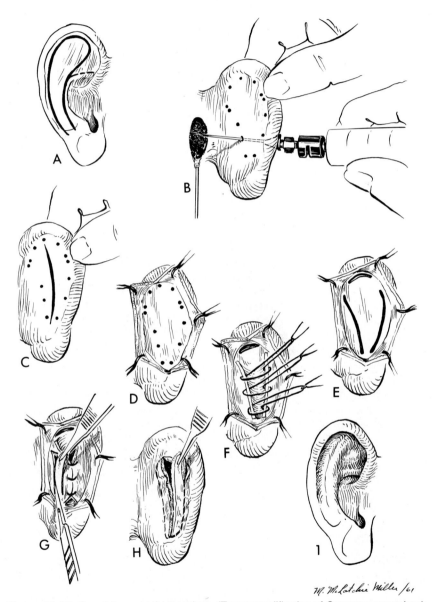

Figure 40–27. Complete corrective otoplasty (Tanzer modification of Converse procedure).

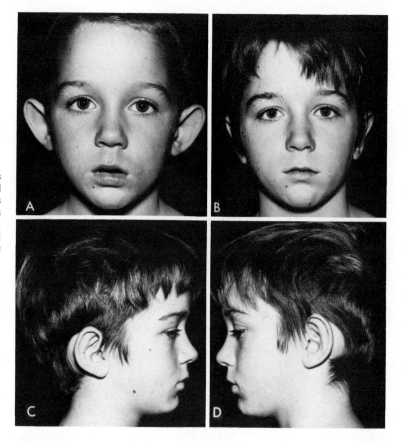

Figure 40–28. *A,* Prominent ears characterized by wide conchae and lack of anthelical folds. Previous treatment of the cartilage by mattress sutures resulted only in recurrence. *B* to *D,* Correction by cartilage tubing to form an anthelical fold, and elliptic excision of excess concha.

helical region through a posterior stab incision near the cauda helicis. The lateral cartilage surface has also been morselized or abraded under direct vision through a lateral incision (Ju, Li, and Crikelair, 1963).

Kaye (1967) advocated an otoplasty method that combines both lateral cartilage scoring and fixation with permanent sutures. He accomplished both of these maneuvers through minimal incisions (Fig. 40–29).

ACQUIRED DEFORMITIES

Total auricular reconstruction in the acquired deformity presents special problems not encountered in microtia. These merit separate consideration.

The lack of skin coverage is much more critical than in microtia, since an existing meatus precludes use of the anterior incision, and extra skin, as usually gained by removing the crumpled microtic cartilage, is not available. This factor compounds the previously mentioned hairline problem. If the existing skin can be used, the cutaneous pocket

is best developed by incisions above and/or below the proposed auricular site. If the local tissues are heavily scarred or restrict the surgeon from developing an ample skin pocket, the repair must be supplemented with fascial flap coverage (see Figs. 40–16, 40–17) (Brent and Byrd, 1983).

Replantation of the Amputated Auricle

Replantation of amputated segments of the auricle was practiced in the seventeenth century. Cocheril (1894) cited the memoirs of Strafford written during the reign of the English King Charles I. To punish Puritan and colonist opposition to the regime, the victim's ear was frequently amputated and nailed to a wooden post. Three of the many victims have been specifically documented: Burton, a minister in the Government; Prynne, a lawyer; and Bartwick, a physician. Earlier, Prynne had published a book that was considered offensive to the Queen and

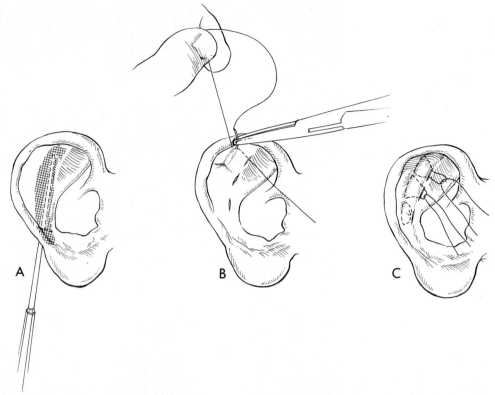

Figure 40–29. The Kaye method to correct flattening of the anthelix. *A,* A subperichondrial tunnel is made on the lateral surface of the cartilage through a medial incision near the cauda helicis; a sharp-tined instrument produces curling by multiple vertical striations. *B, C,* The proper amount of anthelical roll is maintained by several mattress sutures introduced through tiny incisions along the conchal crest and carried across the anthelical fold through holes in the skin. (From Kaye, B. L.: A simplified method for correcting the prominent ear. Plast. Reconstr. Surg., *40:*44, 1967. Copyright © 1967, The Williams & Wilkins Company, Baltimore.)

consequently had his ears amputated. When he appeared before the Tribunal a second time, the presiding judge was surprised to see Prynne with two normal-appearing ears: they were exposed but showed the signs of mutilation. Having been condemned to have his ears amputated a second time, Prynne retrieved the amputated ears, hoping to have them sutured back to their original site as had been done previously. No information is available about the fate of Burton's ears. We know that Bartwick's wife collected his amputated ears and placed them carefully into a handkerchief, hoping to have them replanted. All this took place between 1630 and 1640, long before any reports of replantation of an amputated ear.

Cocheril (1894) cited many examples of successful replantations during the nineteenth century, and stated: "It is difficult to doubt the good faith of these authors: the prestige attached to their names; the clarity of their reports; the official approval given to their reports should suffice to consider them as veracious. The vascularity of the auricle, the rapid healing of wounds of this structure, the fact that the vessels remain gaping, ready to receive nourishing fluid—all militate in favor of the veracity of the reports." The only information missing in all these reports is the size of the amputated parts.

To the modern plastic surgeon, choice of a salvage procedure is influenced by the size of the amputated portion, the condition of the tissues of the amputated segment, and the condition of the stump and surrounding tissues, particularly in the retroauricular area. A clean-cut amputation gives the surgeon a better chance of success. When the ear and its surrounding tissues are mangled and avulsed and bone is exposed, the reconstruction is difficult if not insurmountable. *Small* amputated segments are replaced as composite grafts with some hope of success. Larger amputated segments and subtotal amputation require further consideration.

REPLANTATION OF AURICULAR TISSUE ATTACHED BY A NARROW PEDICLE

Because an ear is richly vascularized and has major vessels extending through its periphery, the partly avulsed auricular tissue can be successfully replaced even though the remaining attachment is tenuous (Figs. 40–30, 40–31).

REPLANTATION OF AURICULAR TISSUE AS A COMPOSITE GRAFT

Even when the piece of auricle is quite large, the completely detached ear tissue may survive when replaced as a composite graft (Figs. 40–32, 40–33), although few successful cases have been reported in the plastic surgery literature (see Fig. 40–36) (McDowell, 1971; Gifford, 1972; Clemons and Connelly, 1973).

REPLANTATION OF AURICULAR CARTILAGE

Because a cartilaginous framework is difficult to reproduce, the salvage and use of denuded auricular cartilage was recommended by Greeley (1944), Suraci (1944),

Conway and associates (1948), and Musgrave and Garrett (1967). Various techniques have been employed to preserve cartilage from an avulsed ear. The skin may be removed and the cartilage buried in an abdominal pocket (Sexton, 1955) or cervical pocket (Conroy, 1972), or placed under the skin of the retroauricular area (Bonanno and Converse, 1974). The latter orthotopic cartilage replantation can be performed only if the regional cutaneous tissues are in satisfactory condition.

Although it is logical, the author finds this procedure futile, since the flimsy ear cartilage almost invariably flattens beneath the snug, discrepant, two-dimensional skin cover. Furthermore, when amputated ear cartilage has been "banked" in the retroauricular region, it hampers later reconstructive attempts by producing an irregular, amorphous structure that is adherent to the overlying regional skin.

REPLANTATION OF THE DERMABRADED AMPUTATED AURICLE

Mladick and associates (1971) and Mladick and Carraway (1973) advocated first derma-

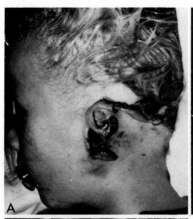
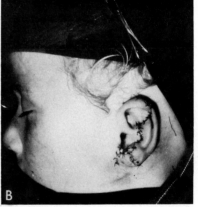
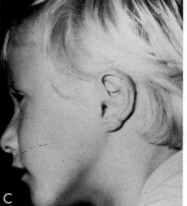

Figure 40–30. Replacement of auricular tissue attached by a narrow pedicle. *A,* Near avulsion of the auricle as a result of a dog bite. *B,* Appearance after repair of the auricular segment, which is nourished by a narrow superior pedicle. *C,* Appearance of the ear one year after the injury. (Patient of Dr. Andries Molenaar.)

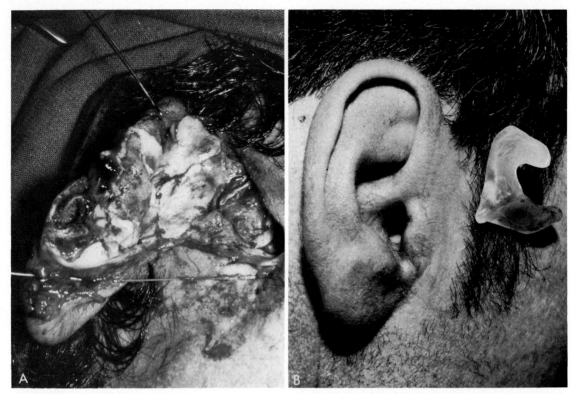

Figure 40–31. Repair of a major auricular avulsion. *A,* The avulsed ear remains attached by a narrow pedicle, which maintains its viability; the canal is transected. *B,* Result after repair of the canal and maintenance of an acrylic mold for four months.

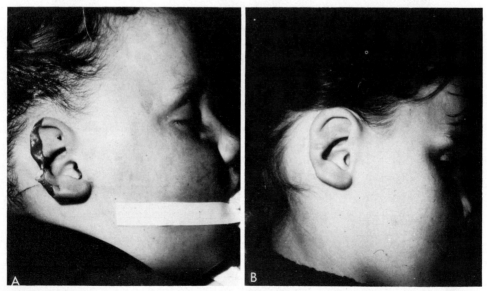

Figure 40–32. Replantation of auricular tissue as a composite graft. *A,* Loss of a portion of the scapha and helix resulting from a dog bite. *B,* The amputated segment was retrieved and sutured in position as a composite graft, with this result two years later. (Patient of Dr. Andries Molenaar.)

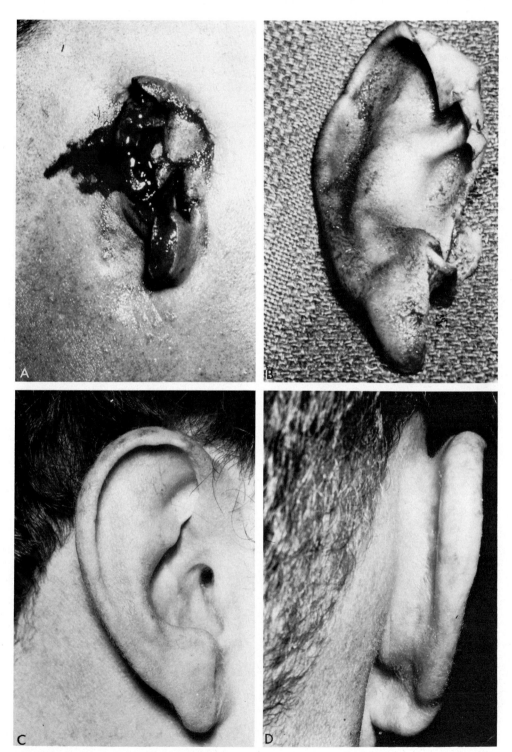

Figure 40–33. Replantation of a totally amputated auricle as a composite graft. *A,* The stump of the amputated auricle 5½ hours after the accident. *B,* The amputated part includes the pinna, the earlobe, and part of the concha. *C, D,* The final result after reattachment. (Courtesy of Doctors Clemons and Connelly, 1973.)

brading and then reattaching the amputated ear to its stump. The reattached ear is then buried in a subcutaneous postauricular pocket, a maneuver that allows revascularization through the exposed dermis of the dermabraded auricle (Fig. 40–34). Several weeks later, the ear is exteriorized by blunt dissection from its covering flap, which is allowed to slide behind the helical rim. At this time, the subcutaneous attachments of the medial auricular surface are left intact. The exposed raw auricular surface is dressed, and epithelization begins within several days.

Rather than separate the medial auricular attachments from their bed several weeks later to allow spontaneous reepithelization, as Mladick originally suggested, the author considers it safer to wait several months before separating the ear frame from the head; at that time the new retroauricular sulcus can be skin grafted as in a classic microtia reconstruction.

REPLANTATION OF THE AMPUTATED AURICLE AFTER REMOVAL OF POSTAURICULAR SKIN AND FENESTRATION OF CARTILAGE

Almost invariably, the replantation of large composite parts is doomed to fail (Grabb

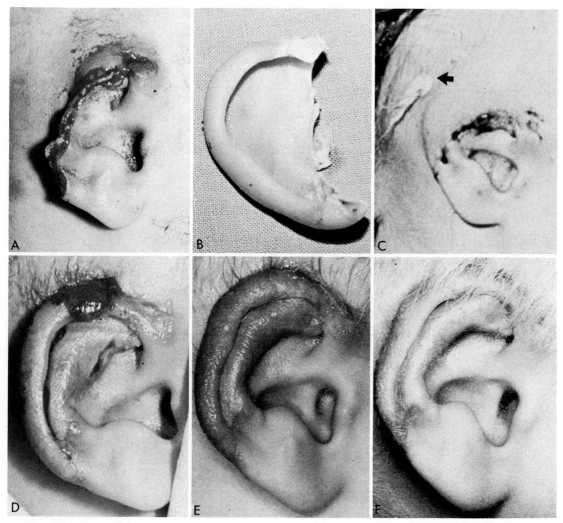

Figure 40–34. Reattachment of the severed auricle by dermabrasion and subcutaneous "pocketing." *A,* The amputated stump. *B,* The severed part. *C,* The dermabraded reattached part is buried in a postauricular pocket; a traction suture *(arrow)* from the helix flattens out the auricle to gain better apposition of the tissues. *D,* The ear has been exteriorized and is almost completely epithelized (see text for details); one granulating area is seen at the superior margin. *E,* One month after injury, the ear has a red flush over the reattached segment. *F,* Appearance at five months. (From Mladick, R., and Carraway, J.: Ear reattachment by the modified pocket principle. Plast. Reconstr. Surg., *51:*584, 1973. Copyright © 1973, The Williams & Wilkins Company, Baltimore.)

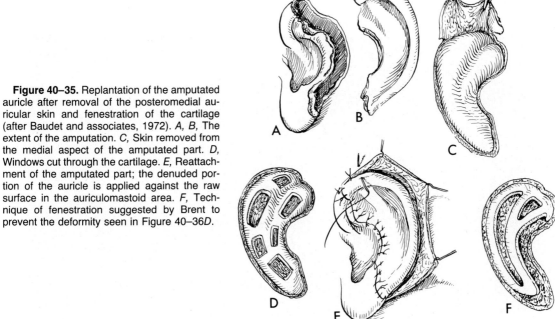

Figure 40–35. Replantation of the amputated auricle after removal of the posteromedial auricular skin and fenestration of the cartilage (after Baudet and associates, 1972). *A, B,* The extent of the amputation. *C,* Skin removed from the medial aspect of the amputated part. *D,* Windows cut through the cartilage. *E,* Reattachment of the amputated part; the denuded portion of the auricle is applied against the raw surface in the auriculomastoid area. *F,* Technique of fenestration suggested by Brent to prevent the deformity seen in Figure 40–36*D.*

and Dingman, 1972), unless one increases the vascular recipient area. Instead of employing dermabrasion to achieve this, Baudet, Tramond, and Goumain (1972) removed the skin from the postauricular portion of the amputated part, fenestrated the cartilage (Fig. 40–35), and placed the auricular segment into a raw area established by raising a flap of retroauricular-mastoid skin (Fig. 40–35*E*). The cartilaginous windows allowed direct contact of the auricular skin with the recipient site, thus facilitating its revascularization. Although some distortion of the superior helical border occurred (Fig. 40–36), the result was satisfactory.

REPLANTING THE EAR CARTILAGE AND IMMEDIATELY COVERING IT WITH A FASCIAL FLAP AND SKIN GRAFT

In selected cases when the wounds are clean, the scalp is intact, and the patient's general condition is stable, one might be tempted to remove the skin of the amputated ear and cover the filleted cartilage immediately with a temporoparietal fascial flap and skin graft. Because the author has routinely observed poor results in filleted ear cartilages that have been subcutaneously banked, he prefers to utilize Baudet's fenestration technique initially (see Fig. 40–35), and to reserve

the fascia for secondary reconstruction should this effort fail.

MICROSURGICAL EAR REPLANTATION

Although there have been several reports of success with microsurgically replanted ears (Pennington, Lai, and Pelly, 1980; Juri and associates, 1987), this procedure tends to fail owing to the small size of the vessels within the amputated ear. Therefore, what initially appears to be a successful replant often fails as venous congestion ensues. However, Mutimer, Banis, and Upton (1987) salvaged one such case by applying leeches to the congested replant.

With this in mind, the author feels that one should accomplish the anastomosis end to side in the temporal vessels rather than sacrifice them for an end to end repair, in order to preserve an axial pattern fascial flap for a future reconstruction if the replant fails.

Deformities Without Loss of Auricular Tissue

IRREGULARITIES IN CONTOUR

The most common post-traumatic auricular deformities without actual tissue loss result

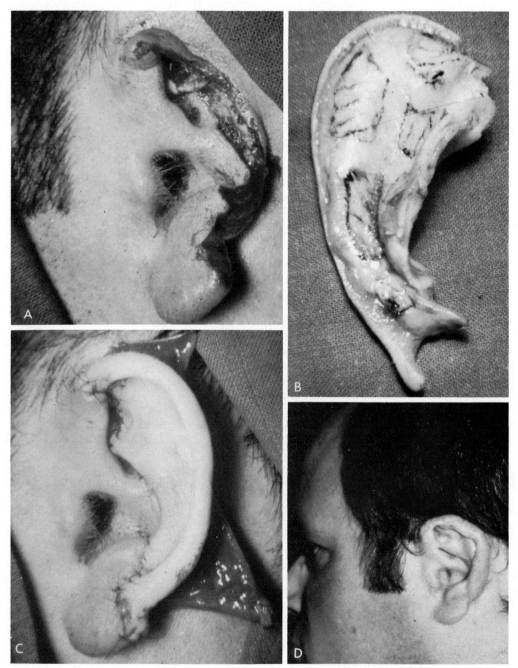

Figure 40–36. Replantation of the amputated auricle after removal of the posteromedial auricular skin and fenestration of the cartilage. *A,* Appearance of the stump of the amputated auricle. *B,* The denuded medial aspect of the cartilage; the outlines of the windows to be cut through the cartilage are indicated. *C,* The auricle immediately after reattachment. *D,* Final appearance. (Courtesy of D. F. J. Baudet.)

from faulty approximation of full-thickness lacerations, which is manifested by distortion and notching of the helical border.

Meticulous approximation of the wound margins is essential when primarily repairing lacerations or secondarily repairing maladjusted tissues. Z-plasties, stepping, halving, or dovetailing of the cartilage edges and soft tissue wounds are important measures in preventing recurrence of contour irregularities.

OTOHEMATOMA: "CAULIFLOWER EAR"

Frequently found in pugilists, this deformity results from a direct blow or excessive traction that produces a hemorrhage. Blood collects between the perichondrium and cartilage and produces a fibrotic clot that thickens and obliterates the ear's convolutions. This is similar to the process that produces thickening of the septal cartilage, which is also common in boxers and wrestlers.

Immediately after the hematoma has occurred, the blood clots and serum must be drained. While simple needle aspiration is almost invariably followed by recurrent fluid collection, a small incision permits evacuation of the hematoma under direct vision. The incision should be long enough to permit retraction, inspection, and the application of a large suction tip for the aspiration of blood clots. Conforming, compressive gauze bolsters are placed on either side of the auricle and are maintained for seven to ten days by horizontal mattress sutures (4-0 nylon), which traverse the bolsters as well as the ear.

Late treatment of the cauliflower ear deformity consists of carving and excising the thickened tissue to improve the auricular contour. Exposure is obtained by raising a skin flap through carefully placed incisions. After completing the carving, similar dressings must be applied to ensure coaptation of the soft tissues to the cartilaginous framework and to prevent hematoma formation.

STENOSIS OF THE EXTERNAL AUDITORY CANAL

The concha is elongated inward by the external auditory canal through an opening, the meatus, through which lacerations may extend and ultimately produce stenosis.

Whenever possible, one must carefully suture circular lacerations involving the canal and keep the canal packed tightly during the healing period. A small, prosthetic appliance should be prepared to maintain patency of the canal. This is made by taking an impression with dental compound and creating a perforated mold of acrylic resin. The prosthetic support should be worn for three or four months until the tendency toward stenosis disappears (Fig. 40–37).

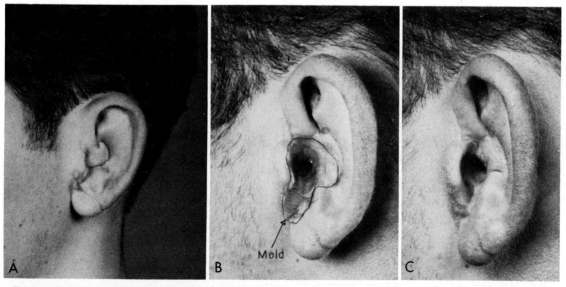

Figure 40–37. Traumatic stenosis of the external auditory canal. *A,* Stenosis of the external auditory canal resulting from laceration. *B,* Acrylic mold worn after skin grafting. *C,* Result obtained; the canal remains patent. (From Converse, J. M.: Reconstruction of the auricle. Plast. Reconstr. Surg., 22:150, 1958. Copyright © 1958, The Williams & Wilkins Company, Baltimore.)

Cicatricial stenosis of the external auditory meatus and canal is remedied by Z-plasties of the cicatricial bands (Steffensen, 1946). In severe stenosis, when the meatus is closed and the canal is filled with scar tissue, the cicatricial tissue must be excised; the skin defect is repaired by means of the skin graft inlay technique, for which a full-thickness retroauricular graft is uniquely suitable.

To facilitate skin grafting, two impressions should be taken of the canal with dental compound: one impression serves to apply the graft firmly within the canal until the skin graft is vascularized; the other is duplicated in clear acrylic and should be worn by the patient for 3 or 4 months to counteract the tendency for secondary contraction of the graft and subsequent stenosis (Fig. 40–37). A detail worth noting is to prepare the mold in such a manner that the distal portion fills the concha; this precaution ensures prosthesis stability.

Deformities With Loss of Auricular Tissue

These deformities may result from loss of skin or cartilage, or full-thickness loss of auricular tissue.

LOSS OF AURICULAR SKIN

Auricular trauma that results only in skin loss is usually secondary to burns. Loss of retroauricular skin results in adhesions between the ear and the mastoid region, whereas skin loss from the anterolateral surface may cause forward folding of the ear. When a burn destroys the skin, the cartilage also becomes involved, the result being a full-thickness defect of the auricle (see Chap. 41 for early treatment of the burned ear). However, partial-thickness burns that are adequately treated may heal with only varying degrees of contraction and thinning of the helical border.

FULL-THICKNESS DEFECTS OF THE AURICLE

For purposes of classification, full-thickness defects of the ear may be divided into six groups: defects (1) of the upper third, (2) middle third, and (3) lower third; (4) partial and (5) total loss; and (6) loss of the lobule.

MAJOR AURICULAR LOSS AFTER TRAUMA

Loss of a major portion of the auricle or the entire ear may result from a razor slash, flying glass, a gunshot injury, flame or radiation burns, or human or dog bites. *Complete* traumatic loss of the auricle is unusual, since a portion of the concha and the external auditory canal are usually preserved even in cases of severe injury. When a large portion of the auricle or the entire ear has been destroyed, a number of obstacles must be surmounted in successive stages. These include (1) a suitable skin covering devoid of hair follicles, (2) a framework of cartilage to maintain the upright position of the reconstructed auricle and to represent its characteristic convolutions, and (3) a covering of skin for the posteromedial aspect of the auricular framework after it is raised from the mastoid area. Additional "retouching" procedures may be necessary to achieve a satisfactory repair of the reconstructed auricle.

SKIN COVERING

The presence of supple and well-vascularized skin is the sine qua non for success in auricular reconstruction. The quality of the residual local soft tissues varies in traumatic defects. When amputation of the auricle is by means of a clean-cut laceration, the local residual skin remains relatively unscarred and thus may be utilized. Likewise, minimally scarred skin following healed partial-thickness burns may be of sufficiently good quality to avoid skin grafting. On the contrary, if the auricle has been avulsed, destroyed by a burn, or injured by a gunshot, the area may show multiple linear or surface scars, necessitating excision and replacement with a skin graft before the auricular reconstruction begins. Should this be necessary, a full-thickness graft from the contralateral retroauricular region or supraclavicular area is most suitable for this purpose, although a thick split-thickness skin graft suffices if the former is not available. It is essential that the skin overlying a cartilage graft has an adequate blood supply and is sufficiently loose to permit insertion of a three-dimensional framework of adequate size. Therefore, the skin graft must be allowed to mature for a number of months before cartilage replacement is undertaken.

Sometimes the local skin is irreparably scarred, or skin grafts have matured inadequately to permit framework placement without supplementing the soft tissue cover. In these cases, a temporoparietal fascial flap must be used (Brent and Byrd, 1983).

First, all thick scars and unusable soft tissues are excised while great care is taken to preserve the temporal vessels, which may be entangled in the scarred tissues. Rib cartilage is harvested and a framework is sculpted as for correcting microtia (see Figs. 40–8, 40–9). Finally, the fascial flap is elevated.

To determine how large a fascial flap is needed for adequate coverage, one must first assess the periauricular skin. At times the scar excision is so extensive that total fascial flap coverage of the framework is necessary. However, at other times the lower portion of the framework can be "pocketed" beneath available skin, and therefore only a variable portion of the upper framework requires fascial flap coverage.

Use of this fascial flap requires a familiarity with the course of the superficial temporal vessels. The artery remains beneath the subcutaneous tissue and within the temporoparietal fascia until a point approximately 12 cm above the anterosuperior auriculocephalic attachment. At this point the artery emerges superficially and interlinks with the subdermal vascular plexus (Byrd, 1980). Consequently, this is the limit of the fascial vascular domain, since continued distal dissection would interrupt the fascial circulation.

After first mapping the vessels with a Doppler flowmeter, exposure to the fascia is gained via a Y-shaped incision that extends superiorly above the proposed auricular region (see Fig. 40–16*A*). The dissection begins just deep to the hair follicles, and continues down to a plane where subcutaneous fat adheres to the temporoparietal fascia. Because initial identification of this plane can be difficult, care must be taken not to damage the follicles or the underlying axial vessels. This is tedious, but once the scalp dissection is accomplished, the inferiorly based temporoparietal fascial flap is easily raised from the underlying deep fascia (aponeurosis) that envelops the temporalis musculature.

The fascial flap is draped over the framework (see Fig. 40–16*D*) and coapted to it by means of suction via a small infusion catheter. The flap is affixed to the peripheral skin in "vest-under-pants" fashion, in order to secure a tight closure. Finally, a patterned, thick split-thickness skin graft is sutured over the fascia-covered framework. The new ear's convolutions are packed with Vaseline gauze, and finally a head dressing is applied.

AURICULAR PROSTHESES

The auricular prosthesis should be reserved for patients in whom surgical reconstruction is impractical or contraindicated, or for whom an experienced surgeon is unavailable.

For the most part, auricular prostheses have no practical value for children, but may be worthwhile for older persons who have undergone ablative cancer surgery or who have extensive burns. Even so, many adults find them undesirable after a short trial experience, as there is always a constant fear of the prosthesis becoming dislodged at embarrassing moments. There is also the psychologic discomfort of wearing an "artificial part." The introduction of osseointegrated percutaneous implants has offered a solution to the retention of ear prostheses (Albrektsson and associates, 1987) (see also Chap. 72).

Additional problems that arise from local skin irritation by the adhesive glue frequently necessitate discontinuance of the prosthesis for a period, which in turn causes the patient further embarrassment. Furthermore, obvious color contrast calls attention to the prosthetic ear in climatic changes where the prosthetic part remains a constant color while the surrounding skin varies as the patient passes from indoor to outdoor environmental surroundings.

When an auricular prosthesis has been elected for the younger patient, a trial period should ensue, on the understanding that surgical reconstruction may be desired later. It is wise to avoid preliminary excision of the microtic lobule or other remnants merely to "gain an improved surface for adherences of the prosthesis," as has been advocated. If the patient desires surgical reconstruction later, which has often been the author's experience, the missing lobule, shortage of skin, and residual scar pose significant surgical handicaps.

Partial Auricular Loss

Most auricular deformities one encounters in everyday practice are acquired *partial* defects. They present the surgeon with an unlimited variety of unique problems whose reconstructions are influenced by the etiology, location, and nature of each residual deformity.

In the management of acute auricular trauma, initial meticulous reapproximation of tissues and appropriate wound care greatly facilitate the reconstructive task ahead. Likewise, the innovative use of residual local tissues in a post-traumatic deformity greatly simplifies the reconstruction and contributes to a pleasing outcome.

STRUCTURAL SUPPORT
Contralateral Conchal Cartilage

A variety of tissues are available to provide the structural support required for an auricular reconstruction. Although the quantity of cartilage needed to fabricate a total ear framework necessitates the use of costal cartilage, one is not always compelled to employ this tissue, especially in a *small*, partial auricular reconstruction. Because it is often possible to use an auricular cartilage graft, which is obtained most frequently from the contralateral concha under local anesthesia (Figs. 40–38, 40–39), the correction of partial losses is less extensive than the procedure to correct total auricular losses.

Auricular cartilage, used as an orthotopic graft in ear reconstruction, is superior to costal cartilage in that it provides a delicate, flexible, thin support.

The conchal cartilage graft can be obtained by a posteromedial incision, as described by Adams (1955) and Gorney, Murphy, and Falces (1971) or through an anterolateral approach, which the author uses more frequently. The latter, performed through an incision several millimeters inside the posterior conchal wall–inferior crus contour line, is a simple method of obtaining a precise graft under direct visual exposure (Brent, 1979).

Ipsilateral Conchal Cartilage

In certain partial reconstructions, it is more advantageous to employ an ipsilateral than a contralateral conchal cartilage graft. However, it is imperative that an intact anthelical strut be present to permit removal of an ipsilateral conchal cartilage graft without subsequent collapse and further deformity of the ear.

An ipsilateral conchal cartilage graft is particularly advantageous when a retroauricular flap is being raised to repair a major defect in the helical rim. Elevation of the flap provides the required conchal cartilage exposure without the necessity of an additional incision, and removal of the cartilage graft places the ear closer to the mastoid region. In effect, this maneuver produces a relative gain in length, thus enabling the flap to cover the cartilage graft after it is spliced to the rim and eliminating the need for a skin graft in the flap donor site.

Furthermore, the ipsilateral concha may be used occasionally as a composite flap of skin and cartilage (see Fig. 40–47). This innovative technique, proposed by Davis (1974), is applicable to defects of the upper third of the auricle, and should be employed only when the anthelical support remains intact.

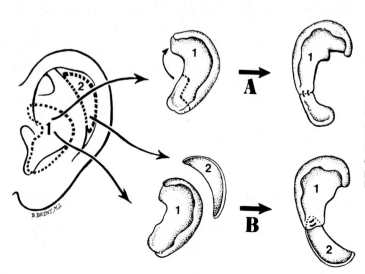

Figure 40–38. The use of auricular cartilage for framework fabrication in major auricular reconstruction. *A,* Sectioning and splicing of conchal cartilage; the concha is rotated 90 degrees (technique of Gorney, Murphy, and Falces). *B,* The combination of conchal and scaphal cartilage; the conchal piece is rotated 90 degrees (technique of Brent.)

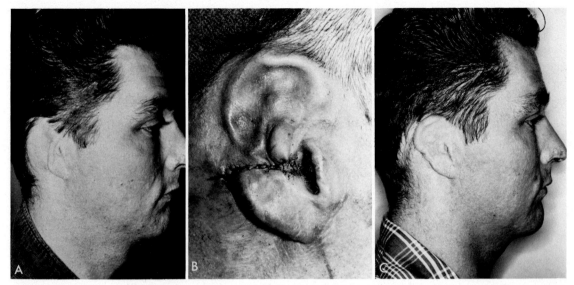

Figure 40–39. The use of auricular cartilage for framework support in the reconstruction of the burned ear. *A,* Burn deformity of the ear. *B,* Appearance after the first stage of reconstruction. *C,* The final result. (From Gorney, M., Murphy, S., and Falces, E.: Spliced autogenous conchal cartilage in secondary ear reconstruction. Plast. Reconstr. Surg., *47:*432, 1971. Copyright © 1971, The Williams & Wilkins Company, Baltimore.)

Composite Grafts

Small to moderate-sized defects may be repaired with composite grafts from the unaffected ear, particularly if the latter is large and protruding (Day, 1921; Adams, 1955; Pegram and Peterson, 1956; Nagel, 1972). One can resect a wedge-shaped composite graft of less than 1.5 cm in width from the scapha and helix of the unaffected ear, and transplant it to a clean-cut defect on the contralateral ear (Fig. 40–40). The success rate of composite grafts can be enhanced by removing a portion of the skin and cartilage, thus converting part of the "wedge" to a full-thickness skin graft, which is readily vascularized by a recipient advancement flap mobilized from the loose retroauricular skin (Brent, 1977). A strut of the helical cartilage is preserved within the graft for contour and support (Fig. 40–41).

Despite a slight inclination toward shrinkage after transplantation, the composite graft offers a simple and expeditious reconstructive technique for partial auricular defects.

SPECIFIC REGIONAL DEFECTS

Helical Rim

Acquired losses of the helical rim may vary from small defects to loss of major portions of the helix. The former usually result from tumor excisions or minor injuries, and are best closed by advancing the helix in both directions as described by Antia and Buch (1967) (Fig. 40–42). The success of this excellent technique depends first on totally freeing the entire helix from the scapha via an incision in the helical sulcus that extends through the cartilage but not through the skin on the posterior surface of the ear. Second, the posteromedial auricular skin is undermined, dissecting just superficially to the perichondrium until the entire helix is hanging as a chondrocutaneous component of the loosely mobilized skin (Fig. 40–42C,D). Extra length can be gained by a V-Y advancement of the crus helicis (Fig. 40–42D,E), and surprisingly large defects can be closed without tension.

Although this technique was originally described for upper third auricular defects (Antia and Buch, 1967) (Fig. 40–43), the author has found that it is even more effective for middle third defects and is equally applicable in repairing earlobe losses. Reconstruction of larger helical defects requires a more sophisticated procedure that recreates the absent rim by using an auricular cartilage graft covered by an adjacent flap, as previously described. Although advancement flaps of local soft tissues (Figs. 40–44, 40–45) have also been employed to provide helical contour, the author finds that these flaps often produce a

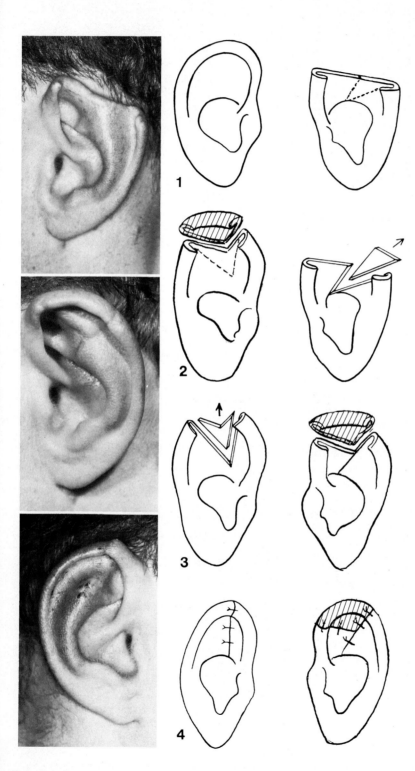

Figure 40–40. Reconstruction of an auricular defect with a composite graft from the contralateral ear. *Left, above,* An auricular defect resulting from a human bite. *Center,* Appearance of the ear three years after reconstruction with a composite graft. *Below,* Appearance of the donor ear 14 days after the surgical procedure. *Right,* The sequence of repair, from the above downward; the donor ear is at the left and the defective ear being reconstructed on the right. (From Nagel, F.: Reconstruction of a partial auricular loss. Plast. Reconstr. Surg., *49*:340, 1972. Copyright © 1972, The Williams & Wilkins Company, Baltimore.)

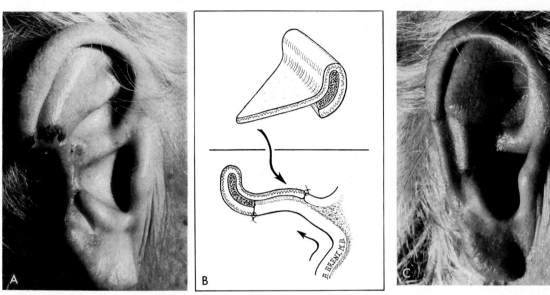

Figure 40–41. Enhancement of composite graft revascularization by decreasing "composite bulk." *A,* Auricular defect with residual chondrodermatitis. *B,* The bulkiness of the composite graft is decreased by removing the posteromedial auricular skin and cartilage while preserving a cartilage strut in the helical rim. A retroauricular flap is advanced to serve as a recipient bed for the remaining anterolateral cutaneous portion of the wedge-shaped graft. *C,* The final result.

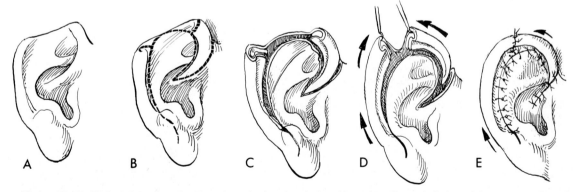

Figure 40–42. Helical defect repaired by advancement of auricular skin and cartilage. *A,* Defect of the upper portion of the auricle. *B,* Lines of incisions through skin and cartilage. *C,* The incisions completed; note the downward extension into the earlobe. *D,* The skin-cartilage flaps mobilized. *E,* The repair completed. (After Antia, N. H., and Buch, V. I.: Chondrocutaneous advancement of flap for the marginal defect of the ear. Plast. Reconstr. Surg. *39:*472, 1967. Copyright © 1967, The Williams & Wilkins Company, Baltimore.)

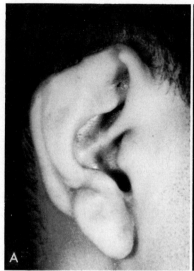
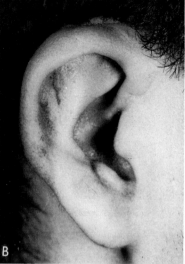

Figure 40–43. *A,* Traumatic defect of the superior helical region. *B,* Repair by helical advancement as illustrated in Figure 40–42. (From Antia, N. H., and Buch, V. I.: Chondrocutaneous advancement of flap for the marginal defect of the ear. Plast. Reconstr. Surg., *39*:472, 1967. Copyright © 1967, The Williams & Wilkins Company, Baltimore.)

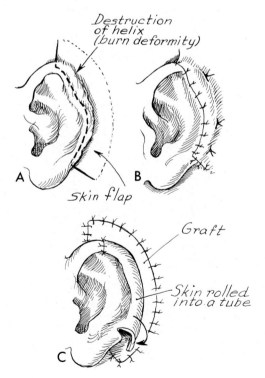

Figure 40–44. Technique for restoring the helical margin. *A,* Outline of the incisions for an advancement flap from the retroauricular area. *B,* The advancement flap sutured in position. *C,* In a second stage, the pedicle of the advancement flap has been sectioned, the flap rolled into a tube, and the resulting defect covered by a split-thickness skin graft. (After Padgett and Stephenson, 1948.)

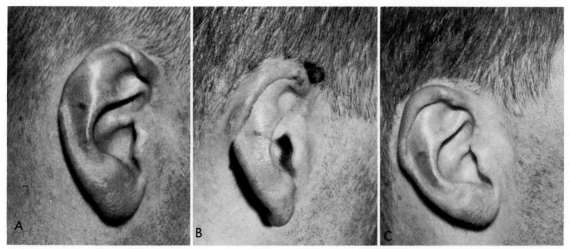

Figure 40–45. Helical reconstruction with a postauricular flap. *A,* Acquired loss of the helical rim. *B,* The postauricular flap in position over the auricular margin. *C,* The completed reconstruction, following division of the flap. (From Lewin, M.: Formation of the helix with a postauricular flap. Plast. Reconstr. Surg., 5:452, 1950. Copyright © 1950, The Williams & Wilkins Company, Baltimore.)

disappointing long-term result unless a strut of cartilage has been incorporated into the repair.

Another sophisticated method of helical reconstruction is the use of thin-calibered tube flaps, which can successfully create a fine, realistic helical rim when meticulous technique is combined with careful case selection (Fig. 40–46). Minor burns often destroy the helical rim yet leave the auriculocephalic sulcus skin intact, thus providing an optimal site for tube flap construction (Steffanoff,

1948) and minimizing the risk of tube migration or failure, and secondary deformity.

Upper Third Auricular Defects

Upper third defects may be reconstructed by four major methods.

1. Minor losses confined to the rim are repaired either by helical advancement, as previously described (see Fig. 40–42), or by a readily accessible preauricular flap.

2. Intermediate losses of the upper third

Figure 40–46. Helical restoration with a fine caliber tube flap. *A,* Migration of the supraclavicular tube flap to the ear with helical loss. *B,* Completion of the helical reconstruction; note the splice of the superior junction by a Z-plasty.

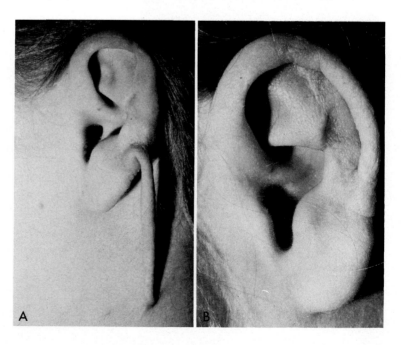

are repaired with a banner flap, as described by Crikelair (1956), which is based antero-superiorly in the auriculocephalic sulcus. This flap should be used in conjunction with a small cartilage graft to ensure a satisfactory long-term result.

3. Major losses in the superior third are most successfully reconstructed with a con-tralateral conchal cartilage graft as classi-cally described by Adams (1955). In this tech-nique, it is imperative that the cartilage graft be anchored to the cartilaginous remnant of the helical root by means of a suture placed through a small incision at that point. This prevents the cartilage graft from "drifting" and ensures helical continuity.

4. If the existing skin is unfavorable for the above technique, the entire concha may be rotated upward as a chondrocutaneous composite flap on a small anterior pedicle of the crus helicis (Davis, 1974). This is a tech-nically demanding procedure that is re-stricted to individual deformities in which a large concha exists (Fig. 40–47).

Middle Third Auricular Defects

Major middle third auricular defects are usually repaired with a cartilage graft, which is either covered by an adjacent skin flap (Fig. 40–48) or inserted via the tunnel pro-cedure (see below). Occasionally, conditions

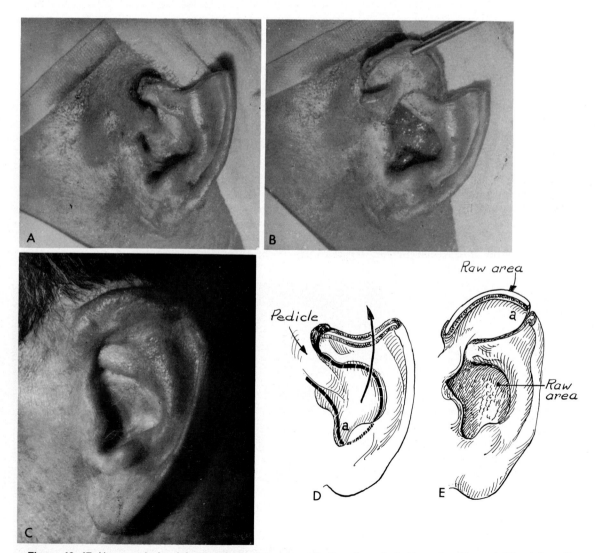

Figure 40–47. Upper auricular defect repaired with a composite flap of conchal skin and cartilage. *A,* The defect. *B,* The composite conchal flap elevated. *C,* The final appearance. *D, E,* Diagram of the procedure, indicating the incisions and the raw surfaces to be grafted. The anterior cutaneous pedicle (crus helicis) maintains the blood supply. (After Davis, 1974.)

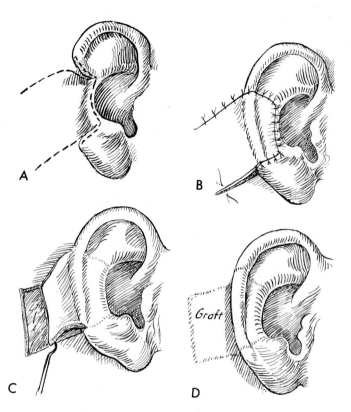

Figure 40–48. Dieffenbach's technique for reconstruction of the middle third of the auricle, drawn from his description (1829–1834). *A,* The defect and the outline of the flap. *B,* The flap advanced over the defect. *C, D,* In a second stage, the base of the flap is divided and the flap is folded around the posteromedial aspect of the auricle. A skin graft covers the scalp donor site.

may favor a specially prepared composite graft, as described previously (see Fig. 40–41).

The tunnel procedure (Converse, 1958) is an effective technique for moderate-sized defects of the auricle (Figs. 40–49, 40–50), and in major defects it has the advantage of preserving the retroauricular sulcus. In this technique, the auricle is pressed against the mastoid area and an ink line drawn on the skin in this area, keeping the line parallel and adjacent to the edge of the auricular defect (Fig. 40–51). Incisions are made through the skin along the ink line, and also through the edge of the auricular defect (Fig. 40–51*C,D*). The medial edge of the auricular incision is sutured to the anterior edge of the mastoid skin incision (Fig. 40–51*E*). A cartilage graft is placed in the soft tissue bed and joined to the edges of the auricular cartilage defect (Fig. 40–51*G, H*). The mastoid skin, which has been undermined, is advanced to cover the cartilage graft, and the edge of the skin flap is sutured to the lateral edge of the auricular skin (Fig. 40–51*I*). A healing and vascularization period of two or three months is permitted, during which time the cuta-neous tunnel behind the auricle must be cleansed with cotton-tipped applicators. The auricle is detached in a second stage, and the resulting elliptic raw areas on the ear and mastoid region are skin grafted (Fig. 40–52).

Middle third auricular tumors are excised and closed either by wedge resection with accessory triangles (see Fig. 40–61), or by helical advancement, as previously described (see Fig. 40–42).

Lower Third Auricular Defects

Lower third losses that encompass more than earlobe tissue present an especially complex challenge, and reconstruction must include a cartilage graft to provide the support necessary to ensure the long-term contour.

Preaux (1971) described an impressive technique for repairing lower third defects by means of a superiorly based flap doubled upon itself, but the author finds that contour and support are created and maintained with less risk by primarily inserting a contralateral conchal cartilage graft subcutaneously in the proposed site of reconstruction.

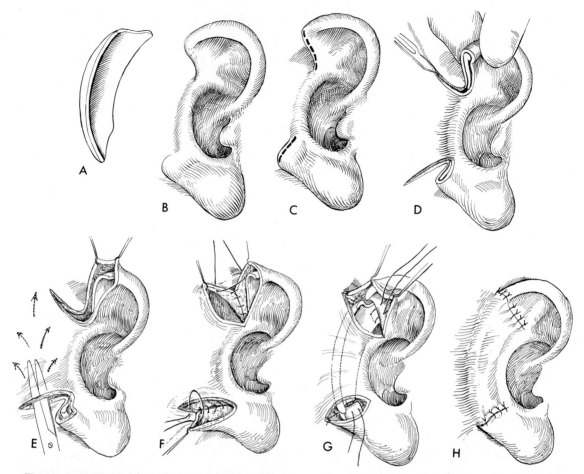

Figure 40–49. Repair of a defect of the middle third of the auricle: the tunnel procedure. *A,* Carved costal cartilage graft. *B,* The defect, *C,* Incisions through the margins of the defect. *D,* Incisions through the edge of the defect are extended backward through the skin of the mastoid area. *E,* The skin of the mastoid area is undermined between the two incisions. *F,* The medial edge of the incision at the border of the auricular defect is sutured to the upper edge of the postauricular incision. A similar type of suture is placed at the lower edge of the defect. *G,* The cartilage graft is placed under the skin of the mastoid area and anchored to the auricular cartilage by catgut sutures. *H,* Suture of the skin incision. (From Converse, J. M.: Reconstruction of the auricle. Plast. Reconstr. Surg., *22:*150, 230, 1958. Copyright © 1958, The Williams & Wilkins Company, Baltimore.)

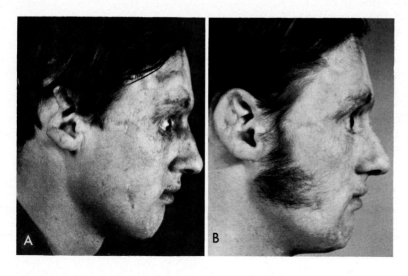

Figure 40–50. Repair of a middle third auricular defect with a carved costal cartilage graft. *A,* Traumatic loss of the middle third of the auricle in a war veteran. *B,* Repair by the technique of Converse illustrated in Figure 40–49. (From Converse, J.M.: Reconstruction of the auricle. Plast. Reconstr. Surg., *22:*150, 230, 1958. Copyright © 1958, The Williams & Wilkins Company, Baltimore.)

Figure 40–51. Repair of a postero-superior auricular defect by the "tunnel procedure" of Converse. *A,* The portion of the ear to be restored. *B,* The auricle is pressed against the mastoid process. *C,* An ink outline is traced on the skin overlying the mastoid process, parallel to the edge of the auricular defect. *D,* Incisions are made along the edge of the defect and through the skin of the mastoid area.

Illustration and legend continued on the following page

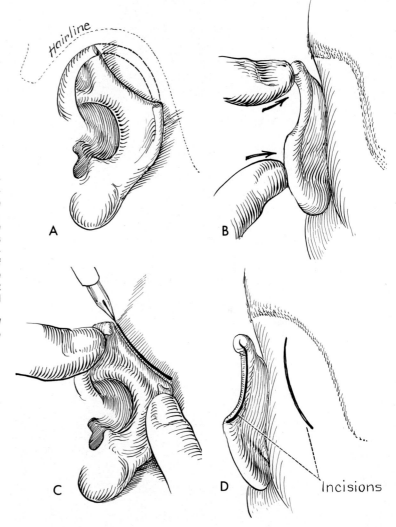

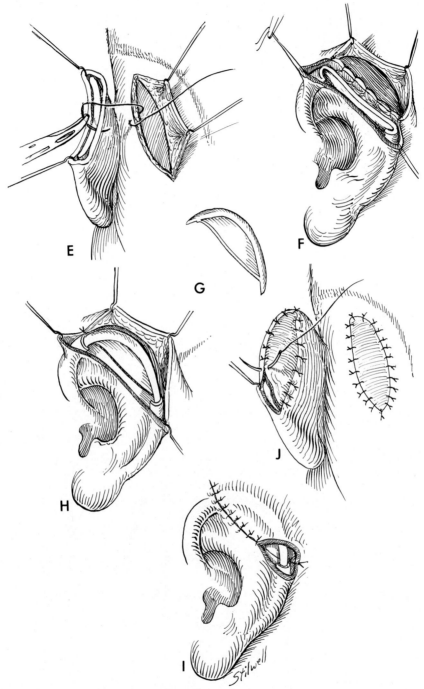

Figure 40–51. *Continued. E,* Suture of the medial edge of the auricular incision to the anterior edge of the mastoid incision. *F,* The suture has been completed. *G,* Costal cartilage graft. *H,* The costal cartilage graft has been embedded. *I,* The skin of the mastoid area is advanced to cover the cartilage graft. *J,* In a second stage, the auricle is separated from the mastoid area, and full-thickness retroauricular grafts from the contralateral ear cover the defects. (From Converse, J. M.: Reconstruction of the auricle. Plast. Reconstr. Surg., 22:150, 230, 1958. Copyright © 1958, The Williams & Wilkins Company, Baltimore.)

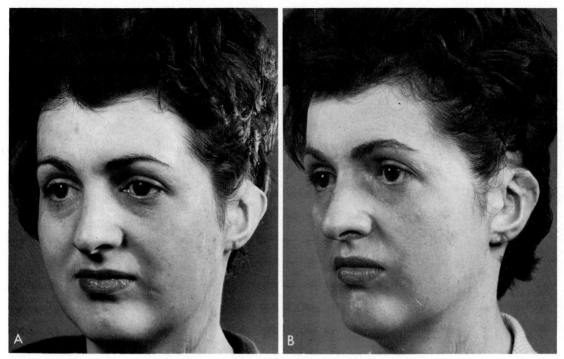

Figure 40–52. A superior auricular defect resulting from a burn. *A,* Preoperative appearance. *B,* The result obtained by the "tunnel procedure" shown in Figure 40–51. (From Converse, J. M.: Reconstruction of the auricle. Plast. Reconstr. Surg., 22:150, 230, 1958. Copyright © 1958, The Williams & Wilkins Company, Baltimore.)

Acquired Earlobe Deformities

Traumatic clefts and keloids that result from ear piercing are the most common acquired defects of the earlobe. Cleft earlobes, usually occurring from the dramatic extraction of earrings, can be repaired most efficiently by Pardue's (1973) ingenious adjacent flap, which is rolled into the apex of the wedge defect, thus maintaining a tract lined with skin that permits further wearing of earrings (Fig. 40–53).

Another common occurrence in everyday practice is the earlobe keloid, which previously was treated with varying degrees of success by irradiation and steroid injections (Cosman and Wolff, 1974; Ramakrishnan, Thomas, and Sundararajan, 1974). Because there is strong evidence that pressure plays an important role in keloid therapy (Ketchum, Cohen, and Masters, 1974; Snyder, 1974), a light pressure-spring earring device may be worth a trial in reducing postexcisional recurrence of earlobe keloids (Brent, 1978).

Construction of an earlobe is rarely re-

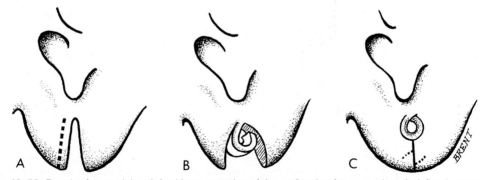

Figure 40–53. Repair of an earlobe cleft with preservation of the perforation for an earring. *A,* A flap is prepared by a parallel incision on one side of the cleft; the other side is freshened by excision of the margin. *B,* The flap is rolled in to provide a lining for preservation of the earring tract. *C,* Closure is completed; a small Z-plasty may be incorporated. (After Pardue, 1973.)

quired in congenital microtia, because the lobe is formed by the repositioning of auricular remnants. However, a portion or the entire lobe may be missing in traumatic deformities of the ear, and a variety of techniques for its reconstruction have been proposed.

As early as 1907, effective techniques (Gavello quoted by Nélaton and Ombrédanne) were devised to repair earlobes with local flaps. In the 1970's and 1980's numerous methods have been developed (Figs. 40–54 to 40–60) (Zenteno Alanis, 1970; Guerrero-Santos, 1970; Preaux, 1971; Brent, 1976).

Tumors of the Auricle

TUMORS

Sebaceous cysts of the auricle are often treated improperly or neglected. Most commonly, they are found on the medial aspect of the ear, particularly in the lobule, and these should be excised in toto during the quiescent period through the medial surface of the lobule, to minimize deformity.

The most common auricular lesion is actinic keratosis, which, like carcinomas, occurs in outdoor workers with fair complexions. Other benign auricular lesions, such as granuloma pyogenicum, beryllium granuloma, verruca contagiosa, verruca senilis, cylindroma, nevus, papilloma, lipoma, lymphangioma, leiomyoma, and chondroma, should be surgically excised. Keloid of the earlobe is common; the treatment of this lesion is also discussed in Chapter 21.

MALIGNANT TUMORS

Over 5 per cent of skin cancers involve the auricle (Arons and Sadin, 1971). The vast majority of these are cutaneous, usually basal cell or squamous cell carcinomas. A minority are malignant melanoma.

When first seen, the cartilage is involved by direct extension in approximately one-third of the cutaneous carcinomas of the auricle. Because of this finding and because cartilage is an excellent barrier to the spread of the tumor, it is thought that the cartilage must be included in the surgical excision (Hoopes, 1974).

The cervical lymph nodes are rarely involved in basal cell carcinoma of the auricle, but are involved in approximately one-third of all squamous cell carcinomas and malignant melanomas.

Most of the malignant lesions are located on the helical rim, and they can be eradicated with a wedge excision (Fig. 40–61) or a helical advancement (see Fig. 40–42). Many of the tumors located on the lateral and medial auricular surfaces can be treated adequately by excision and subsequent skin grafting, or by local flap coverage. Others require definitive reconstructive procedures previously detailed in this chapter. Radiation therapy is of

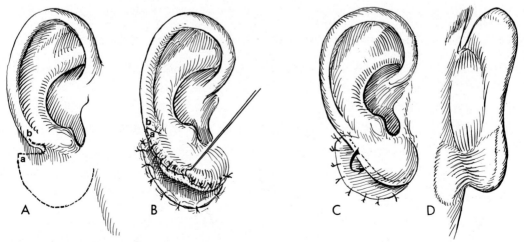

Figure 40–54. Reconstruction of an earlobe. *A,* The design of the flap. *B,* The posterosuperior angle of the flap has been inserted into the lower portion of the helical border. The raw surfaces are covered by full-thickness skin grafts. *C,* As healing takes place, the edge of the flap tends to roll on itself. *D,* The postoperative appearance of the new lobe. (From Converse, J. M.: Reconstruction of the auricle. Plast. Reconstr. Surg., 22:150, 158. Copyright © 1958, The Williams & Wilkins Company, Baltimore.)

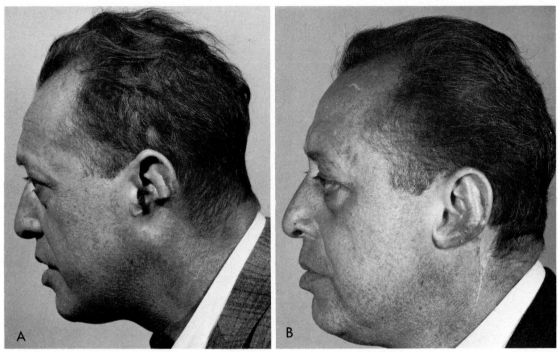

Figure 40–55. *A,* Loss of the lower part of the auricle. *B,* The result obtained with a flap based on the mastoid process and folded on itself. Note the scar of the approximated edges of the flap's donor site. (Patient of Dr. Cary L. Guy.)

Figure 40–56. Reconstruction of the lower portion of the auricle and the earlobe. *A,* The defect and the outline of the lining flap. *B,* The outline of the cover flap and of the fat flap used for fill. *C,* The lining flap is covered by the cover flap, and the fat flap is introduced between them. *D,* The secondary defect is closed by direct approximation. (Courtesy of Dr. J. Davis.)

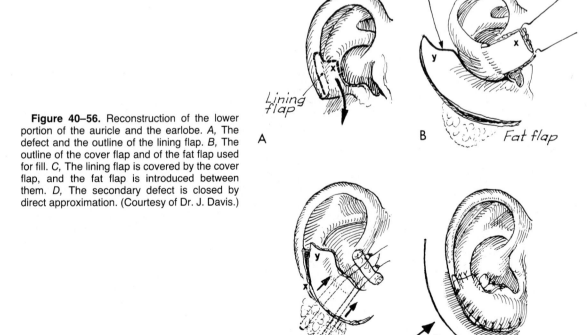

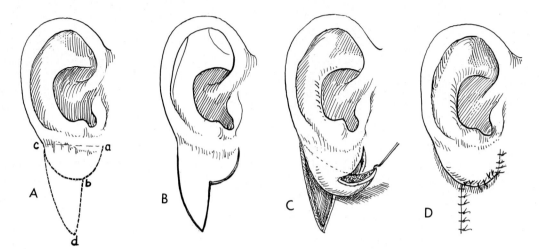

Figure 40–57. Reconstruction of the earlobe. *A,* The curved line *abc* outlines the proposed earlobe as measured on the unaffected contralateral auricle. A vertical flap is outlined; line *bd* is equal in length to line *ab*, and *cd* is equal to *ca*. *B,* Incisions are made through the outlined skin and subcutaneous tissue. *C,* The vertical flap is raised from the underlying tissue as far upward as the horizontal line *ac,* and the apex of the flap is sutured to point *a. D,* The operation completed. (After Zenteno Alanis, 1970.)

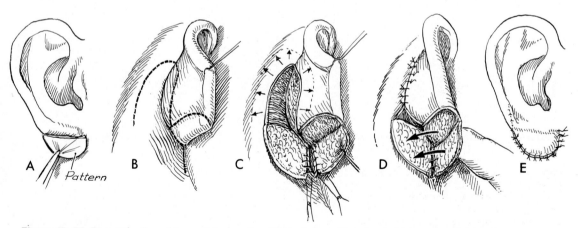

Figure 40–58. Reconstruction of the earlobe by a two-flap technique (Converse). *A,* The pattern of the planned earlobe. *B,* The pattern has been placed on the posteromedial aspect of the auricle and an outline made. The outline of the second flap from the retroauricular area is also shown; note the line of the vertical incision for insertion of the lobe. *C,* Each of the flaps is sutured to an edge of the vertical incision, thus anchoring the new earlobe. *D,* The two flaps are sutured to each other. *E,* The operation completed. (From Kazanjian and Converse.)

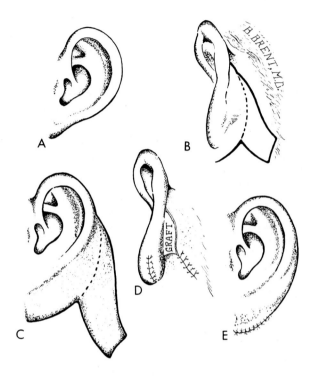

Figure 40–59. Construction of an earlobe with a reverse contoured flap. *A,* The earlobe deficiency. *B,* An auriculomastoid flap outlined. *C,* The elevated flap hanging as a curtain from the inferior auricular border. *D,* The flap folded under and sutured and the mastoid defect closed. A small graft is placed over the auricular donor defect. *E,* The completed earlobe, exaggerated by one-third to allow for shrinkage. (From Brent, B.: Earlobe reconstruction with an auriculo-mastoid flap. Plast. Reconstr. Surg., *57:*389, 1976. Copyright © 1976, The Williams & Wilkins Company, Baltimore.)

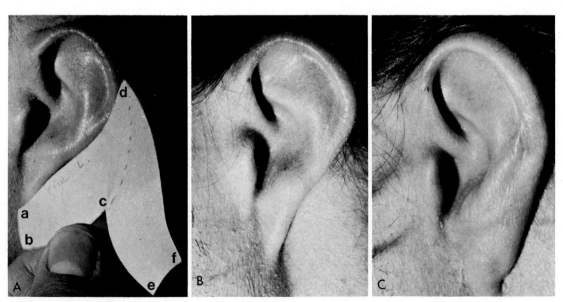

Figure 40–60. Earlobe reconstruction. *A,* The reverse contour pattern, in which *ab* is equal to *ef, bc* to *ce,* and *ad* to *df. B,* Congenital deficiency of lobular tissue. *C,* Completed construction by the technique illustrated in Figure 40–59. (From Brent, B.: Earlobe reconstruction with an auriculo-mastoid flap. Plast. Reconstr. Surg., *57:*389, 1976. Copyright © 1976, The Williams & Wilkins Company, Baltimore.)

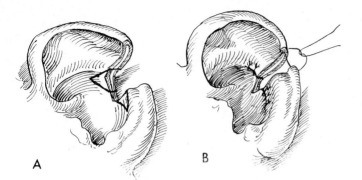

Figure 40–61. Wedge resection of a helical tumor. *A,* The tumor has been excised, and secondary wedges are outlined to facilitate closure of the defect. *B,* Details of the closure.

A

B

no value in managing recurrences and metastases, and is poorly tolerated by the auricle.

When the cancer is large and includes cartilaginous invasion, the ear must be totally excised with surrounding soft tissue. Radical resection of the cervical lymph nodes in continuity with resection of the involved auricle should be performed. At times the only hope of effecting a cure in auricular cancer involves resection of the temporal bone (Parsons and Lewis, 1954; Lewis, 1960; Mladick and associates, 1974).

Patients requiring total auricular ablation are usually older and generally are not candidates for total auricular reconstruction. Often a prosthesis is preferred, but if total ear reconstruction is indicated it is advisable to postpone reconstruction until the threat of recurrence is well past.

MICROTIA AND ATRESIA: INDICATIONS FOR AND TIMING OF MIDDLE EAR SURGERY*

Aural atresia is an absent or incomplete external auditory canal. Concomitant temporal bone malformations are variably associated with aural atresia, such as abnormalities of the middle ear, ossicles, cochleovestibular labyrinth, and facial nerve (Schuknecht, 1974). Along with aural atresia, these malformations can impede the audition of the developing infant.

Two areas are of major concern in the successful management of microtia and aural atresia: cosmesis and the provision of effective sound transmission as early as possible to a functioning cochlea. Meaningful rehabilitation mandates prompt audiologic diagnosis

---

*Contributed by Dr. P. E. Hammerschlag.

to establish hearing during the period of maximal language formation and acquisition, which begins in infancy (McConnell and Liff, 1975; Pollack, 1979). Appropriately chosen bone conduction hearing aids provide sufficient acoustic transmission during the first years of life, which are critical for language development. Nonsurgical auditory rehabilitation also permits more accurate evaluation over time to identify patients best suited for optimal otologic surgical reconstruction.

It must be emphasized that not all patients with atresia are realistic candidates for otologic surgery. Detailed preoperative evaluation is required to identify those who may optimally benefit from aural atresia repair. Reasonably precise assessments usually can be obtained with high resolution CT scanning and expert pediatric audiologic evaluation; these often require supplementary audiometric techniques (Chakeres and Spiegel, 1983).

Diagnosis

The extent to which the sound conduction mechanism (the external auditory canal and ossicles) and the cochlea reserve (the sensorineural component) are impaired is determined by sophisticated audiometry, best performed in a facility experienced in evaluating infants. In addition to behavior observation audiometry (BOA) and conditioned orientation response (COR) techniques, other methods such as ABR (auditory brain stem response) may be used to assess the uncooperative or retarded infant with bilateral atresia or mixed loss (Goldstein, Kendell, and Arick, 1963; Davis, 1965; Lloyd and Cox, 1975). A variation of the latter method found to be helpful in evaluating hearing in bilateral atresia is achieved with simultaneous multielectrode ABR recordings; monaural air conduction as well as mastoid placement bone conduction click stimuli are used with this technique (Finitzo-Hieber, Hecox, and Cone, 1979; Hall and associates, 1984).

If cochlear function is normal, nonsurgical audiologic rehabilitation is begun as soon as possible during infancy. It should be emphasized that a child with only one normal functioning cochlea is amenable only to nonsurgical rehabilitation and otologic surgery is precluded; surgery with potential risk to the labyrinth in a single hearing ear should be avoided (microtia repair does not affect labyrinthine functions).

High resolution CT with targeted views (coronal and axial) of the temporal bone represents a major advance in the preoperative assessment of aural atresia (Turski and associates, 1982). Factors evaluated by CT scanning should cover the presence or absence of stapes, oval window obstruction, pneumatization of the mastoid, the size of the middle ear space, facial nerve anatomy, malleus-incus formation, the incudostapedial joint, an atretic plate, the osseous (cochlea and vestibular) labyrinth, and the external canal. With this information the experienced otologist can identify patients with significant abnormalities that will decrease the likelihood of successful otologic improvement and increase the potential risks of facial paralysis and sensorineural damage. In the uncooperative child detailed CT scans may require sedation or general anesthesia. If necessary, CT and ABR audiometry can be performed during the same general anesthesia in centers prepared for this type of detailed assessment (Jahrsdoerfer and associates, 1985).

Rehabilitation

Infants with bilateral aural atresia are aided as early as possible with bone conduction hearing aids, and entered in an infant hearing rehabilitation program to maximize auditory and language development. Infants with unilateral atresia and normal contralateral hearing usually do not require early amplification of the atretic ear. Although they lack sound directionality associated with binaural hearing, their language development can be normal, in contrast to infants with bilateral atresia. Indeed, it should be emphasized that infants with bilateral atresia should receive amplification well before 4

months of age. Delaying amplification to the second year risks irreversible effects on auditory and language development (McConnell and Liff, 1975). Therefore, the audiometric evaluation must take priority over a CT scan, which latter is really part of a "preoperative" assessment.

Properly selected surgical candidates are those in whom repair of an uncomplicated atresia is anticipated. In such candidates, on the basis of cochlear reserve and radiologic information, otologic surge may achieve a postoperation speech reception threshold of 15 to 25 decibels (within the range of normal hearing) (Jahrsdoerfer, 1978). Adequate middle ear space, satisfactory mastoid pneumatization, reasonable ossicular complex formation, a patent oval window, and evidence of a stapes on CT scan are some of the criteria that suggest a satisfactory candidate for optimal surgical repair of atresia. Other factors leading to sensorineural hearing loss (fenestration for fixed stapes), poor hearing, or facial paralysis may be identified only at surgery. If potential risks are encountered at surgery, the procedure can be safely aborted, and postoperatively the patient can be rehabilitated as a nonsurgical candidate.

Needless to say, repair of aural atresia requires the skills of an experienced otologist for proper preoperative and intraoperative assessment. Effective and safe surgery for aural atresia is beyond the skill of a novice otologist.

Infants with bilateral atresia who are candidates for otologic surgery can undergo the operation between the ages of 4 and 6 years. Bilateral repair of uncomplicated atresia should permit near-normal to normal hearing without the use of hearing aids. Surgical intervention should be planned to allow sufficient time for multistage auricular reconstruction followed by otologic surgery before entering school. The plastic surgeon and otologist must work in concert.

Patients with unilateral atresia (also meeting the above strict preoperative criteria) can undergo surgical repair without urgency. Aural atresia repair may be performed during childhood or later when there is participation by the patient and plastic surgeon in the decision-making process. Unilateral atresia patients may be assisted with an implantable bone conduction hearing device, which is cosmetically superior to the conventional bone conduction hearing aid (Hough and associates, 1987).

Results and Complications

Bellucci (1977) cited his experience with 48 patients in whom surgical repair of atresia improved hearing to near-normal levels (less than 30 decibels) in 45 per cent. His technique included mastoidectomy, tympanoplasty, and fenestration of the horizontal canal for stapes fixation. The best results were with ossicular repositioning in the presence of a mobile stapes. There was a 25 per cent regression in hearing, a finding associated with mastoid cavity infection. Poor results were also noted when there was failure to obtain adequate visualization of the middle ear cleft. In 10 of the 21 patients requiring fenestration, two showed no change from the preoperative level. A 25 per cent regression to beyond near-normal hearing was also observed after fenestration of the horizontal semicircular canal, especially in children. It was hypothesized that children have a high incidence of osteoneogenesis obliterating the fenestration.

These results led Bellucci (1977) to suggest that otologic surgery for atresia be limited to those with binaural atresia, since the likelihood of improving hearing in an ear with unilateral atresia, to provide contralateral hearing to complement the normal hearing ear, was not sufficiently high to warrant surgery. In contrast, patients with the largest conductive deficit (i.e., those with binaural atresia) would benefit most from surgical improvement in hearing.

Subsequent experience suggests that more precise preoperative evaluation can identify patients who could undergo uncomplicated atresia repair without mastoidectomy and fenestration, especially in the hands of experienced otologists, and could obtain normal or near-normal hearing (Jahrsdoerfer and Hall, 1986). With a more consistent success in obtaining near-normal hearing in properly selected patients, it appears that this otologic reconstruction can be considered for those with unilateral atresia as well as bilateral atresia. Nevertheless, surgery for unilateral atresia remains controversial and is performed electively without the same sense of urgency as in patients with bilateral atresia.

As noted earlier, in patients not meeting these more stringent criteria for surgery or in whom the operating surgeon elects to not risk membranous labyrinthine injury (i.e., with fenestration/stapedectomy), benefit can be obtained from such options as bone con-

duction hearing aids, an air conduction aid in a newly reconstructed external ear canal, or an implantable bone conduction hearing device.

Complications of aural atresia repair can include facial nerve paralysis, which has been reported since the advent of surgery for aural atresia (Kiesselbach, 1882). In a series of 202 surgical cases, an experienced otologist noted the incidence of facial paralysis to be less than 2 per cent; in all four patients the facial nerve paresis was transient and occurred after nerve mobilization to improve access to the stapes or oval window (Jahrsdoerfer and Hall, 1986).

Congenital aural atresia associated with syndromic malformations such as the Treacher Collins syndrome probably is associated with the greatest likelihood of abnormal facial nerve anatomy. The incidence of facial paralysis may be reduced with preoperative high resolution CT scanning, which can delineate the course of the facial nerve. Intraoperatively, the operating microscope and facial nerve monitoring systems have further decreased the occurrence of inadvertent facial nerve injury (Hammerschlag, Breda, and Cohen, 1988).

Sensorineural hearing loss can occur with direct injury to the membranous labyrinth from fenestration, stapedectomy, or direct transmission of acoustic trauma from incorrect use of a high speed drill. The incidence of sensorineural hearing loss in one large series was less than 2 per cent and this loss was thought to be secondary to a stapedectomy (Jahrsdoerfer and Hall, 1986).

The incidence of postoperative infection and canal stenosis varies and is based on the experience and technique of the surgeon. A higher incidence of otorrhea is associated with creation of an open mastoid cavity than with those cases not requiring mastoidectomy (Bellucci, 1977). In the latter series the complication rate was less than 1 per cent. Because skin grafts lining the external canal lack cerumen glands, crusting of desquamated debris can occur and lead to otitis externa. This can be avoided by cleansing of the external auditory canal debris at regular intervals after surgery.

Canal stenosis may require revision surgery. If conchal cartilage is present, the cartilage incision for the newly created meatus need only be normal in size. If there is no conchal cartilage, the meatoplasty should be twice normal size to compensate for postoperative contraction. Frequently, edema of the auricular graft occurs after its elevation and mobilization associated with atresia repair; it should resolve within one month upon the return of auricular definition.

Timing of Middle Ear Surgery

Review of the literature reveals the longstanding controversy between plastic surgeons and otologists over which part of reconstruction should come first: auricular reconstruction or atresia repair. Advocates for preliminary auricular reconstruction cite the compromised blood supply after atresia repair as reducing rib cartilage graft viability, and the poor elasticity of scarred scalp skin as interfering with satisfactory graft placement. Most experienced observers cannot recall an optimal auricular reconstruction being performed after atresia repair. The otologist is concerned that the correct site for the new external auditory canal, which cannot be determined until after the atresia repair, may not be identical to that anticipated in the previously reconstructed auricle.

Resolution between those advocating these differing points of view is achieved by close cooperation and planning between the two surgeons. In reality, the otologist can mobilize the previously implanted autogenous rib graft with a postauricular incision, which can be extended to a rhytidectomy type of flap to reposition the auricle over the newly created bony external auditory canal.

Microtia is usually a multistage reconstructive endeavor. The auricle can be elevated from the scalp for final skin graft placement (Aguilar and Jahrsdoerfer, 1988).

Optimal timing for unilateral microtia repair is based on maturation of the rib cartilage donor site and the cooperation of the child. Such repair can usually occur by age 7 years. Elective unilateral atresia repair in properly selected patients can occasionally be carried out in conjunction with the microtia repair, or later when the patient can participate in the decision-making process.

In children with bilateral atresia, there is a greater urgency to improve audition in both ears at an earlier date. The earliest date at which rib cartilage might be considered sufficiently mature for microtia repair is when the patient is 6 to 7 years. In properly selected

candidates, the aural atresia repair can proceed in conjunction with the auricular reconstruction. Alternatively, the child who is not a candidate for otologic surgery can undergo surgical implantation of a bone conductive hearing device after the microtia repair.

REFERENCES

Aase, J. M., and Tegtmeier, R. E.: Microtia in New Mexico: evidence for multifactorial causation. Birth Defects, *13*:113, 1977.

Adams, W. M.: Construction of the upper half of the auricle utilizing a composite concha cartilage graft with perichondrium attached on both sides. Plast. Reconstr. Surg., *16*:88, 1955.

Aguilar, E. A., and Jahrsdoerfer, R. A.: The surgical repair of congenital microtia and atresia. Otolaryngol. Head Neck Surg., *98*:600, 1988.

Albrektsson, T., Branemark, P. I., Jacobsson, M., and Tjellstrom, A.: Present clinical applications of osseointegrated percutaneous implants. Plast. Reconstr. Surg., *79*:721, 1987.

Antia, N. H., and Buch, V. I.: Chondrocutaneous advancement of flap for the marginal defect of the ear. Plast. Reconstr. Surg., *39*:472, 1967.

Arey, L. B.: Developmental Anatomy. 7th Ed. Philadelphia, W. B. Saunders Company, 1974.

Arons, M. D., and Sadin, R. C.: Auricular cancer. Am. J. Surg., *122*:770, 1971.

Baudet, J., Tramond, P., and Goumain, A.: A propos d'un procédé original de réimplantation d'un pavillon de l'oreille totalement séparé. Ann. Chir. Plast., *17*:67, 1972.

Becker, O. J.: Surgical correction of the abnormally protruding ear. Arch. Otolaryngol., *50*:541, 1949.

Becker, O. J.: Correction of the protruding deformed ear. Br. J. Plast. Surg., *5*:187, 1952.

Bellucci, R. J.: Congenital auricular malformations: indications, contraindications, and timing of middle ear surgery: an otologist's viewpoint. *In* Converse, J. M. (Ed.): Reconstructive Plastic Surgery. 2nd Ed. Philadelphia, W. B. Saunders Company, 1977, pp. 1719–1724.

Bhishagratna, K. K. L.: An English Translation of the Susruta Samhita. Calcutta, Wilkins Press, 1907.

Bonanno, P. C., and Converse, J. M.: *In* Kazanjian, V. H., and Converse, J. M. (Eds.): Surgical Treatment of Facial Injuries. 3rd Ed. Baltimore, Williams & Wilkins Company, 1974, p. 1292.

Brent, B.: Earlobe construction with an auriculomastoid flap. Plast. Reconstr. Surg., *57*:389, 1976.

Brent, B.: The acquired auricular deformity. A systemic approach to its analysis and reconstruction. Plast. Reconstr. Surg., *59*:475, 1977.

Brent, B.: The role of pressure therapy in management of earlobe keloids: preliminary report of a controlled study. Ann. Plast. Surg., *1*:579, 1978.

Brent, B.: The versatile cartilage autograft: current trends in clinical transplantation. Clin. Plast. Surg., *6*:163, 1979.

Brent, B.: The correction of microtia with autogenous cartilage grafts. I. The classic deformity. Plast. Reconstr. Surg., *66*:1, 1980a.

Brent, B.: The correction of microtia with autogenous cartilage grafts. II. Atypical and complex deformities. Plast. Reconstr. Surg., 66:13, 1980b.

Brent, B.: Total auricular construction with sculpted costal cartilage. In Brent, B. (Ed.): The Artistry of Reconstructive Surgery. St. Louis, C. V. Mosby Company, 1987, pp. 113–127.

Brent, B., and Byrd, H. S.: Secondary ear reconstruction with cartilage grafts covered by axial, random, and free flaps of temporoparietal fascia. Plast. Reconstr. Surg., 72:141, 1983.

Broadbent, T. R., and Mathews, V. I.: Artistic relationships in surface anatomy of the face. Plast. Reconstr. Surg., 20:1, 1957.

Brown, J. B., Cannon, B., Lischer, C. E., Davis, W. B., and Moore, A.: Surgical substitution for losses of the external ear: simplified local flap method of reconstruction. Surg. Gynecol. Obstet., 84:192, 1947.

Byrd, H. S.: The use of subcutaneous axial fascial flaps in reconstruction of the head. Ann. Plast. Surg., 4:191, 1980.

Chakeres, D. W., and Spiegel, P. K.: A systematic technique for comprehensive evaluation of the temporal bone by computed tomography. Radiology, 146:97, 1983.

Chongchet, V.: A method of anthelix reconstruction. Br. J. Plast. Surg., 16:268, 1963.

Clemons, J. E., and Connelly, M. V.: Reattachment of a totally amputated auricle. Arch. Otolaryngol., 97:269, 1973.

Cloutier, A. M.: Correction of outstanding ears. Plast. Reconstr. Surg., 28:412, 1961.

Cocheril, R. C.: Essai sur la restauration du pavillon de l'oreille. Thèse pour le Doctorat en Médecine. Lille, L. Danel, 1894.

Conroy, C. C.: Salvage of an amputated ear. Plast. Reconstr. Surg., 49:564, 1972.

Converse, J. M.: Reconstruction of the auricle. Plast. Reconstr. Surg., 22:150, 230, 1958.

Converse, J. M.: The absorption and shrinkage of maternal ear cartilage used as living homografts: follow-up report of 21 of Gillies' patients. In Converse, J. M. (Ed.): Reconstructive Plastic Surgery. 2nd Ed. Philadelphia, W. B. Saunders Company, 1977, p. 308.

Converse, J. M., Horowitz, S. L., Coccaro, P. J., and Wood-Smith, D.: The corrective treatment of the skeletal asymmetry in hemifacial microsomia. Plast. Reconstr. Surg., 52:221, 1973.

Converse, J. M., Nigro, A., Wilson, F. A., and Johnson, N.: A technique for surgical correction of lop ears. Plast. Reconstr. Surg., 15:411, 1955.

Converse, J. M., Wood-Smith, D., McCarthy, J. G., Coccaro, P. J., and Becker, M. H.: Bilateral facial microsomia. Plast. Reconstr. Surg., 54:413, 1974.

Conway, H., Neumann, C. G., Golb, J., Leveridge, L. L., and Joseph, J. M.: Reconstruction of the external ear. Ann. Surg., 128:226, 1948.

Cosman, B.: Repair of moderate cup ear deformities. In Tanzer, R. C., and Edgerton, M. T. (Eds.): Symposium on Reconstruction of the Auricle. St. Louis, MO, C. V. Mosby Company, 1974, p. 118.

Cosman, B.: Repair of the constricted ear. In Brent, B. (Ed.): The Artistry of Reconstructive Surgery. St. Louis, MO, C. V. Mosby Company, 1987, p. 99.

Cosman, B., and Wolff, M.: Bilateral earlobe keloids. Plast. Reconstr. Surg., 53:540, 1974.

Crikelair, G. F.: A method of partial ear reconstruction for avulsion of the upper portion of the ear. Plast. Reconstr. Surg., 17:438, 1956.

Cronin, T. D.: Use of a Silastic frame for total and subtotal reconstruction of the external ear: Preliminary report. Plast. Reconstr. Surg., 37:399, 1966.

Cronin, T. D.: Use of a Silastic frame for reconstruction of the auricle. In Tanzer, R. C., and Edgerton, M. T. (Eds.): Symposium on Reconstruction of the Auricle. St. Louis, MO, C. V. Mosby Company, 1974, p. 33.

Curtin, J. W., and Bader, K. F.: Improved techniques for the successful silicone reconstruction of the external ear. Plast. Reconstr. Surg., 44:372, 1969.

Davis, H.: Slow cortical responses evoked by acoustic stimuli. Acta Otolaryngol., 59:179, 1965.

Davis, J.: Reconstruction of the upper third of the ear with a chondrocutaneous composite flap based on the crus helix. In Tanzer, R. C., and Edgerton, M. T. (Eds.): Symposium on Reconstruction of the Auricle. St. Louis, MO, C. V. Mosby Company, 1974, p. 247.

Davis, J. E.: On auricular reconstruction. Internatl. Microform J. Aesthetic Plast. Surg., Otoplasty, 1972-C.

Day, H. F.: Reconstruction of the ears. Boston Med. Surg. J., 185:146, 1921.

Dellon, A. L., Claybaugh, G. L., and Hoopes, J. E.: Hemipalatal palsy and microtia. Ann. Plast. Surg., 10:475, 1983.

Dieffenbach, J. F.: Die operative Chirurgie. Leipzig, F. A. Brockhaus, 1845.

diMartino, G.: Anomalie du pavillon de l'oreille et procédé d'otomiose. Bull. Acad. Med. (Paris), 22:17, 1856–1857.

Dupertuis, S. M., and Musgrave, R. M.: Experiences with the reconstruction of the congenitally deformed ear. Plast. Reconstr. Surg., 23:361, 1959.

Ely, E. T.: An operation for prominence of the auricles. Arch. Otolaryngol., 10:97, 1881.

Erich, J. B.: Surgical treatment of protruding ears. Eye, Ear, Nose Throat Monthly, 37:390, 1958.

Erich, J. B., and Abu-Jamra, F. N.: Congenital cup-shaped deformity of the ears: transmitted through four generations. Mayo Clin. Proc., 40:597, 1965.

Farkas, L. G.: Growth of normal and reconstructed auricles. In Tanzer, R. C., and Edgerton, M. T. (Eds.): Symposium on Reconstruction of the Auricle. St. Louis, MO, C. V. Mosby Company, 1974, p. 24.

Finitzo-Hieber, T., Hecox, K., and Cone, B.: Brain stem auditory evoked potentials in patients with congenital atresia. Laryngoscope, 89:1151, 1979.

Fukuda, O.: Otoplasty of cryptotia. Jpn. J. Plast. Surg., 11:117, 1968.

Fukuda, O.: The microtic ear: survey of 180 cases in 10 years. Plast. Reconstr. Surg., 53:458, 1974.

Furnas, D. W.: Correction of prominent ears by concho-mastoid sutures. Plast. Reconstr. Surg., 42:189, 1968.

Gavello, P.: Quoted by Nélaton, C., and Ombrédanne, L.: Les Autoplasties. Paris, G. Steinheil, 1907.

Gibson, T., and Davis, W.: The distortion of autogenous cartilage grafts: its cause and prevention. Br. J. Plast. Surg., 10:257, 1958.

Gifford, G. H.: Replantation of severed part of an ear. Plast. Reconstr. Surg., 49:202, 1972.

Gillies, H.: Plastic Surgery of the Face. London, H. Frowde, Hodder & Stoughton, 1920.

Gillies, H.: Reconstruction of the external ear with special reference to the use of maternal ear cartilages as the supporting structure. Rev. Chir. Structive, 7:169, 1937.

Goldstein, R., Kendell, D. L., and Arick, B. E.: Electroencephalic audiometry in young children. J. Speech Hear. Dis., 28:331, 1963.

Gorney, M., Murphy, S., and Falces, E.: Spliced autogenous conchal cartilage in secondary ear reconstruction. Plast. Reconstr. Surg., 47:432, 1971.

Gosserez, M., and Piers, J. H.: Invagination congénitale du pavillon de l'oreille. Ann. Chir. Plast., 4:143, 1959.

Grabb, W. C.: The first and second branchial arch syndrome. Plast. Reconstr. Surg., 36:485, 1965.

Grabb, W. C., and Dingman, R. O.: The fate of amputated tissues of the head and neck following replacement. Plast. Reconstr. Surg., 49:28, 1972.

Greeley, P. W.: Reconstruction of the external ear. U.S. Naval Med. Bull., 42:1323, 1944.

Guerrero-Santos, J.: Correction of hypertrophied earlobes in leprosy. Plast. Reconstr. Surg., 46:381, 1970.

Hall, J. W., III, Morgan, S. H., Mackey-Hargadine, J., Aguilar, E. A., III, and Jahrsdoerfer, R. A.: Neuro-otologic applications of simultaneous multi-channel auditory evoked response recordings. Laryngoscope, 98:883, 1984.

Hammerschlag, P. E., Breda, S., and Cohen, N. L.: Intraoperative monitoring for preservation of facial nerve function in cerebellopontine angle surgery. Presented at VI International Symposium on the Facial Nerve, Sao Paulo, 1988.

Hanhart, E.: Nachweis einer einfach-dominanten, unkomplizierten sowie einer unregelmässig-dominanten, mit Atresia auris, Palatoschisis und anderen Deformationen-verbundenen Anlage zu Ohrmuschel-Verkümmerung (Mikrotie). Arch. der Julius Klaus-Stift, 24:374, 1949.

His, W.: Zur Entwickelung des Acusticofacialisgebiets beim Menschen. Arch. Anat. Phys. Anat., Suppl., 1899.

Hoopes, J. E.: Reconstruction of the auricle after tumor resection. In Tanzer, R. C., and Edgerton, M. T. (Eds.): Symposium on Reconstruction of the Auricle. St. Louis, MO, C. V. Mosby Company, 1974.

Hough, J., Vernon, J., Himelick, T., Meikel, M., Richard, G., and Dormer, K.: A middle ear implantable hearing device for controlled amplification of sound in the human: a preliminary report. Laryngoscope, 97:141, 1987.

Jahrsdoerfer, R. A.: Congenital atresia of the ear. Laryngoscope, 88(Suppl. 13):1, 1978.

Jahrsdoerfer, R. A., and Hall, J. W., III: Congenital malformations of the ear. Am. J. Otol., 7:267, 1986.

Jahrsdoerfer, R. A., Yeakley, J. W., Hall, J. W., III, Robbins, K. T., and Gray, L. C.: High-resolution CT scanning and auditory brain stem response in congenital aural atresia: patient selection and surgical correlation. Otolaryngol. Head Neck Surg., 93:292, 1985.

Ju, D. M. C., Li, C., and Crikelair, G. F.: The surgical correction of protruding ears. Plast. Reconstr. Surg., 32:283, 1963.

Juri, J., Irigaray, A., Juri, C., Grilli, D., Blanco, C. M., and Vazquez, G. D.: Ear replantation. Plast. Reconstr. Surg., 80:431, 1987.

Kageyama, M.: Correction apparatus for pocket ear. J.J.M.I., 5:435, 1928.

Kaye, B. L.: A simplified method for correcting the prominent ear. Plast. Reconstr. Surg., 40:44, 1967.

Kessler, L.: Beobachtung einer über 6 Generationen einfach-dominant vererbten Mikrotie 1. Grades. HNO, 15:113, 1967.

Ketchum, L. D., Cohen, I. K., and Masters, F. W.: Hypertrophic scars and keloids. A collective review. Plast. Reconstr. Surg., 53:140, 1974.

Kiesselbach, W.: Versuch zur Anlegung eines ausseren Gehorgangesbei angeborener Missbildung bei der Ohrmuscheln mit fehlender ausserer Gehorgange. Arch. Ohrenh. Leipz., 19:127, 1882, cited in Jahrsdoerfer, R. A.: Congenital atresia of the ear. Laryngoscope, 88(Suppl. 13):1, 1978.

Kirkham, H. J. D.: The use of preserved cartilage in ear reconstruction. Ann. Surg., 11:896, 1940.

Knorr, N. J., Edgerton, M. T., and Barbarie, M.: Psychologic factors in the reconstruction of the ear. In Tanzer, R. C., and Edgerton, M. T. (Eds.): Symposium on Reconstruction of the Auricle. St. Louis, MO, C. V. Mosby Company, 1974, p. 187.

Königsmark, B. W.: Hereditary deafness in man. N. Engl. J. Med., 281:713, 1969.

Letterman, G. S., and Harding, R. L.: The management of the hairline in ear reconstruction. Plast. Reconstr. Surg., 18:199, 1956.

Lewis, J. S.: Cancer of the ear. Laryngoscope, 70:551, 1960.

Lloyd, L. L., and Cox, B. P.: Symposium on sensorineural hearing loss in children: early detection and intervention. Behavioral audiometry with children. Otolaryngol. Clin. North Am., 8:89, 1975.

Longacre, J. J., de Stefano, G. A., and Holmstrand, K. E.: The surgical management of first and second branchial arch syndromes. Plast. Reconstr. Surg., 31:507, 1963.

Longenecker, C. G., Ryan, R. F., and Vincent, R. W.: Malformations of the ear as a clue to urogenital anomalies: report of six additional cases. Plast. Reconstr. Surg., 35:303, 1965.

Luckett, W. H.: A new operation for prominent ears based on the anatomy of the deformity. Surg. Gynecol. Obstet., 10:635, 1910.

Lynch, J. B., Pousti, A., Doyle, J., and Lewis, S.: Our experiences with Silastic ear implants. Plast. Reconstr. Surg., 49:283, 1972.

Matsumoto, K.: The characteristics of cryptotia and its therapy. Jpn. J. Plast. Reconstr. Surg., 20:563, 1977.

May, H.: Transverse facial clefts and their repair. Plast. Reconstr. Surg., 29:240, 1962.

McConnell, F., and Liff, S.: Symposium on sensorineural hearing loss in children: early detection and intervention. The rationale for early identification and intervention. Otolaryngol. Clin. North Am., 8:77, 1975.

McDowell, A. J.: Goals in otoplasty for protruding ears. Plast. Reconstr. Surg., 41:17, 1968.

McDowell, F.: Successful replantation of severed half of ear. Plast. Reconstr. Surg., 48:281, 1971.

McEvitt, W. G.: The problem of the protruding ear. Plast. Reconstr. Surg., 2:481, 1947.

McKenzie, J., and Craig, J.: Mandibulo-facial dysostosis (Treacher Collins syndrome). Arch. Dis. Child., 30:391, 1955.

Minkowitz, S., and Minkowitz, F.: Congenital aural sinuses. Surg. Gynecol. Obstet., 118:4, 1964.

Mladick, R. A., and Carraway, J. H.: Ear reattachment by modified pocket principle. Plast. Reconstr. Surg., 51:584, 1973.

Mladick, R. A., Horton, C. E., Adamson, J. E., and Carraway, J. H.: The core resection for malignant tumors of the auricular area and subjacent bones. Plast. Reconstr. Surg., 53:281, 1974.

Mladick, R. A., Horton, C. E., Adamson, J. E., and Cohen, B. I.: Pocket principle: a new technique for reattachment of a severed ear part. Plast. Reconstr. Surg., 48:219, 1971.

Morestin, H.: De la reposition et du plissement cosmétiques du pavillon de l'oreille. Rev. Orthop., 14:289, 1903.

Musgrave, R. H.: A variation on the correction of the congenital lop ear. Plast. Reconstr. Surg., 37:394, 1966.

Musgrave, R. H., and Garrett, W. S.: Management of avulsion injuries of the external ear. Plast. Reconstr. Surg., 40:534, 1967.

Mustardé, J. C.: The correction of prominent ears using simple mattress sutures. Br. J. Plast. Surg., 16:170, 1963.

Mustardé, J. C.: The treatment of prominent ears by buried mattress sutures: a ten-year survey. Plast. Reconstr. Surg., 39:382, 1967.

Mutimer, K., Banis, J. C., and Upton, J.: Microsurgical reattachment of totally amputated ears. Plast. Reconstr. Surg., 79:535, 1987.

Nagel, F.: Reconstruction of a partial auricular loss. Plast. Reconstr. Surg., 49:340, 1972.

Nauton, R., and Valvassori, G.: Inner ear anomalies: their association with atresia. Laryngoscope, 78:1041, 1968.

Navabi, A.: One-stage reconstruction of partial defect of the auricle. Plast. Reconstr. Surg., 33:77, 1964.

Nélaton, C., and Ombrédanne, L.: Les Autoplasties. Paris, G. Steinheil, 1907.

Ogino, Y., and Yoshikawa, Y.: Plastic surgery for the congenital anomaly of the ear. Keisei Geka, 6:79, 1963.

Ohmori, S., and Matsumoto, K.: Treatment of cryptotia, using Teflon string. Plast. Reconstr. Surg., 49:33, 1972.

Owens, N., and Delgado, D. D.: The management of outstanding ears. South. Med. J., 58:32, 1955.

Paletta, F., Ship, A., and Van Norman, R.: Double spring release in otoplasty for prominent ears. Am. J. Surg., 106:506, 1963.

Pardue, A. M.: Repair of torn earlobe with preservation of the perforation for an earring. Plast. Reconstr. Surg., 51:472, 1973.

Parsons, H., and Lewis, J. S.: Subtotal resection of the temporal bone for cancer of the ear. Cancer, 7:995, 1954.

Peer, L. A.: Reconstruction of the auricle with diced cartilage grafts in a Vitallium ear mold. Plast. Reconstr. Surg., 3:653, 1948.

Pegram, M., and Peterson, R.: Repair of partial defects of the ear. Plast. Reconstr. Surg., 18:305, 1956.

Pennington, D. G., Lai, M. F., and Pelly, A. D.: Successful replantation of a completely avulsed ear by microvascular anastomosis. Plast. Reconstr. Surg., 65:820, 1980.

Pierce, G. W.: Reconstruction of the external ear. Surg. Gynecol. Obstet., 50:601, 1930.

Pierce, G. W., Klabunde, E. H., and Brobst, H. T.: Further observations on reconstruction of the external ear. Plast. Reconstr. Surg., 10:395, 1952.

Pollack, D.: Educational Audiology for the Limited Hearing Infant. Springfield, IL, Charles C Thomas, 1979, pp. 68–88.

Potter, E. L.: A hereditary ear malformation transmitted through five generations. J. Heredity, 28:255, 1937.

Preaux, J.: Un procédé simple de reconstruction de la partie inférieure du pavillon de l'oreille. Ann. Chir. Plast., 16:60, 1971.

Ramakrishnan, K. M., Thomas, K. P., and Sundararajan, C. R.: Study of 1,000 patients with keloids in South India. Plast. Reconstr. Surg., 53:276, 1974.

Reisner, K.: Tomography in inner and middle ear malformations: value, limits, results. Radiology, 92:11, 1969.

Rogers, B.: Berry-Treacher Collins syndrome: a review of 200 cases. Br. J. Plast. Surg., 17:109, 1964.

Rogers, B.: Microtia, lop, cup and protruding ears: four directly inherited deformities? Plast. Reconstr. Surg., 41:208, 1968.

Schuknecht, H. F.: Pathology of the Ear. Cambridge, MA, Harvard University Press, 1974, p. 184.

Sexton, R. P.: Utilization of the amputated ear cartilage. Plast. Reconstr. Surg., 15:419, 1955.

Snyder, G. B.: Button compression for keloids of the lobule. Br. J. Plast. Surg., 27:186, 1974.

Spira, M., McCrea, R., Gerow, F. J., and Hardy, S. B.: Analysis and treatment of the protruding ear. Trans. Fourth Internatl. Congr. Plast. Surg. Amsterdam, Excerpta Medica, 1969, p. 1090.

Stark, R. B., and Saunders, D. E.: Natural appearance restored to the unduly prominent ear. Br. J. Plast. Surg., 15:385, 1962.

Steffanoff, D. N.: Auriculo-mastoid tube pedicle for otoplasty. Plast. Reconstr. Surg., 3:352, 1948.

Steffensen, W. H.: Method of correcting atresia of ear canal. Plast. Reconstr. Surg., 1:329, 1946.

Steffensen, W. H.: Comments on total reconstruction of the external ear. Plast. Reconstr. Surg., 10:186, 1952.

Steffensen, W. H.: Comments on reconstruction of the external ear. Plast. Reconstr. Surg., 16:194, 1955.

Stenström, S. J.: A "natural" technique for correction of congenitally prominent ears. Plast. Reconstr. Surg., 32:509, 1963.

Straith, R. E.: Correction of the protruding ear. Plast. Reconstr. Surg., 24:277, 1959.

Streeter, G. L.: Development of the auricle in the human embryo. Carnegie Contrib. Embryol., 14:111, 1922.

Suraci, A. J.: Plastic reconstruction of acquired defects of the ear. Am. J. Surg., 66:196, 1944.

Tagliacozzi, G.: De Curtorum Chirurgia per Insitionem. Venice, Gaspare Bindoni, 1597.

Takahashi, H., and Maeda, K.: Survey of familial occurrence in 171 microtia cases. Jpn. J. Plast. Surg., 15:310, 1982.

Tanzer, R. C.: Total reconstruction of the external ear. Plast. Reconstr. Surg., 23:1, 1959.

Tanzer, R. C.: The correction of prominent ears. Plast. Reconstr. Surg., 30:236, 1962.

Tanzer, R. C.: An analysis of ear reconstruction. Plast. Reconstr. Surg., 31:16, 1963.

Tanzer, R. C.: Total reconstruction of the auricle. The evolution of a plan of treatment. Plast. Reconstr. Surg., 47:523, 1971.

Tanzer, R. C.: Correction of microtia with autogenous costal cartilage. In Tanzer, R. C., and Edgerton, M. T. (Eds.): Symposium on Reconstruction of the Auricle. St. Louis, MO, C. V. Mosby Company, 1974a, p. 47.

Tanzer, R. C.: Secondary reconstruction of the auricle. In Tanzer, R. C., and Edgerton, M. T. (Eds.): Symposium on Reconstruction of the Auricle. St. Louis, MO, C. V. Mosby Company, 1974b, p. 238.

Tanzer, R. C.: The constricted (cup and lop) ear. Plast. Reconstr. Surg., 55:406, 1975.

Tanzer, R. C.: Microtia. Clin. Plast. Surg., 5:317, 1978.

Taylor, W. C.: Deformity of ears and kidneys. Can. Med. Assoc. J., 93:107, 1965.

Torikai, T.: Anatomy of the auricular muscles and its application to surgical treatment of cryptotia. Jpn. J. Plast. Reconstr. Surg., 25:46, 1982.

Turski, P., Norman, D., DeGroot, J., and Capra, R.: High-resolution CT of the petrous bone: direct vs reformatted images. A.J.N.R., 3:391, 1982.

Washio, H.: Cryptotia—pathology and repair. Plast. Reconstr. Surg., 52:648, 1973.

Webster, G. V.: The tail of the helix as a key to otoplasty. Plast. Reconstr. Surg., 44:455, 1969.

Wildervanck, L. S.: Hereditary malformations of the ear in three generations: marginal pits, preauricular appendages, malformations of the auricle and conductive deafness. Acta Otolaryngol., 54:553, 1962.

Zenteno Alanis, S.: A new method for earlobe reconstruction. Plast. Reconstr. Surg., 45:254, 1970.

41

Joel J. Feldman

Facial Burns

Burn-related deaths and injuries constitute one of the main public health problems in the United States (see also Chap. 23). In 1980, it was estimated that 8111 persons died of thermal injury (fire, hot substances, corrosives, steam, and electrical current). In the same year, it was estimated that 60,900 persons were admitted to hospitals for thermal injury (Frank and associates, 1987). The groups most vulnerable to burn injury are the very young, the elderly, and the physically handicapped. Certain types of work also provide an increased risk of injury due to burns. In the adult population, predisposing causes are responsible for most burns (Maisels and Ghost, 1968; MacLeod, 1970; MacArthur and Moore, 1975). Alcoholism, epilepsy, chronic neurologic and psychiatric diseases, and drug dependency have also been found to be major risk factors (Papp, 1984).

Although the causes of burn injury are numerous, certain patterns appear in nearly every epidemiologic study. Flame burns involving clothing ignition are especially apparent in the data. Feller (1977) reported a series of 4596 cases, 3946 of which involved clothing ignition, as opposed to 650 cases in which clothing was not ignited. The severity and extent of the injury involving clothing ignition was dramatic. The mortality rate for victims whose clothing ignited was four times higher than that of patients whose clothing was not ignited, the area of total burn was nearly 100 per cent greater, the percentage of full-thickness injury was six times greater, and the number of days of hospitalization was 60 per cent greater. Most of the accidents occurred in the home; the common ignitors were open-space heaters, kitchen ranges, and matches. Among elderly victims, the ingestion of alcohol or prescriptive medications is often a causative factor.

Flammable liquids are another frequent cause of burn injury in the United States. Both young and adult males are inclined to use gasoline for cleaning items such as paintbrushes, automobile parts, and bicycle parts. In many cases the gasoline vapors are ignited by the pilot light of a hot water heater or a spark from a metal object. These injuries are generally quite severe and often involve the face.

Industrial burn accidents often involve acid, chemicals, or molten metals, and facial burns are common in this type of accident. The intense heat of a flash burn may injure only the exposed parts of the body, most often the hands and face. Ordinary clothing often provides surprisingly effective protection in flash burn situations.

In many automobile accidents, the gas tank ruptures and the fuel may explode. Facial and hand burns almost invariably result. Pontén (1968) studied burn injuries in 94 automobile accidents and showed that the incidence and severity were greater when the fuel tank was in the front than when it was at the rear of the vehicle.

Facial burns represent between one-fourth and one-third of all burns (Roper-Hall, 1962; Skoog, 1963; Tubiana, 1967a,b). In a review of a large burn unit, Dowling, Foley, and Moncrief (1968) reported that almost 60 per cent of all patients admitted had facial burns. Among young children with burns, scald injuries from hot substances and flame injury from playing with matches are common.

The severity of injury and deformity from facial burns ranges from relatively minor to severe. However, even relatively minor facial disfigurement can have a severe psychologic and social impact on the victim. The basic concerns are for function, comfort, and appearance. From the standpoint of priorities, function is always the most important. Eyelid function is important for the protection of the cornea; function of the lips and mouth is important for eating, speaking, dental hygiene, and the retention of oral fluids; and patent nasal passages are functionally important for comfortable breathing. A mobile neck is important for proper eating, speaking, seeing, and general posture. Facial scarring affects comfort by distorting facial features, limiting the mobility of facial parts and imposing a tight and restrictive sensation. Alteration in facial appearance is caused by the change in color and texture of injured skin, hypertrophic scarring, scar contractures that distort the position of facial features, and the actual loss of the facial parts due either to the thermal injury or to secondary infection and trauma. Scarring not only alters facial expression but also limits it. In cases of facial burn injury, the role of the plastic surgeon is to minimize the final deformity as much as possible.

ACUTE MANAGEMENT OF FACIAL BURNS

Although this chapter is devoted primarily to the late treatment and secondary recon-struction of facial burn deformities, the time to begin thinking of reconstruction is immediately after the burn has taken place. If the surgeon managing the acute injury will not be primarily responsible for the later reconstruction, it is preferable for the reconstructive surgeon to be consulted early on, allowing the needs of reconstruction to enter into the strategic planning of the acute care. The decisions made and the actions taken in the early period may significantly affect the process of later facial repair. For example, the early application of neck splints can help to avoid debilitating neck contractures. Splinting and stretching of the oral commissure may afford some control over oral stenosis. Proper eye care and careful observation can prevent corneal injury from exposure; proper head positioning and timely intervention may prevent destructive chondritis of the ears. If at all possible, the donor sites used for the resurfacing of areas of the body other than the face should be thoughtfully rationed, preserving the best color and texture matched skin for eventual use on the face. It should be remembered that for the patient who survives the burn injury, the long-term quality of life will be determined in large part by the degree of residual facial deformity after reconstruction. The overall quality of the reconstruction in turn is largely dependent on the quality and quantity of unaltered skin in the neck, chest, and shoulder regions, spared not only by the burn injury itself but also by the harvesting of skin grafts by the acute care surgeon.

Most surgeons have historically considered the face "off limits" for excision and grafting in the early postburn period, thus showing a reluctance based on several factors: (1) the frequent difficulty encountered in evaluating the depth of a facial burn injury, (2) the unique value that has been placed on preserving every millimeter of viable facial skin, and (3) the disappointing results obtained in the past with early primary excision (down to fat) and coverage with thin split-thickness skin grafts. However, more recent reports by Engrav and associates (1986) and Heimbach and Engrav (1984) have demonstrated encouraging results with early sequential excision and grafting of facial burns in selected patients. These authors believe that for deep second and third degree facial burns, the approach of allowing spontaneous separation of the eschar followed by delayed grafting on granulation tissue often leads to significant functional and cosmetic abnormality, necessitating major secondary facial reconstruction.

Engrav and associates (1986) debrided the face of loose blisters on admission and carried out twice daily hydrotherapy with debridement thereafter. Topical antibacterial agents were also applied. Some areas of the face that showed superficial burn injury were covered with porcine xenografts. During the period between admission and the tenth day after the burn, large body surfaces and hand lesions were treated. On the tenth day after injury, an evaluation was made of whether the facial burn wounds would be healed later than three weeks following injury. If it was thought that the face would not be healed by three weeks, plans were made for excision and grafting to take place no later than 14 days after injury.

For the excision, the Goulian dermatome was used with a 0.008-inch guard. Excision was carried deep enough for normal tissue to be visualized. If superficial areas of burn were excised as part of the area being grafted, it was found to be important to excise them deeply enough to prevent the wound from reepithelizing and healing underneath the new skin graft, which would result in an area of graft loss. As far as was practical, the face was excised and grafted according to regional esthetic units (see Esthetic Considerations below).

Burns on the ears were debrided conservatively but not excised at this time. Deeply burned areas on the eyelids were excised. Unhealed burns on the anterior and lateral neck were also excised as a final unit if the patient's condition permitted. At the completion of the facial and neck excision, bleeding not controlled by epinephrine-soaked pads was managed by needlepoint electrocauterization. Burned tissue excised from the neck was usually grafted at this time; however, because of the cosmetic importance of an excellent graft take on the face, grafting of the face was delayed for 24 to 48 hours to be certain of hemostasis. During this period, the excised facial wound was covered with allograft as an occlusive biologic dressing. The patient was returned to the operating room, usually 48 hours later, at which time a negative Duplicast impression was made over the biologic dressing to conform exactly to the patient's face. A pressure device of elastomer was then constructed from this mold to be applied over the autografts at the end of the procedure. Engrav and associates (1986) preferred to use thick split-thickness skin grafts (0.018 to 0.025 inches) harvested from the scalp (Berkowitz, 1981), neck, or infraclavicular area (Edgerton and Hansen, 1960) if the intention was to obtain a satisfactory color match with the healed or unburned areas on the face. If the entire face is to be grafted, color match with the unburned areas becomes irrelevant. Thick grafts are important in order to achieve a satisfactory appearance and to minimize contraction. Splinting and pressure devices were applied over the grafts in the operating room. Postoperatively, the devices were removed twice a day, the grafts inspected, and any hematomas removed through small incisions placed in the relaxed skin-tension lines. Patients were fed parenterally or via tubes for three days and asked to refrain from talking. Pressure garments were worn until the wound matured.

Although early tangential excision and the application of thick split-thickness skin grafts can produce gratifying results in selected patients with deep facial burns, Feldman (1986) pointed out that the use of the neck and upper chest as skin graft donor sites for the face may be imprudent, even though grafts from these locations provide a more reliable color match with unburned area on the face. Feldman believed that the neck and upper chest, if unburned, should be left undisturbed during the acute burn period so that they can be used for local or regional flap resurfacing of the face later on; he considered that flap resurfacing of the partially scarred or unilateral scarred face often provided a more normal long-term appearance than even the very best skin grafted face. In any event, there is little if anything to be gained by acutely excising and resurfacing a face with *thin* skin grafts, except the attainment of a closed wound. Thin skin grafts do not prevent contractures from developing, and their ultimate quality (texture and color) is so poor that eventual replacement is almost certain. For most patients with facial burns, it is usually best to aim initially for a healed, closed wound, trying to minimize along the way deformities and contractures, yet anticipating that secondary correction will be required.

PATIENT-SURGEON RELATIONSHIP

Patients who have suffered the physical and psychologic pain of burn injury and disfigurement are in need of a special level of caring from their surgeon. They need not only technical expertise, but also a great deal of the surgeon's time, understanding, and compassion. Facial burn reconstruction usually requires multiple operations over a period of months or years. To move patients through the process of repair requires mutual trust and respect among patients, their families, and the surgeon (Meyer and Knorr, 1977; Macgregor, 1977). An optimistic attitude on the part of the surgeon is crucial to patients' physical and emotional rehabilitation, but optimism must be tempered with realism. Early in the reconstructive process, the surgeon must discuss sensitively but candidly with patients and families not only what can be done, but what cannot be done. It is a prevalent misconception that scars can somehow be erased completely and that a burned face can eventually be returned to normal. While normalcy is the goal, it can never be entirely achieved. For both the patient and the surgeon, realistic expectations are important to the "success" of reconstruction.

The psychologic and social recovery of patients who have suffered facial burns depends on a number of factors: the age and sex of the individual; the size, visibility, and severity of the facial disfigurement; the degree of social support patients receive from relatives and friends; the preaccident personality characteristics; and the degree to which patients believe that they still have opportunities to achieve satisfaction and happiness in life. The separate and combined effects of these factors are different for each patient. However, studies have shown that the rate of psychologic and social recovery depends largely on the extent of cosmetic facial disfigurement. For this reason, the goal of reconstruction should be to restore a normal appearance, and whenever possible to introduce elements of facial beauty.

TIMING THE RECONSTRUCTION

The timing of reconstruction is dependent on a number of factors: physiologic, psychoemotional, and socioeconomic and the condition of the facial scarring as it affects function, comfort, and appearance. The physical health of the patient must be carefully assessed, especially if only a short time has elapsed since the initial burn injury. The psychologic condition of the patient must be considered, including mood (particularly depression or suicidal ideation); the level of cooperativeness; the degree of enthusiasm for or against reconstruction; the level of emotional support (or lack of it) provided by family, friends, and health workers; and the possibility of an ongoing drug dependency.

In many patients, contractures and deformity elsewhere on the body have to be dealt with first for reasons of function and comfort. In terms of the face, scarring that causes contractures of the eyelids, lips, corners of the mouth, and neck may require early intervention. Scars causing little or no contracture can be left longer.

It has been written that definitive correction of facial burn scarring should be delayed for one year or longer after healing of the acute wound—the so-called "waiting period"—until the scars and initial skin grafts have matured. In general, this is a sound principle, since contracture release or facial resurfacing that takes place within an area that is still contracting will undoubtedly yield results that are compromised by some degree of recontracture. Furthermore, the combination of sufficient time (perhaps years), external pressure (splints and elasticized masks), and local steroids will improve many non–contracture-producing scars to a point at which the patient's ultimate appearance is better without having had surgery than would have been achieved by a hasty resurfacing.

This is particularly true of some localized nodules of hypertrophic scar on the upper and lower lips, and patches of scar in the submental region of the neck—scars that are initially raised and red, but cause no significant distortion of adjacent structures. Left alone for several years, the scars often fade and flatten dramatically, leaving an area of skin that has attained a color and texture only slightly different from that of normal skin and certainly better looking than a skin graft patch. Moreover, the naturally "feathered" edges of the burn scar may become less noticeable than the line of a surgical excision scar. If these non–contracture-producing islands of scar do not achieve a desirable level of inconspicuousness, they can be removed completely later on or, after they have matured and become soft and pliable, they can often be improved by partial excision, edge revision, and Z-plasty to relieve residual tightness and contour irregularities. On the other hand, when it is apparent that an area of facial scarring will eventually need to be removed or replaced regardless of the degree of improvement that may take place over time, there is nothing to be gained by allowing the scar to mature if the scar in its entirety is to be discarded later on. This principle applies particularly to scars on the cheeks. Knowing which scars to remove, when to remove them, which scars to leave, and for how long constitutes judgments made on the basis of wisdom gained through experience.

DEVELOPMENT OF A MASTER PLAN

The ultimate quality of a facial reconstruction is only as good as the quality of the initial plan. No matter how well the surgery is performed technically, if the plan is flawed, the result will be flawed; if the plan is excellent—esthetically designed and thoughtfully coordinated—the result has a chance for excellence. A long-range reconstructive strategy should be outlined early in the repair process, especially when dealing with the severe facial burn. The process begins with an unhurried and thorough physical examination, and a leisurely conversation with the patient and family. First impressions are important, in terms both of how the surgeon sees the patient physically and emotionally, and of how the patient "sees" the surgeon. The surgeon should obtain a sense of the patient's priorities, wishes, and expectations, along with an estimate of the time, inconvenience, discomfort, and secondary donor site deformity that the patient is able to accept in the reconstruction. At the time of the initial consultation, excellent quality color photographs should be taken of the patient, including frontal, oblique, and profile views of the head and neck as well as multiple close-up views from different angles of all facial features. Photographs of the chest, trunk, back, and extremities should also be taken to allow the surgeon to remember the availability of various donor sites. The surgeon may formulate in his own mind an approach to the reconstruction of the face, but it is usually best not to go into specific details of the plan for reconstruction with the patient at the time of the initial consultation unless the repair is relatively simple and straightforward. For more complex, multistaged reconstructions, the surgeon should spend time quietly studying the photographs of the patient before arriving at the overall plan for repair. An unhurried, contemplative study of photographs often reveals aspects and nuances of the facial deformity that were unappreciated when the patient was examined in person. In this way, the surgeon sees the overall reconstruction as composed of related and integrated parts: priorities can be ordered, donor sites rationed, complementary procedures combined (e.g., using otherwise discarded tissues to rebuild an adjacent part), and anesthetic opportunities used to the best advantage (e.g., carrying out a flap delay at the time that an unrelated facial area is being worked on). The plan should be put in writing, describing what is to be accomplished at the first operation, at the second, at the third, and so on. The interval between procedures should be determined, and a timetable established for accomplishment of the major components of the reconstruction. The plan must be flexible, since in practice the surgeon must often wait to see the result of one procedure before going on to the next. Before finalizing the initial plan, it is usually best to reexamine the patient at least a second time (since tissues look and feel differently "in the flesh" than they do in photographs), and because the patient's reaction may in itself make the surgeon modify the plan. While the emotional, social, and economic implications of reconstruction should always be considered, the most important factor in choosing between alternative methods of repair is which tactic promises the best result in the long run. The notion that a less complex, albeit less appropriate, procedure saves the patient several operations and reduces time away from school, work, and family can be inaccurate. What appears at first to be a less involved approach frequently produces less than satisfactory long-term results, necessitating multiple unplanned revisions and "touch-up" operations. In time, the simpler methods can end up costing the patient more time and inconvenience than a seemingly more complicated but better designed surgical approach.

ESTHETIC CONSIDERATIONS

The word "esthetic" means "pertaining to a sensitivity to art and beauty." In facial reconstruction, it is a concern for the outline, form, and proportion of facial features; skin color and texture; symmetry; scar positioning; and facial expressivity. The surgeon's esthetic sensibility directly affects how he sees the patient's deformity, how he envisions the final result, and how he designs the operative procedures. Esthetics are involved at every level of presurgical decision making. A basic set of esthetic values should be appreciated when deliberating every case, regardless of the specific conditions.

In the planning of any reconstructive procedure, the functional considerations (vision, opening and closing the mouth, neck mobility, and so forth) take precedence over appearance. However, in the cervicofacial region, the esthetic goals and functional imperatives are, for the most part, inseparable; the disabilities are usually manifest as visible abnormalities. Therefore, it should be understood that, although the focus is on appearance, there is a prevailing (albeit sometimes unwritten) concern for facial function.

The two basic esthetic elements that determine facial appearance are the quality of the facial contours and the quality of the facial skin cover. In terms of restoring a normal appearance to the face after injury, it is probably more important to restore normal facial contour and form than it is to restore a completely normal facial skin cover. Often, the burn injury has produced deformity both of facial contours and of facial cover. The facial features should be rebuilt and reshaped before resurfacing is carried out. In other words, "the restoration should be designed from within outward" (Gillies and Millard, 1957).

Facial Contours

Restoration of facial form means not only restoring normal shape to the facial parts, but also returning them to normal position. Contractures, both major and minor, should be corrected, releasing, relocating, and realigning displaced eyelids, lips, nasal alae, chins, cheeks, and necks. Missing parts need to be rebuilt and contours defined.

In planning the repair, the practiced eye of the surgeon is the best judge of facial architecture, but a helpful exercise is to project the patient's facial photographs onto a screen over which film or tracing paper is applied so that the surgeon can draw out the needed repositioning and reshaping of any deformed facial feature. Reshaping often involves augmenting deficient parts, reducing or excavating other parts, or a combination of both. This type of planning using overlays on photographs is extremely valuable.

In planning the correction of contour deformities, the aim should be not only to reestablish normal form but also to achieve, if possible, a beautiful normal appearance (Millard, 1986). This means that procedures used in cosmetic (esthetic) surgery can and often should be incorporated as part of the reconstructive procedure. For example, neck lipectomy and platysma tightening and contouring procedures can be applied to give a most attractive cervicomandibular contour; alloplastic implants can be used for chin augmentation; cosmetic reduction and augmentation rhinoplasty techniques can be applied to the reconstruction of the nose; and cosmetic blepharoplasty methods can be used to improve the appearance around the eyes. Since the initially burned patient is always somewhat disfigured, any elements of beauty that can be added to the face are desirable.

Form and contour refer to the three-dimensional aspects of the facial features: not only the shape of a feature but the highlights and shadows that result. Contour abnormalities may be either quite apparent (e.g., clearly inadequate projection of the nasal tip or chin) or quite subtle (e.g., the presence or absence of a well-defined upper lip philtrum dimple or the concave sulcus at the junction of the lower lip and chin). It should be remembered that even with the most normal-appearing facial skin cover, the face will never look good if the facial contours are inadequate.

Facial Skin Cover

A scar, by definition, is a permanent mark. For every scar, there are two possible "ideal" fates: either the new scar will mature and fade with time, leaving only an inconspicuous mark that blends unobtrusively with its surroundings, or the area of scarring can be completely excised surgically, leaving only a faint line hidden along a natural skin crease. For some scars, one or the other of these ideal outcomes is attainable. However, in reality many scars need more than just time; because of their size or location, they cannot be simply removed but need to be replaced. In regard to both removal and replacement of facial scarring (see Cheek Resurfacing below), there are elements of surface esthetics to be considered.

Homogeneity

Skin color and surface texture should be uniform within any region of the face, and preferably over the entire face as a whole. Added skin grafts or skin flaps that do not have the same color and texture as the surrounding skin give a patched appearance. Generally, well-matched skin grafts should be added only to a face that will remain permanently graft covered. Well-matched skin flaps should be added to a face that is either flap covered or unscarred. Even a very well matched skin graft will never look completely normal if bordered by normal skin (except perhaps in the upper eyelid). A "skin patch" on the face should be avoided at almost any cost.

Symmetry

Since the face is two-sided and since facial asymmetry is always inherently visually disturbing, what is done to one side of the face should be done to the other side. If only one side of the face is scarred, the aim of reconstruction should be to replace the scarred side with skin that matches as closely as possible the uninjured side. This is usually best done with a skin flap taken from an adjacent area, if available. If both sides of the face are extensively scarred, either a completely skin grafted face or a completely skin flapped face should be the final result of bilateral cheek resurfacing. Edge scars should also be replaced in symmetric positions. If there is visual balance of color, texture, and scar placement, less important visual abnormalities can be overlooked.

Regional Esthetic Units

The face can be envisioned as composed of a number of neighboring geographic territories limited by natural lines, folds, and changes in skin texture, as well as the hairline (Fig. 41–1) (Gonzalez-Ulloa and associates, 1954; Gonzalez-Ulloa, 1956; Stark, 1982). A skin graft or skin flap applied to the face should, if possible, cover an entire esthetic unit, not just part of the unit. In this way, a patched appearance is less apparent, because skin of uniform color and texture covers a complete natural region of the face, and the edge scars are relatively concealed along the boundaries of each region. To cover a complete unit, normal skin may occasionally be sacrificed (Aufricht, 1944). If the facial area to be resurfaced extends into more than one esthetic territory, the involved units should be combined into a single large, composite unit, allowing the largest possible skin graft or flap to be used. This maneuver minimizes the number of seams and gives a more homogeneous appearance to the face. A principle emphasized by Millard (1986) is relevant: "Do not cut a flap or graft to fit a random defect. Make the defect fit the natural aesthetic unit and then fit the flap or graft to that unit!" Although the concept of resurfacing the face according to regional esthetic units should be applied when regional resurfacing of the face is done, there are exceptions to this rule. One exception is when an area of scarring on the cheek is replaced with an adjacent or regional skin flap. In this situation, an available flap may be sufficiently large to replace the entire area of cheek scarring but may not be large enough to cover the entire regional esthetic unit of the cheek. In this situation, it would be acceptable to have the flap edge scar run across the cheek in a less than ideal position in order to obtain surface color and texture homogeneity. Another exception to the rule is when an entire face needs resurfacing. In this regard, the entire face and anterior neck (as seen in most clothing) should be considered a single esthetic unit of uniform color and texture rather than an assemblage of smaller regional subunits. Ideally, total facial resurfacing should be done with a single sheet of skin (either flap or graft). In this way, facial skin homogeneity and symmetry are ensured and visi-

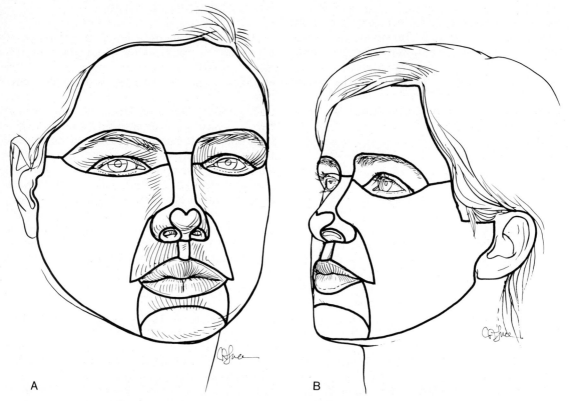

Figure 41–1. Esthetic units of the face. *A,* Frontal view. *B,* Lateral view.

ble seams are minimized. Unfortunately, this type of single sheet total facial resurfacing is rarely possible or practical.

REPAIRING SPECIFIC AREAS

Cheek Resurfacing

Resurfacing entails either scar removal or scar replacement. *Scar removal* involves total scar excision followed by bringing together the unscarred neighboring skin along a linear or curvilinear seam. Scar removal can be a simple procedure if the scar is relatively small in size and located at a distance from mobile structures such as the lips or eyelids. The removal of large cheek scars is often complex, requiring the transposition of large adjacent cheek, cheek-neck, or neck-chest skin flaps. Scar removal and resurfacing with neighboring flaps should be designed so that, with rare exceptions, the flap donor site is closed primarily without a skin graft. Transposition of a neck flap to the cheek in a way that requires skin grafting the neck donor site should be avoided. If, because of size or

location, the cheek scar cannot be completely removed in one procedure, either a staged excision and sequential flap advancement or a skin expansion should be performed—both methods allowing closure of the flap donor site without a skin graft (see below).

Scar replacement involves a substitution: resurfacing all or part of the cheek with either a new skin graft or a skin flap brought to the cheek from a distance (i.e., *not* a neighboring flap). For subtotal facial resurfacing, scar removal is always preferable to scar replacement, since local flap repair imparts a normal or near-normal skin color and texture to the face; replacement tissue (distant flaps or skin grafts) usually matches poorly the unscarred areas on the face. (An exception is an upper eyelid skin graft or retroauricular skin graft to the lower eyelid.) Smith (1944, 1946, 1950) emphasized the importance of using tissue from the vicinity whenever possible for repair. Local skin flaps, Z-plasties (often used to reposition scar in a more favorable location for subsequent removal), and "multiple excision" (removal of scarred areas in stages) were regarded by Smith as the "procedures of choice," whereas skin grafts and distant flaps were termed "procedures of necessity," to be used only when neighboring skin flaps were unavailable, or used simply as temporary wound cover, to be removed subsequently. The author agrees entirely with Smith's point of view.

ESTHETIC CONSIDERATIONS OF CHEEK RESURFACING

The goal in the treatment of cheek scars from burns is the same as that for scars resulting from any other cause: to restore normal function and to make the scarring as visually inconspicuous as possible. As for appearance, there are two basic objectives: *uniformity* and *normalcy*. Of the two, uniformity (i.e., homogeneity and symmetry) of surface color and texture has priority. Of course, the more normal the uniform cover, the better, but harmony overall is more important than trying to restore a normal cover to only one part or scattered parts of the face. The one exception to the rule of achieving complete uniformity of facial color and texture relates to the distribution of the beard in a male patient, since whiskered skin shows a different color and texture from that of nonwhiskered skin. However, the surgeon must always see the face as a whole, even when (and particularly when) only one side or a portion of one side is to be resurfaced. Therefore, if one cheek is scarred and the other is unscarred, the aim of cheek resurfacing should be to match the normal unscarred side as closely as possible. The best match will be achieved with neighboring cheek or neck skin flaps, if these are available. In this setting, any kind of skin graft resurfacing produces a less satisfactory result, even if the graft is taken from a color-matched area in the head and neck area. Even the most optimal full-thickness or thick split-thickness skin graft applied to a cheek will never mimic the normal cheek skin perfectly. For a unilateral cheek resurfacing when the contralateral cheek is unscarred, the best choice (esthetically) is nearly always a skin flap, and the closer the flap is located to the cheek, the better is the match. What McIndoe said in 1949 remains true today: "A severe burn limited to one side of the face can be treated most satisfactorily by a . . . flap designed to produce a half face in one piece." On the other hand, if the entire face is scarred and one or both cheeks need resurfacing, the surgeon must decide whether the final result is to be a skin grafted or a skin flapped face. If sufficient local or regional flap tissue is available to resurface the whole or most of the face, the author prefers a skin flapped face to a skin grafted face, since a softer texture is usually attainable with flaps. However, individual considerations always apply in making the choice, including the availability of unscarred donor site skin, concern for the secondary donor site deformity, the color and texture quality of the skin grafts used on the face in the past, and the patient's acceptance of alternative approaches.

REGIONAL ESTHETIC UNIT OF CHEEK

As illustrated in Figure 41–1, the esthetic unit of the cheek usually has a superior boundary along the junction between the lower eyelid and the cheek, with the line extending up to and just below the lateral canthus. The line extends slightly upward to join the temporal hairline in the lateral forehead region. The lateral boundary runs along the anterior temporal hairline and sideburn, heading in an inferior direction in the preauricular skin crease. A less noticeable scar is often obtained when the lateral scar is placed in a retrotragal position (as is commonly done in a face lift procedure) rather than in front of the ear. The cheek unit extends medially to the nasolabial crease, jogging into the corner of the mouth, and curving downward along a seam separating the lower lip and chin from the adjacent cheek. The cheek unit extends inferiorly to just below the jawline. In certain cases, it is preferable to enlarge the esthetic unit of the cheek to include the lower eyelid, the lateral segment of the upper lip, or both. For example, if the lower eyelid is scarred or has been previously skin grafted, resurfacing both the eyelid and the cheek with the same sheet of skin (either graft or flap) avoids both a color and texture discrepancy and a visible seam between the cheek and the lid. If an ectropion does result, a secondary eyelid release and skin addition can be done, with the eyelid no worse and perhaps better than it would have been if the one-piece cheek-eyelid cover had not been attempted. In most cases, however, it is not appropriate for several reasons to treat the lower eyelid as if it were part of the cheek. The resurfacing flap in a male patient can place hair-bearing skin in the normally hairless lower eyelid; the flap being used to cover the cheek simply cannot reach sufficiently high to cover the eyelid comfortably without tension; and recovering a normal unscarred lower eyelid can unnecessarily risk eyelid ectropion.

As for including the lateral aspect of the upper lip segment in the cheek unit, a small scar along the philtral crest of the upper lip dimple is usually less conspicuous than a scar seam along the nasolabial crease. Therefore, if the lateral upper lip subunit (see section on The Upper Lip below) needs to be resurfaced, and if the skin flap or graft available for cheek resurfacing is sufficiently large to include the lip, the lip might best be covered with the same sheet of skin as used on the cheek, bearing in mind that the two sides of the upper lip should match. Do not skin graft one side of the upper lip if the other side is covered with a flap, and vice versa. If the cheek needs resurfacing but the adjacent upper lip is unscarred, one should consider excising and resurfacing the lip along with the cheek only in female patients, never in males. In males, preserving the ability to grow a mustache is quite important; a medial cheek scar along the nasolabial crease is always preferable to giving up a whiskered upper lip. Figure 41–8 illustrates the enlarged cheek unit (cheek and lower eyelid and lateral upper lip) resurfaced with a one-piece flap transferred to the face from the shoulder on a tube pedicle.

When less than a complete cheek unit is scarred and small areas of normal skin are present within the unit, it is often best to discard the unscarred minority along with the scarred majority so that a one-piece, one-color, one-texture cheek results. This principle is particularly applicable when the cheek is being recovered with a skin graft. On the other hand, when a local or regional flap is being used to resurface an incompletely scarred cheek and there is only sufficient flap available to allow removal of the scarred area alone, it is preferable to accept a less than ideal seam line between the flap and the unscarred cheek skin than it is to choose a larger but less well matched skin graft or distant flap. In terms of esthetic priorities, making a satisfactory skin color and texture match is more important than placing a flap edge scar in an ideal position.

As noted in the discussion on Esthetic Considerations, a face (or face and anterior neck) is really seen by others as a single visual unit, not an assemblage of regional subunits. Thus, when an entire face needs to be resurfaced, it is best (at least theoretically) to resurface the entire face with a single piece of skin—be it flap or graft—to ensure that the skin color and texture are completely uniform throughout, and the edge scars inconspicuous. Figure 41–2 shows a patient who had the entire face and anterior neck (excluding the upper lip, nose, eyelids, and forehead) resurfaced with a large, single full-thickness skin graft. The overall result is satisfactory, although the skin graft did hyperpigment somewhat (it was taken from the lower abdomen and anterior thigh), and it repigmented a second time after an attempt was made to lighten the color by chemical peel. The author has successfully resurfaced the entire face with a single-sheet, full-thickness skin graft in four patients. The procedure is complex, with many potential pitfalls, and requires *extremely careful patient selection*. The caveats and technical details of the procedure have been previously described (Feldman, 1984, 1987a). It must be remembered that the large, full-thickness skin graft donor site must itself be covered with a split-thickness skin graft, and this secondary deformity should be appreciated. Although the objective results have been superior to the more traditional regional unit resurfacing with skin grafts, the surface color and texture of a full-thickness skin graft taken from the torso or extremities is never completely normal. The grafts require approximately two years to achieve their final softness and color. The skin either appears slightly hyperpigmented or displays the original donor site color of the chest or abdomen. In all four patients mentioned above there were some areas of hypopigmentation where epithelial loss had occurred.

A more normal surface texture can be achieved with a single-sheet, thin skin flap. Figure 41–3 illustrates a face resurfaced with a one-piece, wrap-around cervicopectoral flap (Feldman, 1984, 1987a). The skin color and texture of the flap are normal and match the remainder of the face almost perfectly. Facial expressiveness is also preserved with the thin flap. There are, however, negative aspects to the use of a large, random-pattern transposition flap of this type: the precarious nature of the flap's blood supply and the significant secondary skin graft deformity on the

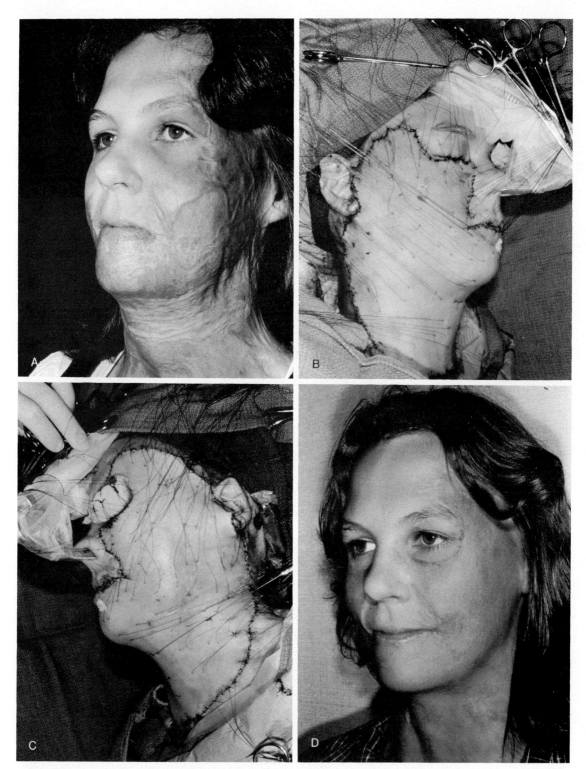

Figure 41–2. Single-sheet resurfacing of the complete face and neck "esthetic megaunit" with a large, full-thickness skin graft. *A,* Preoperative view. *B, C,* Harvest and application of the graft 24 hours after excision of the cervicofacial unit. *D,* Two years postoperatively. (From Feldman, J. J.: Reconstruction of the burned face in children. *In* Serafin, D., and Georgiade, N. G. (Eds.): Pediatric Plastic Surgery. St. Louis, C. V. Mosby Company, 1984.)

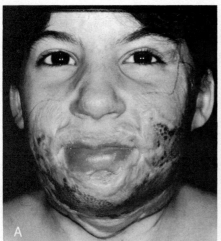

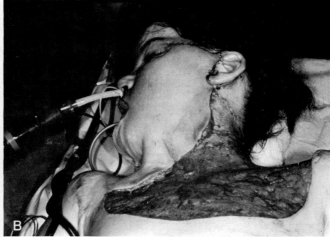

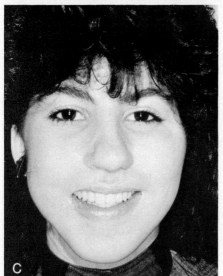

Figure 41–3. Single-sheet resurfacing of the face with a delayed random pattern, single-piece, wrap-around cervicopectoral flap. *A,* Preoperative view. *B,* Intraoperative view after flap transfer. *C,* Final result. Note how naturally the thin flap transmits the normal facial contours during animation. The skin grafted donor site on the anterior chest is concealed by clothing. (From Feldman, J. J.: Reconstruction of the burned face in children. *In* Serafin, D., and Georgiade, N. G. (Eds.): Pediatric Plastic Surgery. St. Louis, C. V. Mosby Company, 1984.)

chest—almost certainly an unacceptable price to pay in a female patient unless the chest and shoulders were already badly scarred. The patient illustrated in Figure 41–3 was treated before the development of skin expansion (see Chap. 13), which might have allowed a nearly comparable resurfacing without disfigurement of the donor area.

REMOVAL OF SMALL CHEEK SCARS

An island of scar or a skin graft patch surrounded by unscarred skin can be directly excised and the defect closed primarily without extensive mobilization of adjacent skin flaps, if a preoperative "pinch test" demonstrates that the skin beside the scar can be brought together by pinching with the surgeon's fingers. Bands of scar can be replaced with a narrower linear scar in this fashion. However, when doing the "pinch test," the surgeon should be certain that there is no resultant distortion of the mobile parts of the face, i.e., the lower eyelid or the corner of the mouth. It is also important that the skin edges after excision be brought together without excess tension, otherwise a widened scar results. The defect remaining after elliptic excision of round or square-shaped scars can often be closed along a line that runs in one of several directions. The direction chosen by the surgeon should avoid distortion of nearby facial features, and place the linear scar parallel to the relaxed skin tension lines of the face in that region (see Chap. 1). However, the shape and location of the scar to be removed often offer little or no choice as to the direction of wound closure, and the surgeon is forced to close the wound along a line that runs against the relaxed skin tension lines. In such a case, it is usually best simply to make a careful linear closure, and if subsequent scar contracture, tenting, or hypertrophy develops, one should consider a secondary surgical revision, i.e., Z-plasty or running W-plasty (Borges, 1973). Segments of scar hypertrophy may also benefit from the application of external pressure, steroid injections, or both.

REMOVAL OF MODERATE-SIZED CHEEK SCARS

If the cheek scar is excessively broad for simple excision and closure, but still occupies one-half to one-third or less of the cheek area, or presents as a band of scar along the jawline region, the scar can often be excised and the defect closed after an extensive undermining of the normal skin on both sides of the scar. The more extensive the undermining of the adjacent skin, the greater can be the stretch and advancement of the flaps, and the easier the closure. It is usually helpful to undermine the flaps beyond the nearest bony prominence in the face and neck area, to release the dermo-osseous and dermofascial connective tissue attachments that limit flap extension. This principle means that for scars to be removed from the middle and lower cheek, the skin superior to the scar should be undermined over the malar eminence as far as the lower eyelid and undermined inferiorly to a point below the mandible in the lower neck. For scars along the jawline, inferior skin flap undermining should extend to a location below the clavicle and suprasternal notch, creating a large flap that is untethered by bony and fascial attachments. An example of a broad band of jawline scar removed and closed after extensive superior and inferior undermining is shown in Figure 41–4.

To assess the risks of extensive skin undermining, an understanding of the blood supply of the skin is required. In simple terms, a random area of skin receives its blood supply from two sources: vertically from perpendicular musculocutaneous perforators, and horizontally (circumferentially) via the subdermal and subcutaneous vascular plexus. Broad areas of skin can survive on either one of the two sources; in general, both systems are not required. Therefore, an island of skin and fat cut circumferentially down to muscle survives completely, even though deprived of its horizontal source (e.g., an island musculocutaneous flap). Likewise, if the skin is extensively undermined (severing the perforators beneath the flap), it still survives if an adequate horizontal blood supply is maintained by avoiding overextensive circumscribing skin incisions; examples include the broad-based skin flap raised during a face lift operation, and the widely undermined flap developed for insertion of a large skin expander. In summary, safe mobilization of random-pattern skin flaps involves a compromise between dividing the vertical and horizontal blood supply. If an extensive skin undermining is performed, the incisions along the sides of the flap should be limited. If more flap transposition and less flap stretch is needed

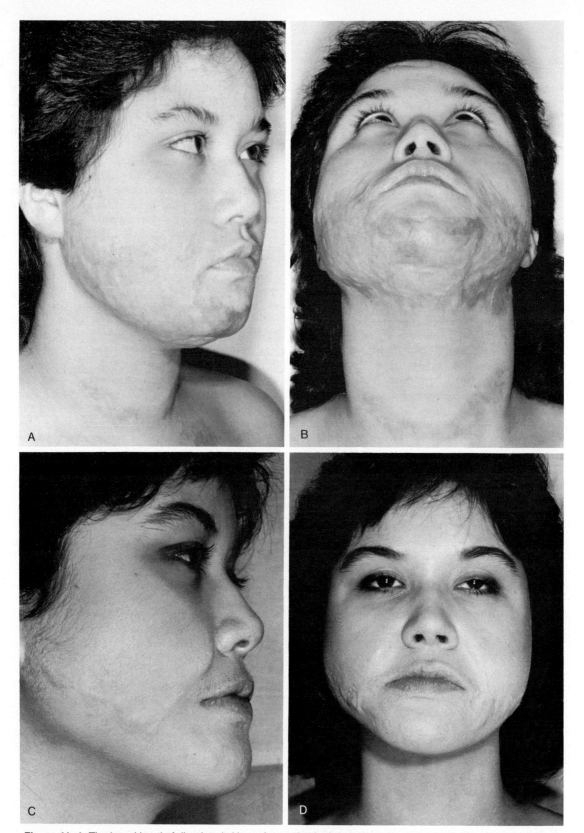

Figure 41–4. The broad band of discolored skin graft covering both lower cheeks and chin *(A, B)* was removed in one stage with direct closure after extensive inferior skin undermining below the clavicles onto the upper chest, superior skin undermining in the cheeks to the lower eyelids, and undermining beneath the unscarred skin in the upper chin. The ascending neck advancement flap and the descending cheek and chin advancement flaps were then joined *(C, D)*.

(requiring incisions that cut across the horizontal blood supply), undermining should be limited.

Moderate-sized scars too large to be removed in one stage can often be removed in two (or more) procedures without the need for skin expanders (see below). In 1915 Morestin described in detail his "gradual reduction method" of progressive stretching of the skin to make up for the deficiency remaining after a "more or less long series of small partial operations." Morestin did not undermine the adjacent skin margins. Each of his excisions was small and closure was "simple." In some cases, the procedures were carried out as often as every three or four days. Like Morestin, Davis (1929) did not undermine the neighboring skin to facilitate closure, believing that "undercutting tends to make more scar, and the tissues do not loosen as readily for the secondary operations." However, Davis removed the maximal amount of lesion that he could at each procedure, and then waited a sufficiently long time between operations to allow the local skin to relax and the scar to soften. Smith's (1946) method of "multiple excision" differed in that he extensively undermined the neighboring unscarred skin, making additional incisions to create various advancement and rotation flaps. The shortest interval between procedures was six to eight weeks. A number of these cases were described in detail and illustrated with photographs showing patients before and after each stage in Smith's book on plastic surgery published in 1950. When there was adequate local skin available for repair, Smith's approach made the removal of both moderate- and large-sized cheek scars possible. Converse, Guy, and Molenaar (1969), Guy and Converse (1987), and Stark (1975, 1984) reported excellent results with staged excision and sequential advancement-rotation neck flaps for resurfacing most of a cheek esthetic unit.

A modification of the *inferomedially based* cervicofacial advancement-rotation flap used for resurfacing moderate- or large-sized cheek areas is the "angle-rotation flap" of Schrudde and Beinhoff (1987). The flap incorporates an "angle" (actually a Burow's triangle) of hairless lower mastoid skin from behind and below the ear that is attached to the main cheek-neck flap. As the flap is transferred superiorly, the small neck "angle" of skin rotates anteriorly and superiorly into a pre-auricular position, and the triangular mastoid donor site closes along a transverse linear seam (after adjacent skin undermining), leaving a scar in an inconspicuous location. If the entire cheek scar cannot be removed in one stage, the flap can be rotated and readvanced several times. Figures 41–5 and 41–6 demonstrate the use of the flap.

For scars in the medial cheek, medial cheek–upper lip area, or medial cheek–lower eyelid area, a *laterally based* ascending cervicofacial flap can be used (Kaplan and Goldwyn, 1978; Mercer, 1988). With its lateral pivot point, the flap glides along the nasolabial fold to cover the medial cheek much more efficiently than a medially based flap. Its disadvantage is the more conspicuous rotation-advancement incision scar along the medial cheek and upper neck. However, if there is already scarring in the lower medial cheek and neck region, this may be the flap of choice.

To limit the necessity for extensive skin undermining or staged removal of lesions, Sasaki (1987a) described a method of intraoperative sustained limited expansion (ISLE) that allows the surgeon to stretch the skin intraoperatively beyond its usual limits using "cyclic loading"—intermittent short periods of skin stretching and relaxation; this maneuver takes advantage of the viscoelastic properties of skin (mechanical creep and stress relaxation) described by Gibson (1977) (see Chap. 7). Sasaki inserted one or more temporary expanders under the skin around the defect and inflated the balloons with saline until the overlying skin was taut and blanched. After three minutes of stretch the expanders are deflated for two minutes. The process is repeated three or four times, and each time a progressively greater volume of saline can be instilled into the expanders as the skin progressively "gives." The average skin gain in the midface is 1.0 to 2.5 cm per expander. Although adjacent skin undermining is limited to that needed to insert the temporary expanders, some ischemia to the flap margins may occur, so that the edges need to be trimmed back until bright red dermal bleeding is seen before wound closure. The recruitment of "extra skin" permits excision and closure of small- to moderate-sized defects that otherwise might have required more extensive flap incisions and undermining. However, ISLE is not a method designed to yield a narrower scar, since skin "stretch-

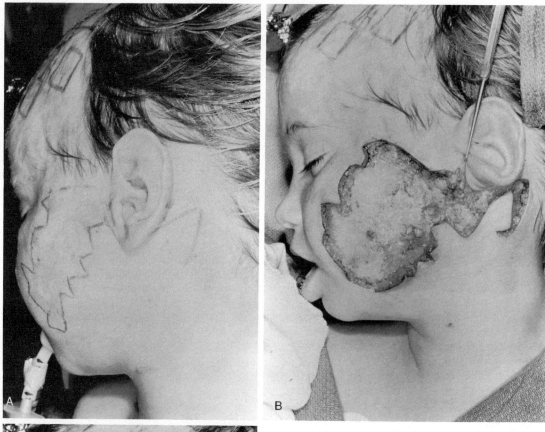

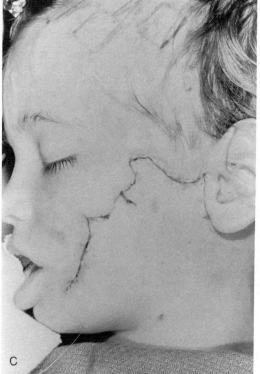

Figure 41–5. The angle-rotation flap (Schrudde). *A,* The cheek scar marked for excision and the cheek-neck flap with the mastoid skin "angle" outlined. *B, C,* After scar excision and flap advancement-rotation. The postauricular flap "angle" rotates to a position in front of the lower ear, and the donor site behind the ear is closed primarily.

back" may result in a wide scar that requires a secondary revision. The technique awaits the test of time.

Another method aimed at limiting the amount of undermining and incision making around an area of skin to be removed, and that also takes advantage of the biomechanical stretch capacity of the skin, has been called "presuturing" (Liang and associates, 1988). The margins of the skin to be removed are approximated under tension with sutures inserted under local anesthesia, the night before surgery or several hours preoperatively. The skin relaxes under the stretch and allows removal and closure of relatively large lesions with little if any skin undermining.

REMOVAL OF LARGE CHEEK SCARS

The distinction between a moderate-sized and a large area of cheek scarring is imprecise, but a large area generally occupies more than one-half to two-thirds of the cheek unit. However, even relatively small scars can be difficult to remove if located in unfavorable positions where skin traction easily distorts an adjacent facial feature or where the neighboring skin is deficient. For the removal of large cheek scars, there are basically two methods from which to choose: (1) staged partial excision with stepwise flap resurfacing and (2) flap expansion prior to total or near-total scar removal. The choice between using a skin expander or sequentially moving a flap depends on individual considerations, including the exact location of the cheek scarring and the geographic relationship of the unscarred local skin being used for flap repair. Although there has been enthusiasm in recent years for skin expansion, the surgeon should remember that generating an "expanded flap" takes at least two procedures: one to insert the expander and one to remove the expander and advance the flap. Often a third operation is needed for adjustments to flap position and scar revisions. The process of skin expansion does carry the potential for complications, patient discomfort, and inconvenience. Although an expanded flap is a larger flap with an enhanced blood supply, the scar tissue capsule that forms around the expander reduces flap skin elasticity and impedes flap movement. Furthermore, expanded neck flaps still require peripheral advancement and rotation incisions to allow the flap to ascend onto the cheek. Expanded flaps also have a tendency to retract somewhat postoperatively, possibly causing a traction deformity of an eyelid, lip, or oral commissure. This information is not designed to say that skin expansion should not often be the procedure of choice, but only to point out that a number of factors need to be considered in making the choice. As a general rule, if the cheek scar can be removed in two (or perhaps three) stages without an expander and with approximately the same amount of secondary incisional scarring, it is probably preferable to do the resurfacing without the expander. If, in addition to an unscarred neck, there is unscarred skin above the jawline in the lower cheek, staged excision and sequential flap advancement is often preferable. On the other hand, when the cheek scarring extends down to or below the jawline, neck skin expansion is usually required to resurface the complete or near-complete cheek esthetic unit. Whereas a nonexpanded skin flap tends to slide primarily in one direction, the expanded skin flap has been enlarged in both height and width, offering a greater potential for complete cheek unit resurfacing. Once transferred onto the cheek, the expanded neck flap can be repositioned on the cheek by means of the usual flap adjustment maneuvers (Fig. 41–7). The use of a skin expander (or expanders) usually provides sufficient flap to accomplish the necessary resurfacing in one stage, but if flap size is insufficient, the once expanded and once transferred flap can be reexpanded and advanced a second time.

STAGED EXCISION WITH SEQUENTIAL FLAP ADVANCEMENT

For most large cheek scars accompanied by a mostly unscarred neck, an inferomedially based advancement-rotation neck flap is used, always closing the donor site primarily. It is the author's opinion that, when the entire ipsilateral neck is unburned, some type of cervicofacial, cervical, or cervicopectoral flap can be designed to resurface the complete cheek unit without the need for a skin graft to cover the flap donor site. Having even a little unscarred cheek skin above the jawline as part of the flap makes the job of total or near-total cheek resurfacing much easier. A modification of Schrudde's "angle-rotation flap" design (see the description above) can be used at the first stage, extending the flap's posterior incision one-third of the way down

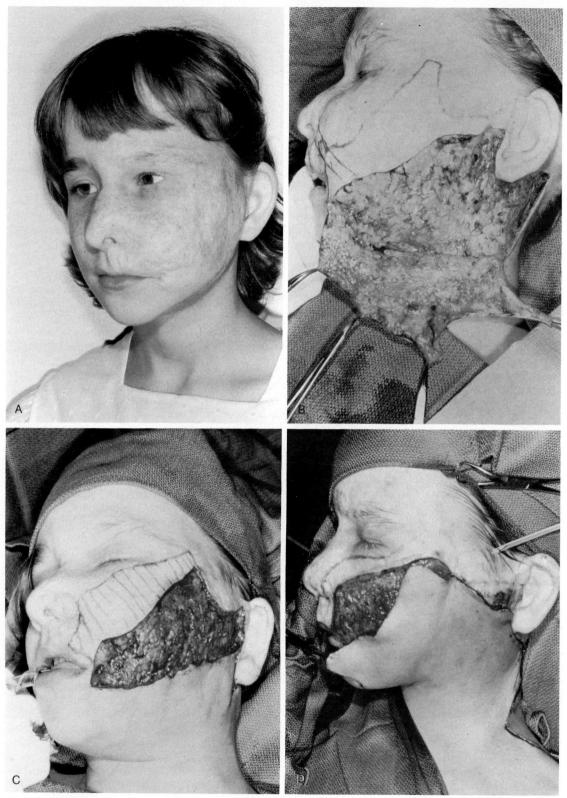

Figure 41–6. Staged cheek scar removal with sequential neck flap advancement. *A,* Preoperative view. *B,* First-stage excision. Note the design of the angle-rotation flap. *C,* Second-stage excision. *D,* Third-stage excision. The flap "dog ear" adjacent to the mouth is unfurled and is ready to be applied to the upper lip.

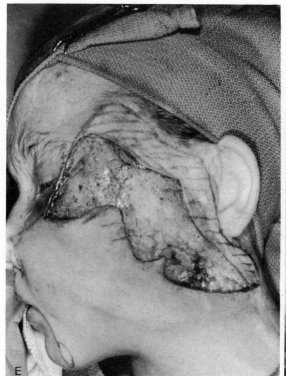
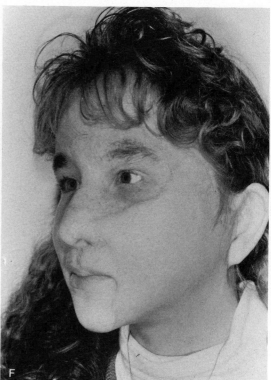

Figure 41–6 *Continued E,* Fourth and final scar excision and superoposterior flap advancement. Note that the flap rotation incision extends down to the supraclavicular area. The absent left nasal ala was reconstructed with an "expendable" cheek-nasolabial scar flap supported with conchal cartilage. *F,* Final appearance.

the lateral neck along the edge of the occipital hairline. The flap is undermined in the subcutaneous plane (above the platysma muscle in the neck). The flap is transposed and laid on top of the cheek scar, which is marked and partially excised. At the first and second stages, it is usually best to move the flap as far medially and superiorly as possible along the nasolabial line toward the inner canthus of the eye. After the flap has been moved to its final position along the medial line of the cheek, it is much easier to shift it backward (like a "face lift") to recover the lateral cheek and temporal areas. At the second or third flap advancement procedure, if the flap does not rotate or ascend "adequately," the lateral neck incision is extended farther in an inferior direction along the occipital hairline. In cases in which only neck skin is available for total cheek coverage, the upper lateral point of the flap at the base of the earlobe must rotate and ascend to the superior side of the nose. To permit this rotation, a perpendicular

back cut of several centimeters aimed anteriorly just above the clavicle is often necessary to allow the flap to reach its intended destination. The back cut aids medial rotation by adding a curve to the straight line in the neck, and the maneuver also assists upward flap advancement by invoking the principle inherent in pantographic expansion (Stark, 1955). The back cut creates a secondary defect, which is closed by wide undermining and advancing the skin over the shoulder and infraclavicular region. At each stage, the surgeon must weigh the benefit to be gained by extending the flap edge incision (i.e., greater flap mobility) against the disadvantages of more incision (with a visibly longer scar and an increased risk to flap blood supply). Figure 41–6 illustrates a case of staged removal of a large cheek scar. Note that the dog-ear that invariably accumulates around the flap's pivot point at the chin was advanced, unfurled, and used to resurface the left lateral upper lip subunit.

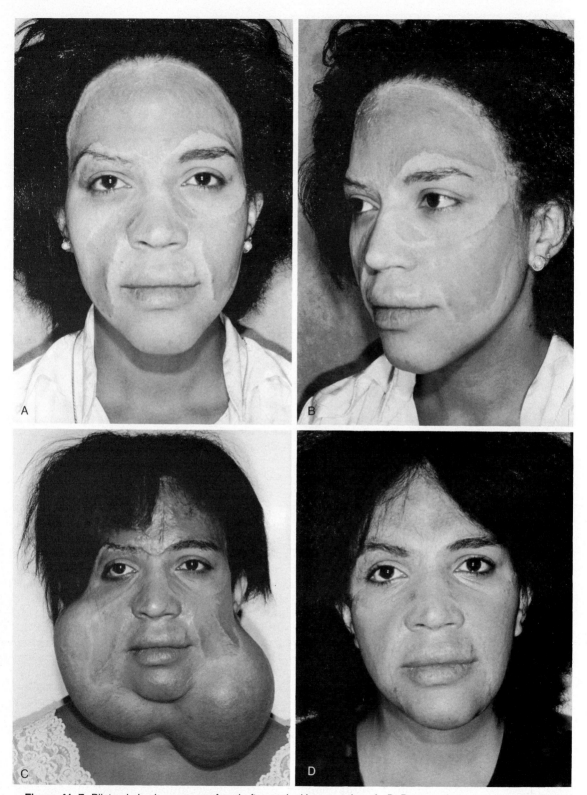

Figure 41–7. Bilateral cheek scars resurfaced after neck skin expansion. *A, B,* Preoperative appearance. *C,* During skin expansion. *D, E,* Postoperative appearance after secondary advancement of the previously transposed flaps. *F,* Left neck expander insertion through a perpendicular incision in the lower cheek scar. Remote filling port insertion through a perpendicular incision behind the occipital hair line. *G,* Immediately before and *H,* immediately after expander removal and flap transposition.

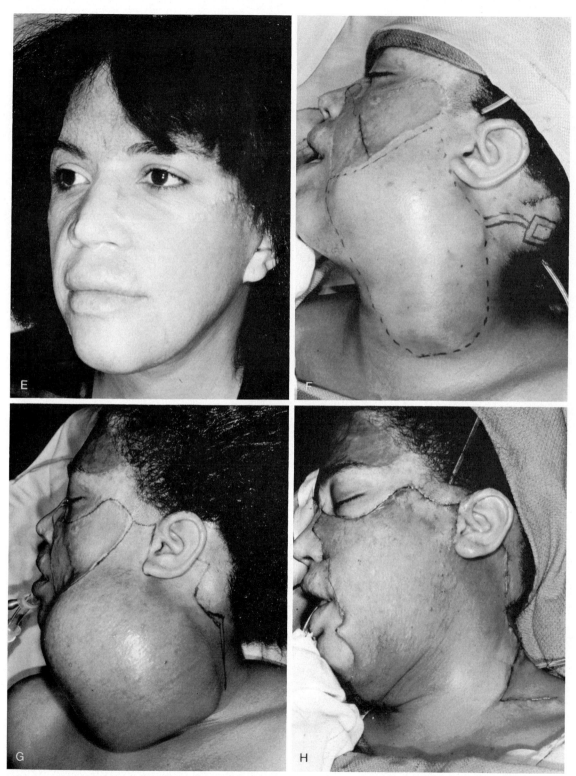

Figure 41–7 *Continued*

EXPANDED SKIN FLAPS FOR CHEEK RESURFACING

When skin expansion is indicated, *medial cheek scars* can be managed by expansion of the lateral cheek skin (Radovan, 1987). If the upper lip is also scarred, expansion of the neck can provide an expanded, laterally based ascending neck flap that can usually cover the medial cheek and upper lip more easily than the more commonly used medially based cheek-neck flap. However, the vertical submandibular neck scar that accompanies the laterally based flap must be acceptable to both patient and surgeon, which is not often the case. To avoid the anterior neck scar, large areas of medial cheek scarring (which cannot be resurfaced by simple advancement of an expanded lateral cheek flap) are usually best managed with a medially based cheek-neck flap that leaves an inconspicuous scar along the preauricular crease and occipital hairline.

Lateral cheek scarring is managed by expansion of either medial cheek skin, upper neck skin, or both. When a large area of the cheek requires resurfacing and the ipsilateral neck is unscarred, a medially based, expanded neck advancement-rotation flap is usually chosen. Whatever unscarred lateral and inferior cheek is present is included in the flap. Expanders have been placed in the cheek and neck over facial nerve branches, major blood vessels, and the trachea without difficulty (Argenta and VanderKolk, 1987). Figure 41–7 illustrates expansion of bilateral cheek-neck flaps to allow complete removal of mismatched skin grafts on both cheeks. Note that the final flap suture lines have been placed along the natural boundaries of the cheek esthetic unit (the nasolabial crease, infraorbital rim, and preauricular-retrotragal line) to make them minimally conspicuous.

For scarring across the lower cheeks and chin in one patient, Marks, Argenta, and Thornton (1987) first placed two side by side skin expanders across the full width of the anterior neck to resurface the lower face and the chin. To correct the remaining eversion of the lower lip without using a skin graft, they subsequently made a transverse incision in the submental area and advanced the flap again in a superior direction as a bipedicle flap to reach the vermilion margin. The flap release defect in the upper neck was in turn closed with a second bipedicle flap from the lower neck.

Nearby areas other than the neck have also been expanded for cheek resurfacing. Marchac and Pugash (1987) preexpanded the hairless lateral forehead, which was transferred to the cheek as a Converse scalping flap (see Chap. 37). The forehead donor site was easily closed primarily without the usual skin graft, and two to three weeks after the flap transfer to the cheek the pedicle was divided and the flap inset. The hair-bearing scalp pedicle was returned to normal position and the hairline reestablished. The forehead skin on the cheek reportedly gave an excellent color and texture match with the remainder of the face, and the vertical donor site scar on the forehead was minimally conspicuous. Marks and associates (1988) described a preexpanded, hair-bearing temporal artery island scalp flap for reconstructing the beard on an entire scarred lateral cheek, with primary closure of the scalp donor site.

The general principles of skin expansion are discussed in Chapter 13. To these, the author would add the following technical considerations.

As emphasized by Sasaki (1987), it is the planning, execution, and postoperative management of procedure no. 1 (the expander insertion procedure) that almost always determine the success or failure of the three-component process of insertion, expansion, and flap transposition. Planning involves selection of the size, shape, placement, and number of expanders to be used. Standard-sized and -shaped expanders are usually satisfactory, but the surgeon should not hesitate to order customized expanders if these would do a better job. Exposed (clear) x-ray film laid on the face and neck can be used to make cut-out patterns that can be given to the manufacturer for precise expander shape construction. Whenever a custom expander is ordered, a standard expander of approximately the same size and shape should also be ordered as a back-up in case a defect is found or created in the custom unit at the time of insertion. Custom expanders should not be ordered with excessive projection as a means of achieving a greater than usual fill volume. The incompletely filled and redundant expander envelope may form a stiff fold that can erode through a thin overlying skin flap. To obtain the needed skin expansion, it is usually preferable to "overfill" a low profile expander than it is to underfill a high profile implant. It has been shown that silicone expanders can safely tolerate volumes considerably in excess of their listed full volume (Hallock, 1987).

One large, properly shaped expander is usually superior to two small adjacent expanders. However, in some cases, two or more expanders grouped together can give the best fit around the area to be removed; multiple expanders can also give differential expansion to specialized areas within the region to be repaired. A round or rectangular expander generates a hemispheric flap that advances mostly from the central portion of the leading edge of the flap, with the expanded skin on the sides of the flap tethered by scar and unable to move forward. For this reason, when the cheek scar to be removed is circular in shape, the use of a crescent-shaped expander (Manders and Wong, 1987) is helpful. The expander straddles the scar, extending halfway around its circumference, so that the skin on the sides of the scar as well as the skin over the dome of the expander is stretched. The advancing edge of the expanded "crescent flap" pivots forward to cover the excision defect "like the handle of a bucket moving from one side of the mouth of the bucket to the other."

The author usually prefers expanders with remote fill ports, rather than those with an integral fill valve, because of the potential injury to a thin skin flap by repeated injections through it into a self-contained valve. Leighton and associates (1988), van Rappard and associates (1988), and Schneider and associates (1988) all demonstrated that the skin over the center of an expander (where the integral fill valves are located) stretches more than the skin at the periphery. This skin is less durable (i.e., has decreased tensile strength and elasticity), making it more easily injured.

Selecting the site of the incisions to be used for expander placement is important. The incision that offers the greatest ease of pocket dissection, hemostasis, and expander positioning is along the edge of the scar-flap junction. However, the *tangentially oriented insertion incision*, which is parallel and close to the forces of expansion, is at risk of dehiscence after the expander inflation begins. To avoid early scar disruption and expander exposure, the surgeon using the tangential incision should (1) position the expander at least 1 to 2 cm away from the incision, (2) close the incision securely in multiple layers, and (3) delay inflation for several weeks or

longer to allow incisional healing to take place. Despite these precautions, incision separation necessitating expander removal can occur, and is probably the most common cause of "expansion failure" (Antonyshyn and associates, 1988; Neale and associates, 1988). The other disadvantage of the tangential insertion incision is that by having to delay inflation for several weeks after insertion, the potential for immediate flap expansion achieved by skin undermining is lost, prolonging the expansion process. In some cases the early development of scar contracture around the uninflated implant can also make subsequent flap expansion more difficult.

The author prefers a *radially oriented insertion incision* (Sasaki, 1985) whenever practical and possible. Placed perpendicular to the forces of expansion, it does not pull apart with flap expansion; thus, expander inflation to the point of tissue tolerance can begin at the time of expander insertion. Immediate initiation of inflation has several advantages: (1) folds in the expander shell are essentially eliminated, lessening the risk of pressure-point flap necrosis; (2) the flap stretch gained by skin undermining is maintained rather than lost; (3) seroma and hematoma formation are minimized; and (4) the overall time for flap expansion is shortened. The radial insertion incision can often be conveniently placed within the cheek scar that is to be removed.

Another favorable incision location when a neck expander is being used is perpendicular and posterior to the occipital hairline (behind the line of a future neck flap rotation incision). The same incision can be used to place both the expander and its remote fill valve; a single carefully placed incision can be used to insert more than one expander and more than one filler port. Although a single incision is often all that is needed for expander insertion, one or more additional radially oriented incisions should certainly be used if it helps to dissect the subcutaneous pocket or to place the expander or its fill port. The incisions should always be placed where they will be permanently concealed (e.g., within the scalp), or permanently camouflaged within a scar that will remain, or placed within the scar that is to be removed. The incisions should not compromise the design or blood supply of the intended flap or other future flaps that may be used for repair of the cheek, neck, or scalp region. The disadvantage of the small radial incision is that dissection of the expander pocket must be done blindly with scissors. For the plastic surgeon experienced in face lift surgery, this is usually a technically simple maneuver. However, hemostasis is difficult or impossible through these small, and at times remote, incisions; therefore, suction drainage of both the expander pocket and the remote fill port pocket should be performed in every case. If a hematoma should develop, there is an increased risk of infection, thick scar capsule formation, or both, which are precursors to expander or fill port exposure.

Before insertion, the expander should be filled with air and immersed under water to check for leaks anywhere in the system. If the entire system (expander, fill valve, and connecting tube) are air-tight, the air is completely removed from the expander, and it is rolled up into a tight "cigarette" and pushed into the prepared pocket with a fingertip or blunt-tipped instrument. Because the expander is more easily inserted when it is rolled tightly, the author prefers an expander without a firm backing. Once inside the pocket, the expander is unrolled by inflating it with saline through the fill valve. If the pocket is too small for a smooth and comfortable expander fit, the expander should be completely deflated and removed, and the pocket adjusted. Attempting to dissect the pocket with the expander in place risks making a hole in the implant. Although the pocket for the expander should be of adequate size, the inferior extent of the pocket dissection should be limited to the desired location for the expander. Skin expanders placed in the cheek, and particularly those in the neck, always slide caudad to the most dependent place in the pocket after the supine patient becomes erect. Gravitational pooling of saline also stretches the skin more over the inferior portion of the expander. For these reasons, the expander pocket should not be overdissected inferiorly or medially. After reinsertion, the expander is again filled until the overlying skin is tightly stretched. This maneuver eliminates the kinks or wrinkles in the expander. A sufficient amount of saline is withdrawn so that the skin is not overstretched and shows satisfactory color and capillary refill. The remote fill valve is positioned in a separate pocket. The pocket for the port should be generous enough for the overlying skin to drape comfortably over the

valve. If the valve pocket is too tight, the port may erode the overlying skin. If it appears that the fill valve could either flip over in the pocket or slide along the connecting tube tunnel toward the expander, it should be fixed to the surrounding tissues with a suture or two placed through the silicone cuff that surrounds the edge of the valve. Generally, the remote fill valve should not be placed inferior to a cheek or neck expander, to prevent the expander from sliding or expanding over the fill port.

During the day and night after expander insertion, the skin overlying the expander should be observed at frequent intervals. If there is any suggestion of duskiness or vascular embarrassment, saline should be withdrawn from the expander until the skin feels relaxed and skin color returns to normal. After a day or two, the withdrawn volume of saline can usually be safely reinstilled.

Postoperative expander inflation usually begins at one week, with weekly inflations thereafter. Twice weekly or more frequent inflations can be carried out if practical and properly monitored. A 23 gauge butterfly needle and tubing is connected to a syringe for inflation. The discomfort of needle penetration can be lessened by first raising a small wheal of lidocaine over the injection port with a 30 gauge needle. Making the inflation procedure as painless as possible is particularly important in children. Jackson and associates (1987) reported a low infection rate with externalization of the remote fill port, and Nahai and McGain (1988) proposed using the disposable trocar that comes with many wound drainage kits as a simple means of tunneling the connecting tube through the subcutaneous tissues and out through the skin. Although the author has yet to employ an externalized port, the method has the obvious advantages of patient comfort and less potential risk of valve damage and fluid leakage from improper needle penetration. The potential disadvantages of the external port are the risks of low grade infection due to motion of the connecting tubing through the skin (particularly if the expander is left in place for several months) and accidental avulsion of the valve (especially in children). Additional experience with externalized filling ports will determine when and how best to use them.

Regardless of the type of valve used, the inflation procedure is the same: at each fill session the expander is inflated until the overlying skin is taut, but not overstretched (a matter of judgment). Slight capillary blanching is acceptable if it lasts no more than five to ten minutes after the completion of inflation. If there is any doubt about the adequacy of skin blood supply, some saline should be withdrawn. Pietila and associates (1988) described a method of "overfilling" the expander at each session to decrease the overall duration of the expansion process. At each session, saline is added to the expander to a point at which subjective parameters such as capillary refill in the skin and tension felt by the patient are at the maximal safe level commonly used clinically. Instead of stopping at that point, the surgeon continues the saline instillation until the dermal capillary blood flow is zero according to a laser Doppler flow meter. Thereafter, saline is withdrawn until visible capillary refill is established and the flow meter shows satisfactory dermal circulation. This "overfilling" at each session resulted in an average volume gain of 59 per cent. However, this author feels that the skin flaps developed over expanders in the cheek and neck are thin to begin with, and usually become thinner as expansion progresses—the result of pressure atrophy on subcutaneous fat. Therefore, although it is appropriate to consider ways of minimizing the period of social embarrassment and inconvenience to the patient by shortening the duration of expansion, in cheek and neck expansion a safe rate of expansion and perhaps more cautious observation must be applied than when the expander is deep to a thicker and less fragile skin flap.

If at any time during the expansion process a kink or fold in the expander shell is seen or felt under the skin, it may be possible to smooth it out with a rapid addition or withdrawal of saline while manipulating the implant. If, however, the kink remains after these maneuvers, the patient should *not* be sent out of the office with the kink present and the overlying skin tense from added saline or pressure necrosis of the skin can easily develop (Manders and associates, 1984a,b). Rather, sufficient saline should be withdrawn so that the skin flap is slightly loose over the fold. Waiting a week before further expansion may allow the scar capsule around the expander to thicken enough to protect the flap over the fold. Saxby (1988) has recommended inverting the "knuckle" by taping it down

firmly with inelastic Micropore tape, thereby eliminating the pressure point on the overlying skin. With the tape on, he immediately proceeds (cautiously) with the inflation regimen until the fold is eliminated by gradual expander distention.

From the onset of expansion, the patient and family should be told to maintain a lookout for an area of skin within the flap that shows even a hint of blue discoloration. This is the sign of a thin spot in the flap, and portends expander exposure. The patient or family should be instructed to see the surgeon immediately if such a spot is seen. The surgeon has two choices: (1) to withdraw saline until the flap is soft, and give the flap time to thicken before attempting slow reexpansion (an approach that can be successful if the flap is not too thin); or (2) if exposure seems imminent, to withdraw some saline and operate immediately, using whatever skin flap expansion has been gained to resurface partially the scarred cheek. It is certainly more prudent to accept a partial success, with the option of reexpanding and completing the reconstruction later on, than to press on in the face of possible expander exposure, risking permanent damage to the flap. In the cheek and neck area, a small hole in the skin over an expander usually becomes a large hole overnight!

The best way to deal with expander exposure is to take steps to prevent it: proper insertion incision placement; dissection of a skin flap with adequate fat padding on its underside; avoidance of hematomas and infection that produce reactive fibrosis and pocket contracture; prevention of shell "knuckles" by not using an expander that requires a large volume of saline to "get the kinks out"; creation of an adequate subcutaneous pocket in which the expander sits comfortably; and avoidance of so rapid an expansion that the flap becomes thin too fast.

There are several rules of thumb by which to gauge the amount of skin expansion necessary to accomplish the resurfacing. One rule suggests that the distance over the dome of the expander attain a length of two (and preferably three) times the distance across the adjacent scar to be removed. Another rule suggests that the curvilinear length over the expander dome minus the flat length across the base of the expander (which also becomes longer as the expander is inflated) should at least equal the distance across the scar to be removed. Experience has taught, however, that none of the mathematical formulas can precisely predict how the expanded skin flap will stretch, slide, and rotate. Thus, the decision regarding how much expansion to attain before operation no. 2 is a matter for the experienced judgment of the surgeon. One rule, however, always applies: it is far better to have too much flap than to have too little.

An expanded cheek flap being used to recover an adjacent area on the cheek can usually move to its new position mostly by advancement. An expanded neck flap with a medial base, however, cannot partially encircle the cheek scar, and it must rotate as well as advance. Therefore, at operation no. 2, the periprosthetic scar capsule that has formed around the expander may severely restrict flap extension. To release the flap from its lining of scar, multiple parallel or perpendicular cuts can be made through the scar to the underlying fat (as is done to the galea aponeurotica to extend a scalp flap), care being taken to avoid injury to the network of blood vessels lying superficial to the capsule. It is this dilated subcutaneous vascular plexus, and not the small network of vessels within the scar capsule itself, that has primarily enhanced the perfusion of the expanded flap. For this reason, the scar capsule around an expander can be completely removed without detriment to the flap (Mahoney, 1988). In actual practice, however, capsulectomy significantly increases the risk of injury to the extracapsular vessels; as shown by Hardesty and associates (1988), multiple capsulotomies at 1 cm intervals produce as much additional flap stretch as a total capsulectomy. However, even capsulotomies must be carefully performed. A cut made a little too deeply through scar across the base of the flap can destroy even the most robust specimen.

Expanded flaps being transferred from the lower cheek to the upper cheek, or from the neck to the cheek, have a propensity to retract downward, causing distortion of the lower eyelid or corner of the mouth. To prevent ectropion, the flap must be sufficiently large and loose to be inset without causing traction on mobile facial features. When the flap is brought up to the lower eyelid, it is best to anchor it well above both the lateral (and medial) canthi, perhaps deepithelizing a portion of the flap laterally to tuck under the skin in the temporal region for added support. Sasaki (1987c) used scattered buried sutures between the dermis on the underside of the flap and the recipient bed, progressively adding sutures from the base of the flap out to the distal edge. The small "dimples" in the flap from the sutures disappear with time. Flaps that have remained expanded for many months (e.g., three to six months) also show less tendency to retract than flaps that have been rapidly expanded.

SCAR REPLACEMENT WITH A REGIONAL TUBE PEDICLE SKIN FLAP

In cases in which cheek resurfacing is best done with flap tissue, but insufficient skin is available for adjacent local flaps, the surgeon should look outside the immediate neighborhood to the chest, shoulder, and back region where adequate-sized areas of undamaged or minimally scarred skin may be present. An area of skin on the shoulder or upper chest can be expanded, and with the enhanced blood supply that results from the expansion process, transferred to the neck and lower cheek on a narrow (medial) pedicle (4 cm wide), as described by Spence (1988). In the case reported by Spence, the expansion also allowed concomitant primary closure of the flap donor site over the shoulder without a skin graft. However, a flap sufficiently large to cover most, if not all, of the cheek may not permit closure of the donor site without a skin graft, and a longer and more reliable pedicle may be needed to carry the skin paddle from the donor site to the face. In this situation, a most useful tool is a delayed random-pattern *direct tube pedicle flap*. The longitudinal vessels within the skin tube dilate over time so that the skin tube becomes the physiologic equivalent of an "axial" pedicle. Although less expeditious, the advantage of a delayed interpolated tube pedicle over a true axial-pattern (direct cutaneous) flap or a microvascular free flap is that the location of the tube pedicle flap donor site is not restricted to those few places where direct cutaneous vessels are found. With appropriate surgical delays, the tube flap can have a size and thinness determined by the surgeon and not by the vascular anatomy inherent in the axial flap design. A delayed direct tube pedicle can do, at times, what no other flap may be able to do: safely bring skin from any random area in the upper torso to the face. Careful planning is the key to success. A pattern of the cheek area to be covered is made from a thin adhesive foam (Reston), and the pattern is placed on the skin of the shoulder, chest, or upper back donor site to be certain that enough unscarred skin is present to cover the cheek area. It is best to carry excess skin to the face so that the flap can be inset without tension. A separate rectangular strip of foam is cut to simulate the tubed pedicle that will carry the skin paddle. The real skin tube (actually a cylinder) (Borges, 1988) will be constructed from a relatively narrow bipedicle flap. Pinching the skin together along the intended axis of the tube determines how wide a pedicle can be made that will still allow primary closure of the surrounding skin beneath the skin tube; often this is a width of only about 4 cm. One end of the foam strip representing the tubed pedicle is attached (by the adhesive backing) to the cheek pattern on the donor site, and the other end is attached to the lateral neck (the base of the pedicle). The composite paddle-pedicle pattern is transferred to the face, where both the position and the angle at which the pedicle joins the cheek pattern along the lateral jawline are adjusted to give the best fit. The length of the tube and its "take-off" position at the base on the neck may also have to be modified. The flap pattern is then transferred to the donor site on its attached pedicle to make sure that the pedicle's reach is long enough, and to be certain that the pattern of the cheek will fit completely into the available donor site. This process of moving the pattern flap back and forth from donor site to cheek is repeated as many times as needed to make the necessary adjustments so that the flap reaches and fits as it should. If the "planning operation" cannot be made to work perfectly by using the pattern flap, the surgical procedure will not work properly, in which case the surgeon should consider expanding the donor site, expanding the pedicle, seeking a different flap altogether, or using a skin graft for the resurfacing.

At the initial procedure, the tubed pedicle is constructed as a bipedicle flap with a length-to-width ratio of approximately 2:1. A longer tube with a 3:1 length-to-width ratio can be safely made if a small skin bridge is maintained centrally along one side. The bridge is divided at the subsequent procedure. If a long tube pedicle is required, two bipedicle tubes are constructed with a common intervening base of skin that has not been undermined containing intact musculocutaneous perforators. Subsequently, the two tubes are joined in stages. At each stage in the multistaged preparation of the flap, in addition to constructing the tubed pedicle, the large skin paddle is sequentially delayed by progressively lifting separated sections of the paddle, and either rolling a narrow segment into a tube, or turning under a square segment to line itself. Progressive tubing or folding under portions of the flap along with staged skin grafting of the flap donor site, has several advantages: it preserves the flap's augmented perfusion gained by the "delay phenomenon"; it avoids repeated elevations of areas that have already been delayed; and it makes the final transposition stage of the fully prepared flap easier, since the flap donor site will have been completely closed. For efficiency, as many different areas of the large paddle as safely possible should be tubed or rolled at the first procedure, leaving intact non-undermined skin segments that are 2 to 3 cm long between the "delayed" segments for maintenance of blood supply. In essence, a network of branched and serially oriented unipedicle and bipedicle flaps are created within the area of the main flap, and at subsequent surgical stages the smaller flaps are joined together to create one large flap supplied by only the proximal pedicle (Gillies and Millard, 1957). A small skin bridge of 1 or 2 cm should be left somewhere over the shoulder area and it should not be divided until the time has come for flap transposition. The little skin bridge not only keeps the tubed flap from dangling (which risks congestion and twisting), but also acts as an important "safety valve" that may provide vascular inflow or egress to keep a severely ischemic or congested flap alive. A day or two before flap transposition is scheduled, whatever blood supply is provided by the distal skin bridge is temporarily interrupted by a rubber band tourniquet. If the distal flap continues to look pink and well perfused with the tourniquet in place, the flap can be safely incised and moved as planned. If, however, the distal flap appears dusky with the tourniquet on, the rubber band is removed, and either more time is allowed to pass before repeating the tourniquet test, or half of the skin bridge is incised before again attempting the tourniquet test a week later. The art of fabricating a tube pedicle flap lies in designing a sequence of flap delays that is both expeditious and safe.

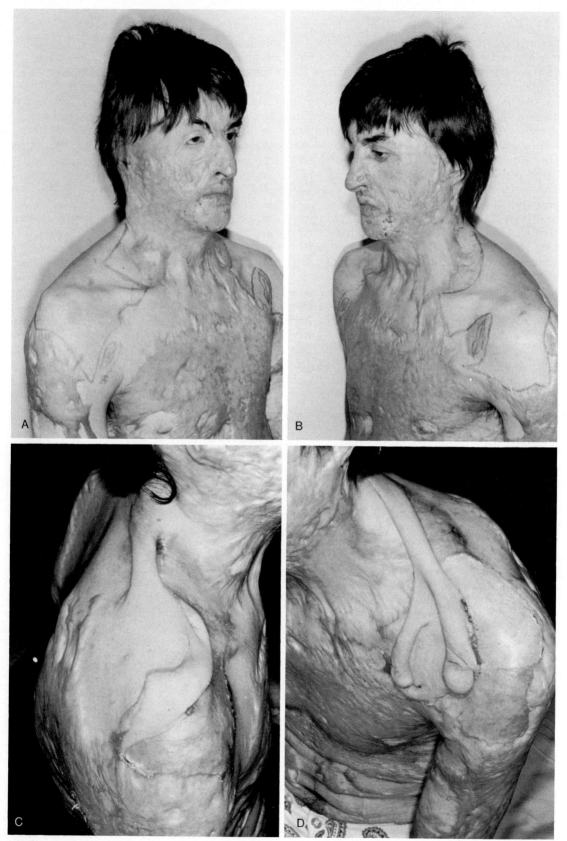

Figure 41–8. Regional tube flaps for facial resurfacing. *A, B,* Preoperative views showing the flaps outlined. *C,* After first delay of the right shoulder flap. *D,* After second delay of the right shoulder flap.

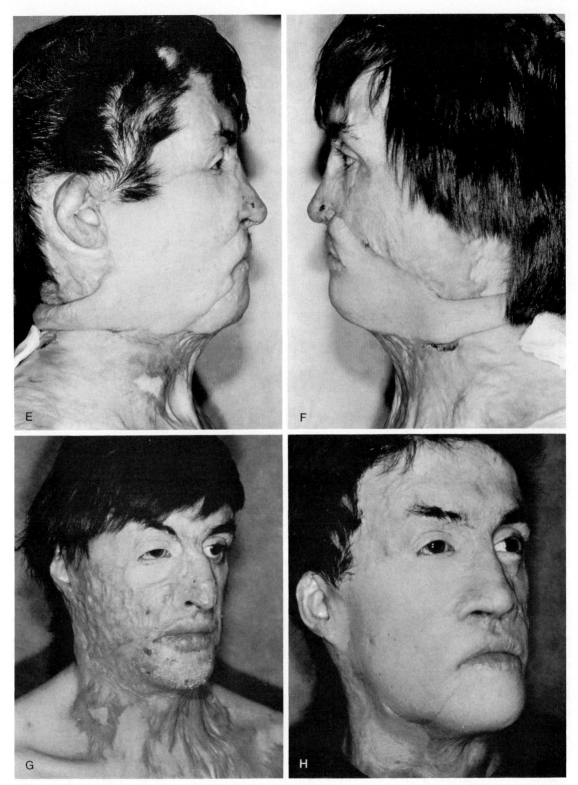

Figure 41–8 *Continued E, F,* Flaps transposed to the face and before the pedicles have been divided and inset onto the anterior neck. *G,* Preoperative view. *H,* Postoperative view. Note that the flap covers the enlarged cheek esthetic unit, including the lower eyelid and half of the upper lip. The chin and the other half of the upper lip were covered with a flap from the left shoulder.

When the flap is transferred to the cheek, its folded and tubed paddle must be opened completely by removing scar from the fatty undersurface and along the flap edges. Enough scar and subcutaneous fat should be excised to make the flap thin and to restore normal skin elasticity. The facial recipient site should not be excised until the flap has been opened, thinned, and tacked on the cheek in the position in which it will lie. Bright red bleeding from the distal flap edges means that the entire flap should survive; a dark (blackish) color of the blood means almost certainly that some portion of the distal end will not survive, and the flap must be trimmed until red bleeding is observed. This is another reason to have prepared an oversized flap, one that will allow some undernourished distal skin to be discarded, leaving sufficient flap remaining to cover the cheek as desired. When the flap is placed and inset on the cheek, tension must be avoided to prevent eyelid or lip displacement, and to avert vascular insult to the flap. Subcuticular suturing is done to avoid suture marks, and drains are always placed beneath the flap. After two to three weeks with the flap on the cheek, the pedicle can be divided. If the tube is to be opened and draped into the neck, it may be safer to partially divide the original pedicle at its base as a surgical delay and complete the separation a week or two later.

Figure 41–8 illustrates bilateral shoulder tube pedicles used to transport the only remaining unscarred skin on the shoulders, upper chest, and upper back to the face. Five preliminary surgical delays were carried out at the time that the nose, right ear, right scalp, and eyelids were being reconstructed. Note that the flap brought to the right side of the face covered the enlarged cheek unit, including the lower eyelid and right upper lip. The flap from the left upper chest was just large enough to replace the scar on the lower cheek, left upper lip, and lower lip-chin unit. The flap-covered face has a uniform color and texture, reveals normal facial contours, and displays normal animation.

SCAR REPLACEMENT WITH A SKIN GRAFT

When using a skin graft on the cheek (or anywhere else on the face) as the final resurfacing material, the aim must be to *avoid a patched appearance.* Pursuant to this end, the surgeon should first ask whether a skin graft is, indeed, what is best for the patient (see Esthetic Considerations above), and if so, how much of the cheek should be resurfaced, what type of graft should be used, and what should be the graft donor site. Particularly when using a skin graft (i.e., not a flap) on the cheek, it is often preferable to cover the full esthetic cheek unit for purposes of homogeneity of cheek color and texture and to camouflage the graft edge scars. *The fewer graft pieces used, the better.* A 4 inch wide Padgett electric dermatome piece or a 4 inch wide Reese drum dermatome skin graft may cover most or all of a small cheek. The 5 inch wide Padgett drum dermatone may be better for a larger cheek. When skin grafts are used to cover both cheeks, the two cheek grafts should be balanced as to outline (i.e., mirror-image units). The color of the graft to be added should match the color of the skin that will remain on the rest of the face as closely as possible, and the donor site should be chosen with this in mind. For example, if the remainder of the face is covered with abdominal skin grafts, the cheek to be recovered should also have its graft taken from the abdominal donor site. To achieve a more normal cheek skin color, the lower neck and periclavicular area is often the preferred donor site (Edgerton and Hansen, 1960). However, the secondary donor site deformity created in this esthetically important area should be carefully considered before choosing this location. If used, the area can be "puffed up" with saline injected subcutaneously with a 25 gauge spinal needle inserted at a distance away to make the skin surface flat and firm for the dermatome. In appropriate adult patients, thick split-thickness grafts taken from the scalp may provide the desired skin color. Regardless of the donor site, however, it should be "thick" to minimize contraction. In adult patients, a split-thickness graft 0.018 to 0.022 inch thick should be used for resurfacing. A thinner graft should be harvested in young children who have thinner skin, or from a previously "cropped" donor site in a patient with extensive body scarring.

A full-thickness skin graft usually contracts less than a thick split-thickness skin graft, maintains a more normal surface texture, maintains better the skin color of the donor site, and perhaps develops less hyperpigmentation after transplantation than the split-thickness graft. For these reasons, a full-thickness skin graft may at times be preferable to a split-thickness graft. However, the disadvantages of the full-thickness skin graft are a greater risk of incomplete graft "take," the greater difficulty of finding a donor site of appropriate color and size to cover a large portion (if not all) of a cheek, and the possible need for coverage of the donor site with a split-thickness graft. The surgeon must balance the advantages and disadvantages in each patient before deciding on a thick split-thickness or full-thickness skin graft. Argenta and associates (1988) have described the expansion of full-thickness skin graft donor sites to allow the harvesting of larger grafts with primary closure of the donor site.

The cheek scar to be replaced is usually excised at the dermis-fat interface. Intradermal excision with a dermatome or by dermabrasion is recommended by some, but is not generally favored by the author because of the greater risk of incomplete graft "take" associated with "overgrafting." Rather, the scarred skin is removed at the level of the fat, using needletip electrocautery to minimize bleeding. Many years of experience with the "electric knife" have demonstrated that skin graft "take" is not compromised by its use, and in fact a dry recipient "bed" with less risk of hematoma increases the chance of total graft survival. For this reason, if the recipient site is bleeding after excision despite a concerted effort at stable hemostasis, rather than chance an incomplete graft "take," consideration should be given to covering the excised area with an occlusive dressing and delaying the application of the graft for a day or two. Once applied, the graft should be carefully tailored and sutured into position, with precise edge to edge approximation. The graft should not overlap the surrounding skin. Some type of secure pressure dressing is usually preferred for a split-thickness graft, but is essential for a full-thickness skin graft (Clodius, 1977). A simple tie-over bolster dressing of Xeroform gauze and cotton secured with a wrap-around-the-head stretch bandage works nicely. Some surgeons also prefer to remove the dressing 24, 48, or 72 hours later to inspect the graft for evidence of hematomas, seromas, or purulent fluid beneath the graft, in the hope of aspirating the fluid and salvaging the overlying portion of graft. However, the author considers that with rare exceptions, there is usually little if anything to be gained by early dressing removal, and something more to be lost when pressure, protection, and immobility are surrendered prematurely. The dressing is usually left on for seven days for a split-thickness graft, and ten days for a full-thickness graft. Two weeks after grafting, the graft is usually sufficiently stable to allow application of external compression with an elasticized garment (e.g., Jobst) or customized splint (e.g., Orthoplast), which can help to prevent hypertrophy of the graft edge scars in susceptible patients.

SCAR REPLACEMENT WITH DISTANT FLAPS OR MICROVASCULAR FREE FLAPS

Flaps transferred to the face from outside the region (e.g., from the abdomen, groin, scapula, arm, or forearm) on tubed pedicles with intermediate carriers (an almost extinct procedure) or by a one-stage microvascular procedure may be an appropriate choice for facial resurfacing when local and regional flaps are unavailable. The disadvantage of these flaps taken from a distance is that they have an abnormal color that does not match a normal face. Unless thinned, either en route or after arrival, they appear bulky and may mask facial expressivity. McIndoe (1949) stated: "the patient tends to smile beneath his graft (sic)." To avoid a most unpleasant "flap patch" on the face, the full esthetic unit of the cheek should be covered. Most important, it should be clearly understood that transferring the flap onto the face alive is not itself the objective of repair—as complex as it alone may be; rather, molding and fitting the living flap so that it fits the face pleasingly is the goal. This usually requires several additional operative procedures after the flap has been placed on the cheek. Unless both the patient and the surgeon are prepared to invest the necessary time for revisions, the procedure should not be undertaken.

The Upper Lip

Second and third degree burns of the upper lip that have either healed by secondary intention or have been skin grafted often leave the lip vertically or horizontally deficient or visibly deformed from scarring (see also Chap. 38). Scar contracture of the lip and the oral commissure produces varying degrees of interference with eating, drinking, speaking, oral hygiene, and facial expressiveness. However, not all burn scars on the upper lip require surgery. Islands of hypertrophic scar resulting from second degree burns that are not producing contracture of the lip are often best left untreated until they have matured. External pressure from elasticized garments or splints, and perhaps the judicious use of steroid injections, may speed the maturation process. Given sufficient time, these scars often flatten and fade acceptably into their surroundings, although this may require several years. Nonetheless, it is often best in the long run to give the islands of scar a chance to improve on their own, rather than prematurely excising them and replacing the skin of the upper lip with a skin graft or skin flap of a different color and texture and with new edge scars. After the islands of scar have softened and flattened, they can often be improved by partial excision using local flaps and Z-plasties.

THE UPPER LIP ESTHETIC UNIT AND SUBUNITS

The upper lip has two anatomic components of different color: the *vermilion*, with its lateral segments and central tubercle; and the *skin-covered lip* above, with its lateral lip segments and central philtral dimple. The complete regional esthetic unit of the skin-covered lip is the area between the two nasolabial creases, from the vermilion margin up to the nostril sills and columella base, including the small nasojugal triangles of skin surrounding the alar lobules. The lateral lip segments are mirror-image components, reflecting the inherent symmetry of the upper lip. Therefore, when resurfacing the lip, both lateral segments should be given identical skin color and texture. The central philtrum is an esthetic subunit whose shape, length, and depth are important elements. If the philtral dimple is undamaged or its shape and vertical dimension are only slightly altered, it should always be left alone, and only the lateral lip segments resurfaced. As mentioned above in the discussion on Cheek Resurfacing, if the lateral upper lip subunit is scarred and the adjacent cheek is being resurfaced with either a skin flap or a skin graft, it may be best to resurface the upper lip with the same sheet of skin that covers the cheek, remembering that the two lateral

lip segments should be covered with identical types of tissue (both either skin graft or skin flap). In male patients the whiskered upper lip displays a color and texture not found in the hairless lip of females or in a lip that is covered with nonwhiskered skin. For this reason, a minimally scarred upper lip in a male should rarely, if ever, be excised and resurfaced with anything but a whiskered skin flap. Most men prefer to have some scarring of the upper lip rather than abandon the potential to grow even a meager mustache.

The choice of resurfacing material for the lip (skin graft or skin flap) depends in large part on what has been used to resurface the adjacent cheeks. The new lip cover should be chosen to blend as unobtrusively as possible with its surroundings (with the possible exception of adding a new mustache to a hairless lip in a male patient).

SKIN GRAFTING THE UPPER LIP

Skin graft resurfacing of a scarred upper lip (rather than skin flap resurfacing) is done (1) when the cheeks are to be permanently skin grafted and a grafted upper lip would seem to blend better than one covered with a flap; (2) as an initial approach to the correction of contracture and deformity, leaving open the option for subsequent flap resurfacing of the lip or cheek-lip complex; (3) if one side of the lip has already been skin grafted and is to be left skin grafted, i.e., to obtain overall symmetry of lip cover and texture; and (4) if the desired flap is unavailable or impractical.

A graft for the upper lip should be either a thick split-thickness (0.016 to 0.020 inch) or a full-thickness skin graft. The type of graft depends on donor site availability, donor site disfigurement, and the desired color of the graft that will match best with the rest of the face. The author generally prefers a thin full-thickness skin graft, which seems to provide a somewhat better texture and has less tendency for contraction than a thick split-thickness graft. The full-thickness skin graft donor site can almost always be closed primarily. The periclavicular skin usually yields a satisfactory color match with the nonburned facial areas. In Caucasian patients, if a slightly pinkish-colored graft is desirable, the retroauricular skin can be used. Preexpansion of the retroauricular skin may permit the harvesting of an adequate-sized graft and still allow closure of the donor site without a secondary skin graft. In older patients with facial skin laxity, a full-thickness skin graft from either the submental area or the pre-auricular area can provide a graft of desirable color and texture, with primary closure of the graft donor site. In patients who have had the rest of the face skin grafted with grafts taken from the abdomen or thighs, a full-thickness skin graft from the inguinal region or lower abdomen often blends well.

SCAR EXCISION AND SKIN GRAFT PLACEMENT

The technical aspects of resurfacing the upper lip have been described by Feldman (1987b, c). It is important that a complete lateral lip subunit be resurfaced, so that the superior border of the graft is placed high inside the nostril sill and wrapped tightly around the alar base. The little triangle of nasojugal skin beside the alar lobule should be included with the resurfacing. A well-designed Cupid's bow vermilion margin should also be outlined. A reasonably normal central lip dimple should be preserved. If it is scarred, however, central lip tissue can be elevated as a superiorly based flap and used to elongate a short columella. Scarred skin flaps elevated with a thin layer of fat and cut from the lateral lip segments and based superiorly can also be used to rebuild the alar lobules and nostril margins. When the upper lip is being resurfaced, the surgeon should always consider using scarred skin flaps for nasal base reconstruction. The needletip electric knife is useful for excising the upper lip scar. It is important that sufficient subdermal scar and soft tissue bulk be removed from the lip before laying on the new skin cover so that an unpleasant profile convexity to the lip (rather than a pleasing concave pout) is avoided.

A pattern of the excised lip is made by pressing a dry gauze sponge against the lip. The pattern, modified so that an overlong upper lip is not created, is transferred to the selected donor site. If a full-thickness skin graft is being used, it is harvested with a No. 15 scalpel blade, leaving a thin layer of deep dermis over the subcutaneous fat (in essence, this is a very thick split-thickness skin graft). The margins of the donor site can be undermined and closed primarily. The skin graft is carefully sutured into position with interrupted silk sutures that are left long at the nostril sills and columella base superiorly, and along the vermilion margin inferiorly. The sutures are cut short along the lateral edges of the graft. A tie-over "mustache" type of bolster dressing is constructed by using the long sutures from above and below. The bolster is given compression and secured with a gauze bandage that wraps circumferentially around the upper lip and occiput. The dressing is left in place for seven to ten days.

RECONSTRUCTION OF THE PHILTRUM

The reconstruction of a well-defined and lasting philtrum dimple in a diffusely scarred or skin grafted upper lip requires a rigid frame that can resist flattening. A composite skin-cartilage graft from the ear has proved to be the best way of constructing the dimple in the burned lip. The method was originally described by Schmid (1955, 1964) for secondary reconstruction of the philtrum in the bilateral cleft lip. The author (1984, 1987) has modified the technique for the burned lip. The graft is usually harvested from the fossa triangularis of the ear, but can also be taken from the concha. The cupped cartilage portion of the graft is trimmed back so that only enough cartilage remains to maintain the concave shape of the graft. Having a 1 to 2 mm cuff of full-thickness skin bordering the cartilage helps to ensure complete vascularization of the composite graft. The recipient site is prepared by excavating the soft tissues in the central upper lip, and often excising some central vermilion to create a little trough between the peaks of the Cupid's bow. The skin of the composite graft should extend from the vermilion trough below to the columella base above. A narrow dimple looks better than one that is too wide. The composite graft can be sutured into place with interrupted 5-0 silk sutures on fine needles left long to create a small tie-over bolster dressing. If the composite graft is being set into the central lip at the same time that the lateral lip segments are being resurfaced with skin grafts, the lateral edges of the composite graft can be sutured to both the medial edges of the lateral lip grafts and the deepithelized philtral columns with interrupted 6-0 chromic catgut sutures. The composite graft is covered with the same tie-over "mustache" bolster that is used to apply pressure to the lateral lip grafts. Figure 41–9 shows a patient

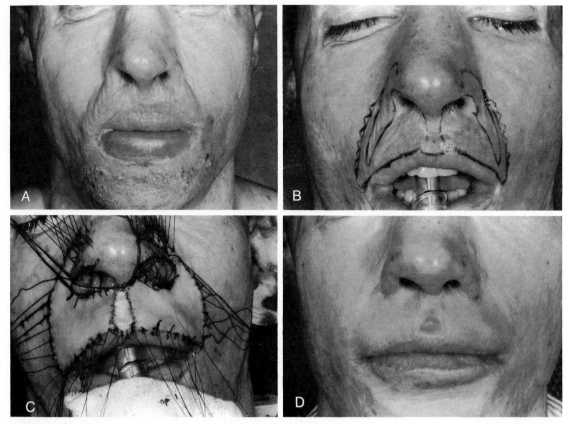

Figure 41–9. Upper lip resurfacing. *A,* Preoperative view. *B,* Scar-fat flaps from the lateral lip area outlined, to be used for rebuilding the alar bases and nostril margins. The columella-based central lip scar-fat flap is outlined for columella elongation. *C,* Lateral lip subunits (including nasojugal triangles adjacent to the nose) covered with thick split-thickness skin grafts. The philtral dimple reconstructed using a composite skin-cartilage graft from the ear. *D,* Postoperative appearance.

who had the lateral lip segments resurfaced with full-thickness skin grafts and the central dimple recreated with a composite skin-cartilage graft from the ear. A scar flap from the central upper lip was used to elongate the columella, and the scar of the lateral lip segments was fashioned into flaps to rebuild the alar margins.

SKIN FLAP RECONSTRUCTION OF THE UPPER LIP

In the uncommon situation in which the upper lip is badly scarred but the adjacent cheek is spared, some type of nasolabial or cheek flap can be used to recover the lateral lip segment. Jackson (1987) described the use of medial cheek skin expansion to generate sufficient medial cheek skin to resurface the upper lip with inferiorly based nasolabial flaps that still permit closure of the flap donor sites along the nasolabial lines. As mentioned

above in the discussion on Cheek Resurfacing, large, medially based advancement-rotation flaps from the lower cheek and neck invariably develop a dog-ear of excess flap tissue in the region of the lower lip and chin. The dog-ear can be unfurled and used to resurface the lateral upper lip area when the cheek flap is transferred upward as a secondary or tertiary procedure. In male patients, reconstruction of a mustache may be desirable. Marks and associates (1988) used a long, unilateral, superficial temporal artery island scalp flap to reconstruct the full mustache by tunneling the axial pedicle beneath the cheek skin and using preliminary scalp expansion to allow easy closure of the donor site. Walton and Bunkis (1983) reported a one-stage method of transferring a free occipital hair-bearing scalp flap to the lip with microvascular anastomoses. An occipital donor site was chosen because it seemed less vulnerable to male pattern baldness. Schmid (1954) described a bipedicle submandibular neck flap for mustache reconstruction, with primary closure of the upper neck donor site. Upper neck skin expansion can also be used to generate sufficient whiskered skin to be carried from the neck to the lip on a narrow skin pedicle (perhaps best delayed) based in the lower cheek just above the jawline. Hyakusoku and associates (1987) described a prefabricated hair-bearing neck island flap for mustache reconstruction. A long strip of superficial temporalis fascia containing the superficial temporal artery and vein was tunneled under the cheek skin to the jawline, where the superficial temporal vessels were anastomosed with the facial vessels, implanting the distal end of the vascular-fascial leash beneath the chin skin. Three weeks later, a bearded skin island flap was designed on the implanted vascular bundle and transferred through a subcutaneous cheek tunnel to the lip. For "patching-in" a section of mustache, a free hair-bearing scalp graft can be used, as demonstrated by Brent (1987).

VERMILION ADJUSTMENTS

Improvements in the appearance of the vermilion portion of the lip, either along the mucocutaneous line of the Cupid's bow or along the free border, can often be made at the time of lip resurfacing; they can also be done as independent procedures. In 1932 Gillies designed the so-called "Cupid's bow operation," which involved superior advancement of the undermined vermilion to recreate the Cupid's bow outline and to bring more vermilion into view. The Cupid's bow procedure is done at the same time as resurfacing of the upper lip. Notches and irregularities of the free border of the vermilion can be improved by Z-plasty, V-Y plasty, or local vermilion flap transpositions (see Chap. 38). A thin vermilion can be augmented by using Kesselring's technique (1985) of tunneling a deepithelized dermal strip.

The Lower Lip and Chin

Wound healing and skin graft contraction in the lower lip and chin area frequently produce eversion or ectropion of the lower lip, presenting as a protrusion of rolled-down lip vermilion and mucosa. Blunting of the sulcus between the lip and the chin adds to the

deformity and can make the chin appear small. An associated neck contracture that also obscures the cervicomental angle adds to the "pseudomicrogenia." Ectropion of the lower lip interferes with lip seal and may cause drooling. Associated scarring at the oral commissures may limit the ability to open the mouth. Eversion of the lower lip can be most distressing to the patient, both functionally and esthetically, and its correction should have a high priority.

In some patients a purely extrinsic neck scar can transmit a pull on the lower lip, causing distortion when the neck is in the neutral or extended position. In this situation, correction of the neck contracture eliminates the tug on the lip. However, if the patient's neck is placed in flexion and an upward push on the skin around the chin fails to restore the lip to a normal position, an intrinsic lip contracture exists that cannot be corrected by a neck scar release alone. In this case, more skin must be added to the lip or lip-chin area.

Except as a temporary measure to relieve lip eversion in the early postburn period, a simple scar release and skin graft addition—rather than a complete esthetic unit or subunit excision—should not be performed. Precise placement of the edges of a skin graft or skin flap to the lower lip and/or chin area is esthetically very important. The lower lip subunit is composed of two areas: the colored vermilion, and the narrow strip of skin lying transversely between the vermilion margin and the curved upper border of the chin prominence between curved lines running from the corners of the mouth downward to the sides of the chin. The small lower lip skin subunit below the vermilion is dumbbell shaped, the small isthmus of skin above the chin being quite narrow. Most attempts at resurfacing only the lower lip subunit produce a less than ideal esthetic result because the lower border of the graft or flap almost invariably winds up lying too low, i.e., across the chin prominence rather than in the depth of the lip-chin sulcus, which is only 1 cm below the central lip vermilion margin. For this reason, if the chin area is also scarred, the lower lip and chin should be resurfaced as a combined esthetic unit, placing the lower edge of the graft or flap below the mandibular border in the shadow of the chin. If the small lower lip subunit is to be resurfaced with a skin graft and the chin resurfaced with a skin flap (an unusual combination), it is best to resurface the lower lip subunit first, with the graft extending down onto the chin, and to apply the flap in a second stage, trimming away some of the excess graft over the chin and placing the upper edge of the flap precisely along the upper border of the chin prominence. In this way the small lower lip subunit is precisely covered by the skin graft, and the chin subunit is precisely covered by the flap. The combined lower lip-chin area is confined between a pair of lines that resemble parentheses, the lines extending from the corners of the mouth downward and cupping around the chin. When resurfacing either the lower lip or the lower lip-chin area alone, it is best not to extend the graft or flap beyond this area into the cheek region (as is commonly done).

When resurfacing the lower lip and chin, the area to be excised and recovered is outlined. The vermilion margin is outlined, often excising some vermilion to give a smooth and symmetric vermilion border. The area over the chin prominence is outlined as an oval to be deepithelized, to maintain the maximal chin projection. If the cheeks are skin grafted and the lower lip-chin region is also to be skin grafted, the lateral vertical borders of the lip-chin unit should be drawn as darted zigzag lines. The interdigitation of the skin grafts leaves a less conspicuous seam. Often, concomitant scar releases and small local flap transpositions are carried out at the oral commissures to correct commissure tightness. The outline of the lower lip resurfacing should be designed so as not to interfere with the small reconstructive procedures at the commissures.

The area over the chin prominence is deepithelized first, and the lower lip scar is removed with the needletip electric knife. Some subcutaneous fat and muscle tissue should be excised just above the chin prominence to create a deep and well-defined sulcus between the lip and chin. A strip of orbicularis muscle should also be excised just below the vermilion edge in order to prevent an unattractive transverse bulge (rather than the desired concavity). The recontouring of the lower lip and chin is a sculptural procedure, and the surgeon should use the needletip electric knife to carve out the contours. If the chin is small, a silicone chin implant is frequently helpful to add anterior chin projection. This can easily be done after the overlying lower lip and chin scar has been removed, so that the soft tissues over the chin can stretch to accommodate the implant. The silicone implant is inserted through the submental approach, creating a supraperiosteal pocket of adequate size. The implant should be positioned in the pocket so that it rests along the anteroinferior border of the mandible, and should be anchored in place with absorbable sutures to the periosteum. The muscle layer is carefully reapproximated over the implant. If there is fullness in the neck region below the chin, a submental lipectomy and plication of the medial borders of the platysma should be carried out to improve the esthetic contours of the anterior neck. If a skin graft is used to cover the lower lip and chin area, it should be taken from a donor site that gives a satisfactory color match with skin grafts that already cover or will cover the cheeks. A thick split-thickness skin graft is generally used. If only the small lower lip subunit is being resurfaced, a full-thickness skin graft can be harvested, with primary closure of the donor site. If the cheeks are unscarred or covered by a skin flap, it is usually best to cover the lower lip and chin area with a color-matched skin flap rather than a skin graft. At times, the flap covering the chin will be part of the larger cheek flap, as shown in Figures 41–3 and 41–8. At other times, a separate flap must be developed to cover only the lower lip-chin region. When this type of flap is used, it is important that the flap be anchored above the corners of the mouth on both sides so that there is a support sling for the vermilion margin, avoiding any downward tension on the lip from the flap. A safe maneuver is to overlap the vermilion margin with excess flap, so that the vermilion edge can be precisely inset at a secondary procedure, without risk of lower lip eversion, and with certainty that there will be sufficient flap to slide comfortably into a deepened lip-chin sulcus after an aggressive secondary defatting of the flap has been done. Figure 41–10 shows a lower lip and chin resurfaced with a delayed interpolated flap from the upper arm. At times, the chin alone can be resurfaced by creating a broad ascending neck advancement flap. This can be done by an extensive undermining of the neck skin, as shown in Figure 41–4, or by using a skin expander in the neck.

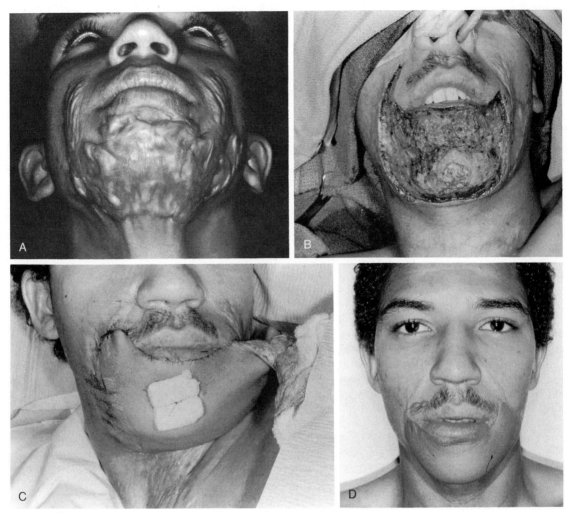

Figure 41–10. Chin and lower lip resurfacing with a delayed interpolated flap from the upper arm. *A,* Preoperative appearance. *B,* Lip-chin unit scar excised and soft tissue sculpting accomplished. *C,* Superiorly based upper arm flap turned back and rotated into position. Note the "sling" effect of the flap anchored above the corners of the mouth to support the lower lip vermilion. *D,* After pedicle division and flap defatting over the lower lip as far down as the lip-chin sulcus. The left side of the flap beyond the lateral border of the desired lip-chin esthetic unit should be excised with medial advancement of the cheek.

The Neck

Scarring of the neck produces problems with function and appearance (see also Chap. 39). The concave and highly mobile anterior neck with its thin skin cover is particularly prone to flexion contractures that can range from minimally restrictive to crippling mentosternal synechiae. An upper neck contracture often exerts a pull on the face above, causing extrinsic distortion of the lower lip, ear, nose, and cheek and possibly the lower eyelid. Scar contracture of the neck may also make endotracheal intubation for anesthesia difficult. Preoperative consultation with the anesthesiologist is recommended if there is a possibility that intubation may be difficult. This is particularly true if the anterior neck contracture is associated with scar contractures around the mouth. The surgeon and anesthesiologist should together formulate a plan for safe management of the airway, including the specific sequence of steps to be taken if intubation becomes problematic. The fiberoptic bronchoscope may be helpful for intubating the awake but well-sedated patient with a severe neck flexion contracture. Infrequently, scar contracture release may first be necessary under local anesthesia with the patient heavily sedated. Once the neck can be adequately extended, endotracheal intubation can be safely carried out and general anesthesia administered.

Severe anterior neck contractures can usually be prevented with proper splinting of the neck and timely surgical intervention in the acute phase after injury (see Chap. 23). The patient whose neck has been burned should be positioned in bed without pillows so that the neck is maintained in extension. Often, some type of soft collar or bulky dressing is helpful. A padded but rigid neck extension splint should be used if contracture begins to develop.

Surgical intervention is either made early to obtain a closed neck wound or to relieve early scar contracture; or made later as a more definitive treatment for an established contracture or to improve the appearance of the neck. In the acute or intermediate phase after burn injury, if the neck area is incompletely healed or the patient's overall condition is poor, definitive resurfacing of the neck with the best quality skin flaps or skin grafts available should be postponed, and less desirable skin grafts should be used to obtain wound closure or to improve neck function and patient comfort temporarily by skin addition. At the early procedures, neck scar releasing incisions should not transgress into the nonburned lateral neck skin, which would compromise the later use of lateral neck skin flaps. The relatively thin split-thickness skin grafts, applied in the early phase, can be expected to contract even with proper neck splinting, but if they are used specifically as a temporary approach to scar release and wound closure, their application can be justified.

The definitive or late phase treatment of neck scarring is directed at either vertical or horizontal bands of scar or broad areas of anterior neck scarring. Vertical bands are usually best treated with Z-plasties or various interdigitated local skin flaps that reorient the resulting scars into more favorable transverse or oblique directions. When Z-plasties are carried out, there are always two choices of design, depending on the orientation of the side limbs of the Z. The proper design is one that places the side limbs along the relaxed skin tension lines of the neck (i.e., as close to transverse rather than vertical as possible). The Z-plasty flaps should be cut thickly, with

subcutaneous fat on the undersurface of the flaps, particularly at the distal tips. Z-plasties carried out within scar can be done successfully if the flaps are incised as described. However, some flap tip necrosis is often seen. These areas usually heal satisfactorily with a smoother, more comfortable neck than would have been achieved with only a skin graft addition. Small skin grafts always contract despite splinting and result in both a functional and an esthetic disappointment. Figure 41–11 illustrates a local interdigitated flap for the treatment of vertical linear bands on the neck. Horizontal bands of scar can usually be removed in one or more stages with extensive skin undermining and adjacent flap advancement (see Fig. 41–4). This technique is discussed below in the section on Ascending Neck-Chest Advancement Flaps.

Broad areas of neck scarring with contracture are treated by transverse incisional release (i.e., without scar excision) and skin addition (skin graft or skin flap), or by scar excision followed by skin addition. The choice between scar release or scar excision depends on the quality of the neck skin surface.

Irregular, hypertrophic scars should be excised. Flat, smooth, but tight neck scars can be simply released. From the standpoint of appearance, resurfacing of the complete esthetic unit of the anterior neck with a single piece of skin (either a graft or flap) of uniform color and texture gives a better result. From a functional point of view, large thick skin grafts generally seem to contract less than do narrow thick skin grafts. The reason for this is unclear, but nonetheless it is a phenomenon repeatedly observed.

The general approach to neck scarring is the same as that for the cheek; i.e., small- to moderate-sized areas of scarring should be removed and the defect closed with local skin flaps. The large areas of neck scarring should be replaced with either regional skin flaps or thick skin grafts. In certain cases, a combination of local skin flaps and thick split-thickness skin grafts is appropriate. If neck scar contracture release is carried out rather than scar excision, a single releasing incision is made transversely at the tightest point of neck scarring, or two transverse releasing incisions can be made—one in the region of the hyoid bone to produce a desirable definition of the cervicomandibular angle, and a second releasing incision in the supraclavic-

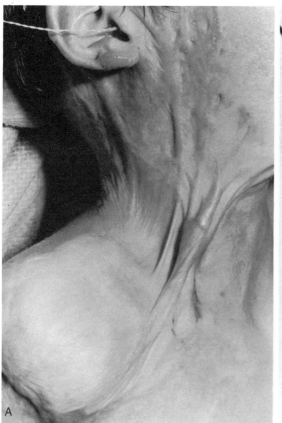

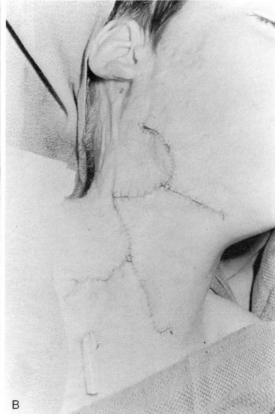

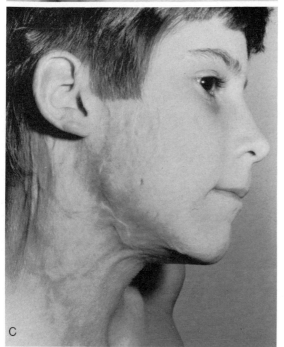

Figure 41–11. Correction of a vertical linear neck scar band with local interdigitated skin flaps. *A,* Preoperative appearance. *B,* After flap transposition. *C,* Postoperative appearance. (From Feldman, J. J.: Reconstruction of the burned face in children. *In* Serafin, D., and Georgiade, N. G.: Pediatric Plastic Surgery. St. Louis, C. V. Mosby Company, 1984.)

ular region to enhance neck extension. This leaves two areas to be covered with skin, with an intervening bridge of scarred skin over the central neck. After the initial releasing incisions are made with the scalpel, it is helpful to use the needletip electric knife for the deeper scar release so that a meticulous hemostasis is maintained.

If the platysma is not heavily involved with scar, it should not be incised. If the platysma is involved, it should be lightly cut at different levels so that a smooth, flat bed is left for coverage by a graft or flap. While postoperative neck function is of primary importance, the appearance of the neck must be kept in mind at all times. Unfortunately, neck scar releasing incisions are often made too deeply at one level, creating an unsightly transverse cleft in the neck. The releasing incisions should extend across the full width of the anterior neck scar, with the lateral ends of the incisions designed as a reclining Y to avoid vertical graft edges that are prone to recurrent contracture. The unscarred lateral neck skin should not be incised unless the surgeon is absolutely certain that this neck skin will not be subsequently used for flap harvesting. If the surgeon is certain of this, the lateral, vertical margins of the wound on each side of the neck can be interrupted by making one arm of a Z-plasty and transposing it from a vertical to a transverse position, with the other arm of the Z-plasty formed by the skin graft. To obtain the optimal postoperative appearance of the neck, a submandibular and submental lipectomy is often useful, removing the subcutaneous fat overlying the platysma muscle. This maneuver helps to define the jawline and the cervicomandibular angle. Vertical midline plication and paramedian platysma plication also is often helpful in improving neck contour before a skin graft or skin flap is applied. When large areas of the neck are to be resurfaced with a skin graft, meticulous hemostasis is essential; if not, delayed skin grafting at 24 to 48 hours is prudent. The most common reason for graft loss is hematoma formation. Split-thickness skin grafts used for definitive neck resurfacing should be thick (0.018 to 0.022 inch) to reduce the tendency for secondary graft contraction. The Reese dermatome is helpful in taking a large graft (4 × 6 inches) of uniform thickness. The Padgett electric dermatome can be used to harvest longer lengths of skin.

The fewer the number of graft pieces used, the better. Careful edge to edge approximation of the graft to the recipient wound margin should be done to avoid unattractive ridges around the graft. The grafts can be secured with either interrupted or running sutures, scattered interrupted silk sutures being left long to tie over a large gauze and cotton bolster dressing. The tie-over sutures usually are placed only superiorly and inferiorly along the wound edges and not along the lateral margins on each side, since the bolster seems to conform better to the neck if it is wrapped on circumferentially with a gauze bandage. This appears to hold the sides of the dressing down in position better than sutures on the sides. The tie-over bolster dressing is preferred to the "open treatment," when definitive grafting is done, in order to ensure graft contact with the irregularities of the bed and to discourage small hematomas and seromas. If the cotton is moistened with saline, it allows the dressing to mold more precisely to the underlying neck contours, but cotton should be dry and soft over the larynx (thyroid cartilage) to prevent pressure necrosis or abrasion in this area. The sutures above and below should not be tied so tightly that they pull upward on the skin graft, which could cause some tearing or tenting of the graft; the sutures should be used only to hold the bolster in position. The wrap-around gauze bandage is what should be used to compress the cotton dressing against the skin graft and the underlying bed.

Postoperatively, the neck should be maintained in extension. This is often done with either a small, soft towel or a blanket roll placed transversely beneath the shoulders. In the immediate postoperative period, sandbags placed on either side of the head can be used to prevent patients from turning the head from side to side until they are sufficiently awake to be cooperative. Flexing the entire back of the bed upward allows patients to see and take oral fluids and soft foods by mouth while still maintaining the neck in extension. Some surgeons have advocated the removal of the neck dressing 24 to 48 hours after surgery to examine for hematomas, seromas, or infection, but the author believes that there is more to be gained and less to be lost by leaving the dressing intact and undisturbed for seven to ten days. If there are small hematomas or seromas or purulence beneath the graft, their removal a day or two after graft application rarely improves graft "take" in these areas. On the other hand, early removal of the dressing may permit fluid extravasation beneath a precariously adherent graft, allow for microvascular congestion within a thick skin graft, expose the graft to external trauma, and allow the patient an undesired amount of early neck mobility. Unless neck grafting is done in the acute phase for simple wound closure in a contaminated environment (in which case early examination of the graft may well be appropriate), the dressing should be left in place for seven to ten days. When the bolster dressing is removed, it is important that the neck be immediately resplinted to prevent graft contraction (see Chap. 39). A contoured and customized rigid splint is preferable. While it is being fabricated, a soft neck extension splint can be worn. The neck splinting should be carried out even if there are some raw spots on the graft. When the rigid neck extension splint is applied, it should be removed at frequent intervals during the first 24 to 48 hours to ensure that it is not eroding or abrading the skin graft. Modification of the splint may be necessary to avoid trauma to the new graft. The customized rigid neck extension splint must be worn continuously day and night for a minimum of six months after neck skin grafting. After that time, it may be possible to discontinue the splint for periods, but at the earliest sign of contracture the splint must be reapplied and again worn continuously until the tendency for contracture and graft shrinkage has passed. A gradual weaning from the splint is the usual course; it often needs to be worn for a year or longer.

For the treatment of neck contractures from scar covering the entire anterior neck, Cronin (1961) demonstrated the effectiveness of total scar excision, delayed skin grafting with a thick split-thickness skin graft, and the prolonged postoperative use of a custom-fitted collar to maintain extension, molding, and pressure on the skin grafted neck. However, for subtotal neck scarring, Cronin recommended the use of local flaps, when available, rather than thick skin grafts, believing that flaps contract less than splinted skin grafts. It is the author's opinion that regional flaps to the neck behave better in terms of function and appearance than skin grafts.

LOCAL AND REGIONAL SKIN FLAPS FOR NECK RESURFACING

Local and regional skin flaps used to replace neck scar provide a good color and texture match with the unscarred areas on the neck—the exception, of course, being the absence of the beard in flaps harvested from outside the whiskered neck area itself. Skin flaps do not contract as do skin grafts, and so require no postoperative neck splinting, an added comfort and convenience to the patient. The long-term result of a flap reconstruction of the neck is therefore more predictable than that of a skin graft. Often, there is an adequate amount of unscarred skin in the neighborhood of the neck (i.e., the lateral neck, upper chest, shoulders, and upper back) to permit neck resurfacing with matched and pliable skin (Janvier and Colin, 1972). If the neck scarring is contained within the anterior borders of the sternomastoid muscles, with the surrounding skin unscarred, the entire central anterior neck can often be resurfaced by using bilateral flaps with primary closure of the flap donor sites, thus avoiding the secondary deformity of a skin graft at the donor site.

VERTICAL TO TRANSVERSE FLAP TRANSPOSITION

A neck that is tight in the vertical direction (the usual situation) may have sufficient laxity in the horizontal direction to permit the use of unilateral or bilateral vertical neck flaps transposed from the sides across the neck, to correct the vertical deficiency and allow the flap donor sites to be closed primarily (Mir y Mir, 1969; Jabaley, Cat, and Lac, 1971). The unscarred skin on one or both sides of the neck is pinched with the surgeon's fingers to determine how wide a flap can be taken that still allows closure of the flap donor site. The superiorly based flap is elevated and rotated into a transverse position. The neck scar is released or excised and the flap inset. When bilateral flaps are used, crisscrossing the triangular flaps in the central neck gives wider coverage and also avoids vertical seams. A Z-plasty along the vertical line of the donor site should be performed either at the time of flap transposition or at a later time to interrupt the vertical scar, which could contract or hypertrophy. A dog-

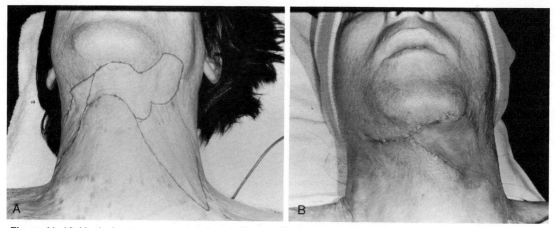

Figure 41–12. Vertical-to-transverse neck flap. *A,* Submandibular skin graft outlined for excision and a superiorly based vertical left neck flap marked. *B,* After a secondary procedure to remove a small remaining patch of right submental skin graft. The vertical neck scar resulting from the earlier flap donor site closure is inconspicuous in this patient.

ear at the flap rotation point may also be trimmed later on. Figure 41–12 illustrates a vertical-to-transverse flap transposition for removal of the upper neck skin graft.

BILOBED FLAPS

Two V-shaped lobes are designed on the neck, chest, or shoulder, the design depending on the distribution of unscarred or minimally scarred skin and surrounding tissue laxity. The two lobes are designed with a common base located superiorly on the lateral neck or upper shoulder region. The width of each lobe is determined by pinching the skin with the fingers to make sure that the donor sites will close. At times the more posterior lobe is used to fill the defect remaining after transposition of the anterior lobe. In some cases it may be possible to bring both lobes together so that they lie side by side on the anterior neck, with both lobe donor sites closed primarily. To be certain that this is possible, the skin bordering the prospective lobes should be pinched with the fingers of both of the surgeon's hands at the same time to ensure that there is enough stretch in the intervening tissues between the two lobes to allow the two donor sites to close simultaneously. If not, one or more of the lobes will have to be repositioned or reduced in width. If the anterior neck between the medial edges of the sternocleidomastoid muscles is scarred and the lateral neck and shoulder region is unscarred on both sides, bilateral bilobed flaps can provide total or near-total anterior neck

resurfacing. For the bilobed flap, the anterior lobe often extends inferiorly on the lateral neck into the infraclavicular region, or a wide lobe can be taken from the loose skin anterior to the deltopectoral groove, leaving a linear donor site scar in the anterior axillary fold. The posterior lobe is often designed as a transverse shoulder flap extending onto the deltoid area. The anterior lobe (cervicopectoral lobe) often rotates 90 degrees, and the shoulder lobe frequently turns nearly 180 degrees. One or more dog-ears invariably develop around the rotation points, and these are trimmed at a later time. The flaps should be incised, transferred, interdigitated, and sutured in place over the neck scar, and the donor site(s) are closed before the neck scar is excised, so that an accurate measure of the amount of scar that can be removed and resurfaced can be made. Figure 41–13 illustrates a patient who underwent bilateral bilobed flap reconstruction for resurfacing the anterior neck.

LATERALLY BASED ADVANCEMENT FLAPS

Pennant-shaped and laterally based flaps of unscarred skin can often be designed and transferred medially across the neck as another method of shifting normal skin from the lateral to the anterior neck region. In order to allow the flaps to expand completely, the attachments of the skin to the underlying sternocleidomastoid muscles must be cut. The distal ends of the flaps are overlapped, one

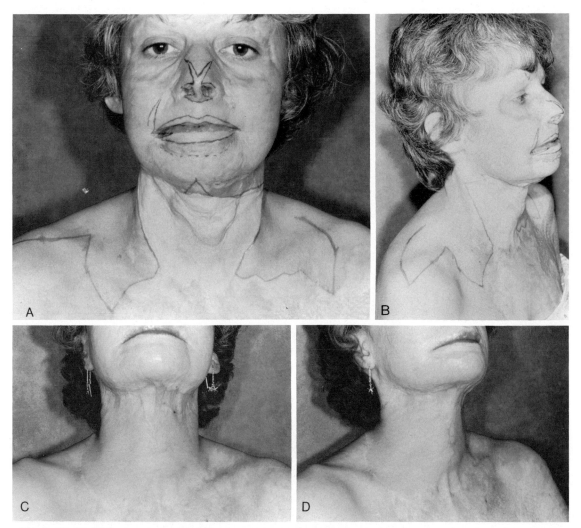

Figure 41–13. Bilobed neck-shoulder flaps for anterior neck resurfacing. *A, B,* Preoperative views with flaps outlined. Note the "skeletonized" neck covered with hypopigmented skin grafts. *C, D,* Postoperative views with the interdigitated bilateral bilobed flaps covering the neck. The flap donor sites were closed primarily without skin grafts.

above the other, to give an interdigitated closure in the front of the neck (Fig. 41–14).

COMBINATION OF LOCAL FLAPS AND SKIN GRAFTS

When the entire anterior neck needs to be resurfaced, but a limited amount of local flap tissue is available, bilobed flaps or laterally based flaps from each side can be used in combination with skin grafts. The rationale for this combination is that some skin flap is better than none. Usually it is better to position the better looking and more stretchable flap tissue in the central portion of the neck, and the less pleasing and more inelastic skin grafts above (in the submental area) and below (in the supraclavicular area) (Fig. 41–

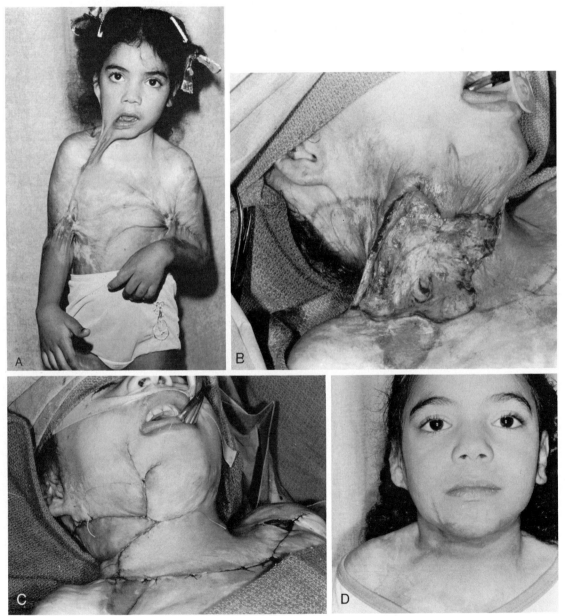

Figure 41–14. Laterally based neck advancement flaps. *A,* Preoperative view with a neck scar bridging from the jaw to the axilla. *B,* After scar excision, with a laterally based right neck flap outlined above the defect and a laterally based left neck flap outlined below the defect. *C,* After flap advancement and crisscross closure. Note the small skin gap at the left shoulder where the flap was back-cut. This was dressed and allowed to close secondarily. The pleated scar along the jaw line was excised and closed primarily. *D,* Postoperative view.

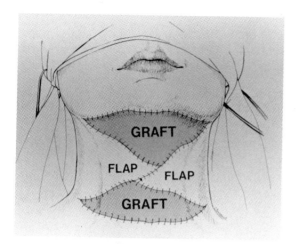

Figure 41–15. Combined use of lateral neck advancement flaps and skin grafts for neck resurfacing. The better looking and more elastic flaps are crisscrossed over the more visible central neck, and the skin grafts are placed in the less conspicuous shadow areas below the chin or above the clavicles. When possible the submandibular skin graft should be excised later.

15). When flaps and grafts are used together, there are many seams and edges. All the join lines should be oriented transversely or obliquely in order to avoid scars that might hypertrophy or contract.

SHOULDER FLAPS

Unilateral or bilateral "random-pattern" skin flaps based superiorly in the mastoid-occipital region (Mutter, 1842) can be used effectively for neck resurfacing. Anterior trapezius musculocutaneous flaps have also been used, but the author finds that the incorporation of a small amount of muscle at the base of the flap does not significantly augment the blood supply to the main random-pattern portion of the flap, and risks injury to the spinal accessory nerve (XI). For these reasons, the anterior trapezius musculocutaneous flap is not recommended. Shoulder flaps with a width of 5 cm can usually have their donor sites closed primarily with a linear scar along the anterior border of the trapezius muscle. Wider flaps (used in the patient shown in Fig. 41–16) need to have the flap donor site covered with a split-thickness skin graft, or the donor site can be "expanded." Long random-pattern shoulder flaps should have a preliminary delay or two. There is always a large dog-ear at the flap rotation point, which uselessly takes up a significant

length of the proximal flap, and is one reason why a transverse shoulder flap is not an efficient flap for neck resurfacing. If bilateral shoulder flaps are used, they should be interdigitated to avoid a vertical scar along the front of the neck, which invariably contracts and hypertrophies. Shoulder flaps raised just above the muscular fascia are often thick and usually require several subsequent debulking procedures for flap thinning, repositioning, and dog-ear excision. The author prefers to use bilobed flaps (as described above) if available, with one narrow lobe coming from the shoulder region and one from the upper chest, rather than using one wide-lobed shoulder flap, which is more difficult to transfer and may require an undesirable skin graft or skin expansion at the donor site.

ASCENDING NECK-CHEST ADVANCEMENT FLAPS

Scars lying transversely across the neck can often be removed and replaced with unscarred skin from the lower neck and upper anterior chest by using an ascending advancement flap. If the scar is narrow, it can be excised and the defect closed in one procedure. Broader scars require repeated partial excisions and sequential flap advancement. The patient shown in Figure 41–17 had the entire skin grafted area on the neck removed and replaced with flap skin from the anterior chest in three successive procedures at intervals of two weeks. At each procedure additional undermining of the anterior chest skin was carried out in a plane superficial to the pectoral fascia (eventually reaching the areolae of the breast) with staged excision. The older method of creating a large transverse bipedicle flap, using a releasing incision at the inferior border of the flap with the insertion of a skin graft below the flap, is unnecessary. Sequential advancement is a procedure that takes advantage of both the viscoelastic properties of skin and the "delay" phenomenon in bringing a broad mobilized flap of skin into an adjacent area. In a sense, it is a form of skin expansion without use of a subcutaneous expander implant.

EXPANDED SKIN FLAPS

See the discussion on skin expansion in the above section on Cheek Resurfacing. The placement of expanders under unscarred

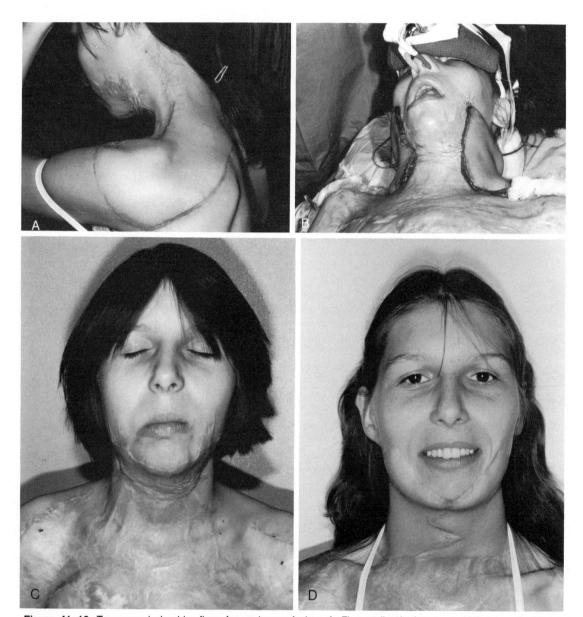

Figure 41–16. Transposed shoulder flaps for neck resurfacing. *A,* Flap outlined after a surgical delay. *B,* Bilateral shoulder flaps temporarily tacked to the sides of the neck prior to anterior neck and lower cheek scar excision. *C, E,* Preoperative views. *D, F,* Postoperative views after flap defatting and midline zigzag flap closure. In this case the wide flap donor sites had to be skin grafted. Use of "expanded" flaps would permit primary closure of the shoulder donor sites.

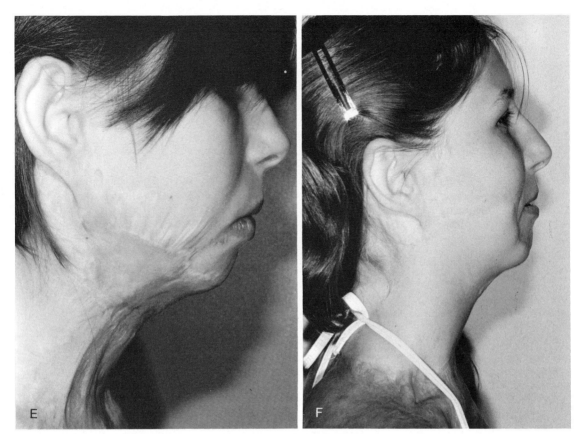

Figure 41–16 *Continued*

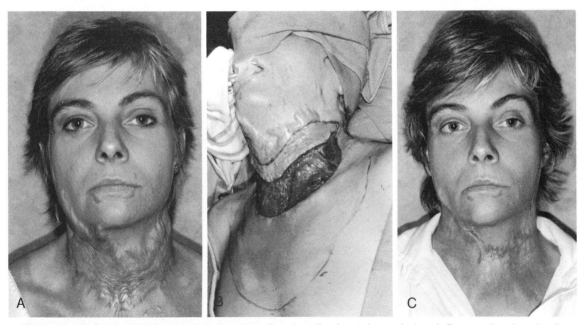

Figure 41–17. Sequential advancement of an ascending chest flap for neck resurfacing. *A,* Preoperative view showing rippled and pigmented skin graft covering most of the anterior neck. *B,* At the first procedure, through a transverse incision along the lower edge of the neck scar, the anterior chest skin was undermined to the superior aspect of the breasts and the chest flap advanced upward, allowing removal of one-third to one-half of the neck scar. *C,* After the last of three flap advancements done at two week intervals. The chest skin flap had been undermined down to the areolae of the breasts. All the neck scar was removed. A final scar revision is planned.

areas of the neck, shoulders (Spence, 1988), chest, and upper back can provide enlarged flaps for neck coverage.

TUBE FLAPS

Regional tube flaps harvested from areas of the chest, upper arms, or back that are not immediately adjacent to the neck can be used effectively for neck resurfacing. The method used is the same as that discussed in the section on Cheek Resurfacing. Fahmy (1985) extensively used and described the use of tube flaps from the back in the treatment of anterior neck contractures.

MICROVASCULAR FREE FLAPS

Free flaps can be used for replacement of neck scar by means of microvascular techniques if local or regional flap tissue is unavailable and if it is considered that coverage by a distant flap has advantages over a skin grafted neck. Microvascular free flaps taken from a distance have, of course, a different color and texture surface from that of normal neck skin. It is important that a sufficiently large flap be applied to the neck so that the visible esthetic area of the neck in clothing is completely covered with the flap, to avoid a patched appearance. Unfortunately, the dorsalis pedis and forearm free flaps, which are relatively thin and have a better color than lateral thigh, groin, or parascapular flaps, are of limited size and cannot cover the entire anterior neck (Kobus, 1988). Free flaps are really not "one-stage procedures," because they always require one or more secondary procedures for defatting and peripheral scar revision (Fig. 41–18).

The Nose

Because the nose is central and projecting, it is commonly injured in facial burns. The disfigurement associated with distortion of the alar margins, nasal tip, and columella is particularly distressing. Other than an altered surface texture or discoloration, the skin burned nose may look normal for several weeks after injury. Only when the eschar separates and the wound begins to heal by contraction and reepithelization does the deformity insidiously but relentlessly begin to appear. Surface wound contraction produces

elevation of the alar margins and nasal tip; over time, more and more nostril and vestibule are visible on frontal view. A scarred and shortened columella can be pulled tight by the retracting forces. If the upper lip is also burned (as is commonly the case), the angle between the columella and the lip may flatten to an almost straight line on profile view. Full-thickness skin injury to structures around the nasal base and tip that leaves cartilage exposed to desiccation, as well as deeper burns with direct cartilage thermal injury, imposes an even greater deformity. On the dorsum of the nose, however, the thermal injury usually involves only skin, and the underlying skeleton and nasal lining most often escape injury. The healing of extensive central facial burns with or without skin grafts may leave the nose looking flat, with apparent loss of dorsal nasal support, but dorsal projection is usually restored after the taut overlying scar has been removed.

Appropriate correction of the nasal burn deformity depends on both an accurate diagnosis of the problem and an understanding that the nasal repair must be seen in the context of the repair of the rest of the face. In terms of diagnosis, a careful study of the patient's photographs with overlay drawings helps to delineate the amount of nasal tip that needs to be rebuilt, and also displays abnormalities of dorsal height, malposition of alar lobules, and the relationship of the nose and columella to the upper lip. An innovative approach to the nasal reconstruction should develop as a result of leisurely examination of clinical photographs. As for the nose in relation to the rest of the face, it should be kept in mind that the skin covering the nose should match the skin color and texture that will either remain permanently or will be surgically placed on the rest of the face. If the face is to remain skin grafted, the nose should be grafted with matched skin. If the face is to be skin flapped, it may be best to apply a skin flap to the nose of similar color and texture. When nasal resurfacing is indicated, with either graft or flap, the complete esthetic unit of the nose or the appropriate esthetic subunits (see Fig. 41–1) should be covered so that a patched effect is minimized. In rare cases in which the nasal tip region is uninjured and only the dorsum of the nose is scarred, only the dorsal esthetic subunit need be resurfaced from the radix to the cephalic border of the alar cartilages. When the dor-

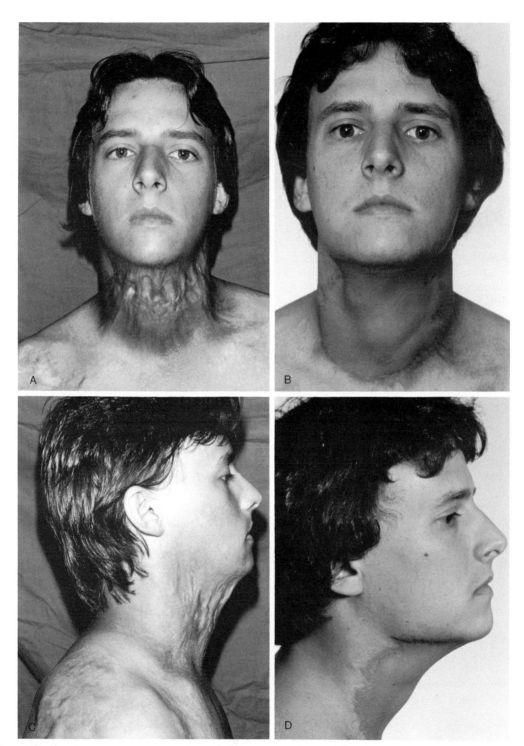

Figure 41–18. Microvascular free groin flap for neck resurfacing. *A, C,* Preoperative views. *B, D,* Postoperative views after several flap defattings. (Courtesy of Dr. Donald Serafin. From Feldman, J. J.: Reconstruction of the burned face in children. *In* Serafin, D., and Georgiade, N. G. (Eds.): Pediatric Plastic Surgery. St. Louis, C. V. Mosby Company, 1984.)

sum is unscarred but the nasal tip or alae require resurfacing, it may be appropriate to resurface only these subunits. In most cases, however, the complete esthetic unit of the nose should be resurfaced with a single sheet of uniform skin. If the alar margins are minimally retracted and the nasal tip has adequate projection, margin releasing incisions made just above the alar edges allow the margins to roll down prior to total nasal scar excision and resurfacing. If the nasal tip lacks projection, and if both the tip and the bridge of the nose require resurfacing, the dorsal soft tissues can be deepithelized and advanced distally as a flap toward the tip, or the tip-based flap(s) can be turned backward to augment the tip before laying on the graft or flap (Feldman, 1984). If cartilaginous nasal tip augmentation is required for rebuilding a tightly scarred tip, a thin skin flap cover will be required.

When a midline forehead flap is available, it is usually the preferred choice (see Chap. 37). If only a narrow flap is required for dorsal resurfacing, the forehead donor site can be closed directly. If only the nasal tip needs cover, the midline forehead flap can be somersaulted over backward in two stages, as described by Juri and associates (1985). When a wider midline forehead flap is required for either nasal bridge coverage or nasal tip and alar coverage, a subcutaneous forehead skin expander is an excellent technique of generating a sufficiently large flap to permit both total nasal resurfacing and primary closure of the forehead donor site (Adamson, 1988; Manders, Farvey, and Davis, 1986; Bolton, Chandrasekhar, and Gottlieb, 1988). Even if the forehead has been skin grafted or is scarred but the underlying frontalis muscle layer is intact, an expanded forehead flap can be used to provide a new nasal cover with a color and texture that matches the scarred or grafted face. The tissue expander should be inserted into a subgaleal (subfrontalis) position, and not placed in a subcutaneous pocket where the thin overlying skin flap can be more easily eroded by a knuckle in the expander shell. The dissection of a subcutaneous pocket is also more difficult, and hematoma formation is a risk. The reason given by some authors for placement of the midline expander in the subcutaneous plane is that without the muscle layer, a thinner flap can be generated that drapes more easily over the nasal framework. However, the scar tissue capsule that forms around the subcutaneous expander often requires excision in the distal portion of the flap to thin the flap adequately. The subcutaneous position offers little benefit and far greater risk than the subfrontalis position. When using an expanded forehead flap, a longer and broader flap than may appear necessary should be generated by the expansion, not only because the flap undergoes immediate contraction after the expander has been removed, but also because "extra" flap is usually needed to cover a newly augmented nasal tip and nasal base. A Doppler probe is useful for tracing the supratrochlear artery alongside the nose. After the vessel location has been marked, the flap can be elevated on a narrow pedicle to give the flap adequate mobility. It is best to include an axial vessel in the flap's pedicle, but McCarthy and associates (1985) demonstrated with injection studies in cadavers that the median forehead flap can be adequately supplied without incorporating the supratrochlear vessels. This was confirmed clinically by Guan, Wang, and Zhang (1988), who successfully used expanded skin grafted median forehead flaps on narrow random-pattern pedicles. Nonetheless, it is safer to include a pulsatile vessel in the base if possible. Expanded forehead flaps usually remain stiff and edematous for several months after surgery, so that both patient and surgeon should expect a waiting period before final nasal contours begin to appear. A patient in whom total nasal resurfacing was accomplished with an expanded forehead flap is illustrated in Figure 41–19. In this case, nasal tip augmentation was achieved with distal advancement of a delayed and deepithelized dorsal flap and onlay conchal cartilage grafts, over which the forehead flap was applied. Feldman (1988) discussed the use of an eccentric forehead flap when only one side of the forehead is available.

When flap coverage of the nose is required, but the forehead is so deeply scarred that a forehead flap is not available, the Tagliacozzi flap from the upper arm can be used, as described by Miller (1985). Once on the nose, if the skin color of the arm flap is not a good match with the rest of the face, the skin can be removed and replaced with a better color-matched skin graft. This type of distant flap, however, is not commonly needed for the treatment of the burned nose. Even in patients who appear to have considerable alar

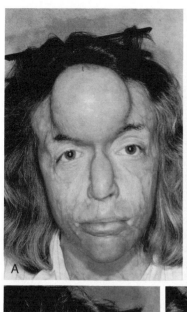
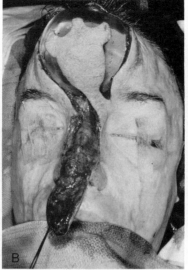
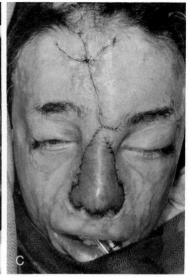

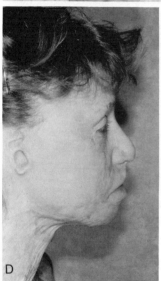
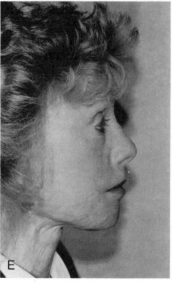

Figure 41–19. Nasal reconstruction with an expanded, previously skin grafted midline forehead flap. To provide the needed augmentation to the tightly scarred nasal tip, flap coverage was necessary. *A,* The expander in a subfrontalis muscle pocket introduced through a radial incision in the frontal scalp. *B,* A previously delayed total dorsal nasal flap is hinged at the nasal tip before being deepithelized and contoured to provide soft tissue augmentation for the tip. A conchal cartilage graft was added on top of the deepithelized flap to provide additional tip support. The forehead flap has been incised with a narrow pedicle containing the angular artery. *C,* Forehead flap transposed for complete nasal esthetic unit resurfacing. The forehead donor site was closed primarily. *D, E,* Preoperative and postoperative profiles.

margin and tip loss, local tissues can usually be redistributed to make up for what seems to be missing. Retracted alae can be corrected at the same time as an upper lip resurfacing, using scar-covered lip flaps that are based superiorly at the alar lobule and rotated into releasing incisions along the nostril margins. The scarred flaps should be elevated with some underlying subcutaneous fat to preserve a subdermal blood supply. To ensure their survival, they are best "delayed" a week or two before transposition. Scarred flaps from the upper lip can also be used to rebuild the alar lobule itself, or advanced upward from the central lip to elongate a shortened columella. If the cheek is to be resurfaced, naso-

labial flaps can be used for both alar lobule and alar margin reconstruction (Spear, Kroll, and Romm, 1987; Hauben and Sagi, 1987). For the notched alar margin, various types of local advancement-rotation flaps can be used (Juri and associates, 1985; Thompson and Sleightholm, 1985). If the retracted alar margin is smoothly arched and the nose is skin graft covered, a composite skin-cartilage graft harvested from the posterior aspect of the ear can be used. The alar margin is released with a curved skin incision in the alar crease that extends medially into the tip as far as needed. If further downward mobilization of the margin is required, the incision is deepened between the lateral crus of the alar cartilage and the caudal border of the upper lateral cartilage, leaving the underlying mucous membrane intact. The nasal lining can then be undermined superiorly and peeled away from the deep surface of the upper lateral cartilage. The lining is incised transversely across the area where the upper lateral cartilage slips beneath the nasal bone. The nasal lining is then pulled inferiorly. A long, crescent-shaped composite skin-cartilage graft from the ear is used to fill the defect. The graft sits on the repositioned but intact nasal lining, with the "releasing window" in the lining concealed beneath the skin and cartilage above. The remaining raw surface within the nose reepithelizes in a short time (Ohura, 1974). Major defects of the alar nasi that involve all layers (skin, cartilage support, and internal lining) require other methods of repair (Burget, 1985; Burget and Menick, 1985, 1986; Barton, 1988; Millard, 1988) (see also Chap. 37).

Many of the deformities to the nasal base (alar margins, columella, and nasal tip) associated with burns can be repaired by the same techniques that are applied to the cleft lip nasal deformity (see Chap. 56). The overall esthetic result of facial reconstruction can often be enhanced by incorporating a "cosmetic rhinoplasty" (see Chap. 35).

The Ear

Isolated burns of the ears are uncommon and usually result from either thermal or chemical contact injury. However, when associated with burn injury to other areas of the body, burns of the ear are common. Over a seven-year period, 52.7 per cent of all patients admitted to the U.S. Army Institute of Surgical Research Burn Unit (Mills and associates, 1988) sustained burns of one or both ears. Two types of thermal damage to the external ear can occur. The first type is partial- or full-thickness burn with or without direct thermal injury to the cartilage. Superficial second degree burns of the thin skin covering the ear usually heal with little if any deformity. Hypertrophic scars or keloids, however, may develop in certain patients with an underlying genetic proclivity. In third degree burns, the ear skin exposes segments of underlying auricular cartilage, leading to desiccation of the cartilage and areas of focal necrosis. Whether by direct thermal

injury or by desiccation, the eschar of nonviable skin and cartilage usually separates with an underlying fibrovascular tissue bed that ordinarily heals without infection. Depending on the location and extent of the injury, the ear heals with either a localized and minor deformity or a severe deformity. When the injury to skin and cartilage is extensive, severe deformity usually cannot be prevented. However, a successful salvage of the ear cartilage using a platysma musculocutaneous flap was reported by McGrath and Ariyan (1978). Within four hours after admission, the patient (who had a contact burn of the skin covering the entire anterior aspect of the ear) was taken to the operating room, where the skin over the anterior ear surface was excised and the flap applied. Thirteen days later the bulk of the flap was removed, leaving a thin layer of platysma muscle covering the cartilage (the "crane principle"). The platysma muscle on the cartilage was then covered with a split-thickness skin graft. Other authors have suggested using an immediate turn-over temporoparietal fascial flap to salvage the ear cartilage, but the surgeon must be mindful that the fascia may represent the last best option for secondary ear reconstruction (see below), and therefore may prudently not wish to sacrifice the fascia in an attempt at acute salvage. The compromise, however, might be to use the postauricular fascia as a turn-over flap, saving the superior temporoparietal fascia for later use if necessary.

The second type of auricular cartilage damage is suppurative chondritis, which involves secondary infection of the cartilage. In the burn population studied by Mills and associates (1988), this process most commonly occurred three to five weeks after the burn. These authors found that it was not possible to predict which burned ears would develop chondritis with infection occurring in both superficial partial-thickness burns and full-thickness injuries. They observed that most patients with full-thickness burns of the ear and exposed cartilage did not develop chondritis. In ears with partial-thickness injury, suppurative chondritis at times developed even after reepithelization had occurred. Ninety-five per cent of the cultures yielded *Pseudomonas* and 55 per cent yielded *Staphylococcus*. Suppurative chondritis is typically characterized by dull ear pain that increases in intensity in a matter of hours. The ear becomes warm, erythematous, swollen, and exquisitively tender, particularly when pressure is applied behind the ear in the auriculocephalic angle. Inflammation usually starts along the helix or anthelix and may progress to involve the entire ear. A fluctuant area is sometimes noted on the anterior surface of the ear and may drain spontaneously. Drainage may expose necrotic cartilage in the abscess cavity. Tenderness subsides with drainage of the abscess, but may recur with the spread of the infection.

Suppurative chondritis of the ear is better prevented than treated. The most important preventive measure is strict avoidance of pressure on the injured ear (Grant, Finley, and Coers, 1969) and effective topical chemotherapy to control bacterial proliferation, primarily from *Pseudomonas* species. Systemic antibiotic prophylaxis does not appear to influence the course.

During the study interval from 1967 to 1984 reported by Mills and associates (1988), the incidence of suppurative chondritis decreased from 20 to less than 3 per cent in patients with burns of one or both ears. The crucial factors causing the improvement related to the avoidance of pressure and the use of topical mafenide acetate burn cream (see Chap. 23).

A number of approaches are advocated for the treatment of suppurative chondritis. Wanamaker (1972) used polyethylene drains both anteriorly and posteriorly for antibiotic irrigation with polymyxin B solution every two to three hours for four to five days. Greminger and associates (1980) advocated iontophoresis, the migration of charged ions of antibiotics in an electric field. Gentamicin-soaked gauze was placed on the infected ear along with an electrode, and another electrode was placed on the back. A current of 10 to 15 mA was applied for 20 to 60 minutes twice a day. Stroud (1963, 1978) reported that excision and drainage usually resulted in reappearance of the infection in one to two weeks. This occurred because the cartilage of the ear prevented collapse of the abscess cavity obliterating the dead space. Stroud proposed excision of the abscess cavity and underlying necrotic cartilage, leaving the posterior skin intact. Subsequent wound granulation and epithelization could then take place. However, no comparisons of the recurrence or duration of the disease were reported. Spira and Hardy (1963) recommended an extensive incision, filleting the ear open, with drainage and moist packing immediately upon diagnosis. Treatment at the Institute of Surgical Research (Dowling, Foley, and Moncrief, 1968; Mills and associates, 1988) consisted of either formal debridement with incision and bivalving of the ear and excision of all nonviable cartilage, or (as is now more common) prompt local debridement of infected tissue after early recognition of the process. These authors believed that early diagnosis and treatment were essential to limit the progression of infection and necrosis and to minimize deformity. When chondrectomy was necessary, the complete removal of all nonviable cartilage was critical in preventing recurrence. A single layer of fine-mesh gauze soaked in antibacterial solution was placed between the skin flaps of the ear to reduce the risk of progressive infection. Light dressings were applied over the ear without pressure. The gauze was changed daily until secondary closure was achieved.

After the burned ear has healed and the deformity has been established, questions arise as to whether reconstruction should be undertaken and, if so, when. In some women in whom the deformity is confined to the superior aspect of the ear, concealment of the deformity by the hair may be an appropriate long-term solution. In many patients with more important functional and esthetic deformities elsewhere on the face and body, these other areas need to repaired before ear reconstruction is addressed. However, the surgeon should remember that ear reconstruction is often a multistaged undertaking, and therefore the stages of repair can and often should be carried out at the same time that other areas are being worked on. In this way, ear reconstruction can be accomplished in large part without operative procedures dedicated solely to ear repair. In cases of total or near-total loss of an ear, the use of an ear prosthesis may be considered by some patients if the prostheses are artistically fabricated and psychologically acceptable to them. The external prosthesis can be either a short- or long-term solution to the problem of total ear loss in selected patients. Many patients, however, do not accept the wearing of an artificial ear and prefer autogenous tissue reconstruction. The technical advances of the use of the fascial turn-over flap and skin expansion now permit a satisfactory ear reconstruction in situations of total ear loss in a scarred environment. These methods are described below.

The repair of ear deformities from burns employs the same surgical techniques as those used to repair acquired deformities from other forms of trauma and tumor excision. Brent (1977) described a systematic approach to repair of the acquired ear deformity; a detailed description may be found in Chapter 40. Some personal preferences, however, will be presented in specific regard to the burned ear. The most common ear deformities associated with burns involve the periphery of the ear (the helix, anthelix, and lobule). Localized defects of the helix and scapha, as occur after tumor excision (but are uncommon after burns), can be repaired by advancing superior and inferior chondrocutaneous helical rim flaps based on the postauricular skin, as described by Antia and Buch (1967). The disadvantage of this method, however, is that the ear is made somewhat smaller as a result. When the helical rim alone has been damaged and lacks the normal rolled edge over a long portion, and when the scapha is present for support, a thin skin tube flap migrated to the ear in stages can recreate a delicate helical roll. If the postauricular skin is undamaged, a tube constructed just posterior to the auriculocephalic sulcus provides a rim of excellent color match, with a hidden donor site scar. Goldstein and Stevenson (1988) described a modification to the construction of the postauricular tube flap that allows the flap to tube itself, reducing the chance of vascular compromise from tight suturing. When the skin behind the ear is scarred and unavailable for construction of the tube flap, the next best donor site is the lower supraclavicular neck. Davis (1987) recommended that the narrow skin tube be long enough to be transferred from the lower neck to the ear in a single movement, and Converse (1974) suggested opening the flap and radically defatting it before inserting it along the edge of the helical border. If the flap is not opened and defatted completely, it tends to flop forward in an unesthetic and unnatural fashion. Although construction of a helical edge roll with a tube flap is a time-consuming, multistaged procedure, the steps involved in the tubing and migration of the flap are often relatively simple procedures that are part of a larger, overall surgical process to repair other parts of the face or body.

For segmental defects that involve more than the rim of the helix, the author generally prefers a two-stage procedure that involves replacement of the missing cartilage elements with autogenous cartilage, anterior cartilage covering with a delayed local skin flap, and posterior cartilage covering with either the turn-over fascial flap and skin graft (Fig. 41–20) or a hairless superficial temporal artery island flap harvested from an area of burn alopecia in the temporoparietal region (Fig. 41–21). Ipsilateral or contralateral conchal cartilage grafts can be used to replace the missing helical and anthelical elements, but rib cartilage is generally preferred because its stiffness resists flattening and distortion from contraction of the new skin cover, and the rib cartilage framework can be augmented and supported to give a desirable helical projection. At the first stage, the glabrous skin (which may be scarred) in the mastoid region behind the segment to be reconstructed is elevated in a lateral to medial direction up to the posterior edge of the remaining anthelix or conchal cartilage. The flap is replaced in its original position with a small suction drain beneath it to prevent hematoma formation. This "surgical delay" prepares the flap for draping over the new segmental cartilage framework. Often, the inferior aspect of the mastoid skin flap is cut in a V shape (Fig. 41–20B) so that when the flap is later advanced medially, the triangular extension of the flap fits into a vertical releasing incision over the lower helical rim or upper lobule area (Fig. 41–20D). The V-shaped donor site is closed in a V-Y fashion. Two to three weeks after the surgical delay has taken place, the second procedure is undertaken. The anteriorly based mastoid skin flap is reelevated, this time extending the undermining medially beyond the remaining cartilage remnant so that the new rib cartilage piece can be accurately spliced into place. An accurate pattern of the cartilage to be added is made and transferred to the region of the sixth and seventh rib synchrondrosis, and the curved rib cartilage piece is cut out so that it maintains the desired curved shape on its own without having to be sutured to any type of base block or to the cartilage of the ear in order to maintain its shape. The rib cartilage is accurately sculpted so that it has a delicate helical rim. The cartilage frame is fitted into a skin pocket anteriorly at the superior otobasion and into a skin pocket

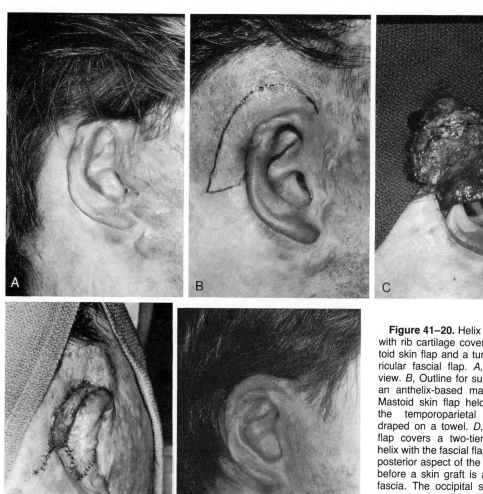

Figure 41–20. Helix reconstruction with rib cartilage covered by a mastoid skin flap and a turnover postauricular fascial flap. *A,* Preoperative view. *B,* Outline for surgical delay of an anthelix-based mastoid flap. *C,* Mastoid skin flap held forward and the temporoparietal fascial flap draped on a towel. *D,* The mastoid flap covers a two-tier rib cartilage helix with the fascial flap covering the posterior aspect of the cartilage graft before a skin graft is applied to the fascia. The occipital scalp was advanced anteriorly to the auriculocephalic sulcus. *E,* Postoperative appearance.

inferiorly alongside the lower helical cartilage remnant. A second crescent-shaped piece of cartilage may be added deep to the helical rim piece to increase the projection of the new helix. The skin flap is advanced "centripically" and draped over the cartilage framework. The mastoid skin is undermined posteriorly and a rectangular flap of postauricular superficial temporalis fascia is elevated in a lateral to medial direction, the vascular base left attached along the auriculocephalic groove (Fig. 41–20*C*). The fascial flap is turned back to cover the posterior aspect of the rib cartilage framework (Fig. 41–20*D*). The occipital scalp is advanced medially as much as possible to bring the hairline close to the ear and to minimize the area

that has to be covered by a skin graft. A subcutaneous suction drain is placed beneath the occipital scalp flap to prevent hematoma formation. In cases in which the temporoparietal area above the ear is hairless as a result of the burn injury, a narrow superficial temporal artery skin island flap can be used for posterior coverage for the cartilage graft, in lieu of the skin grafted turn-over fascial flap (Fig. 41–21).

Many methods have been designed for repair of the deformed earlobe; Brent (1977) and Feldman (1984) described a number of these. Not infrequently, the anteroinferior aspect of the ear lobule is pulled inferiorly by scarring to the adjacent cheek. This deformity can often be corrected simply by converting

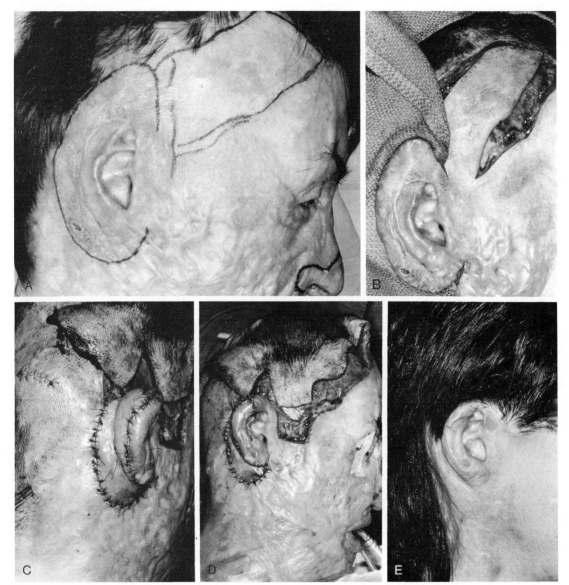

Figure 41–21. Helix reconstruction with a delayed mastoid scar flap and a hairless arterial scalp flap. *A,* Scarred periauricular skin outlined for elevation as the first of two delays. The skin-grafted temporofrontal area that will be covered with a hair-bearing expanded scalp flap is outlined as an arterial island flap. *B,* The mastoid skin flap draped over a towel and the arterial flap elevated. *C, D,* The mastoid flap rolled to form a new helix and earlobe, and the arterial flap used both to line the posterior aspect of the ear and to cover the mastoid flap donor site. Although not used in this case, insertion of a rib cartilage framework beneath the mastoid flap would provide better contour support. *E,* Postoperative view.

the scar band into a superiorly based flap of scar and subcutaneous fat that is turned upward and forward into a vertical scar releasing incision to recreate the anterior border of the lobule (Fig. 41–22). Either the flap donor site is closed in a direct linear fashion or the closure line is broken by a Z-plasty. When the lobule has been totally lost and the adjacent cheek is being resurfaced, a simple method that is often successful is to incise a thick and oversized earlobe from the local scar tissue and line the undersurface of the lobule with a skin graft. The lobule should purposely be made too large, in the expectation that it will shrink as the graft contracts; an earlobe made too large can always be made smaller. The lobule flap donor site is covered either with a skin graft or with the skin flap being used to resurface the cheek. Another method that can work well for total lobule reconstruction is that described by Davis (1974, 1987). It involves the turn-over of an inferiorly based skin flap from the lower portion of the helical-anthelical remnant to create a posterior lining for the new lobe, and elevation of an inferiorly based postauricular mastoid skin flap for the anterior lobule surface. A fat flap side extension based along the inferior edge of the mastoid flap is dissected subcutaneously from beneath the skin below the mastoid flap, and the fat flap is turned under the mastoid flap to provide subcutaneous bulk for the new earlobe. Davis called this method a "fat sandwich." The neck and

mastoid skin below the recreated earlobe are undermined and advanced upward in "face lift" fashion to close the mastoid flap donor site. When a skin tube flap is being used to recreate a helical rim roll, the tube flap can also be used to augment or recreate the ear lobule.

When most or all of an ear has been destroyed by the burn injury, one of two reconstructive strategies can be applied, depending on the condition of the skin in the mastoid and periauricular area. If the skin is scarred, tight, and fragile, a turn-over temporoparietal fascial flap can be used to cover a carved autogenous rib cartilage framework, with a color-matched skin graft placed on top of the fascial layer (see also Chap. 40). This method was originally described by Tegtmeier and Gooding (1977) and popularized by Brent (1980) and Brent and Byrd (1983). The fascial flap usually includes the posterior branch of the superficial temporal artery and its accompanying veins, so that it is an axial-pattern flap. However, when the superficial temporal artery has been damaged or is otherwise unavailable, a random-pattern fascial flap can be used successfully. The quality of the reconstructed ear depends largely on the artistic quality of the fabricated rib cartilage framework. A smooth, thin, rounded, and highly projecting helix is of particular importance. The skin graft applied to the fascia should also provide a satisfactory color match with the remaining portions of the ear and

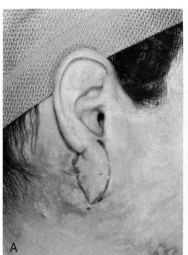 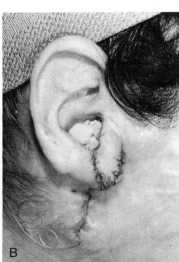 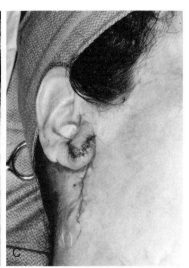

Figure 41–22. *A* to *C,* Earlobe repair with two flaps, a posterosuperiorly based flap turned forward to line the back of the new lobe, and a small anterosuperiorly based flap made from the other flap's dog-ear that is lifted and adjusted to reconstruct the front of the lobe.

the entire periauricular area. Yoshimura, Nakajima, and Kami (1987) suggested using a split-thickness skin graft from the nearby scalp for coverage. The scalp graft provides a very good color match with the unscarred areas in the facial region, the donor site heals quickly and relatively painlessly, and the donor site scar becomes hidden after the scalp hair has regrown.

As mentioned above, the key to quality ear reconstruction is to have a well-defined, projecting, three-dimensional rib cartilage framework over which a very thin skin flap can be draped. If the local skin is pliable, it can be expanded to accommodate the cartilage framework. The skin ideally should be unscarred, soft, and elastic (as is found in an unoperated microtia); however, in burned ears this is rarely the case. Nonetheless, even periauricular areas that have been previously scarred or skin grafted can be expanded if sufficient time has elapsed for the skin and underlying soft tissues to have matured, so that a detectable tissue plane exists between the skin and the underlying deeper tissues. The surgeon can evaluate this by manipulating the skin back and forth beneath his fingers; if there is motion, this indicates a dissectable tissue plane into which a skin expander can be inserted. Another helpful maneuver in determining whether a tissue expander can be accommodated is to inject saline into the subcutaneous plane. If the skin flap balloons up easily, this also suggests that a subcutaneous tissue expander can be accommodated. If, however, the tissues appear to be scarred and tight, it would be hazardous to attempt the expansion method. The expander should be inserted in a subcutaneous position and not beneath the superficial temporalis fascia. The fascia is then available for use if the expander fails. If the skin flap under which the expander lies is thin and fragile, a slow process of expansion is necessary, with careful ongoing observation of the skin. It is particularly important to avoid folds or knuckles in the expander shell, which can easily erode through the thin overlying skin flap. For this reason, an expander with a low initial fill volume that can be "overfilled" is better than one that has an initial redundancy in the expander shell. Figure 41–23 illustrates a case in which an expander was inserted beneath pliable skin grafted soft tissue in the periauricular area for ear reconstruction. The rectangular expander was inserted through a radial incision, with its anterior edge tucked underneath the conchal remnant. The rib cartilage framework was inserted through a remote superior incision at the time of cheek and lateral forehead resurfacing and hairline reconstruction with expanded regional flaps. When the remaining ear cartilage remnants are contracted and deformed, a curved incision (through the expanded flap) following the line of the anthelix and conchal rim can be made to remove the expander. The deformed cartilage can be excised or repositioned, and the rib cartilage framework accurately positioned and spliced to the original ear cartilage remnants. Brent (1980) and O'Neal, Rohrich, and Izenberg (1984) reported successful use of the skin expander in ear reconstruction.

When the local skin cannot be expanded and ipsilateral turn-over fascial flaps are also unavailable owing to extensive deep scarring in the scalp, ear reconstruction can be achieved using the microvascular transfer of a contralateral temporoparietal fascial flap, as reported by Brent and Byrd (1983) and Brent and associates (1985).

The Eyelids

Eyelid burns occur in less than 10 per cent of all thermal injuries (Tubiana, 1967b). However, a large percentage of patients admitted to hospitals with burns involving the face also have burns of the eyelids (Huang, Blackwell, and Lewis, 1978). Most of these are the result of exposure to dry heat from fires, and not of direct contact with hot materials or chemicals. The severity and extent of the eyelid injury depend on the nature, intensity, and duration of exposure to the heat source. Reflex blinking and squinting of the eyelids in response to irritating smoke or the heat of a fire often protect not only the cornea but also the eyelid margins and the pretarsal portion of the lids. Flash heat from a nearby gun fire or electrical explosion may not allow time for reflex blinking. In this situation, the open upper lids tend to suffer less injury than the lower lids, cornea, and conjunctiva. If the exposure to the heat has been brief but not instantaneous (as in an explosion from gasoline vapor), the patient may have sufficient time to close the eyes reflexively (protecting the cornea), but not

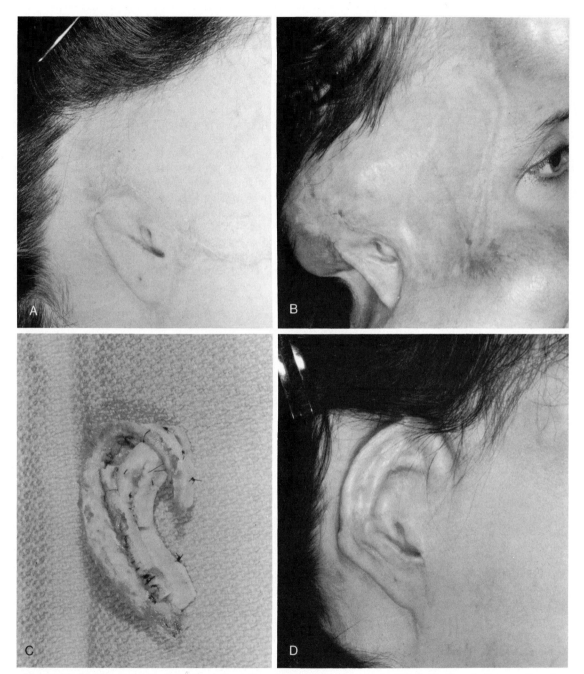

Figure 41–23. Ear reconstruction with a rib cartilage framework under an expanded skin flap. *A,* Preoperative view. Pliable periauricular tissues indicated a dissection plane for placement of the expander. *B,* Multiple expanders inflated for ear, cheek, lateral forehead, and temporal hairline reconstruction. *C,* Three-tiered rib cartilage framework to maintain ear projection. *D,* Postoperative appearance before final adjustments for lobe and tragus position.

enough time to squint tightly to protect the lids themselves (Mustardé, 1979). Exposure to dry heat (as in a house fire) produces a variable pattern of eyelid injury. If the exposure is neither long nor intense, a second degree burn of the eyelid skin may result. A more intense heat of longer duration may cause a full-thickness burn of the eyelid skin and at times the underlying orbicularis muscle. Direct thermal injury to the deeper structures of the eyelids (i.e., the levator muscle mechanism and tarsus) is uncommon. Aside from chemical burns, the most severe eyelid injuries occur in patients who lie unconscious or semiconscious for a period exposed to a source of heat. In these patients, total destruction of all layers of the eyelid may result, in association with direct injury to the globe. Because of the thinness of the eyelid skin and the inherent mobility of the eyelid margins, deformity of the eyelid can result from seemingly superficial burns.

The acute management of eyelid burns includes an early examination of the lids and globe, preferably before lid swelling makes this difficult. Even if significant edema is present, the lid should be retracted and briefly inspected. Foreign bodies (contact lenses in particular) should be looked for and removed. Whenever possible, a baseline examination by an ophthalmologist who will continue to follow the patient is helpful at this early stage. Gentle eyelid and eyelash hygiene should be instituted to minimize crusting, and topical ophthalmic antibiotic ointments and artificial tears should be applied frequently. An early reactive conjunctivitis from the noxious fumes of a fire is frequently observed for several days immediately after a burn; however, the appearance of delayed conjunctivitis several weeks or months after the burn is almost invariably secondary to progressive conjunctival exposure from either an intrinsic or an extrinsic wound contracture. Mild to moderate conjunctivitis is itself not worrisome, but should alert the surgeon to the possibility of concomitant corneal exposure, which is serious. The drying of the cornea can lead to ulceration, scarring, or perforation, with loss of vision. The upper eyelid is responsible for moistening the cornea; therefore, when there is an upper eyelid ectropion, the potential for corneal dehydration is present. Patients who show any degree of conjunctivitis or who have any difficulty closing the eyelids should undergo

a daily examination to assess the adequacy of lid closure, not only while awake, but more important, while asleep. Frequently an awake patient with eyelid ectropion can demonstrate complete coverage of the iris by voluntary squinting and a Bell's phenomenon (upward rolling of the globe in attempted closure of the lids). However, this observation can give the physician a false impression that the cornea is adequately protected. At night, with the patient asleep, when the voluntary component of lid closure is lost, the cornea may well become partially exposed. In cases in which there is only the risk of but little or no actual exposure keratitis, the application of a combination of ointment and artificial tears may suffice for nocturnal protection. "Homemade" moist covering chambers (Hupp, Galanos, and Laterman, 1987) or the commercially available plastic bandage bubble can also be tried. A soft contact lens may be useful, but these tend to become dislodged on upward gaze or collect debris on the surface. Random-fit scleral shells (Constable and Carroll, 1970) can also be worthwhile in selective patients if they are carefully monitored. Nonetheless, if at any time there is doubt concerning the adequacy of nonsurgical measures of corneal protection, upper eyelid contracture release and grafting should be carried out without hesitation (Sloan and associates, 1976). The surgeon should be prepared to release and regraft as needed to ensure this protection. It is far better to release and graft too early or once too often than to wait too long and discover a corneal injury. However, if the cornea appears to be safely protected, it is usually best to delay a minimum of three months, or better yet, six months or longer, before grafting the eyelid, until most of the eyelid and regional contraction has subsided (Silverstein and Peterson, 1973).

Although tarsorrhaphy has been advocated for corneal protection in the past, it is now generally felt that tarsorrhaphy has many more disadvantages than benefits; therefore, it is *not* endorsed by most authorities (Converse, 1979; Miller, 1979; Burns and Chylack, 1979). Tarsorrhaphy does not prevent lid retraction and is not an appropriate substitute for timely skin grafting. The eyelid margins can be severely and permanently deformed by tarsorrhaphy, and some of the most difficult eyelids to repair are those that have undergone this procedure.

As emphasized by Converse and associates (1977), the distinction should be made between an *intrinsic* and an *extrinsic* eyelid ectropion or a combination of the two. A correct diagnosis is important. Attempting to correct an *intrinsic* contracture (scarring within the lid itself) by adding skin outside the lid will fail; an inappropriate release and grafting within the lid for a purely *extrinsic* ectropion will unnecessarily introduce a deforming patch into a normal eyelid and may not completely correct the primary contracture in the adjacent cheek, neck, or forehead.

When an upper and lower eyelid contracture exists on the same side, the more severe contracture of the two is usually corrected first. This assumes, however, that the upper lid contracture is not creating a risk of corneal exposure. If so, the upper lid should always be operated on first. In cases of combined upper and lower ectropion in which healing of the periorbital burn has pulled the lateral portion of the upper eyelid below the transcanthal line, causing an "antimongoloid" slant to the lateral eye (and again, if exposure keratitis is not an issue), the lower eyelid should be operated on first, carrying the lower eyelid releasing incision obliquely upward across the scar pulling downward on the lateral canthal area and lateral upper eyelid. Later, with the lateral upper lid properly repositioned, the upper lid itself can be released and grafted (Feldman, 1979).

Both the upper and lower eyelid on the same side can be released and grafted at the same time if both contractures are minimal and stable. In most cases, however, only one eyelid at a time should be released to ensure that a necessary "overcorrection" can be accomplished to prevent recurrence of the contracture. Although releasing and grafting of bilateral eyelid ectropions is occasionally performed, it is rarely carried out in young children who may become frightened by the relative blindness imposed by bilateral dressings. In certain cases of modest lower eyelid ectropions, however, bilateral release and grafting can be done, allowing the patient to see out through narrow slits above compact dressings.

Surgical release of the upper eyelid is done either with an incision that runs a few millimeters above the eyelash margin (Fig. 41–24) or with an incision above the tarsal plate (Fig. 41–25), depending on the condition of the pretarsal eyelid skin. Either incision extends temporally beyond the lateral canthal region (but staying above the transcanthal line) as far as necessary to obtain a complete release of the lateral upper lid. Medially, the releasing incision is brought to the nose. The supratarsal releasing incision is used only when the lid scarring is primarily in the superior upper eyelid, either when the pretarsal skin is unscarred or when a previously applied skin graft is smooth over the pretarsal area and the eyelid margin does not require additional unrolling. When the supratarsal incision is used, the eyebrow is usually displaced upward, and therefore if the eyebrow is in a normal position or slightly elevated to begin with, it is preferable to use the juxtamarginal incision rather than the supratarsal incision. In cases in which the eyebrow is absent and the pretarsal skin is smooth, the supratarsal incision is appropriate.

When either incision is used, it may be helpful to make the lateral and/or medial ends of the incision Y shaped, which not only allows the introduction of more skin laterally and medially but also helps to prevent postoperative scar contracture in these areas. Temporary traction sutures placed above and below the outlined releasing incision are helpful. After infiltration of local anesthetic solution with epinephrine, the incision should be made superficially just down to the orbicularis muscle with the scalpel. The needletip electric cautery can be used to undermine the scarred skin superiorly just at the interface of the skin and orbicularis muscle so that the wound opens up and releases the contracture (Fig. 41–24*B*). If at all possible, the orbicularis muscle should be kept intact to provide a smooth bed for the skin graft. Often, however, the orbicularis is involved in the scarring and needs to be released as well, but this should be done by painting lightly across the muscle with the needletip cautery at various points while downward traction is maintained on the upper lid, so that a deep crevice is not created in the lid. Although it has been suggested (Falvey and Brody, 1978) that the levator aponeurosis may need to be incised in order to achieve a full release, this is almost never required (except perhaps in the rare case of a deep chemical or contact burn), and in fact care should be taken not to divide the levator. The author has seen unnecessary iatrogenic eyelid ptosis produced by both intentional and unintentional tran-

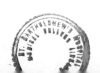

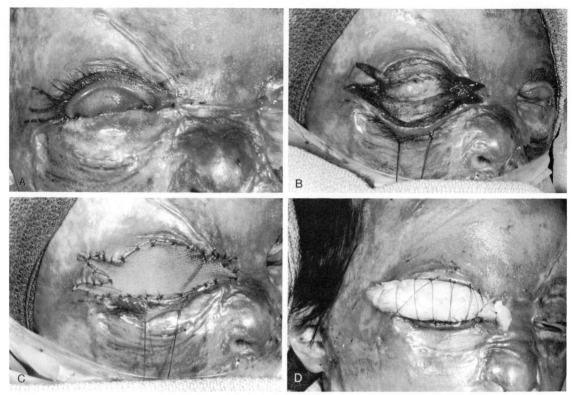

Figure 41–24. Upper eyelid release with a supraciliary incision. *A,* Preoperative view of a scar-everted upper lid and a fishtailed supraciliary incision marked. The releasing incisions should never be carried laterally below the level of the transcanthal line. *B,* Complete release through the preseptal orbicularis muscle with the septum orbitale visible. The upper lid margin can now be pulled downward to reach the infraorbital rim. *C,* The skin graft held with fine absorbable sutures. *D,* Bolster dressing "laced on" with to-and-fro running mattress sutures.

section of the levator aponeurosis. In the vast majority of upper eyelid burns, scarring involves only the skin or the orbicularis muscle. When the upper eyelid is fully released, it should be possible to pull the upper lid margin sufficiently far down so that it reaches the infraorbital rim (Fig. 41–24B). Meticulous hemostasis is essential and this can easily be achieved by doing the dissection with the needletip cautery. Thin, hairless, full-thickness skin grafts from the retroauricular or supraclavicular areas can be used in the upper eyelids for a satisfactory color match with the unburned surrounding periorbital skin. Sometimes, however, these donor sites either are unavailable because of the burn injury or should be saved for use in the more visible lower eyelid. Thicker full-thickness skin grafts should not be used on the upper eyelids because they do not drape and fold well and they give the upper lid a bulky, unattractive appearance. Usually, a medium-thickness (0.014 to 0.016 inch) split-thickness skin graft should be used for the upper eyelid, purposely stretching the eyelid release incision wide apart to introduce sufficient skin so that with the anticipated wound and graft contraction there will still be an adequate amount of skin left in the lid to allow complete lid closure. The donor site for the split-thickness skin graft should be chosen so that the color matches the surrounding periorbital skin. In some cases, a split-thickness skin graft from the scalp may do quite well.

The author has found it easiest and most convenient for both surgeon and patient to suture the graft in place with interrupted and running 6-0 chromic catgut sutures (which do not have to be removed) and "lace on" a narrow and compact lubricated gauze and cotton dressing with a zigzag running 5-0 nylon suture that is tied to itself (Falvey and Brody, 1978). The laced-on dressing is small enough to permit the patient some vision, and is easily removed by simply cutting the nylon suture, a feature that is particularly advantageous in children. The dressing is usually left in place for one week.

The releasing incision for correction of an intrinsic lower eyelid ectropion is subciliary, approximately 2 mm beneath the eyelash margin. It extends medially below the medial canthus and usually continues over to the nose. Laterally, the incision is carried upward and outward far enough to give complete release to the lateral canthal area (Fig. 41–26). As with the upper lid, after the releasing incision is made through the skin to the orbicularis muscle, the remainder of the dissection can be carried out with the needletip electric cautery. With traction sutures placed along the gray line of the eyelid margin to give upward traction, the skin below the releasing incision is lightly undermined with the cautery to produce the release. A deep incision through the orbicularis muscle should be avoided to prevent the all too common iatrogenic depression that is seen along the infraorbital rim. The release of the lower

lid should be completely smooth, avoiding contour irregularities. Light touches with the needletip cautery in the orbicularis muscle release the scar within the muscle without penetrating through deeply. The eyelid margin itself often needs to be unfurled to allow the conjunctiva to roll back against the globe. To do this, the narrow strip of skin above the incision and below the eyelash margin needs to be undermined as far as the hair follicles. Unless this is done, portions of everted conjunctiva may remain and become keratinized, leaving a red "granulating" spot along the eyelid margin. If the lacrimal punctum remains everted, epiphora may also persist. As with the upper lid, "overcorrection" is aimed for. The full esthetic unit of the lower lid should always be covered, with the skin graft extending from the eyelid margin above to the infraorbital rim below, and from medial to lateral canthus (Fig. 41–26B). Less than a full esthetic unit coverage gives a patched appearance. Vincent and Carraway (1987) emphasized the three basic principles for the

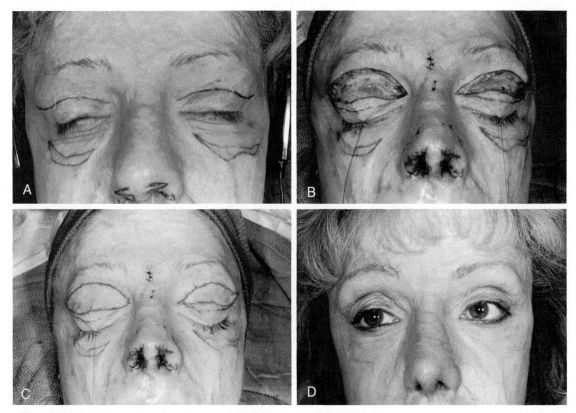

Figure 41–25. Upper eyelid release with a supratarsal incision. *A,* Preoperative view, showing tight lids with acceptably smooth pretarsal skin grafts. *B, C,* After incisional scar release across the full width of the lid and skin graft insertion. *D,* Postoperative appearance.

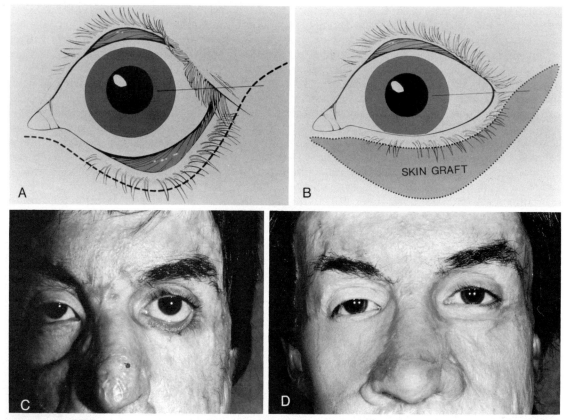

Figure 41–26. Correction of an intrinsic lower eyelid scar ectropion. *A,* Subciliary release incision carried laterally above the level of the lateral canthus. *B,* Skin graft provides sling support for the lid margin and covers the complete esthetic unit of the lower eyelid. *C,* Preoperative appearance of a left lower eyelid ectropion. *D,* Postoperative view.

successful use of grafts in the lower eyelids: (1) a "sling" effect at the canthal areas, (2) an elliptic shape for the graft, and (3) overcorrection of the contracture by at least 20 per cent. They also pointed out the need to evaluate the lacrimal system when the injury involves the medial lower eyelid.

The best skin graft for the lower eyelid is a full-thickness graft from the upper eyelid. Often, however, the upper lids have also been burned and scarred, or the lower lid requires more skin than the upper lids can safely donate. In this situation, a retroauricular full-thickness skin graft usually provides an excellent color match with an unburned adjacent cheek. If the amount of skin needed for the lower lid is large and the area behind the ear relatively small, preexpansion of the retroauricular donor site with a subcutaneous skin expander can be done. The retroauricular skin graft may, however, be too pink in color (in Caucasian patients) for a satisfactory match if the cheek has been skin grafted. In

this situation, a hairless full-thickness graft from the supraclavicular area may be more appropriate. The important point, however, is that the eyelid skin match the color of the cheek. In the lower eyelid, unlike the upper lid, a thicker and more rigid graft can be used, since the graft will not be called upon to drape and fold into a palpebro-orbital sulcus. If a full-thickness skin graft is used, it is important that it be taken from a truly hairless area. Full-thickness grafts from the lower abdomen or inguinal region, although appearing relatively hairless, often grow fine hairs after transplanted, presenting a very unpleasing appearance. If the truly glabrous, thin full-thickness skin grafts are unavailable for lower lid grafting, it is better to use a medium to thick split-thickness skin graft for the eyelid resurfacing. It should be remembered, however, that, both for upper and lower eyelids, the best and most appropriately colored and textured skin grafts should be saved for the final definitive eyelid repair, and not sacrificed at an early temporary procedure that will almost certainly need to be repeated later.

In cases of lower eyelid contracture associated with an unburned upper eyelid, a laterally based upper eyelid transposition skin flap can be used, as originally described by Denonvilliers (1856) and modified by Joseph (1931) (Fig. 41–27). To determine the width of the upper lid flap that will allow the patient to close the upper eyelid completely, the skin of the upper lid should be pinched with the small forceps with the upper lid closed. Including orbicularis muscle in the flap helps to ensure its viability. If the upper eyelid is inadequate for a flap and the eyebrow is low or ptotic, a laterally based transposition flap taken from above the eyebrow and transferred into the lower lid can accomplish both lower eyelid reconstruction and an appropriate elevation of the brow (Fig. 41–28), a method first described by Langenbeck (1843) and subsequently by Kreibig (1940). The flap should be sufficiently long to resurface the entire lower eyelid. Because it is a thin, random-pattern flap with a narrow base, a preliminary delay may be prudent. The flap, taken from above the brow, should *not* include frontalis muscle, to avoid postoperative inability to elevate the eyebrow. A superiorly based flap in the medial canthal region at the top of the nasolabial fold (Blasius, 1842) can also be transferred to resurface the lower eyelid and provide sling support for the eyelid margin in cases in which the medial paranasal cheek is unscarred and hairless. The flap donor site can be closed directly with a scar along the nasolabial crease. Rougier and associates (1981) and Wolfe (1978) described using this "nasojugal" transposition flap in conjunction with an upper lateral cartilage chondromucosal graft from the nose for total reconstruction of a full-thickness lower eyelid defect. For cases in which the upper lid is normal and the lower lid needs both skin and muscle, Siegel (1987) described lower lid repair with a modified (bipedicle) Tripier flap. For patients in whom only additional skin is needed in the lower eyelid and the lower eyelid and malar regions are unscarred, Antonyshyn and associates (1988) reported the use of a small, cigar-shaped, subcutaneous skin expander placed across the lid through an incision in one of the lateral crow's foot

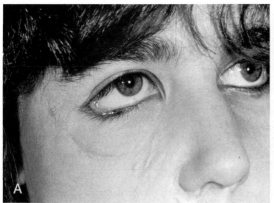
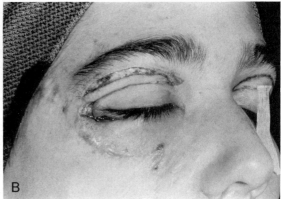
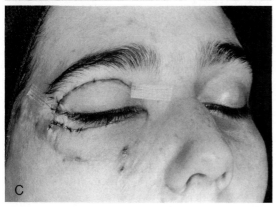

Figure 41–27. Lower eyelid ectropion corrected with an upper eyelid musculocutaneous transposition flap. *A,* Preoperative appearance. *B,* Intraoperative view. *C,* At completion of procedure.

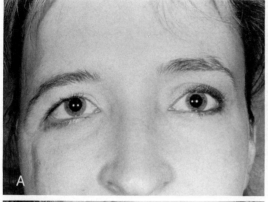
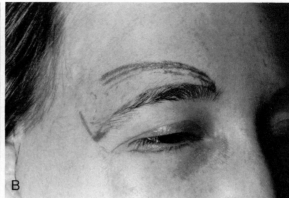
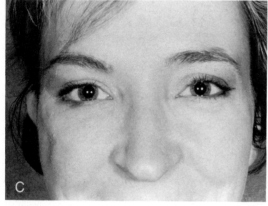

Figure 41–28. Lower eyelid ectropion and brow ptosis simultaneously corrected with a transposition flap from above the brow to the lower lid. *A,* Preoperative appearance. *B,* Outline of flap. *C,* Postoperative appearance.

lines. In the six patients who underwent the expansion procedure, four demonstrated considerable improvement. However, the authors did not include photographs of any of the patients in their report, so the place for localized tissue expansion for the correction of cicatricial ectropion will have to await more detailed reports. Flap reconstruction of the lower eyelid is also discussed in Chapter 34.

Medial epicanthal (nasoethmoido-orbital) scar bands can be partially or completely relieved by extending the medial portions of the upper and lower eyelid releasing incisions across the vertical bands onto the lateral wall of the upper nose. The horizontal-Y or fishtail bifurcation of the incision is sometimes an aid in interrupting the scar as well. The epicanthal bands can also be corrected by using Converse's (1967, 1977) double-opposing Z-plasties, which use all the tissue present in the medial canthal area. Many of the procedures described for correction of the congenital medial epicanthal fold are inappropriate for correction of the burn scar epicanthal fold because they involve the excision of skin (already in short supply in the burned eyelid) along with skin flap interdigitation.

All epicanthal scar bands are not the same, however, and an eclectic and innovative approach is best. The procedure described by del Campo (1984) should be considered. Lateral epicanthal scar bands can be relieved by some type of Z-plasty if the scarring is not too extensive (Tajima and Aoyagi, 1977). The method involves transposing a superiorly based transposition flap containing the scar band into a transverse releasing incision and closing the donor site with a small W-plasty.

The Eyebrows

Absence (either partial or total) of the eyebrows or distortions in their position alter the character of the face. The shape and position of the eyebrows can express surprise, anger, sadness, fatigue, annoyance, relaxation, and a spectrum of other emotions. Without eyebrows, the face usually does not look normal. To the viewer, there is a vague but displeasing lack of expression. The burn patient with missing eyebrows is often unaware of the improvement in appearance that eyebrow reconstruction could make (Brody,

1985). Surgeons can often demonstrate, both to themselves and to the patient, the anticipated change in appearance that eyebrow reconstruction would make by drawing in the brows on a frontal view photograph of the patient. Eyebrow repair or reconstruction can be an important "finishing touch" in the overall reconstruction of a burned face. The significance of the eyebrows should not be underappreciated by the surgeon. For female patients, however, a partially or totally absent eyebrow may be acceptably simulated with a cosmetic pencil. Some women, however, do not like the look of a penciled eyebrow, and most male patients find that solution unacceptable. Nonetheless, the surgeon should be aware that an eyebrow reconstruction that is poorly done technically, placing the new brow in an inappropriate position or resulting in hair growth in a disturbing direction, can make the patient look worse rather than better. Unless the surgeon is willing to pay close attention to the details of proper eyebrow reconstruction, the reconstruction should not be undertaken.

There are two choices for eyebrow repair: (1) single or multiple strip composite scalp grafts (Fig. 41–29) or (2) a hair-bearing superficial temporal artery island flap (Fig. 41–30). The choice depends primarily on the type of eyebrow the surgeon wants to reconstruct. A wider, fuller, and bushier eyebrow (or fill-in eyebrow segment) can be achieved more reliably with a superficial temporal artery island flap, whereas a thin, less dense eyebrow can be more simply reconstructed with a composite graft. If one eyebrow is normal and the other requires total reconstruction, the choice of method depends on the type of eyebrow needed for symmetry. The same principle applies to subtotal eyebrow reconstruction; a bushy wide segment is best added with the island flap, and a thin sparse segment perhaps best added by a composite graft. In most women requiring bilateral total eyebrow reconstruction, a thin eyebrow may look best if the patient is able to add a little density to the brows with a cosmetic pencil, if needed. For this reason, the best first approach toward eyebrow reconstruction is

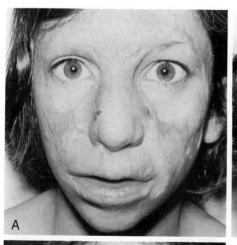
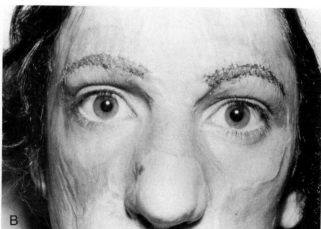
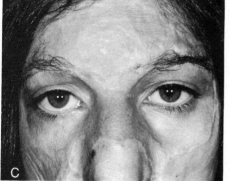

Figure 41–29. Bilateral eyebrow reconstruction with composite scalp strip grafts. *A,* Preoperative appearance. *B,* Five days after graft transposition. *C,* Postoperative view.

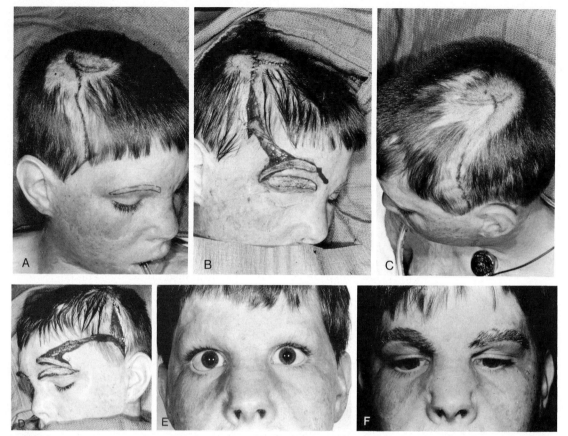

Figure 41–30. Island scalp flap for eyebrow reconstruction. *A, B,* Outline and transposition of right side flap. *C, D,* Left side flap. The flaps were tunneled subcutaneously to the recipient sites. *E, F,* Preoperative and postoperative views.

often the composite graft technique. In a male requiring bilateral total eyebrow reconstruction, the choice depends on the type of brow that would look best on that individual. In the author's experience, the superficial temporal artery island flap gives a more reliably complete eyebrow than the composite graft, although other authors have had a different experience (Pensler, Dillon, and Parry, 1985). The success of either method depends in large part on how the procedure is carried out technically. Reports describing the superficial temporal artery island flap method as unreliable indicate to the author not an inherent problem with the method itself, but inexperience with the technique on the part of the reporter. Other considerations influencing the choice of eyebrow repair are the availability of the superficial temporal vessels on the ipsilateral side, and an awareness that, if the composite graft approach is not successful and the superficial temporal vessels are intact, the island flap method can always

be used as a secondary back-up procedure. Because of this, when the composite scalp grafts are taken, the donor sites should be selected so that they do not cut across the path of the superficial temporal vessels, thereby eliminating the option of using the island flap later.

There are important guidelines that should be applied to eyebrow reconstruction regardless of the method used: any release and skin grafting that is needed for the upper eyelids should be carried out before eyebrow reconstruction. If the eyebrows are inappropriately reconstructed first and the eyelids subsequently operated on, the eyebrows can easily be repositioned into an inappropriately high location by the tissue release in the eyelid-eyebrow region. The eyebrow to be reconstructed should be drawn out preoperatively with the patient sitting in the upright position, aiming for symmetry with an existing eyebrow on the contralateral side or positioning bilateral new eyebrows so that they look best on that particular patient. In doing this, it should be understood that some change in position takes place when the scar in the brow region is incised and opened. At surgery, it is usually best simply to make a releasing incision that allows the somewhat tight tissues to open, rather than to excise a strip of skin at the recipient site. An incision rather than excision adds a little more tissue to the upper eyelid region where it may be needed. Undermining the superior and inferior skin margins opens the recipient site the desired amount. It is important that the new eyebrow(s) be brought medially enough; a common mistake is failure to extend the eyebrow toward the midline sufficiently. It should also be appreciated that placing an eyebrow a little too low is always better than putting it a little too high. A low eyebrow can always be lifted with skin excision above the brow, whereas a brow that is too high may be difficult to reposition lower without producing unwanted traction on the eyelid. A slightly low eyebrow also looks better than the brow that has been placed too high and gives a startled appearance.

The direction of hair growth within the constructed eyebrow is also important. When a unilateral eyebrow repair is being done, the intact contralateral brow is the guide for the direction of hair growth in the different segments of the eyebrows. Generally speaking, however, the hair in the fuller medial portion of the eyebrow grows upward and slightly outward. The hairs in the central two-thirds lie flat and are directed mostly laterally and slightly upward. In the lateral portion of the brow, the hairs usually grow outward and curve somewhat downward.

When a composite graft is being used for the eyebrow repair, a pattern of the planned eyebrow made from a piece of x-ray film can be used to select the most appropriate donor site within the scalp. A location within the ipsilateral temporal region or occipital region supplies a graft with the hairs running in the desired direction. The surgeon must remember that cutting across the superficial temporal vessels should be avoided. In selecting the donor site, it is often helpful to clip, but not shave, the hair so that the direction of hair growth within the scalp can be more easily visualized. It is usually best to open and prepare the recipient site first. Whether this is done under local or general anesthesia, a local anesthetic solution with epinephrine can be used in the brow recipient site for purposes of local hemostasis. A meticulous hemostasis should be obtained with the needletip cautery to minimize devascularization in the recipient bed. The recipient site should be opened deeply enough so that the composite graft edges sit at the same height as the wound edges, and the recipient site should be opened only wide enough to accept the strip so that the edges of the graft and the recipient site sit snugly together without sutures.

It has been recommended that the composite strip graft be no wider than 5 mm to ensure complete revascularization of the graft (Pensler, Dillon, and Parry, 1985). Other authors have suggested that a narrow strip graft of 4 to 5 mm be used at the first operation and a second strip added later to augment the reconstructed eyebrow. Brent (1975) reported the use of two narrow strip grafts separated by a narrow intact strip of skin that was subsequently excised, the two strips being merged later. The author prefers, however, to use a composite graft of whatever width will make the ideal eyebrow, even if the width is 1 cm. With meticulous attention to technical detail, the entire width of the composite graft may "take" completely. If not, small hairless segments of the composite graft can be either excised or filled in secondarily with another strip graft; it seems best to try initially for a one-piece eyebrow. When taking the composite graft, the incisions around the periphery should be beveled away from the graft circumferentially to ensure that a maximal number of uninjured hair bulbs are included in the graft. The incisions are generally extended through the underlying galea aponeurotica. After the graft is completely free, the galea and excess fat on the undersurface of the graft can be carefully trimmed away so that the graft is not thicker than it needs to be, at the same time leaving some tissue on the undersurface of the hair follicles so that they are not exposed. After the graft is harvested, it is immediately inserted into the prepared and completely "dry" recipient site. The graft should be sutured into place with a combination of interrupted and running 6-0 chromic catgut sutures with a fine needle so that a perfect and snug approximation of the edges is achieved. The fine dissolvable suture seems preferable to a nondissolvable suture that may be difficult to remove under the crusting that forms around the edges of the graft. Antibiotic ointment should then be applied over the composite graft, followed by a nonstick lubricated gauze and cotton light compression dressing that is wrapped circumferentially around the head. Some surgeons prefer an "open technique" that leaves the composite graft exposed, but the author favors a compression dressing to discourage hematoma and seroma formation in the recipient bed, as well as to discourage vascular congestion within the composite graft. The patient should be told that after two or three weeks the hairs within the composite graft will fall out as the follicles go into their "rest phase." Approximately three months after surgery, new hair growth should reappear. The patient should also be informed that eyebrows reconstructed with hair-bearing scalp grow long hair that needs to be trimmed periodically.

When the superficial temporal artery island flap is employed, a Doppler probe can be used to trace the peripheral branches of the superficial temporal artery beyond the point where they can be palpated. The posterior branch of the superficial temporal artery is usually chosen since it provides a vascular pedicle within the hair-bearing scalp that is sufficiently long to reach comfortably to the recipient site. The flap procedure should be "planned in reverse" so that the surgeon is certain that the vascular pedicle is long enough to reach its destination. The x-ray film pattern of the eyebrow should be oriented in any direction necessary at the end of the vascular pedicle so that the hairs within the reconstructed eyebrow run in the appropriate direction.

At surgery, subcutaneous infiltration of the scalp along the course of the superficial temporal vessels not only provides hemostasis, which makes the dissection of the vascular pedicle easier, but also helps to locate the dissection plane between the subcutaneous fat and the superficial temporoparietal fascia in which the vessels run. The incision is made along the course of the outlined vascular pedicle and extended up to outline the scalp island flap. The superficial temporal artery and its accompanying veins are not skeletonized but rather included within a broad strip of superficial temporalis fascia, so as to avoid injury to the vessels themselves. The anterior branch of the superficial temporal artery must often be divided distal to its take-off from the main superficial temporal artery in order to give the axial pedicle of the main superficial temporary artery and the posterior

branch sufficient mobility. Careful hemostasis along the cut edges of the superficial temporalis fascia should be carried out to avoid hematoma formation within the subcutaneous tunnel in which the fascial pedicle will lie. A generous subcutaneous tunnel leading from the preauricular area to the brow recipient site should be made so that there is no constriction of the pedicle within the tunnel.

The placement of suction drains both within the subcutaneous forehead tunnel and under the scalp donor site is important. Once in position, the island flap is sutured and dressed as described for the composite graft. As with the composite graft, it is not uncommon for the hairs within the superficial temporal artery island flap to fall out after several weeks and regrow after two to three months. If careful dissection of the vascular pedicle is done, if the subcutaneous forehead tunnel is not too tight, if the pedicle is not placed under tension, and if hematoma in the subcutaneous forehead tunnel is avoided, the island flap for eyebrow reconstruction should be eminently successful.

The Forehead

The treatment of forehead scarring, as with scars elsewhere on the face, depends on the size and location of the scar and the condition of the skin of the adjacent face, brows, nose, and scalp. Small scars surrounded by essentially unburned skin can be excised and closed with respect to the relaxed skin tension lines of the forehead. Scars too large to be removed at one procedure can often be serially removed in one or more procedures. Burn or skin graft scars isolated to the lateral forehead region may be removed by using an ascending cheek advancement-rotation flap, hinging back the lateral eyebrow on a medial base to allow passage of the flap (Juri, Juri, and Cerisola, 1982). For scars not amenable to serial excision or local advancement-rotation flaps, skin expansion can be used. Coleman (1987) used expanded lateral forehead-temporal flaps to resurface the central skin grafted forehead.

If most or all of the forehead has been badly scarred or skin grafted and is in need of resurfacing to improve the surface texture or color, a single-piece resurfacing should be carried out, covering the entire esthetic unit of the forehead from the hairline above to the eyebrows below, and between the eyebrows to the root of the nose. It is important that small strips of skin not be left above the eyebrows, in the glabellar region, or along the edge of the hairline. Scar excision should actually extend into the edge of the eyebrows and into the hairline, beveling the incisions away from the hair follicles in the eyebrows and scalp (Fig. 41–31). In this way, hair growth occurs just at or even through the edge scar, minimizing the scar's visibility. The forehead is usually best resurfaced with a medium split-thickness skin graft harvested as a single piece to cover the full forehead, and taken from a donor site that will give a satisfactory color match with the remainder of the face. Finucan, Budo, and Clarke (1984) suggested that a split-thickness graft from the scalp provided a good color match with an unburned or relatively unscarred face. The Padgett electric dermatome is a useful instrument for harvesting a long strip of split-thickness skin 4 inches wide, usually adequate to cover the complete esthetic unit of most foreheads.

Pigmentation abnormalities in the forehead scar or skin graft are not uncommon. If the forehead scar or skin graft is hyperpigmented, one approach to correction that may be successful is to resurface the forehead with a decolorized split-thickness skin graft from a previously harvested split-thickness skin graft donor site (Lopez-Mas and associates, 1972). It is important, however, that the new skin graft be protected at all times from the sun by using a chemical sunscreen and mechanical sun block for at least four to six months after transplant surgery. For cases of hypopigmentation of the scar or skin graft (so-called leukoderma), Erol and Atabay (1988) reported successful use of dermabrasion followed by application of a thin split-thickness skin graft from the gluteal region. After this procedure, patients are warned to protect the graft from sunlight to prevent hyperpigmentation. Although the treatment of hyperpigmentation with depigmented skin grafts and of hypopigmentation with pigmented skin grafts can sometimes be successful, these procedures are somewhat unpredictable in terms of controlling skin graft and scar pigmentation in all patients.

Scalp Alopecia

Scalp alopecia is a common sequela of burns that involve the facial region. It was estimated that one-quarter of the children who suffer burn injuries of the head and neck area have concomitant burns of the scalp resulting in alopecia (Huang, Larson, and Lewis, 1977). Young children with relatively thin scalp skin are particularly prone to alopecia from scald injuries. There is considerable variability in the extent and distribution of burn baldness, although alopecia in the frontal, temporal, and parietal areas is more common than hair loss in the occiput. Hairless areas of small to moderate size can be concealed most of the time by clever hair styling; on occasion, however, even these can cause significant embarrassment to the patient when

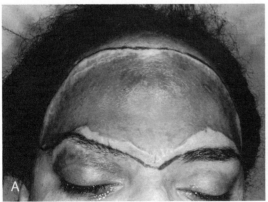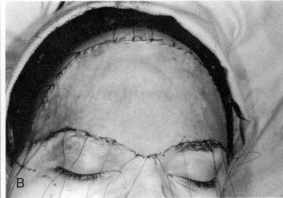

Figure 41–31. Forehead resurfacing. *A,* Previously applied skin graft resulting in portions of color-mismatched skin and conspicuous edge scars above the eyebrows and below the frontal hair line. *B,* Complete forehead esthetic unit resurfaced with new skin graft placed inferiorly as close to the eyebrows as possible, and superiorly just behind the hairline, with beveled incisions in the subcutaneous fat to avoid contour abnormalities.

the bald spot is suddenly revealed to others by a gust of wind or during swimming. Large areas of hair loss are more difficult to conceal, and frequently a top priority of patients undergoing reconstruction for head and neck burns is the correction of scalp alopecia. Although this is commonly done to improve the appearance, many patients also have problems with unstable scar or thin skin grafts covering burned areas of the scalp that break down, bleed, or become infected. Because the hair-bearing scalp is a unique tissue, only other areas of the scalp can be used to replace hairless areas. The currently accepted approach to burn scalp alopecia can be stated simply: small scars surrounded by flexible, hair-bearing scalp are treated by simple excision in one, two, or at most three staged procedures. Larger areas of alopecia not readily amenable to a limited series of partial excisions are treated with scalp expansion (Buhrer and associates, 1988). Scalp reconstruction is also discussed in Chapter 31.

There are basically two ways of approaching serial excision of hairless scalp scar, the choice depending on local conditions (Vallis, 1982). If the bald area is pliable and well vascularized and has a substantial amount of underlying subcutaneous tissue, a central ellipse within the scar can be removed. When the scalp is especially flexible, a fishtail extension at one end of the ellipse can be incorporated (e.g., in the occipital region) to increase the amount of scar excised (Bell, 1982). By manually pushing and sliding the scalp over the skull, an estimate of the width of the scar that can be safely removed is made and the pattern drawn. The procedure is begun with an incision on one edge of the ellipse, followed by extensive undermining of the scar and the scalp on both sides of the pattern in the loose areolar plane between the galea and the pericranium. Parallel relaxing incisions in the galea produce additional stretch and permit more advancement of the scalp. Excision of the scar is begun at one end, removing and closing portions of the patterns in sequence so that the surgeon is not committed to a certain width of excision until the last moment. This maneuver allows for removal of the maximal amount of scar consistent with reasonable tension on the closure. Depending on the flexibility of the scalp, a scar width of up to 3 cm can be excised in the first operation. Smaller amounts can be removed in subsequent pro-

cedures, usually spaced at intervals of four to 12 months. The greater the amount of tension on the closure, the greater is the widening of the scar along the line of closure. This type of anticipated "stretch-back" can sometimes considerably reduce the benefit of scalp excisions for the reduction of alopecia. According to Nordström (1984), most of the stretch-back occurs during the first eight postoperative weeks and is completed by 12 weeks. It is important for the surgeon to be aware of the stretch-back phenomenon, both for correct planning of the surgical program and for predicting the final result.

When the hairless scar is tightly adherent to the underlying bone with little subcutaneous tissue present, the serial excision should be made along the periphery of the scar. The normal hair-bearing scalp on each side is widely undermined and stretched over the yet to be excised scar edges. The precise amount of overlap is marked and the delineated strips are removed. The central portion of the scar remains attached to the skull beneath. A strip up to 1.5 cm in width can be excised from each border at the initial procedure. The principal variable is scalp flexibility: the tighter the scalp, the more are the stages that may be required. Between procedures the patient is encouraged to massage the scalp to prepare for the next excision.

The advent of tissue expansion revolutionized the treatment of scalp alopecia. Argenta (1984) and Manders and associates (1984a) were the first to publish reports of the successful use of expanded scalp flaps for the treatment of alopecia. Before that time, areas of alopecia that could not be removed by serial excision or various large scalp rotation or rotation-advancement flaps (Dingman and Argenta, 1982) were treated by hair-bearing transposition flaps in order to redistribute the existing hair to the periphery of the scalp (particularly along the forehead), so that the remaining hairless areas could be more easily camouflaged by hair styling or a hairpiece (Paletta, 1982). Today, it is thought that an area of up to 30 per cent of the total scalp surface can be removed in two procedures, one to place the expander and the second to remove the expander and advance the expanded flaps (Buhrer and associates, 1988). For larger defects or for patients in whom insufficient hair-bearing scalp tissue has been generated at the initial procedure, the expander can be left beneath the expanded flap for subsequent secondary reexpansion (Manders, 1983). Previously expanded or transposed flaps can also be reexpanded at a later time (Leighton and associates, 1986). A hairless area of 50 per cent or more of the scalp can be replaced with hair-bearing scalp by means of serial expansions. Expansion increases the distance between the hair follicles, and the interfollicular distance can be increased by a factor of 2 before there is noticeable thinning of hair concentration in the donor scalp (Manders and associates, 1984b; Sasaki and Pang, 1984). Significant hair growth occurs even during expansion.

The largest expander that can be placed safely beneath the adjacent hair-bearing scalp should be chosen. The use of multiple expanders placed around the hairless scar is recommended for large defects to facilitate the reconstruction and to decrease the duration of expansion (Sasaki, 1986).

The expanders are placed in the subgaleal space and best positioned immediately adjacent to the defect to be reconstructed. However, they should not be placed under thin, scarred scalp, since these areas are particularly prone to erosion from a fold in the expander shell. In planning scalp expansion, the entire scalp should be carefully examined for hidden patches of burn scar or forgotten incision scars, either of which might significantly influence the placement, size, and shape of the expanders used. It is helpful to wet the hair and part it with a comb in various directions so that the entire scalp is thoroughly surveyed. It is particularly disconcerting to discover at the time of expander insertion previously undetected scalp scars that make the planned expansion risky and the blood supply to the planned flaps precarious. The incision used for insertion of the expander can be either parallel and adjacent to the scars to be removed or perpendicular and more remote from the scar. The placement of the incision at the edge of the scar avoids additional scars and provides direct access to the area of implant placement, but it is more prone to disruption as expansion progresses. The radial remote incision (Sasaki, 1985) lessens the risk of wound dehiscence and also can be used to place the remote filler port, as described above in the section on the use of expanders for check resurfacing. An epinephrine solution injected along the marked incision line, as well as in the subgaleal space, makes for an almost bloodless dissection. Long, curved, blunt-tipped instruments such as a long vascular clamp and the angled Kazanjian zygomatic arch elevator are helpful in dissecting over the curve of the scalp. A malleable retractor can also be bent to conform to the shape of the skull for aid in dissection. Sterilized templates of the expanders, made from x-ray film, help to guide the extent of the subgaleal dissection. The tunnel for the connecting tubing between the expander and the remote filler port should be made so that the tubing does not lie beneath the incision where it may become exposed, and the remote filler port should be positioned where it not only is accessible and comfortable for the patient but also is placed beneath skin that is durable. Thus, it will not be prone to breakdown by being stretched over the port (Neale, 1988).

Expansion usually proceeds at weekly or biweekly intervals over a period of six to 12 weeks. As a general guideline when expanded advancement flaps are being used, the distance over the hemispheric dome of the expander must at least equal the distance across the base of the expander plus the width of the defect to be covered. However, in practice, more expansion than this simple formula suggests should be achieved because more flap will be required to move over the curve of the skull. When rotation is added to the advancement, precise formulas are not helpful. The clinical judgment of the surgeon should determine when the expansion process is complete and reconstruction can be undertaken. Leonard and Small (1986) suggested that both for advancement flaps and rotation flaps the flap edge incisions should be several centimeters up on the side walls of the expanded flap, rather than along the peripheralmost edge of the expanded tissue. The flap will then advance or rotate more easily, and the remaining "skirt" of tissue left along the edges will fall into place to close the secondary defect. Regarding the blood supply to the expanded flaps, Leonard and Small (1986) also suggested that if the flap has a broad base it may safely be planned as a randompattern flap, but if a back cut into the base is proposed that narrows the base considerably, a major artery (such as the superficial temporal or occipital artery) should be incorporated in the flap base. Other authors have not specifically endorsed the requirement for a named artery in the base of an expanded scalp flap, but nonetheless it is helpful to inspect the scar capsule on the undersurface of the flap at surgery after the expander has been removed, and to identify the large caliber vessel or vessels frequently seen entering the flap at the base. When making rotation incisions and back cuts into the base of the flap, the important feeding vessels should be carefully preserved. Releasing incisions made through the scar capsule and galea should be made only if the flap or flaps do not advance or rotate into position easily. Capsulotomies can be helpful, but should be done carefully to avoid injury to the blood vessels lying just superficial to the galea. A great deal of tension should be avoided on flap closure. Sasaki (1985) suggested placing some sutures between the dermis of the flap and the pericranium to minimize tension across the incisions.

When a large area of the scalp is hairless so that there is no real possibility of completely resurfacing the scalp with hair-bearing skin even with serial expansions, the final scalp expansion can involve a transposition flap to provide an anterior (frontal) hairline or a complete peripheral fringe. A microvascular free flap (Ohmori, 1980; Juri and Juri, 1981) can be used to provide forward hair growth along the frontal hairline to conceal the flap edge scar better (see Chap. 31). Preexpansion of these flaps before rotation or free transfer may significantly increase the surface area of the flaps, improve viability, and minimize closure difficulties in the donor site (Leighton, 1986). Figures 41–32 and 41–33 illustrate a case of scalp expansion for alopecia.

Reconstruction of the temporal "sideburn" is important in both men and women. If the temporal area above the ear is hair-bearing and only a small high sideburn is required, as is usually the case in a female patient, some type of one- or two-stage local transposition flap can be used (Juri, Juri, and Colnago, 1981; Fodor and Liverett, 1984). A superficial temporal artery island flap in the temporal or temporoparietal area can also be used for sideburn reconstruction, transferring the flap straight downward so that the direction of the hair growth in the sideburn is appropriate.

To construct an adequate sideburn in a male patient, temporal or parietal scalp expansion can be useful to generate a sufficiently large transposition flap for both sideburn reconstruction and easy closure of the flap donor site. The proper direction for hair growth in the sideburn, however, must always be kept in mind. Sideburn hair should grow downward and backward. For this reason, an anteriorly based temporo-occipital flap above and behind the ear that is transposed forward into the preauricular position will likely transfer the direction of hair growth forward. Anteriorly growing hair within the sideburn can be a particular nuisance to the patient. It cannot be easily combed backward when it is either grown long or clipped short. Therefore, to maintain the same hair growth direction as one finds above and behind the ear, which is downward and backward (as it should be in the sideburn) the expanded temporo-occipital flap is often best moved in two stages: first, a downward rotation on a posteroinferior pedicle, with the expanded flap overlapping the upper ear; and a week or two later, the flap can be safely incised around the ear (narrowing the initial pedicle appreciably), so that the hair growth in the sideburn remains in the same initial direction, i.e., downward and backward. Sideburn reconstruction can also be incorporated in the design of a large expanded advancement-rotation flap being used to cover the entire frontotemporal area. Careful planning is necessary to ensure that when the rectangular extension at the end of the flap that is to be used for sideburn reconstruction is transferred into position, the direction of hair growth within the new sideburn is correct. If, because of the direction of hair growth within the expanded flap or because of the way in which the flap has to be transferred, the proper sideburn hair growth direction cannot be ensured by using the large expanded flap, it is better not to carry out the sideburn reconstruction as part of the correction of the scalp alopecia. Instead, sideburn reconstruction should be deferred and performed as an independent procedure later when the proper direction of hair growth within the reconstructed sideburn can be assured.

The Oral Commissure

Burn scars at or around the corner of the mouth often produce functional oral disability and visual distortion of the lips. The cause of the scarring is usually either a thermal burn involving the central face or an electrical burn that occurs when a child puts a "live"

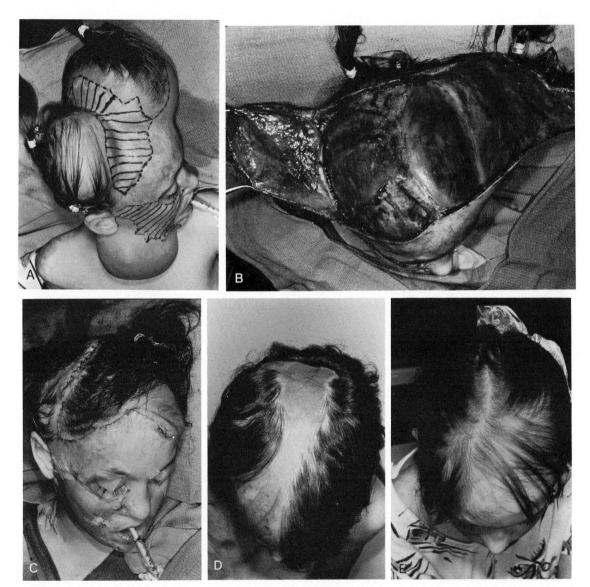

Figure 41–32. Scalp expansion with multiple expanders. *A,* Area of scalp alopecia (striped). *B,* Expanders removed and flaps elevated. *C,* Left side flap advanced for reconstruction of the right anterior hairline, and right side flap used to close the parieto-occipital defect. *D,* Preoperative and *E,* postoperative views.

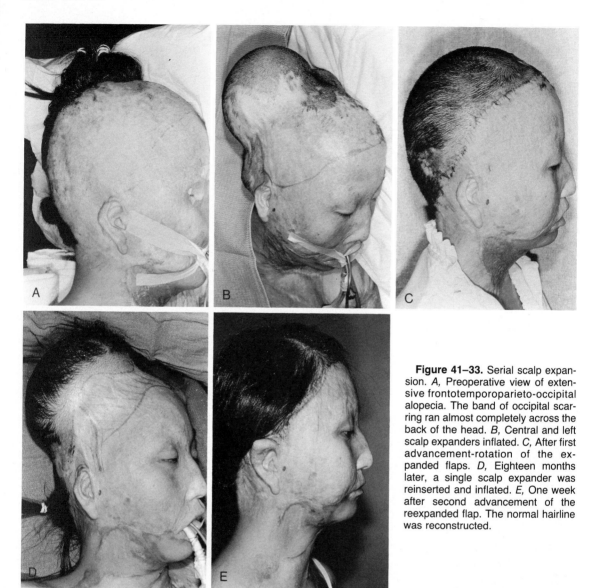

Figure 41–33. Serial scalp expansion. *A,* Preoperative view of extensive frontotemporoparieto-occipital alopecia. The band of occipital scarring ran almost completely across the back of the head. *B,* Central and left scalp expanders inflated. *C,* After first advancement-rotation of the expanded flaps. *D,* Eighteen months later, a single scalp expander was reinserted and inflated. *E,* One week after second advancement of the reexpanded flap. The normal hairline was reconstructed.

extension cord into the mouth. Both causes of perioral injury produce similar characteristics of contracture, but there are also differences. In most of the thermal burns the scarring is more superficial and widespread. Although the injury in electrical burns is more localized, it also is usually much deeper, often involving muscle and mucosa. Regardless of the cause, however, the scar at the corner of the mouth, even one of small size, can narrow the oral opening and inhibit the remarkable elasticity that normally characterizes this area (Fogel and Stranc, 1984).

Since oral stenosis and microstomia in thermal burns are commonly associated with scarring in neighboring areas around the mouth, it usually makes sense to release the tethering scars at the oral commissures at the same time that other procedures are performed, such as when an upper lip, lower lip, or cheek is being released and resurfaced (Anderson and Kurtay, 1971). A reconstructive procedure at the corner of the mouth in these situations can often be a simple one that adds little additional operating time. A transverse or slightly upward incision is made through the scar from the contracted commissure outward to a point in line with, or somewhat lateral to, the pupil of the eye. A small triangle of subcutaneous scar is often removed. If the underlying orbicularis muscle is also tight, it should also be incised. The mucosal lining is mobilized and advanced to the new commissure. Overcorrection is recommended because the opening invariably contracts somewhat (Parks, Baur, and Larson, 1977). Postoperatively, a dynamic expander is useful in helping to prevent recontracture (Colcleugh and Ryan, 1976). Some patients, however, refuse to wear the appliance, and in many recontracture develops to an extent even with splinting. Postponing oral and perioral surgery until the local and regional scars have matured reduces the need for repeated operations on the commissures. However, from a practical point of view, other considerations that concern function, comfort, and appearance make early (and commonly repeated) commissuroplasty appropriate. The subject is also discussed in Chapter 38.

The surgeon should be aware that in extensive face and neck burns, patients' difficulty in opening the mouth can be caused by a tight scar other than one at the corners of the mouth. In these patients, the tight cheek and neck scars also have to be released before the mouth can be opened completely.

Many procedures to deal with oral commissure contractures have been described, and some are quite intricate: various Z-plasties, along with vermilion, muscle, and mucosal transposition and advancement flaps, have been proposed (Szlazak, 1951; Smith, 1954;

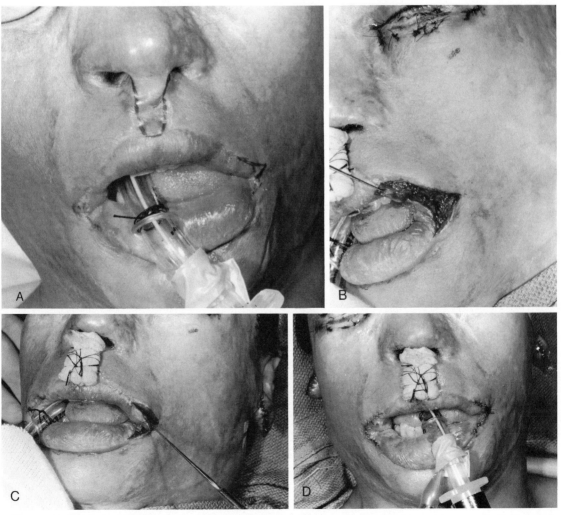

Figure 41–34. Oral commissuroplasty. *A,* Triangular scar excision outlined at both commissures. *B, C,* Superiorly based mucosal flap adjacent to the excision defect elevated to be rotated and advanced to the new commissure, forming the lateral vermilion of the upper lip. The new lateral lower lip vermilion was reconstructed by undermining and advancing outward a buccolabial mucosal flap. *D,* Completed procedure.

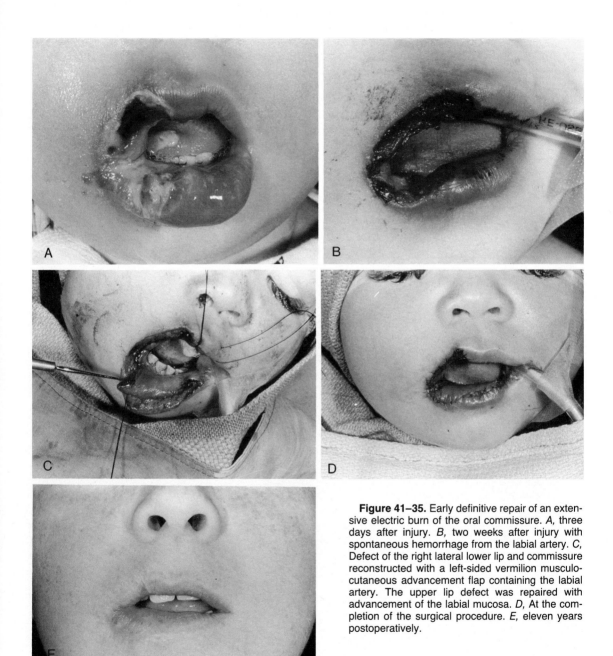

Figure 41–35. Early definitive repair of an extensive electric burn of the oral commissure. *A,* three days after injury. *B,* two weeks after injury with spontaneous hemorrhage from the labial artery. *C,* Defect of the right lateral lower lip and commissure reconstructed with a left-sided vermilion musculocutaneous advancement flap containing the labial artery. The upper lip defect was repaired with advancement of the labial mucosa. *D,* At the completion of the surgical procedure. *E,* eleven years postoperatively.

Mühlbauer, 1970; Fairbanks and Dingman, 1972; Fernandez-Villoria, 1972; Converse, 1972, 1975; Converse and Wood-Smith, 1977; Su, Manson, and Hoopes, 1980). Some of the methods work nicely for some patients some of the time. However, none of the methods can completely guarantee a satisfactory long-term result. In this location, the vagaries of scar contraction often compromise even the best-conceived and best-executed procedure. An example of one type of commissure surgery is shown in Figure 41–34.

Most electrical burns of the lips and commissure should be managed acutely with careful observation and gentle wound hygiene. The wounds are allowed to heal on their own, and if necessary a surgical repair is made a year or several years later when the scar is soft and the deformity is stable (Su, Manson, and Hoopes, 1980). Not infrequently, what first appears to be a fairly extensive injury heals with minimal disfigurement. If bleeding from a labial artery occurs or is imminent, necessitating early operative intervention, the anesthetic opportunity can be used to excise the necrotic tissue and close the wound. If the defect is not extensive, simple undermining and advancement of the labial and buccal mucosa can be carried out. When more extensive tissue destruction has occurred, a definitive repair can be undertaken that will significantly lessen primary wound contraction (Ortiz-Monasterio and Factor, 1980). Later, only minor revisions may be required. Figure 41–35 illustrates the use of a half-lip advancement flap to reconstruct the other half of the lower lip and commissure. In cases of extensive loss of vermilion adjacent to the commissure, a flap taken from the undersurface of the tongue can be used for lower lip repair (Zarem and Greer, 1974; Ortiz-Monasterio and Factor, 1980).

When planning the correction of an established perioral electrical burn deformity, the surgeon should refer to the contralateral uninjured side of the mouth to guide the design for commissure placement and lip recontouring. Symmetry is the most important surgical objective. There is no routine way of carrying out the repair. A careful, detail-conscious analysis of the deformity will dictate what needs to be done. In addition to elongating the corner of the mouth if necessary, the plan should aim at removing white scars from the red vermilion and red scars in the white portion of the lips. Notching along the vermilion margin should be eliminated. Bulky areas should be thinned and depressed spots should be augmented. To adjust and redistribute the red and white lips usually requires a combination of various kinds of flaps such as asymmetric Z-plasties, V-Y and Y-V advancements, lip-switch flaps, and mucosal rotation flaps (Cosman, Gong, and Crikelair, 1968; Hogan and Converse, 1971; Watson, 1973; Kawamoto, 1975; Juri, Juri, and de Antueno, 1976; Balch, 1978; Wustrack and Silsby, 1978; Vecchione, 1979; Juraha, 1988). Every effort should be made to correct or improve the deformity without adding any new scars to the visible white areas of the lip. It is also important to assess the degree of deformity preoperatively with the patient's mouth closed and opened. Often the contours of the mouth are nearly normal with the lips in repose, with the stomal distortion only apparent during speech or eating when the commissural scar is required to stretch.

REFERENCES

Adamson, J. E.: Nasal reconstruction with the expanded forehead flap. Plast. Reconstr. Surg., *81*:12, 1988.

Anderson, R., and Kurtay, M.: Reconstruction of the corner of the mouth. Plast. Reconstr. Surg., *47*:463, 1971.

Antia, N. H., and Buch, V. I.: Chondrocutaneous advancement flap for the marginal defect of the ear. Plast. Reconstr. Surg., *39*:472, 1967.

Antonyshyn, O., Gruss, J. S., Zuker, R., and MacKinnon, S. E.: Tissue expansion in head and neck reconstruction. Plast. Reconstr. Surg., *82*:58, 1988.

Argenta, L. C.: Controlled tissue expansion in reconstructive surgery. Br. J. Plast. Surg., *37*:520, 1984.

Argenta, L. C., Marks, M. W., Iacobucci, J. J., Holson, M., and Austad, E. D.: Expanded full-thickness grafts. Presented at the 59th Annual Meeting of the American Society of Plastic and Reconstructive Surgeons, Toronto, Canada, October, 1988. Plast. Surg. Forum, *11*:176, 1988.

Argenta, L. C., and VanderKolk, C. A.: Tissue expansion in craniofacial surgery. Clin. Plast. Surg., *14*:143, 1987.

Aufricht, G.: Evaluation of pedicle flaps versus skin grafts in reconstruction of surface defects and scar contractures of the chin, cheeks, and neck. Surgery, *15*:75, 1944.

Balch, C. R.: Modification of cross-lip flap. Plast. Reconstr. Surg., *61*:457, 1978.

Barton, F. E.: Aesthetic aspects of nasal reconstruction. Clin. Plast. Surg., *15*:155, 1988.

Bell, M. L.: Scalp reduction. Clin. Plast. Surg., *9*:269, 1982.

Berkowitz, R. L.: Scalp—in search of the perfect donor site. Ann. Plast. Surg., *7*:126, 1981.

Blasius, E.: Rhinoplastik. Z. Dt. Ges. Med., *19*:145, 1842.

Bolton, L. L., Chandrasekhar, B., and Gottlieb, M. E.: Forehead expansion and total nasal reconstruction. Ann. Plast. Surg., 21:210, 1988.

Borges, A. F.: Elective Incisions and Scar Revision. Boston, Little, Brown & Company, 1973.

Borges, A. F.: When is a flap tubed? (correspondence). Plast. Reconstr. Surg., 82:203, 1988.

Brent, B.: Reconstruction of the ear, eyebrow, and sideburn in the burned patient. Plast. Reconstr. Surg., 55:312, 1975.

Brent, B.: The acquired auricular deformity: a systematic approach to its analysis and reconstruction. Plast. Reconstr. Surg., 59:475, 1977.

Brent, B.: The correction of microtia with autogenous cartilage grafts. I. The classic deformity. Plast. Reconstr. Surg., 66:1, 1980.

Brent, B.: Restoration of thermally injured facial features. In Brent, B. (Ed.): The Artistry of Reconstructive Surgery. St. Louis, C. V. Mosby, Company, 1987, pp. 439–445.

Brent, B., and Byrd, H. S.: Secondary ear reconstruction with cartilage grafts covered by axial, random, and free flaps of temporoparietal fascia. Plast. Reconstr. Surg., 72:141, 1983.

Brent, B., Upton, J., Acland, R. D., Shaw, W. W., Finseth, F. J., et al.: Experience with the temporoparietal fascial free flap. Plast. Reconstr. Surg., 76:177, 1985.

Brody, G. S.: Discussion of Pensler, J. M., et al.: Construction of the eyebrow in the pediatric burn patient. Plast. Reconstr. Surg., 76:434, 1985.

Buhrer, D. P., Huang, T. T., Yee, H. W., and Blackwell, S. J.: Treatment of burn alopecia with tissue expanders in children. Plast. Reconstr. Surg., 81:512, 1988.

Burget, G. C.: Aesthetic restoration of the nose. Clin. Plast. Surg., 12:463, 1985.

Burget, G. C., and Menick, F. J.: The subunit principle in nasal reconstruction. Plast. Reconstr. Surg., 76:239, 1985.

Burget, G. C., and Menick, F. J.: Nasal reconstruction: seeking a fourth dimension. Plast. Reconstr. Surg., 78:145, 1986.

Burns, C. L., and Chylack, L. T., Jr.: Thermal burns: the management of thermal burns to the lids and globes. Ann. Ophthalmol., 11:1358, 1979.

Clodius, L.: Excision and grafting of extensive facial haemangiomas. Br. J. Plast. Surg., 30:185, 1977.

Colcleugh, R. G., and Ryan, J. E.: Splinting electrical burns of the mouth in children. Plast. Reconstr. Surg., 58:239, 1976.

Coleman, D. J.: Use of expanded temporal flaps to resurface the skin grafted forehead. Br. J. Plast. Surg., 40:171, 1987.

Constable, J. D., and Carroll, J. M.: The emergency treatment of the exposed cornea in thermal burns. Plast. Reconstr. Surg., 46:309, 1970.

Converse, J. M.: Burn deformities of the face and neck. Surg. Clin. North Am., 47:323, 1967.

Converse, J. M.: Orbicularis advancement flap for reconstruction of the angle of the mouth. Plast. Reconstr. Surg., 49:99, 1972.

Converse, J. M.: Discussion of reconstruction of burned ears. In Tanzer, R. C., and Edgerton, M. T. (Eds.): Symposium on Reconstruction of the Auricle. St. Louis, C. V. Mosby Company, 1974, p. 203.

Converse, J. M.: The "over and out" flap for restoration of the corner of the mouth. Plast. Reconstr. Surg., 56:575, 1975.

Converse, J. M.: Ectropion. In Feller, I., and Grabb, W. C. (Eds.): Reconstruction and Rehabilitation of the Burned Patient. Ann Arbor, MI, National Institute for Burn Medicine, 1979, p. 142.

Converse, J. M., Guy, C. L., and Molenaar, A.: The treatment of giant hairy pigmented nevi of the face. Br. J. Plast. Surg., 22:302, 1969.

Converse, J. M., McCarthy, J. G., Dobrkovsky, M., and Larson, D. L.: Facial burns. In Converse, J. M. (Ed.): Reconstructive Plastic Surgery. 2nd Ed. Philadelphia, W. B. Saunders Company, 1977, p. 1595.

Converse, J. M., and Wood-Smith, D.: Techniques for the repair of defects of the lips and cheeks. In Converse, J. M. (Ed.): Reconstructive Plastic Surgery. 2nd Ed. Philadelphia, W. B. Saunders Company, 1977.

Cosman, B., Gong, K., and Crikelair, G. F.: Horizontal cross-lip flap with pedicle at commissure: case report. Plast. Reconstr. Surg., 41:273, 1968.

Cronin, T. D.: The use of a molded splint to prevent contracture after split skin grafting on the neck. Plast. Reconstr. Surg., 27:7, 1961.

Davis, J.: Discussion of traumatic deformities of the auricle. In Tanzer, R. C., and Edgerton, M. T. (Eds.): Symposium on Reconstruction of the Auricle. St. Louis, C. V. Mosby Company, 1974, pp. 246–247.

Davis, J.: Aesthetic and Reconstructive Otoplasty. New York, Springer-Verlag, 1987, p. 357.

Davis, J. S.: Removal of wide scars and large disfigurements of skin by gradual partial excision with closure. Ann. Surg., 90:645, 1929.

del Campo, A. F.: Surgical treatment of the epicanthal fold. Plast. Reconstr. Surg., 73:566, 1984.

Denonvilliers, C. P.: Blepharoplastie. Bull. Soc. Chir. Paris, 7:243, 1856.

Dingman, R. O., and Argenta, L. C.: The surgical repair of traumatic defects of the scalp. Clin. Plast. Surg., 9:131, 1982.

Dowling, J. A., Foley, F. D., and Moncrief, J. A.: Chondritis in the burned ear. Plast. Reconstr. Surg., 42:115, 1968.

Edgerton, M. T., and Hansen, F. C.: Matching facial color with split-thickness skin grafts from adjacent areas. Plast. Reconstr. Surg., 25:455, 1960.

Engrav, L. H., Heimbach, D. M., Walkishaw, M. D., and Marvin, J. A.: Excision of burns of the face. Plast. Reconstr. Surg., 77:744, 1986.

Erol, O. O., and Atabay, K.: Treatment of hypertrophic scar leukoderma due to burn using dermabrasion and thin skin graft. Presented at the Symposium on Recent Advances in Burn Injuries, Istanbul, Turkey, 1988.

Fahmy, M.: Sculpture in Reconstructive Plastic Surgery. Madrid, Diaz de Santos, S. A., 1985.

Fairbanks, G. R., and Dingman, R. O.: Restoration of the oral commissure. Plast. Reconstr. Surg., 49:411, 1972.

Falvey, M. P., and Brody, G. S.: Secondary correction of the burned eyelid deformity. Plast. Reconstr. Surg., 62:564, 1978.

Feldman, J. J.: The antimongoloid lateral eyelid burn deformity. Plast. Surg. Forum, 2:77, 1979.

Feldman, J. J.: Reconstruction of the burned face in children. In Serafin, D., and Georgiade, N. (Eds.): Pediatric Plastic Surgery. St. Louis, C. V. Mosby Company, 1984, p. 552.

Feldman, J. J.: Discussion of Engrav, L. H., et al.: Excision of burns of the face. Plast. Reconstr. Surg., 77:750, 1986.

Feldman, J. J.: Single sheet resurfacing of the burned face and neck. In Brent, B. (Ed.): The Artistry of Reconstructive Surgery. St. Louis, C. V. Mosby Company, 1987a, p. 327.

Feldman, J. J.: Secondary repair of the burned upper lip. Perspect. Plast. Surg., *1*:31, 1987b.

Feldman, J. J.: Reconstruction of the philtrum with a composite skin-cartilage graft. Perspect. Plast. Surg., *1*:110, 1987c.

Feldman, J. J.: Second opinion: burn reconstruction (a case analysis). Perspect. Plast. Surg., *2*:147, 1988.

Feller, I.: Personal communication to D. L. Larson, 1975. *In* Converse, J. M., McCarthy, J. G., Dobrkovsky, M., and Larson, D. L. (Eds.): Facial burns. Reconstructive Plastic Surgery. 2nd Ed. Philadelphia, W. B. Saunders Company, 1977, p. 1595.

Fernandez-Villoria, J. M.: A new method of elongation of the corner of the mouth. Plast. Reconstr. Surg., *49*:52, 1972.

Finucan, T., Budo, J., and Clarke, J. A.: Partial thickness scalp grafts: clinical experience of their use in resurfacing facial defects. Br. J. Plast. Surg., *37*:468, 1984.

Fodor, P. B., and Liverett, D. M.: Sideburn reconstruction for postrhytidectomy deformity. Plast. Reconstr. Surg., *74*:430, 1984.

Fogel, M. L., and Stranc, M. F.: Lip function: a study of normal lip parameters. Br. J. Plast. Surg., *37*:542, 1984.

Frank, H. A., Berry, C., Wachtel, T. L., and Johnson, R. W.: The impact of thermal injury. J. Burn Care Rehab., *8*:260, 1987.

Gibson, T.: The physical properties of skin. *In* Converse, J. M. (Ed.): Reconstructive Plastic Surgery. 2nd Ed. Philadelphia, W. B. Saunders Company, 1977, p. 70.

Gillies, H., and Millard, D. R., Jr.: The Principles and Art of Plastic Surgery. Boston, Little, Brown & Company, 1957.

Goldstein, J. A., and Stevenson, T. R.: Reconstruction of the ear helix: use of self-tubing pedicle flap. Ann. Plast. Surg., *21*:149, 1988.

Gonzalez-Ulloa, M.: Restoration of the face covering by means of selected skin in regional aesthetic units. Br. J. Plast. Surg., *9*:212, 1956.

Gonzalez-Ulloa, M., Castillo, A., Stevens, E., Alvarez Fuertez, G., Leonelli, F., and Ubaldo, F.: Preliminary study of the total restoration of the facial skin. Plast. Reconstr. Surg., *13*:151, 1954.

Grant, D. A., Finley, M. L., and Coers, C. R., III: Early management of the burned ear. Plast. Reconstr. Surg., *44*:161, 1969.

Greminger, R. F., Elliott, R. A., Jr., and Rapperport, A.: Antibiotic iontophoresis for the management of burned ear chondritis. Plast. Reconstr. Surg., *66*:356, 1980.

Guan, W. X., Wang, E. Y., and Zhang, D. S.: Skin grafted forehead flap for total nasal reconstruction in severe post burn facial deformity. Eur. J. Plast. Surg., *11*:57, 1988.

Guy, C. L., and Converse, J. M.: Nevus excision and serial facial resurfacing. *In* Brent, B. (Ed.): The Artistry of Reconstructive Surgery. St. Louis, C. V. Mosby Company, 1987, pp. 359–364.

Hallock, G. G.: Maximum overinflation of tissue expanders. Plast. Reconstr. Surg., *80*:567, 1987.

Hardesty, R. A., Theodoro, T. D., Bartell, T., Young, V. L., and Mustoe, T. A.: "Something for nothing?" Tissue expansion and enhancement. Presented at the 59th Annual Meeting of the American Society of Plastic and Reconstructive Surgeons, Toronto, Canada, October, 1988. Plast. Surg. Forum, *11*:40, 1988.

Hauben, D. J., and Sagi, A.: A sample method for alar rim reconstruction. Plast. Reconstr. Surg., *80*:839, 1987.

Heimbach, D. M., and Engrav, L. H.: Surgical Management of the Burn Wound. New York, Raven Press, 1984.

Hogan, V. M., and Converse, J. M.: Secondary deformity of the unilateral cleft lip and nose. *In* Grabb, W. C. (Ed.): Cleft Lip and Palate. Boston, Little, Brown & Company, 1971.

Huang, T. T., Blackwell, S. J., and Lewis, S. R.: Burn injuries of the eyelids. Clin. Plast. Surg., *5*:571, 1978.

Huang, T. T., Larson, D. L., and Lewis, S. R.: Burn alopecia. Plast. Reconstr. Surg., *60*:763, 1977.

Hupp, S. L., Galanos, A. N., and Laterman, A.: A simple moisture chamber for the early treatment of corneal exposure in patients with facial burns. J. Burn Care Rehab., *8*:115, 1987.

Hyakusoku, H., Okubo, M., Umeda, T., and Fumiiri, M.: A prefabricated hair-bearing island flap for lip reconstruction. Br. J. Plast. Surg., *40*:37, 1987.

Jabaley, M. E., Cat, N. D., and Lac, N. T.: Use of local flap for burn contracture of the neck. Plast. Reconstr. Surg., *48*:288, 1971.

Jackson, I. T.: Editor's perspective on Feldman, J. J.: Secondary repair of the burned upper lip. Perspect. Plast. Surg., *1*:68, 1987.

Jackson, I. T., Sharpe, D. T., Polley, J., Costanzo, C., and Rosenberg, L.: Use of external reservoirs in tissue expansion. Plast. Reconstr. Surg., *80*:266, 1987.

Janvier, H., and Colin, B.: Traitement par lambeaux de voisinage des rétractions cutanées, séquelles de brulures des faces antérieures et latérales du cou. Ann. Chir. Plast., *17*:26, 1972.

Joseph, J.: Nasenplastik und sonstige Gesichtsplastik. Leipzig, C. Kabitsch, 1931.

Juraha, Z. L.: Reconstruction of the lower lip with two flaps from the upper lip hinged on the superior labial vessels. Br. J. Plast. Surg., *33*:87, 1988.

Juri, J., and Juri, C.: Aesthetic aspects of reconstructive scalp surgery. Clin. Plast. Surg., *8*:243, 1981.

Juri, J., Juri, C., Belmont, J. A., Grilli, D. A., and Angrigiani, C.: Neighboring flaps and cartilage grafts for correction of serious secondary nasal deformities. Plast. Reconstr. Surg., *76*:876, 1985.

Juri, J., Juri, C., and Cerisola, J.: Contribution to Converse's flap for nasal reconstruction. Plast. Reconstr. Surg., *69*:697, 1982.

Juri, J., Juri, C., and Colnago, A.: The surgical treatment of temporal and sideburn alopecia. Br. J. Plast. Surg., *34*:186, 1981.

Juri, J., Juri, C., and de Antueno, J.: A modification of the Kapetansky technique for repair of whistling deformities of the upper lip. Plast. Reconstr. Surg., *57*:70, 1976.

Kaplan, I., and Goldwyn, R. M.: The versatility of the laterally based cervicofacial flap for cheek repairs. Plast. Reconstr. Surg., *61*:390, 1978.

Kawamoto, H. K.: Correction of major defects of the vermilion with a cross-lip vermilion flap. Plast. Reconstr. Surg., *64*:315, 1975.

Kesselring, U. K.: Lip augmentation. Presented at the 18th Annual Meeting of the American Society for Aesthetic Plastic Surgery, Boston, April 17, 1985.

Kobus, K.: Free transplantation of tissues: problems and complications. Ann. Plast. Surg., *20*:55, 1988.

Kobus, K., and Stepniewski, J.: Surgery of post-burn neck contractures. Eur. J. Plast. Surg., *11*:126, 1988.

Kreibig, G.: Vereinfachte Operationmethoden zum Ersatz der Augenlider. Stuttgart, Enke, 1940.

Langenbeck, B.: Handbuch der Anatomie. Gottingen, Dietrich, 1843.

Leighton, W. D., Johnson, M. L., and Friedland, J. A.:

Use of the temporary soft-tissue expander in posttraumatic alopecia. Plast. Reconstr. Surg., 77:737, 1986.

Leighton, W. D., Russell, R. C., Marcus, D. E., Eriksson, E., Sachy, H., and Zook, E. G.: Experimental pretransfer expansion of free-flap donor sites. I. Flap viability and expansion characteristics. Plast. Reconstr. Surg., 82:69, 1988.

Leonard, A. G., and Small, J. O.: Tissue expansion in the treatment of alopecia. Br. J. Plast. Surg., 39:42, 1986.

Liang, M. D., Briggs, P., Heckler, F. R., and Futrell, J. W.: Presuturing—a new technique for closing large skin defects: clinical and experimental studies. Plast. Reconstr. Surg., 81:694, 1988.

Lopez-Mas, J., Ortiz-Monasterio, F., Viale de Gonzalez, M., and Olmedo, A.: Skin graft pigmentation: a new approach to prevention. Plast. Reconstr. Surg., 49:18, 1972.

MacArthur, J. O., and Moore, F. D.: Epidemiology of burns: the burn-prone patient. J.A.M.A., 231:259, 1975.

Macgregor, F. C.: A social science approach to the study of facial deformities and plastic surgery. *In* Converse, J. M. (Ed.): Reconstructive Plastic Surgery. 2nd Ed. Philadelphia, W. B. Saunders Company, 1977, p. 565.

MacLeod, A.: Adult burns in Melbourne: a 5-year survey. Med. J. Aust., 2:772, 1970.

Mahoney, J. L., Morris, S. F., Pang, C. Y., Lofchy, N. M., and Kaddoura, I. L.: The importance of capsular blood flow to the viability of random-pattern skin flaps raised on expanded skin in the pig. Presented at the 59th Annual Meeting of the American Society of Plastic and Reconstructive Surgeons, Toronto, Canada, October, 1988. Plast. Surg. Forum, 11:151, 1988.

Maisels, D. O., and Ghost, J.: Predisposing causes of burns in adults. Practitioner, 201:767, 1968.

Manders, E. K.: Reconstruction of the scalp by tissue expansion. Presented at the Symposium on Tissue Expansion, Ann Arbor, MI, 1983.

Manders, E. K., Farvey, J. A., and Davis, T. S.: Total nasal coverage using expanded forehead flaps. Plast. Surg. Forum, 9:174, 1986.

Manders, E. K., Graham, W. P., III, Schenden, M. J., and Davis, T. S.: Skin expansion to eliminate large scalp defects. Ann. Plast. Surg., 12:305, 1984a.

Manders, E. K., Schenden, M. J., Furrey, J. A., Hetzler, P. T., Davis, T. S., and Graham, W. P., III: Soft-tissue expansion: concepts and complications. Plast. Reconstr. Surg., 74:493, 1984b.

Manders, E. K., and Wong, R. K. M.: Flap design in soft tissue expansion presented at Instructional Course: refinements in tissue expansion—pearls, perils, and pitfalls. Presented at the Annual Meeting of the American Society for Plastic and Reconstructive Surgeons, Atlanta, GA, 1987.

Marchac, D., and Pugash, E.: Expanded scalping forehead flap for coverage of giant congenital nevi of the face: a report of three cases. Eur. J. Plast. Surg., 10:2, 1987.

Marks, M. W., Argenta, L. C., and Thornton, J. W.: Burn management: the role of tissue expansion. Clin. Plast. Surg., 14:543, 1987.

Marks, M. W., Freidman, R. J., Thornton, J. W., and Argenta, L. C.: The temporal island scalp flap for management of facial burn scars. Plast. Reconstr. Surg., 82:257, 1988.

McCarthy, J. G., Lorenc, Z. P., Cutting, C., and Rachesky, M.: The median forehead flap revisited: the blood supply. Plast. Reconstr. Surg., 76:866, 1985.

McGrath, M. H., and Ariyan, S.: Immediate reconstruction of full thickness burn of an ear with an undelayed myocutaneous flap. Plast. Reconstr. Surg., 62:618, 1978.

McIndoe, A.: Total facial reconstruction following burns. Postgrad. Med., 6:187, 1949.

Mercer, D. M.: The cervicofacial flap. Br. J. Plast. Surg., 41:470, 1988.

Meyer, E., and Knorr, N. J.: Psychiatric aspects of plastic surgery. *In* Converse, J. M. (Ed.): Reconstructive Plastic Surgery. 2nd Ed. Philadelphia, W. B. Saunders Company, 1977, p. 549.

Millard, D. R., Jr.: Cleft Craft—The Evolution of its Surgery. Vol. II. Bilateral and Rare Deformities. Boston, Little, Brown & Company, 1977, p. 445.

Millard, D. R., Jr.: Principalization of Plastic Surgery. Boston, Little, Brown & Company, 1986.

Millard, D. R., Jr.: Various uses of the septum in rhinoplasty. Plast. Reconstr. Surg., 81:112, 1988.

Miller, T. A.: Burns of the face: burns around the eyes. *In* Artz, C. T., Moncrief, J. A., and Pruitt, B. A., Jr. (Eds.): Burns: A Team Approach. Philadelphia, W. B. Saunders Company, 1979.

Miller, T. A.: The Tagliacozzi flap as a method of nasal and palatal reconstruction. Plast. Reconstr. Surg., 78:870, 1985.

Mills, D. C., Roberts, L. W., Mason, A. D., McManus, W. F., and Pruitt, B. A.: Suppurative chondritis: its incidence, prevention, and treatment in burned patients. Plast. Reconstr. Surg., 82:267, 1988.

Mir y Mir, L.: Fisiopathologia y Tratamiento de las Quemaduras y sus Secullas. Barcelona, Spain, Cientifico-Medica, 1969, pp. 321–333.

Morestin, H.: La reduction graduelle des difformités tegumentaires. Bull. Mém. Soc. Chir. Paris, 41:1233, 1915. Translated from French by Converse, J. M. *In* McDowell, F. (Ed.): The Source Book of Plastic Surgery. Baltimore, Williams & Wilkins Company, 1977.

Morris, M. W., Friedman, R. J., Thornton, J. W., and Argenta, L. C.: The temporal island scalp flap for management of facial burn scars. Plast. Reconstr. Surg., 82:257, 1988.

Mühlbauer, W. D.: Elongation of mouth in post-burn microstomia by a double Z-plasty. Plast. Reconstr. Surg., 45:400, 1970.

Mustardé, J. C.: Reconstruction of the eyelid. *In* Feller, I., and Grabb, W. C. (Eds.): Reconstruction and Rehabilitation of the Burned Patient. Ann Arbor, MI, National Institute for Burn Medicine, 1979, p. 136.

Mutter, T. D.: Cases of deformity from burns, relieved by operation. Am. J. Med. Sci., 5:66, 1842.

Nahai, F., and McGain, L.: A method for the exteriorization of tissue expander tubing. Plast. Reconstr. Surg., 82:723, 1988.

Neale, H. W., High, R. M., Billmire, D. A., Carey, J. P., Smith, D., and Warren, G.: Complications of controlled tissue expansion in the pediatric burn patient. Plast. Reconstr. Surg., 82:840, 1988.

Neumann, C. G.: The expansion of an area of skin by progressive distention of a subcutaneous balloon. Plast. Reconstr. Surg., 19:124, 1957.

Nordström, R. E.: "Stretch-back" in scalp reductions for male pattern baldness. Plast. Reconstr. Surg., 73:422, 1984.

Ohmori, K.: Free scalp flap. Plast. Reconstr. Surg., 65:42, 1980.

Ohura, T.: Reconstructive surgery of the nose in non-Caucasians. Clin. Plast. Surg., 1:93, 1974.

O'Neal, R. M., Rohrich, R. J., and Izenberg, P. H.: Skin expansion as an adjunct to reconstruction of the external ear. Br. J. Plast. Surg., 37:517, 1984.

Ortiz-Monasterio, F., and Factor, R.: Early definitive treatment of electric burns of the mouth. Plast. Reconstr. Surg., 65:169, 1980.

Paletta, F. X.: Surgical management of the burned scalp. Clin. Plast. Surg., 9:167, 1982.

Papp, T.: Predisposing causes of burns in adults: evaluation of 47 patients who suffered repeated burn accidents. Bull. Clin. Rev. Burn Injuries, 1:63, 1984.

Parks, D. H., Baur, P. S., Jr., and Larson, D. L.: Late problems in burns. Clin. Plast. Surg., 4:547, 1977.

Pensler, J. M., Dillon, B., and Parry, S. W.: Reconstruction of the eyebrow in the pediatric burn patient. Plast. Reconstr. Surg., 76:434, 1985.

Pietila, J. P., Nordström, R. E., Virkkunen, P. J., Voutilainen, P. E., and Rintala, A. E.: Accelerated tissue expansion with the "overfilling" technique. Plast. Reconstr. Surg., 81:204, 1988.

Pontén, B.: Burns in automobile accidents. Scand. J. Plast. Surg., 2:104, 1968.

Radovan, C.: Tissue expansion. In Brent, B. (Ed.): The Artistry of Reconstructive Surgery. St. Louis, C. V. Mosby Company, 1987, pp. 389–393.

Roper-Hall, M. J.: Immediate treatment of thermal and chemical burns. In Troutman, R. C., Converse, J. M., and Smith, B. (Eds.): Plastic and Reconstructive Surgery of the Eye and Adnexa. Washington, Butterworths, 1962, p. 1991.

Rougier, J., Tessier, P., Hervolt, S., Woillez, M., Lekieffre, M., and Derome, T.: Chirurgie Plastique Orbito-Palpebrale. Paris, Masson et Cie., 1974. English translation by Wolfe, S. A.: Plastic Surgery of the Orbit and Eyelids. New York, Masson Publishing, 1981, p. 346.

Sasaki, G. H.: Tissue expansion: guidelines and case analysis. Booklet by Dow Corning Wright, Arlington, TN, 1985.

Sasaki, G. H.: Refinements of tissue expansion. In Jurkiewicz, M. J., Krizek, T. J., Mathes, S. J., and Ariyan, S. (Eds.): Plastic Surgery: Principles and Practice. St. Louis, C. V. Mosby Company, 1986.

Sasaki, G. H.: Intraoperative sustained limited expansion (ISLE) as an immediate reconstructive technique. Clin. Plast. Surg., 14:563, 1987a.

Sasaki, G. H.: Refinements of tissue expansion. In Jurkiewicz, M. J., Krizek, T. V., and Mathes, S. J. (Eds.): Plastic Surgery: Principles and Practice. St. Louis, C. V. Mosby Company, 1987b.

Sasaki, G. H.: Refinements in tissue expansion—pearls, perils, and pitfalls. Instructional Course presented at the Annual Meeting of the American Society of Plastic and Reconstructive Surgeons, Atlanta, GA, 1987c.

Sasaki, G. H., and Pang, C. Y.: Pathophysiology of skin flaps raised on expanded pig skin. Plast. Reconstr. Surg., 74:59, 1984.

Saxby, P. J.: Inelastic tape to treat problems of tissue expansion. Br. J. Plast. Surg., 41:666, 1988.

Schmid, E.: Plastic operations for partial or total losses of the lip. Plast. Reconstr. Surg., 14:138, 1954.

Schmid, E.: Die Anwendung des Haut-Knorpeltransplantates nach König unter besonderer Berücksichtigung der Spaltplastik. Fortschr. Kiefer Gesichtschir., 5:301, 1955.

Schmid, E.: The use of auricular cartilage and composite grafts in reconstruction of the upper lip, with special reference to reconstruction of the philtrum. In Broadbent, T. R. (Ed.): Transactions of the Third International Congress of Plastic Surgery. Amsterdam, Excerpta Medica, 1964, p. 306.

Schneider, M. S., Borkow, J. E., Cruz, I. T., Marrangoni, R. O., Schaffer, J., and Grove, O.: The tensiometric properties of expanded guinea pig skin. Plast. Reconstr. Surg., 81:398, 1988.

Schrudde, J., and Beinhoff, U.: Reconstruction of the face by means of the angle-rotation flap. Aesth. Plast. Surg., 11:15, 1987.

Siegel, R. J.: Severe ectropion: repair with a modified Tripier flap. Plast. Reconstr. Surg., 80:21, 1987.

Silverstein, P., and Peterson, H. D.: Treatment of eyelid deformities due to burns. Plast. Reconstr. Surg., 51:38, 1973.

Skoog, T.: Surgical Treatment of Burns. A clinical report of 789 cases. Stockholm, Almqvist & Wiksell, 1963.

Sloan, D. F., Huang, T. T., Larson, D. L., and Lewis, S. R.: Reconstruction of eyelids and eyebrows in burned patients. Plast. Reconstr. Surg., 58:340, 1976.

Smith, F.: Symposium on plastic surgery: planning the reconstruction of the face. Surgery, 15:1, 1944.

Smith, F.: Multiple excision and Z-plasties in surface reconstruction. Plast. Reconstr. Surg., 1:170, 1946.

Smith, F.: Plastic and Reconstructive Surgery: A Manual of Management. Philadelphia, W. B. Saunders Company, 1950.

Smith, L. K.: Correction of microstomia. Plast. Reconstr. Surg., 14:302, 1954.

Spear, S. L., Kroll, S. S., and Romm, S.: A new twist to the nasolabial flap for reconstruction of lateral alar defects. Plast. Reconstr. Surg., 79:915, 1987.

Spence, R. J.: Clinical use of a tissue expander–enhanced transposition flap for face and neck reconstruction. Ann. Plast. Surg., 21:58, 1988.

Spira, M., and Hardy, S. B.: Management of the injured ear. Am. J. Surg., 106:678, 1963.

Stark, R. B.: The pantographic expansion principle as applied to the advancement flap. Plast. Reconstr. Surg., 15:222, 1955.

Stark, R. B.: Resurfacing the face. Clin. Plast. Surg., 2:577, 1975.

Stark, R. B.: Resurfacing the face. Clin. Plast. Surg., 9:27, 1982.

Stark, R. B.: Total Facial Reconstruction. New York, Gower Medical Publishing, 1984.

Stroud, M. H.: The simple treatment for suppurative perichondritis. Laryngoscope, 73:556, 1963.

Stroud, M. H.: Treatment of suppurative perichondritis. Laryngoscope, 88:176, 1978.

Su, L. T., Manson, P. N., and Hoopes, J. E.: Electrical burns of the oral commissure. Ann. Plast. Surg., 5:251, 1980.

Szlazak, J.: Correction of microstomia. Plast. Reconstr. Surg., 8:71, 1951.

Tajima, S., and Aoyagi, F.: Correcting post-traumatic lateral epicanthal folds. Br. J. Plast. Surg., 30:200, 1977.

Tegtmeier, R. E., and Gooding, R. A.: The use of a fascial flap in ear reconstruction. Plast. Reconstr. Surg., 60:406, 1977.

Thompson, H. G., and Sleightholm, R.: Isolated nasoocular cleft: a one-stage repair. Plast. Reconstr. Surg., 76:534, 1985.

Tubiana, R.: Thermal burns of the face and eyelids. In

Smith, B., Converse, J. M., Obear, M., and Wood-Smith, D., (Eds.): The Second International Symposium of the Manhattan Eye, Ear and Throat Hospital on Plastic Surgery of the Eye and Adnexa. St. Louis, C. V. Mosby Co., 1967, p. 187.

Vallis, C. P.: Surgical treatment of cicatricial alopecia of the scalp. Clin. Plast. Surg., 9:179, 1982.

van Rappard, J. H., Molenaar, J., van Doorn, K., Sonneveld, G. J., and Borghouts, J. M.: Surface-area increase in tissue expansion. Plast. Reconstr. Surg., 82:833, 1988.

Vecchione, T. R.: Reconstruction of the oral mucocutaneous junction. Plast. Reconstr. Surg., 63:430, 1979.

Vincent, M. P., and Carraway, J. H.: Eyelid reconstruction—principles and use of skin grafts. Presented at the 56th Annual Meeting of the American Society of Plastic and Reconstructive Surgeons, Atlanta, GA, November, 1987. Plast. Surg. Forum, 10:197, 1987.

Walton, R. L., and Bunkis, J.: A free occipital hair-bearing flap for reconstruction of the upper lip. Br. J. Plast. Surg., 36:168, 1983.

Wanamaker, H. H.: Suppurative perichondritis of the auricle. Trans. Am. Acad. Ophthalmol. Otolaryngol., 76:1289, 1972.

Watson, A. C.: An innervated muco-muscular flap for the correction of defects of the vermilion border of the lip. Br. J. Plast. Surg., 26:355, 1973.

Wolfe, S. A.: Eyelid reconstruction. Clin. Plast. Surg., 5:525, 1978.

Wustrack, K. O., and Silsby, J. J.: Reconstruction of incompetent oral commissures with dermal-muscle flaps from the lips. Plast. Reconstr. Surg., 62:118, 1978.

Yoshimura, Y., Nakajima, T., and Kami, T.: Scalp graft for elevation of the reconstructed auricle. Plast. Reconstr. Surg., 80:352, 1987.

Zarem, H. A., and Greer, D. M., Jr.: Tongue flap for reconstruction of the lips after electrical burns. Plast. Reconstr. Surg., 53:310, 1974.

42

Daniel C. Baker

Facial Paralysis

This chapter is devoted to a single cranial nerve, but the treatment of facial paralysis is not in the realm of any one specialty. The intracranial, intratemporal, and extratemporal lesions of the facial nerve require the skill and cooperation of the neurosurgeon, the neurologist, the ophthalmologist, the otolaryngologist, and the plastic surgeon. It is only through the close interchange of ideas among these specialists that advances in facial rehabilitation will continue to occur.

Some of the methods of treatment of facial paralysis are controversial, and some are still being developed. The surgeon must employ a number of concepts depending on the etiology, the time interval, the wound characteristics, and the availability and necessity of neuromuscular substitution.

The patterns of facial paralysis vary in the degree of involvement and duration, and no single surgical method can correct a complex combination of axonal and muscular degeneration. Careful preoperative selection of patients based on sound judgment of what can and cannot be achieved by the proposed surgical technique is paramount to a successful operation and a satisfied patient. A combined surgical approach often yields maximal results. The fact that the totally paralyzed face can never be made normal by any of the current methods of reconstruction does not detract from the measured and recognized success of these techniques.

Although much of the recent progress has its origins in the past, the fundamental advances that have been made are associated with an improved understanding of nerve-muscle physiology and rehabilitation of the neuromuscular system. Nerve grafts, crossovers, muscle transfers, free muscle and nerve-muscle grafts, and microneurovascular muscle transfers are the principal methods being developed. All of these techniques concentrate on dynamic reconstruction.

The lifetime work of Bell (1821) was not only of importance for neurology as a whole but also for the study of facial paralysis (Fig. 42–1). In 1814 he sectioned the facial nerve of a monkey with resultant facial paralysis, and demonstrated that the nerve was responsible for facial expression. "On cutting of the respiratory nerve on the face of a monkey, the very peculiar activity of his features on that side ceased altogether. The timid mo-

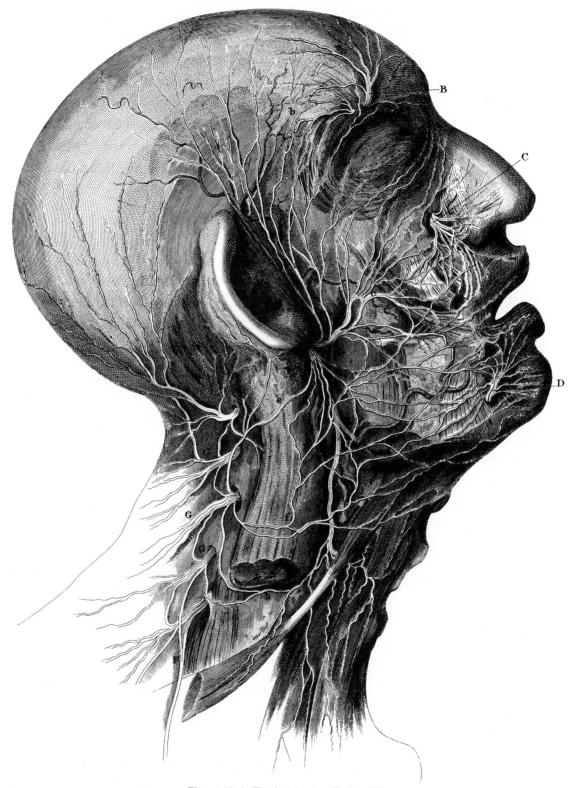

Figure 42–1. The facial nerve (Bell, 1821).

tions of his eyelids and eyebrows were lost, and he could not wink on that side; and his lips were drawn to the other side, like a paralytic drunkard, whenever he showed his teeth in rage. I suspect that the influence of passion, as that of smiling or laughing, is lost in consequence of affections that do not destroy the entire power of the nerve."

Almost 100 years ago, Drobnik (1896) was the first to perform an anastomosis of the facial and spinal accessory nerves to restore facial expression. However, it was not until 1927 that Sterling Bunnell carried out the first successful facial nerve graft. This was followed by the highly successful experimental work of Ballance (1924) and Ballance and Duel (1932) on bridging large intratemporal facial nerve defects in monkeys with free autogenous nerve grafts. Bunnell (1937) bridged defects of the extratemporal facial nerve with free autogenous nerve grafts in one case of resection of a parotid tumor and in another following trauma.

Despite these early successful results, there were few reports of facial nerve repair or grafting in the parotid or cheek area before 1950. In fact, there was considerable pessimism regarding the rationale of facial nerve grafting. Much of the incentive for facial nerve repair and grafting was a direct result of trauma during World War II as well as the facial paralysis resulting from radical operations for cancer of the parotid gland.

Much of the general acceptance of extratemporal facial nerve surgery within the past 30 years is due to the extensive work of Lathrop (1953, 1956, 1963, 1964) and Conley (1975). Conley (1955, 1957, 1961, 1975) especially has been a strong advocate of immediate reconstruction and nerve grafting after ablative procedures, and popularized muscle transfers and nerve crossovers to rehabilitate the paralyzed face.

In the past two decades the work of Smith (1971) and Anderl (1973, 1977a,b, 1985) on crossface nerve grafting has contributed greatly to a renaissance in facial paralysis reconstruction. Most recently the efforts of Harii (1979, 1988), Harii, Ohmori, and Torii (1976), O'Brien and Morrison (1987), Terzis (1987), and Manktelow (1984, 1987) with microneurovascular muscle transfers for facial paralysis have added another dimension to the armamentarium of reconstructive techniques that can be offered to the patient with a paralyzed face.

ANATOMY

Intratemporal Facial Nerve

The facial nerve trunk is formed by the fibers from the supranuclear and infranuclear pathways from the facial nucleus. It leaves the pons, crosses the subarachnoid space to the internal auditory meatus, and enters the facial canal of the temporal bone. Within the facial canal, three branches arise. The most proximal branch is the greater superficial petrosal nerve arising at the level of the geniculate ganglion. It supplies secretomotor fibers to the lacrimal gland and conveys taste from the soft palate, as well as deep pressure sense and pain from the muscles and facial bones. The second branch is the nerve to the stapedius muscle, which provides a dampening effect upon sound vibrations reaching the inner ear. The last branch within the temporal bone is the chorda tympani nerve, which arises approximately 5 mm proximal to the stylomastoid foramen and provides secretomotor fibers to the submaxillary and sublingual glands, and taste fibers from the anterior two-thirds of the tongue.

Extratemporal Facial Nerve

A fundamental knowledge of the surgical anatomy of the parotid gland and facial nerve is essential for the surgeon reconstructing facial paralysis patients. It is important to remember that in infants the facial nerve lies more superficially as it exits the stylomastoid foramen because the mastoid process is not yet completely developed.

The parotid gland is paired and situated immediately inferior and anterior to the lower part of the ear ("parotid" is derived from two Greek words meaning "near the ear") (Fig. 42–2). Its superior limit is at the zygoma; the inferior limit is below the angle of the mandible. It extends anteriorly to a variable extent over the masseter muscle; it is bordered posteriorly by the external auditory meatus, the mastoid and styloid processes, and the sternocleidomastoid and posterior digastric muscles. The deep portion of the gland extends along the bony external auditory meatus behind the ascending ramus toward the base of the skull. The parotid (Stensen's) duct is approximately 6 cm long

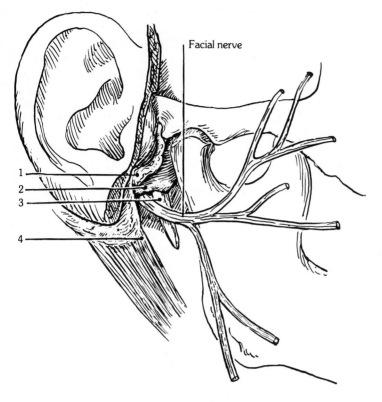

Facial nerve

Figure 42–2. The critical landmarks in identifying the facial nerve's main trunk are: 1, The "conchal cartilaginous pointer"; 2, the tympanomastoid sulcus; 3, the styloid process; 4, the superior border of digastric muscle's posterior belly. These should be identified before searching for the main trunk of the seventh cranial nerve. (From Baker, D. C.: Facial reanimation by hypoglossal-facial nerve anastomosis. *In* Brent, B. (Ed.): The Artistry of Reconstructive Surgery. St. Louis, MO, C. V. Mosby Company, 1987, p. 298.)

and opens into the mouth by a small orifice opposite the maxillary second molar. The direction of the duct corresponds to a line drawn across the face from the lower part of the concha to midway between the free margins of the upper lip and nasal ala, approximately one fingerbreadth below the zygoma. The fascia of the gland is attached to the zygomatic arch above, and to the fascia of the masseter and sternocleidomastoid muscle below. In different regions about the parotid the fascia varies in thickness and fixation as it comes into contact with various muscles, bone, cartilage, blood vessels, and nerves.

The larger superficial segment of the gland, which makes up 70 to 80 per cent of the entire gland, lies lateral to the facial nerve branches, and the smaller deep portion lies medial to these branches. The portion of the gland embraced near the origin of the two major nerve divisions is called the isthmus. There is evidence, from a developmental point of view, that the parotid is anatomically collar-button shaped, with two lobes and a connecting short, slender isthmus; from a surgical point of view, the lobes seem more or less fused, yet are separable with careful surgical technique. In addition, the deep lobe has a retromandibular portion of variable size

that hooks around the posterior portion of the mandible and extends medially into the loose areolar tissues of the upper lateral pharyngeal area in close relation to the internal carotid artery and internal jugular vein.

The facial nerve emerges from the skull through the stylomastoid foramen and passes 0.5 to 1.5 cm inferiorly with a slight anterolateral inclination to enter the parotid gland (Fig. 42–2). The facial nerve branches are given off after it has entered the parotid, with the exception of muscular rami to the occipital, auricular, posterior digastric, and stylohyoid muscles. In this short passage from foramen to gland, the nerve passes anterior to the posterior belly of the digastric muscle and lateral to the styloid process, external carotid artery, and posterior facial vein. Shortly after entering the gland and at a point posterior and slightly medial to the ramus of the mandible, the nerve splits into two main divisions, the *temporofacial* and the *cervicofacial* portions (Fig. 42–3). The two divisions sub-branch to form five main branches: the *temporal, zygomatic, buccal, mandibular,* and *cervical.* The terminal nerve branching (the so-called "pes anserinus," meaning "goose's foot") and possible anastomotic connections are complex. Although many dissections have been performed (Miehlke, Stennert, and Chilla, 1979) to establish the usual patterns, position, and variations of the nerve branches (Davis and associates, 1956), they are relative and cannot be relied on for the specific anatomy of the nerve in the individual patient.

On the basis of clinical experiences with 2000 parotidectomies, Baker and Conley (1979) found that each facial nerve has its own complex and varied anatomic pattern. The main trunk is the most consistent portion of the nerve, usually with a bifurcation within the parotid gland. There can be a trifurcation, however, with the addition of a buccal branch (and occasionally a quadrification, or rarely a plexiform design of the branches) (Fig. 42–4). As the main trunk and its divisions run anteriorly in the gland, they become more superficial, but almost all branching and connecting occur within the parotid gland. To injure the nerve within the gland, the dissection must be carried into the parenchyma of the gland; thus, it is the more distal parts that are at greatest risk.

The temporal division has many connections within its own branches, as well as with those of other nerves in the face. It has five to seven branches, usually consisting of one to the frontal area, two to the orbital area, three to the zygomatic area, and two to the buccal area. The zygomatic branch is the largest and most important, while the frontal branch has the smallest number of connections and is a terminal branch in 85 to 90 per cent of cases. Clinical experience, corroborated by cadaver studies (Davis and associates, 1956; Miehlke, Stennert, and Chilla, 1979), demonstrates that connections between the major divisions are frequent (occurring in 70 to 90 per cent of patients).

The cervical division is almost always the smallest and usually has three to five branches: one buccal, three mandibular, and one cervical. All the branches are approximately the same size, and there are frequent interconnections.

The ramus mandibularis is a delicate branch, perhaps most vulnerable to injury in a face lift, and connects with the other branches in only 10 to 15 per cent of cases. The nerve branches anterior to the parotid gland lie just beneath the superficial masseteric fascia, while the mandibular and cervical branches always (or nearly always) lie deep to the platysma muscle (Fig. 42–5). Theoretically, as long as the dissection remains superficial to this anatomic landmark, the nerve branches cannot be injured during the elevation of a skin flap or removal of excessive subcutaneous fat. However, the development of the platysma is variable, and in some older individuals it may be so thin and atrophic that it is difficult to identify it. Another anatomic point is that, although the nerve branches are relatively superficial for part of their course, they always enter the innervated muscles deeply on the lateral undersurface.

MANDIBULAR BRANCH

The popularization of rhytidectomy techniques for resection of submental and submandibular fat external to the platysma muscle, and the transection of this muscle to

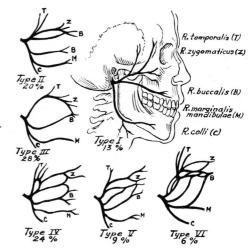

Figure 42–3. Various types of branching of the facial nerve.

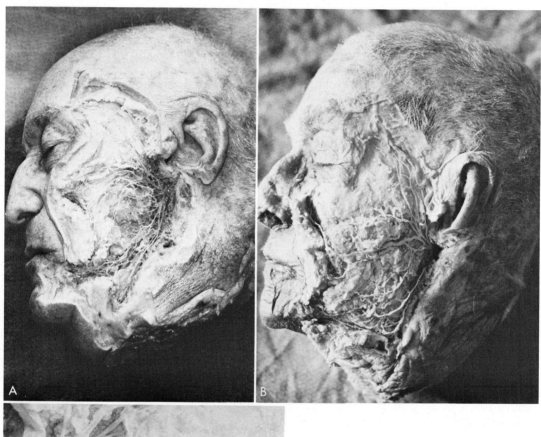

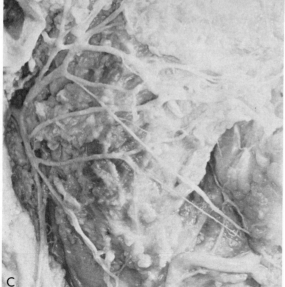

Figure 42–4. Anatomy of the facial nerve (dissected with the operating microscope). *A*, A complex specimen showing multiple connections between the major branches. *B*, Specimen showing a simpler pattern of distribution with two extraplanar branches arising from the main buccal trunk and descending into the lower portion of the face. *C*, Dissection of the right facial nerve. Note the single extraplanar branch arising from a buccal nerve, crossing over two other large branches, and finally intermingling with some of the upturning offshoots of the marginal mandibular nerve. (Courtesy of Drs. A. L. Rhoton and W. Lineweaver.)

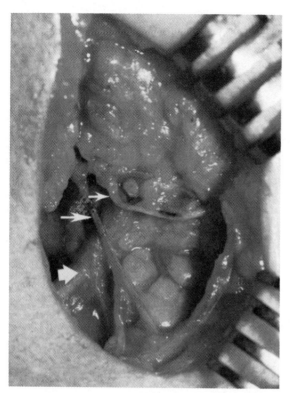

Figure 42–5. The lowest marginal mandibular branch *(upper arrow)* and the cervical branch *(middle arrow)* passing over the facial vein *(lower arrow)* and beneath the platysma. (From Baker, D. C., and Conley, J.: Avoiding facial nerve injuries in rhytidectomy. Plast. Reconstr. Surg., 64:782, 1979.)

create a flap, require the surgeon using them to be careful to avoid injury of the mandibular division of the facial nerve and its branches.

In 1962 Dingman and Grabb presented a study on the mandibular ramus of the facial nerve, based on the dissection of 100 facial halves. They reported that posterior to the facial artery the mandibular ramus ran above the inferior border of the mandible in 81 per cent of their specimens. In the other 19 per cent, the nerve or one or more of its branches ran in an arc, the lowest point of which was 1 cm or less below the inferior border of the mandible. Anterior to the facial artery, all the branches of the mandibular rami were above the inferior border of the mandible. However, these authors also noted that in many specimens fine branches could be seen running along the lower border of the mandible, some up to 2 cm below it, and that every one of these branches terminated in the platysma.

The above study has been a great aid to surgeons. However, it is important to remem-ber that the dissections were performed on cadavers, and in fixed specimens the tissues are stiff, contracted, less mobile, and shrunken. In clinical experiences with parotidectomies and radical neck dissections, Baker and Conley (1979) found that the mandibular branch of the facial nerve has been 1 to 2 cm below the lower border of the mandible in almost every instance. In some individuals with lax and atrophic tissues, the branches were even 3 to 4 cm below the lower border. It is also important to remember that on the operating table when one extends the neck of the patient, this maneuver draws the nerve even lower (Freeman, 1977).

Although the descending cervical division innervates the main body of the platysma muscle at a much lower level, the mandibular division also innervates the upper and anterior portion of the muscle in at least half the patients. Any surgical intervention in this region, or any surgical maneuver deep to the platysma muscle for the removal of fat, can put this nerve in jeopardy. Approximately 15 per cent of the patients have a connection between the mandibular division and the buccal division (from the upper segment of the facial nerve); in these, the functions of the mandibular nerve may return to a certain degree after it is divided. In the remaining patients, however, injury to this nerve may leave a permanent deficit. The latter may be a subtle one if only the platysma muscle branches are affected, but it is a conspicuous deficit if the entire mandibular division is involved.

MIDFACIAL BRANCHES

The facial nerve lies on the external surface of the buccal fat pad and its thin fascia, and delicate nerve branches also lie just under the fascia of the masseter muscle at this level (Fig. 42–6). Dissection in this area must be done cautiously, and plication sutures through the masseteric fascia carry a risk of injury to facial nerve branches.

Studies by Mitz and Peyronie (1976) of the SMAS have demonstrated that anatomic dissection in a plane deep to the SMAS over the parotid can be efficacious in a rhytidectomy. In this region the facial nerve is well protected by the overlying gland. These authors stressed, however, that anterior to the parotid area the SMAS is thin, and surgical dissection of the SMAS in this area may be dan-

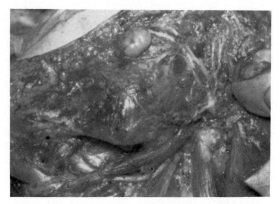

Figure 42–6. The fascia covering the buccal fat pad has been incised, and fat is seen protruding between branches of the facial nerve. Note the fine branches lying on top of the masseter muscle. (The cervical and marginal mandibular branches have been sacrificed in a total parotidectomy for melanoma.) (From Baker, D. C., and Conley, J.: Avoiding facial nerve injuries in rhytidectomy. Plast. Reconstr. Surg., *64*:783, 1979.)

gerous and difficult. Patients with scant subcutaneous tissue or small parotid glands do not have much protection of the nerve branches at this location.

The SMAS (Fig. 42–7) becomes thin in the anterior part of the cheek and suture fixation of the SMAS anterior to the border of the masseter muscle and parotid gland has not been satisfactory.

In the pretragal area and over the parotid gland a dissection of the SMAS is relatively safe, but anterior to the parotid such a dissection becomes difficult and dangerous. Mitz and Peyronie (1976) emphasized that injury to the facial nerve branches may occur (1) when the SMAS is thin, (2) when the retrofascial dissection is carried excessively forward (beyond the anterior border of the parotid gland), and (3) when the superficial parotid lobe is small, leaving the nerves unprotected.

VASCULAR SUPPLY

The main blood supply of the extratemporal facial nerve at the stylomastoid foramen is a branch from the stylomastoid artery off the postauricular artery. The stylomastoid artery exits via the stylomastoid foramen where it runs in close approximation to the main trunk of the facial nerve. It is at this location that the inexperienced surgeon may transect the artery, causing the operative field to fill with blood. Attempts to clamp the "bleeder"

can result in injury to or even transection of the facial nerve. It is at this location that iatrogenic injuries often occur.

Venous drainage about the facial nerve and parotid gland generally parallels the arterial system. The position of the posterior facial vein is important clinically in that it is lateral to the superficial temporal artery and medial to the facial nerve; inferiorly it serves as a reliable landmark for branches of the facial nerve. The cervicofacial division of the facial nerve crosses the posterior facial vein and gives at least one branch to the lateral wall of the vein. The cervical branch descends into the neck to innervate the middle and lower portions of the platysma muscle. The ramus mandibularis is in occasional association with this branch, but is usually separate and anterior to it where the posterior facial vein exits from the inferior part of the gland. The ramus mandibularis may supply a branch to the upper portion of the platysma muscle.

Facial Muscles

There are 17 paired facial muscles (Fig. 42–8) innervated by the seventh cranial (facial) nerve (Table 42–1). The muscles control the movements of the soft tissues of the face. The facial nerve branches innervating these muscles enter in the deeper, more posterior portion of the muscle (Pansky and House, 1964). The muscular fibers penetrate the dermis to insert immediately below the basal epidermal layer. The muscles also interdigitate with the subcutaneous fascia and often with the adjoining muscles. The daily use of these muscles in the emotional and physiologic functions of the face establishes the inevitable pattern of skin lines and wrinkles.

The group of muscles in the upper part of the face are those about the orbit and forehead. The frontalis muscle has inferior extensions interdigitating with the skin about the eyebrows and muscle fibers of the upper borders of the procerus, corrugator, and orbicularis oculi. The latter muscle is divided into orbital, preseptal, and pretarsal components and is responsible for closing the eye. The frontalis muscle elevates the eyebrows, causing horizontal forehead wrinkles depicting the emotions of surprise, doubt, suspicion, and curiosity. Movement of the procerus and corrugator supercilii muscles produce the horizontal and vertical wrinkles in the gla-

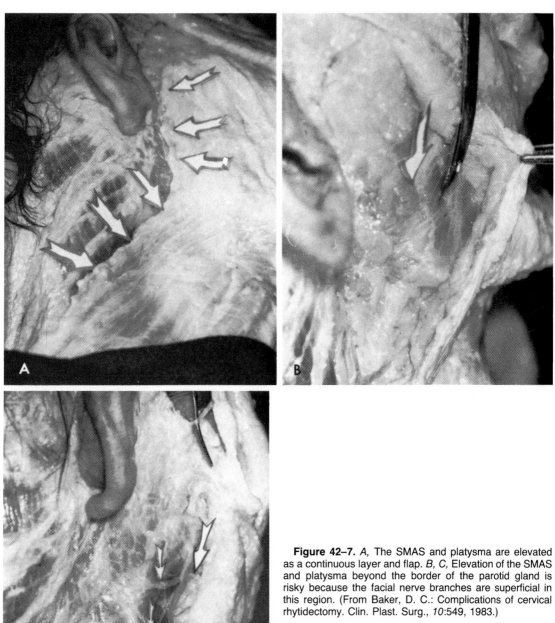

Figure 42–7. *A,* The SMAS and platysma are elevated as a continuous layer and flap. *B, C,* Elevation of the SMAS and platysma beyond the border of the parotid gland is risky because the facial nerve branches are superficial in this region. (From Baker, D. C.: Complications of cervical rhytidectomy. Clin. Plast. Surg., *10*:549, 1983.)

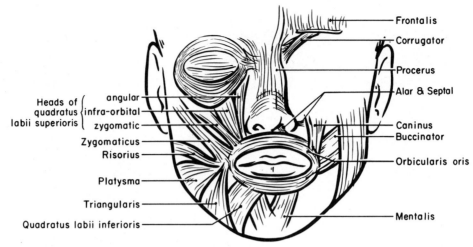

Figure 42–8. The muscles of facial expression: the deeper mimetic muscles on the right side, the more superficial on the left. (This drawing does not show the interweaving fibers of the various muscles to form the orbicularis oris, but regards them as individual muscles seemingly attached to a central raphé. Close examination at the time of surgery shows that the muscles interweave to form the orbicularis oris, which is actually a composite muscle.)

bellar region. The nerve supply to the muscles of the upper third of the face arises from the supraorbital and temporal branches of the facial nerve.

The facial muscles inserting in the nasal pyramid (nasalis, depressor septi nasi, procerus, anterior and posterior dilator nares) contribute little dynamic action to facial movement except in wrinkling of the nose. Their nerve supply is from the infraorbital and buccal branches of the facial nerve.

Perhaps the most important group of muscles in the face consists of those controlling movements of the lips and cheeks. The elevator muscles of the lips (levator labii superioris, levator anguli oris, zygomaticus major and minor, and levator labii superioris alaeque nasi) interdigitate and interlace intimately with the orbicularis oris muscle. They are innervated primarily by the zygomatic and buccal divisions of the facial nerve.

The orbicularis oris muscle provides a

Table 42–1. Muscles of Facial Expression

A. Scalp
1. Frontalis: raises brows and wrinkles forehead as in surprise
2. Occipitalis: with above in raising eyebrows (insignificant physiologic function)

B. Ear
1. Anterior auricular: draws ear up and forward
2. Superior auricular: draws ear up
3. Posterior auricular: draws ear back

C. Eye
1. Orbicularis oculi: sphincter of eye; closes lids; compresses lacrimal sac
2. Corrugator: draws eyebrows downward and medially as in frowning or suffering

D. Nose
1. Procerus: draws medial angle of eyebrow downward
2. Anterior and posterior dilator nares: enlarge nares in hard breathing and anger
3. Depressor septi: constricts nares
4. Nasalis: draws alar wings toward septum and depresses cartilage

E. Mouth
1. Levator labii superioris: raises upper lip

2. Levator labii superioris alaeque nasi: raises lip and dilates nares
3. Zygomaticus minor: with 1 and 2 above, forms nasolabial furrow; deepened when in sorrow
4. Levator anguli oris: with 1 to 3 above, expresses contempt or disdain
5. Zygomaticus major: draws angle of mouth up and back as in laughing
6. Risorius: retracts angle of mouth
7. Depressor labii inferioris: draws lip down and back as in irony
8. Depressor anguli oris: depresses angle of mouth
9. Mentalis: elevates and protrudes lower lip
10. Platysma: retracts and depresses angle of mouth
11. Orbicularis oris: a complex muscle with layers, some parts intrinsic to the lips, the others derived from the following facial muscles: buccinator, levator anguli oris, depressor anguli oris, zygomaticus major and minor; closes lips, protrudes lips, and presses lips to teeth
12. Buccinator: compresses cheek, holds food under teeth in mastication, important in blowing when cheeks are distended with air

Adapted from Pansky, B., and House, E.L.: Review of Gross Anatomy. New York, Macmillan Company, 1964.

sphincter about the oral cavity and lips, and is complemented by extensive interdigitation with all the elevator and depressor muscles of the middle and lower thirds of the face. This confluence of muscles allows for an almost limitless variety of individual facial movement and expressions.

Any surgeon treating facial paralysis should understand the musculature about the mouth, lower lip, and neck (Fig. 42–9) and its innervation. The marginal mandibular branch innervates the depressor anguli oris, the depressor labii inferioris, and the mentalis, as well as part of the orbicularis oris and the risorius.

According to Romanes (1964), the risorius is a thin and flat muscle, in part a continuation of the platysma on the face and in part a separate muscle. It originates from the parotid fascia and inserts into the skin at the angle of the mouth. The function is to retract the angle of the mouth laterally to produce a sardonic expression (although there is some doubt that the muscle is always present).

The depressor anguli oris is a triangular muscle arising from the mandible and inserting at the modiolus labii at the corner of the mouth and the lateral part of the lip, where its fibers are continuous with the orbicularis and risorius. The muscle draws the lower lip downward and laterally in an expression of sadness or disgust.

The depressor labii inferioris also originates from the oblique line of the mandible, and it inserts into the skin of the lower lip (blending with the orbicularis oris). It runs deep and medial to the depressor anguli oris. The function is to draw the lower lip downward and laterally, and to evert the vermilion border (as in expressing irony) (Hueston and Cuthbertson, 1978).

The mentalis arises from the mandible below the incisor teeth and inserts into the skin of the chin. Contraction protrudes and elevates the lower lip and wrinkles the skin of the chin, expressing doubt or disdain.

The orbicularis oris is a complex muscle formed by the contributions from the other muscles converging on the mouth. In the lower lip, the deeper fibers are derived from the buccinator. This muscle may be supplied in part by the marginal mandibular branch, as well as by the buccal branch of the facial nerve.

The platysma muscle arises from the upper deltoid and pectoral regions, and inserts on the lower cheek and corner of the mouth

where it interdigitates with the depressor muscles (Fig. 42–10). As noted by Huber (1931), the platysma and depressor labii inferioris are derived from the primitive sphincter colli muscle, and they have a common insertion at the modiolus. In lower animals, such as the horse, the platysma serves to jerk the skin of the neck for pest control. In man the platysma may be a strong depressor of the lower lip; in certain individuals with a well-developed platysma, this muscle can be seen as constantly active during chewing, swallowing, talking, and other facial expressions. This muscle is supplied by the cervical branch of the facial nerve; not infrequently, however, branches from the marginal mandibular branch supply the anterior portion of the muscle.

Rubin (1974) categorized three basic types of human smile, each dependent on the relative strength of the individual muscle groups about the mouth (Fig. 42–11).

Ellenbogen (1979) emphasized that the platysma muscle is important in the "full denture" smile, in which the lower teeth are exposed and the vermilion everted. He correctly noted that severing one or all cervical branches of the facial nerve in cutting a platysmal flap can give the appearance of a palsy of the marginal mandibular branch. The deformity is not as severe, of course, as that caused by cutting the entire mandibular division (with a paresis of all the depressors of the lower lip).

ETIOLOGY

A patient presenting with facial paralysis is a diagnostic challenge. Facial paralysis

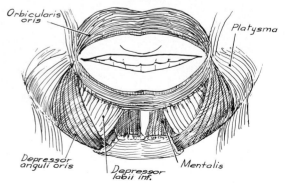

Figure 42–9. The circumoral and depressor muscles of the lower lip. (From Baker, D. C., and Conley, J.: Avoiding facial nerve injuries in rhytidectomy. Plast. Reconstr. Surg., 64:784, 1979.)

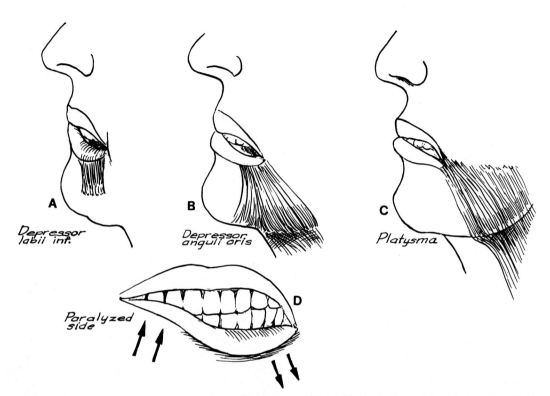

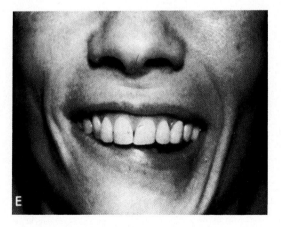

Figure 42–10. *A,* The action of the depressor labii inferioris is to evert the vermilion border and also to move the lower lip downward and laterally. *B,* The action of the depressor anguli oris moves the lower lip downward and laterally. *C,* The action of the platysma also moves the lower lip downward and laterally. Temporary weakness of this muscle following transection of the platysma may be confused with marginal mandibular nerve injury. *D,* The deformity produced by palsy of the marginal mandibular branch results primarily from the inaction of the depressor muscles. The elevators may accentuate this deformity by pulling the inert lower lip upward and laterally. (The platysma is a significant depressor in only a small percentage of individuals.) *E,* Typical deformity of marginal mandibular nerve paralysis. The paralyzed side is flattened and elevated. (From Baker, D. C.: Complications of cervical rhytidectomy. Clin. Plast. Surg., *10*:550, 1983.)

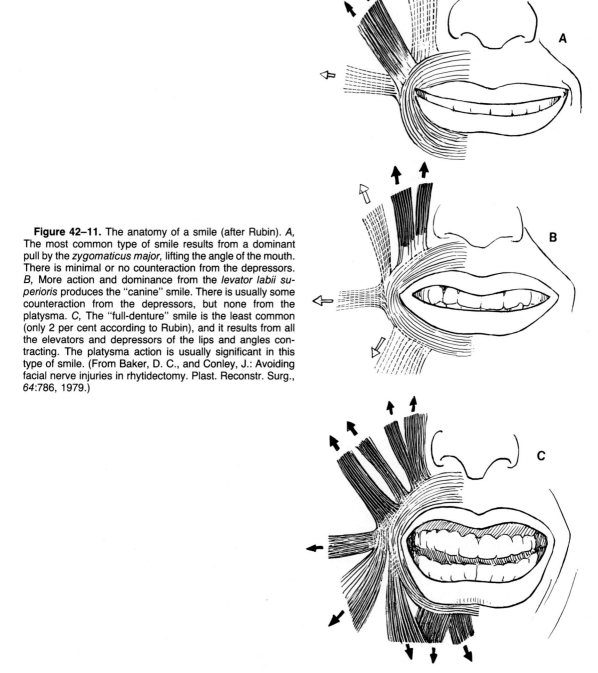

Figure 42–11. The anatomy of a smile (after Rubin). *A,* The most common type of smile results from a dominant pull by the *zygomaticus major,* lifting the angle of the mouth. There is minimal or no counteraction from the depressors. *B,* More action and dominance from the *levator labii superioris* produces the "canine" smile. There is usually some counteraction from the depressors, but none from the platysma. *C,* The "full-denture" smile is the least common (only 2 per cent according to Rubin), and it results from all the elevators and depressors of the lips and angles contracting. The platysma action is usually significant in this type of smile. (From Baker, D. C., and Conley, J.: Avoiding facial nerve injuries in rhytidectomy. Plast. Reconstr. Surg., *64:*786, 1979.)

usually represents a manifestation of any number of disorders or abnormalities. May (1986), reviewing the medical literature from 1900 to 1983, listed over 75 causes under the following categories: birth, trauma, neurologic, infection, metabolic, neoplastic, toxic, iatrogenic, and idiopathic.

The various etiologic factors involved may be broadly classified into three major groups:

> *Central or intracranial region*
> Vascular abnormalities
> Central nervous system degenerative diseases
> Tumors of the intracranial cavity
> Trauma to the brain
> Congenital abnormalities and agenesis
> *Temporal bone region*
> Bacterial and viral infections
> Cholesteatoma
> Trauma
> Longitudinal and horizontal fractures of the temporal bone
> Gunshot wounds
> Tumors invading the middle ear, mastoid, and facial nerve
> Iatrogenic causes (surgical injury)
> *Parotid gland region*
> Malignant tumors of the parotid gland
> Trauma (lacerations and gunshot wounds)
> Iatrogenic factors (surgical injury)
> Primary tumors of the facial nerve
> Malignant tumors of the ascending ramus of the mandible, the pterygoid region, and the skin

Every effort should be made to determine an etiology since many of the causes of facial paralysis are treatable.

DIAGNOSIS

Patients with isolated facial nerve dysfunction can usually be properly diagnosed by obtaining a medical history, performing a careful physical examination, and conducting a few select tests of facial nerve function (May, 1979). A careful history should be taken of the onset and duration of the paralysis, exposure to infection, medication, and trauma. Slow, gradual onset of facial paralysis may be suggestive of a tumor, whereas rapid onset suggests infection or Bell's palsy. May (1986) summarized the steps in the diagnostic evaluation of facial palsy (Table 42–2).

Table 42–2. Diagnostic Evaluation of Facial Palsy

History*
Physical examination*
Topognostic tests
    Hearing* and balance tests
    Schirmer test*
    Stapes reflex*
    Submandibular flow test
    Taste test*
Electrical tests
    Maximal stimulation test (MST)
    Evoked electromyography (EEMG)*
    Electromyography (EMG)
Radiographic studies
    Plain views of mastoid and internal auditory canal
    Pluridirectional tomography of temporal bone
    Computerized tomography of brain stem, cerebellopontine angle, temporal bone, skull base; contrast sialography of parotid
    Chest radiographic survey to detect sarcoidosis, lymphoma, carcinoma
Surgical exploration
Special laboratory tests
    Lumbar puncture (cerebrospinal fluid) to detect meningitis, encephalitis, Guillain-Barré syndrome, multiple sclerosis, meningeal carcinomatosis
    Complete white blood cell count and differential to detect infectious mononucleosis and leukemia
    Mono spot test to detect infectious mononucleosis
    Heterophil titer to detect infectious mononucleosis
    Fluorescent trepanemal antibody titer to detect syphilis
    Erythrocyte sedimentation rate to detect sarcoidosis, collagen vascular disorders
    Urinary and fecal examinations:
        Acute porphyria: elevated porphyrins and urinary porphobilinogen
        Botulism: *C. botulinum* toxin in stool specimen
        Sarcoidosis: urinary calcium
    Serum cryoglobulins and immune complexes to detect Lyme disease
    Serum globulin level to detect sarcoidosis
    Serum and urinary calcium determinations to detect sarcoidosis
    Serum angiotensin-converting enzyme level to detect sarcoidosis
    Serum antinuclear antibody test (ANA) and rheumatoid factor (RF) to detect collagen vascular disorders (periarteritis nodosa)
    Bone marrow examination to detect leukemia, lymphoma
    Glucose tolerance test to detect diabetes mellitus

*Performed routinely. The other studies are ordered depending on the suspicion raised by the history and physical examination or abnormalities noted in the routine tests.
After May, M.: The Facial Nerve. New York, Thieme Medical Publishers, 1986.

Examination of facial nerve function begins with initial observation of the patient at rest. Muscular tone and symmetry should be noted. Twitches and spasms may represent evidence of partially returning or misdirected nerve fibrils. The lines of facial expression, including the nasolabial fold, should be observed. Motor function is tested by asking the patient to wrinkle the forehead, close the eyelids tightly, show the teeth, pucker the lips, and grimace. The platysma muscle and depressors can be tested by having the patient draw the lower lip and corner of the mouth downward. Paralysis of the buccinator and orbicularis oris muscles results in speech impairment, drooling, and inability to whistle or puff out the cheeks.

Location of the Lesion

There are two varieties of facial nerve motor weakness. Supranuclear paralysis involves the upper motor neuron or corticobulbar pathways (Fig. 42–12). A distinguishing feature is the preservation of the orbicularis oculi and frontalis muscles associated with a paralysis of the lower facial muscles contralateral to the side of the lesion. A unilateral upper motor neuron lesion does not affect muscle function of the forehead or eye because the lower motor neuron supplying the upper facial muscles receives upper motor neuron innervation from both sides of the cerebral cortex. Central types of facial paralysis result from a lesion invading the motor

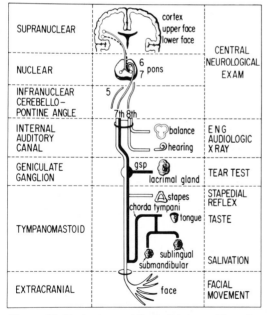

Figure 42–12. Anatomy of the facial nerve. The column on the left indicates the anatomic levels that can be identified by applying the tests indicated in the right column. (From May, M.: Facial paralysis: differential diagnosis and indications for surgical therapy. Clin. Plast. Surg., 6:277, 1979.)

area supplying the face or the corticobulbar projections through the internal capsule, cerebral peduncle, or pons. The most common etiology is vascular or neoplastic, and other neurologic deficits are usually present.

Lesions of the facial nucleus deep in the pons, or of the facial nerve in its intratemporal or extratemporal portion, result in weakness of the entire ipsilateral half of the face, including the forehead. Vascular and neoplastic lesions most commonly cause lesions of the facial nerve nucleus.

Diagnosis of the site of intratemporal lesions of the facial nerve requires assessment of the function of the three major branches of the facial nerve arising within the temporal bone. The most proximal branch is the greater superficial petrosal nerve supplying secretomotor fibers to the lacrimal gland and taste from the soft palate (Fig. 42–13). The modified Schirmer's test is the standard measure to assess lacrimal gland function, and an abnormal test suggests damage to the greater superficial petrosal nerve. The nerve to the stapedius muscle arises next above the chorda tympani, exerting a protective dampening effect on sound vibrations reaching the inner ear. Loss of the stapedius branch of the facial nerve manifests as intolerance to loud sounds such as high-pitched voices and the clashing of dishes. The chorda tympani nerve supplies secretomotor fibers to the anterior two-thirds of the upper half of the tongue. Function may be tested by applying galvanic current and noting a metallic taste on the normal side of the tongue and the sensation of electric shock on the affected side. Application of a bitter solution is not perceived by a tongue lacking chorda tympani innervation. Salivary flow tests are no longer thought to be reliable prognostic or topognostic indicators (May, 1986).

PATHOLOGY

The facial nerve contains 10,000 fibers of which approximately 7000 are myelinated and innervate the facial muscles (Crumley, 1980). The remaining 3000 fibers are secretomotor and sensory fibers. Virtually all the latter fibers leave the main trunk of the facial nerve proximal to the stylomastoid foramen. This means that the extratemporal portion of the facial nerve is made up primarily of motor axons supplying the muscles of facial expression.

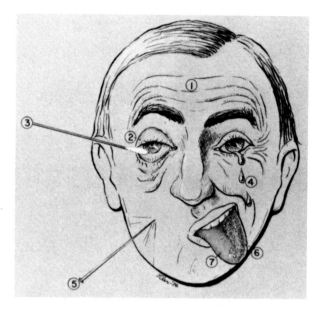

Figure 42–13. Neurologic signs in patients diagnosed as having Bell's palsy. 1, Intact forehead; 2, miosis; 3, loss of corneal sensation; 4, loss of tearing; 5, loss of sensation; 6, deviation of tongue; and 7, loss of taste papillae. (From May, M., and Hardin, W.: Facial palsy: interpretation of neurologic signs. Laryngoscope, *88*:279, 1978.)

When an axon is injured, histologic and biologic changes take place in the cell body and in the axon both proximal and distal to the site of injury. Axonal injuries may also lead to muscular aberrations and degeneration, which subsequently interfere with return of function. The distance from the cell body to the site of injury determines the degree of injury to the entire neuron. Axon interruption close to the motor end plate in the facial muscle is of much less consequence than intracranial and intratemporal injuries. Clean surgical transections produce less cell body disruption than do crushing injuries. Younger patients generally have a better chance of prompt and complete return of facial movement after peripheral nerve injury.

Classification (Seddon, 1943) of nerve injury (see Chap. 19) helps to explain and predict the outcome of the injury.

In *neurapraxia* only the myelin sheath is affected; the conduction of impulses is blocked but axoplasmic transport continues. The nerve distal to the site of the lesion has abnormal voluntary motor function but retains normal electrical stimulability. This usually occurs for several days after trauma and disappears spontaneously and completely.

In *axonotmesis* axonal continuity is lost, resulting in wallerian degeneration distally. Although the neural element is separated and damaged, the myelin sheath remains intact. Spontaneous but incomplete recovery may be expected. If the endoneural tube is also disrupted, aberrant regeneration of axonal sprouts may randomly enter distal endoneural tubes.

In *neurotmesis* all components of the peripheral nerve are transected. The epineural sheath is disrupted, allowing axon sprouts outside the nerve sheath to produce neuromas.

Muscle

After denervation the facial muscles undergo a complex series of biochemical and histologic changes. According to Crumley (1985) these changes allow the muscle to survive for a longer period of time without innervation, while making it biochemically attractive to axon sprouts. In humans this state usually lasts 18 to 24 months, during which time the muscle seeks reinnervation by retaining its motor end plate substructure and elaborating substances that attract axons (Crumley, 1985).

If the muscle is not reinnervated, it undergoes atrophy with disappearance of contractile elements and eventual replacement of the entire muscle by collagenous and fatty tissue. Proper electrophysiologic and anatomic assessment of muscle viability in facial paralysis is essential in deciding on the proper reconstructive procedure. The best results in facial reanimation occur when existing viable facial muscles can be reinnervated.

However, after significant atrophy of the facial muscles, new muscle tissue must be transferred to accomplish facial reanimation.

Electrodiagnostic Tests

A variety of electrical tests can evaluate facial nerve function and assess the integrity of various facial nerve branches (Esslen, 1973, 1977) (see Chap. 19). The purposes of electrical tests are to determine the location of the nerve injury and the extent of damage, to differentiate central from peripheral lesions, and to prognosticate recovery or progression of paralysis. Since the facial nerve retains its conductivity for approximately 72 hours after nerve transection, most tests demonstrate evidence of nerve injury only after that lag period. It is essential to perform the first electrodiagnostic test as soon as possible to serve as a baseline.

CONDUCTION TEST

The facial nerve is maximally stimulated at the angle of the mandible when a recording electrode is placed in the frontalis or orbicularis muscles. Latency of the distal muscle potential is measured from onset of stimulus, first on the normal then on the abnormal side. Latency greater than 3.8 msec is considered abnormal. If normal response is obtained only with a current twice the normal threshold, nerve conduction is said to be absent. The length of latency period suggests the nature of nerve injury: neurapraxia, axonotmesis, or neurotmesis.

STRENGTH-DURATION CURVES

Strength-duration curves are graphic measurements of nerve and muscle excitability. Two variables are measured: the amount of current required to cause a minimal perceptible contraction, and the threshold of contraction at progressively shorter durations. In normal muscle, fine intramuscular nerves respond. In denervated muscle, the response is that of a direct muscle stimulation. During reinnervation, a broken curve is obtained that shows elements of both muscle and nerve stimulation. The curve roughly demonstrates a quantitative determination of the degree of reinnervation.

CHRONAXIE

Chronaxie is the duration of a stimulus (twice the minimal stimulus acting over an infinite period of time) that evokes a mechanical muscle twitch (rheobase). Normal chronaxie is less than 1 msec. Any pathologic process that impairs conductivity of lower motor neurons produces an abnormal chronaxie. It takes a longer stimulus to obtain a direct reaction from muscle fibers. This is a gross test, and there has to be substantial nerve damage before the nerve shows an abnormality.

The maximal stimulation test (MST) and nerve excitability test (NET) are used for early evaluation of facial nerve damage. Both sides of the face are tested and the response from the involved side is compared with that of the normal side. These tests may be employed approximately 72 hours after injury and are helpful in making an early prognosis in Bell's palsy, or in determining the degree of compression of the nerve by trauma or tumors (May, 1986).

ELECTROMYOGRAPHY

Electromyography is a technique of recording muscle potentials without external stimulation (Figs. 42–14, 42–15). It can determine nerve muscle pathways and intrinsic muscle pathology. By the insertion of needle electrodes in the facial muscles, the electrical interference is recorded. Normal muscle at rest does not have electrical potentials. Fibrillation in a muscle at rest indicates denervation. After partial voluntary muscle contraction, motor unit potentials of 500 to 800 mV in amplitude and 4 to 8 msec in duration are generated. On maximal contraction all motor neurons fire simultaneously, but asynchronously, in a pattern known as the interference pattern. Two weeks after complete nerve transection, fibrillation is seen in muscles at rest, although no change is observed in voluntary contraction. In partial nerve laceration, fibrillation is seen in muscles at rest. On slight voluntary contraction, multiple polyphasic potentials appear, with some giant forms, as evidence of reinnervation. On maximal voluntary contraction, the number and size of potentials remain approximately the same. In myopathy, the characteristic finding is low voltage and an inability to recruit additional motor units on voluntary contraction.

MUSCLES	FIBRILLATION	FASCICULATION	VOLUNTARY MOTOR UNIT POTENTIALS
Rt. frontalis Lateral portion	2 Plus	0	From 25 to 50% of the total normal number are seen during attempted voluntary contraction by the patient; most of these potentials are "nascent" polyphasic potentials of the type seen during earliest reinnervation (see graph).
Medial portion	Trace to 1 Plus	0	Only one or two giant, rapid-firing polyphasic potentials present during attempted maximal voluntary contraction.
Rt. orbicularis oculi (Corrugator portion)	0	0	Normal
Lt. frontalis	0	0	Normal

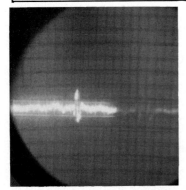

Figure 42–14. Electromyographic study of reinnervation of the right frontalis muscle. The inset shows polyphasic voluntary motor unit potentials.

ELECTROMYOGRAPHY			
MUSCLES	FIBRILLATION	FASCICULATION	VOLUNTARY MOTOR UNIT POTENTIALS
Rt. Frontalis	0 (gritty sensation on needle electrode insertion)	0	None seen
Lt. Frontalis	"	0	None seen
Rt. Zygomaticus	0	0	Essentially normal in form and in total numbers.
Lt. Zygomaticus	0	0	About 25% of the expected normal number were seen during what appeared to be maximal voluntary contractions; these potentials were relatively normal in form.
Rt. Orbicularis Oris	0	0	Essentially normal in form and in total numbers.
Lt. Orbicularis Oris	0	0	Same as left zygomaticus (above).
Rt. Depressor Anguli Oris	0	0	Essentially normal in form and in total numbers.
Lt. Depressor Anguli Oris	0	0	Same as left zygomaticus (above), except about 50% of the expected normal number were present.

COMMENT: This examination confirms the clinical impression of total paresis of the frontalis muscles bilaterally. Further, the gritty sensation on electrode insertion suggests fibrous replacement of muscle has occurred.

Figure 42–15. Electromyographic report on a child with facial paralysis before masseter muscle transposition.

ELECTRONEUROGRAPHY

Electroneurography is a means of measuring peripheral nerve conduction and recording compound action potentials of a given muscle (Hughes, 1982). This test can be performed only if the facial nerve on the other side of the face is uninjured. The test is useful in quantitating the degree of nerve dysfunction.

In acute facial nerve trauma, nerve conduction testing and electroneurography are the tests most helpful in determining the degree of denervation in the first week after trauma. Intensity-duration curves at 15 days after trauma provide better information as to the degree of denervation. To assess the degree of reinnervation, the most sensitive test is electromyography. Reinnervation patterns are detected in electromyography weeks before clinical evidence of facial movement can be seen.

Spontaneous Regeneration

For the past 20 years, the concept of "spontaneous return of movement" to the face by accessory neural pathways has challenged the surgeon. None of the various mechanisms that have been proposed to explain this phenomenon has been completely satisfactory. The most popular theory is open-field regeneration based on chemotaxis, with regrowth of single or multiple nerve filaments. It seems unlikely, however, that a nerve would redirect and regrow through several centimeters of scar tissue to rejoin peripheral branches. In addition, this phenomenon has not been demonstrated during surgical reexploration of patients who have had spontaneous facial nerve recovery.

In 1955 Conley reported two cases of spontaneous return of movement, noting that the intimate proximity of the facial nerve and the trigeminal nerve presents the possibility that the trigeminal nerve may assume some of the physiologic duties of the facial nerve. Martin and Helsper (1957) proposed the trigeminal nerve as the source of reinnervation; 28.5 per cent of their patients had some return of motion. However, this figure was not sufficiently high to justify nonrepair in view of the excellent results achieved with facial nerve grafting.

Contralateral innervation has been demonstrated by electrical testing in approximately 45 per cent of individuals; it occurs primarily in the regions of the mentum and the orbicularis oris and oculi, where there is bilateral circular anatomy of the muscle groups. Studies by Nishimura, Morimoto, and Yanagihara (1977) demonstrated that in normal individuals the facial nerve extends several centimeters beyond the midline, a finding representing a possible source of contralateral facial nerve regeneration.

Muscular or myoneurotization, the theory that nerves from nonparalyzed muscle transplants might invade and reinnervate paralyzed muscles, was first advanced in 1911 by Lexer and Eden. In 1915 Erlacher reported on muscular neurotization in experiments with guinea pigs; subsequently there have been some clinical references to myoneurotization (Figs. 42–16, 42–17). It has been postulated that outgrowing motor axons spread rapidly along the endoneural tubes of degenerated nerves and into denervated muscle fibers to form motor end plates. As pointed out by Miller and associates (1978), removal of investing muscle fasica is an important requisite for myoneurotization to occur. Therefore, in a radical parotidectomy, which should include a cuff of masseter muscle, the possibility for masseter muscle axonal ingrowth into the mimetic muscles is indeed significant. Transposing and implanting the remaining masseter muscle enhances this possibility.

Other accessory neural pathways for "spontaneous return" exist owing to the connection of the peripheral part of the facial nerve with 12 other nerve systems. Conley (1973) demonstrated the greater superficial petrosal nerve and geniculate ganglion as a potential route. It is obvious that there is more than one mechanism involved in the "spontaneous return" phenomenon. Usually an interval of six to 12 months is required before effective movement is observed, evidence indicating that a regrowth or rerouting process has occurred.

SURGICAL RECONSTRUCTION

Many factors must be considered in the evaluation of patients with facial paralysis. Surgical exploration may also be necessary for complete assessment of the neural and muscular status in patients presenting with partial, segmental, or complete paralysis.

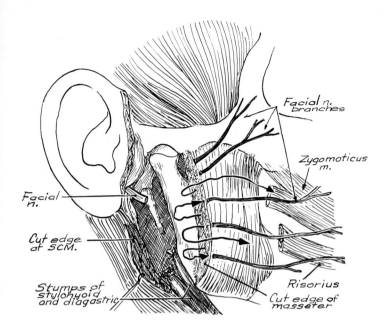

Figure 42–16. Representation of the ideal circumstances for myoneurotization. Freshly denervated mimetic muscles (vascular supply intact) come into contact with transposed masseter muscle (neurovascular supply intact). Living muscle is interdigitated with living muscle. (From Baker, D. C., and Conley, J.: Regional muscle transplantation for rehabilitation of the paralyzed face. Clin. Plast. Surg., 6:324, 1979.)

The goals of rehabilitation of the paralyzed face should be the following: (1) normal appearance at rest; (2) symmetry with voluntary motion; (3) restoration of oral, nasal, and ocular sphincter control; (4) symmetry with involuntary motion and controlled balance in expressing emotion; and (5) no loss of other significant functions. No surgical technique can accomplish all of these goals, and no single routine approach is suitable for all patients. The choice of a corrective procedure requires a detailed analysis of the etiology, duration, and extent of the deformity as well as the overall prognosis. Dynamic reconstruction and neural reconstitution are always preferable to static methods except under special circumstances.

By applying physiologic principles with clinical and diagnostic evaluation, the appropriate surgical procedure and alternatives can be planned to correspond with the duration and extent of the facial paralysis.

Two essential elements are required for facial movement: an intact facial nerve and healthy facial muscles. If the facial muscles are healthy, the requirements for reinnervation are (1) a viable ipsilateral facial nerve nucleus, (2) a proximal nerve segment capable of supporting axonal regeneration, and (3) a distal nerve segment through which axons may regenerate to the facial muscles. However, significant muscular degeneration may preclude reanimation without the trans-

fer of new muscular tissue to the face. There is often a combination of neural and muscular deficit requiring transfer of both elements for reanimation.

Injury and repair may be divided into three stages: (1) immediate (0 to three weeks), (2) delayed (three weeks to two years), and (3) late (over two years).

Lacerations and iatrogenic injuries of the facial nerve are best repaired immediately. At the time of the initial injury the elasticity of the nerve may permit closure of minor gaps without the use of grafts. In addition, the anatomy is not distorted by scarring and fibrosis. It is within the first three weeks after injury that the neural and muscular elements have the best chance of complete recovery.

After three weeks the cell body and proximal nerve segment are usually capable of regeneration for up to two years. During this period the endoneural tubules are preserved and they can guide regenerating axons to the facial muscles. Although the facial muscles undergo histologic changes and degeneration, the muscles are capable of restoring near-normal function if the regenerating nerves reach them. During this period the surgical procedure of choice should be one that will bring in new neural input to the existing facial muscles, i.e., nerve grafting or nerve crossover procedures.

After two years of denervation, muscle

MUSCULAR NEUROTIZATION

Intimate contact between host muscle+muscle contact

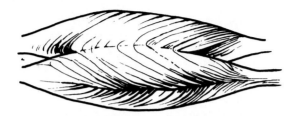

NEURAL NEUROTIZATION

Nerve to nerve suture

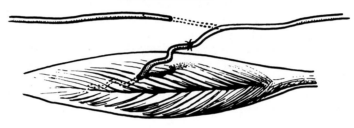

Nerve implantation into the muscle

with Cross face nerve implantation

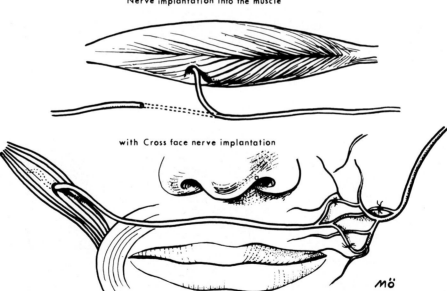

Figure 42–17. Schema of muscular and neural neurotization. Muscular neurotization requires intimate contact between the host muscle and muscle graft. Neural neurotization of the muscle can be accomplished either by nerve to nerve suture or by direct implantation of the nerve into the muscle. The lowest drawing shows crossface nerve grafting in combination with muscle transplantation. (Courtesy of Dr. G. Freilinger.)

atrophy and fibrosis occur, albeit to a variable degree. The extent may be evaluated by electromyography to demonstrate the absence of potentials, and biopsy to demonstrate the absence of muscle fibers (Crumley, 1985). Significant muscle atrophy requires the transfer of new muscle to the face, either by regional muscle transfers or by distant microvascular muscle transfers.

Direct Nerve Repair

In the primary repair of a severed facial nerve, careful realignment should be attempted to reestablish the original relationship of the nerve ends (Figs. 42–18, 42–19). Fascicles, as well as epineural vessels and other identifying anatomic landmarks, can be aligned. The traditional technique of peripheral nerve repair using epineural sutures remains the most popular. The basic principles used in peripheral nerve repair also apply to the facial nerve: (1) microsurgical technique, instrumentation, and sutures (9–0, 10–0 nylon); (2) avoidance of tension at the suture line; (3) use of the smallest number of fine caliber sutures that will precisely coapt the nerve by epineural or interfascicular repair; and (4) adequate preparation of nerve ends by resecting contused tissue or excess epineurium.

INTRANEURAL TOPOGRAPHY AND SYNKINESIS

In 1972 Millesi, Berger, and Meisal introduced the technique of microsurgical interfascicular and perineural nerve repair. The advantages of the Millesi (1977a, 1979) technique of fascicular or interfascicular coaptation are, theoretically, to unite corresponding fascicles or fascicle groups, thereby reducing the outgrowth of axons in the wrong direction. This would be a great advantage in facial nerve repair or grafting, in order to eliminate or minimize the amount of synkinesis or mass movement that normally follows regeneration. Synkinesis is the unintentional muscular movement of one portion of the face that occurs while another part of the face moves voluntarily. Most commonly,

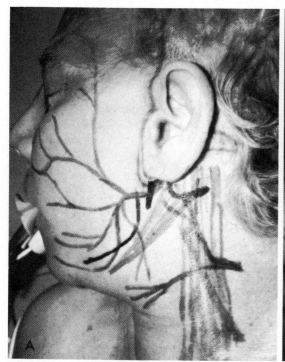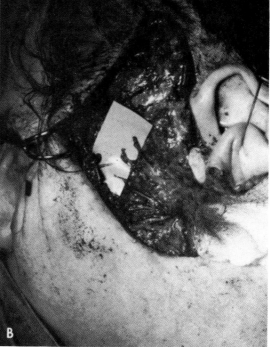

Figure 42–18. *A*, Preoperative markings on the patient in Figure 42–19, who sustained transection of all branches of the upper division of the facial nerve during a rhytidectomy. *B*, Intraoperative findings of multiple transections and neuromas. The nerve endings were liberated, the neuromas resected, and the nerves reapproximated without grafting. (From Baker, D. C.: Complications of cervicofacial rhytidectomy. Clin. Plast. Surg., *10*:554, 1983.)

there is an upward movement of the oral commissure and upper lip during blinking or winking of the eye, and closure of the eye during talking and smiling. According to Crumley (1980), the former is more common and more severe because the orbicularis oculi muscle is innervated by a greater number of facial neurons than are the orbicularis oris and elevators of the lip. The cervical and marginal mandibular branches also participate in mass movements, but to a lesser extent than the buccal and zygomatic branches, undoubtedly because of fewer anastomoses among the branches.

Elimination of synkinesis is possible only if the nerve fibers supplying a certain muscle group are concentrated in a specific area of the cross section of the facial nerve. The spatial orientation of the facial nerve, however, is still a matter of dispute. Sunderland (1977) believed that the nerve fibers are more or less diffusely distributed, whereas May (1973) and Miehlke (1958, 1977) believed that discrete fasciculi may be present proximal to the stylomastoid foramen. Theoretically, if a fascicular pattern exists, nerve grafting of individual fasciculi should result in selective reinnervation of facial muscles with less evidence of mass movement.

According to May (1977a), the temporal division of the facial nerve contains fibers that primarily terminate in muscle groups in the upper face, whereas the cervical division primarily innervates muscles in the lower face. Theoretically, repair of a defect just distal to the bifurcation into two main divisions, by suturing grafts from the proximal segment of the lower trunk and upper trunk to the distal segment, should give ideal results with minimal or no synkinesis. May reported such a case of a gunshot injury to the face that transected both upper and lower divisions of the facial nerve. The defect was repaired with interposition nerve grafts using the Millesi technique. Although the patient had excellent return of facial motor function, the movement was still associated with the complications of facial reinnervation: tics, spasm, synkinesis, and obvious persistent facial weakness. It was concluded that, although the spatial anatomy of the facial nerve has been documented clinically and experimentally, what has seemed theoretically possible could not be achieved clinically.

Sunderland (1977) extensively reviewed the problem of mass movement in facial nerve repair, and Sade (1975) emphasized the propensity of the regenerating facial nerve to deviate, split, and shift from the original axone-plate relationship, seeking out denervated muscle groups without relationship to the nerve's central origin. These are only some of the reasons for the synkinesis that occurs in the complex reinnervation of the facial muscles.

Extratemporal Nerve Grafting

According to Baker and Conley (1979), the primary indication for facial nerve grafting is to reconstruct a defect of the facial nerve in order to reconstitute this system without tension (see also Chap. 67). This principle applies primarily to cases in which there has been loss of the main trunk or peripheral divisions of the facial nerve secondary to trauma, scarring, and resection from tumors. By far the most common use of extratemporal facial nerve grafting is in the treatment of tumors of the parotid gland. The following relative classification outlines the indications for resection and preservation of the facial nerve in the treatment of parotid tumors (see also Chap. 67):

Relative Indications for Facial Nerve Resection
1. High-grade malignant tumors
2. Large malignant tumors occupying a major portion of the parotid gland
3. Malignant tumors of the deep lobe
4. Malignant tumors presenting with facial paralysis
5. Recurrent malignant tumors
6. Certain recurrent, benign, mixed tumors compromising the facial nerve

Relative Indications for Preservation of the Facial Nerve
1. All benign tumors and cysts
2. Early low-grade malignant tumors of the lateral lobe (some may require segmental resection of the facial nerve, total parotidectomy, and postoperative irradiation)
3. Recurrent mixed tumors (some may require segmental resection of the facial nerve and total parotidectomy)

Facial nerve grafting is best done immediately in cases of clean traumatic injuries or in ablative procedures for cancer before scar-

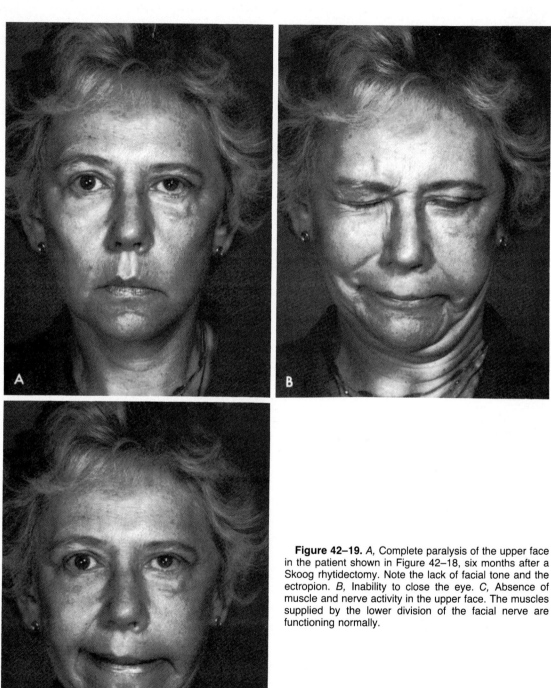

Figure 42–19. *A,* Complete paralysis of the upper face in the patient shown in Figure 42–18, six months after a Skoog rhytidectomy. Note the lack of facial tone and the ectropion. *B,* Inability to close the eye. *C,* Absence of muscle and nerve activity in the upper face. The muscles supplied by the lower division of the facial nerve are functioning normally.

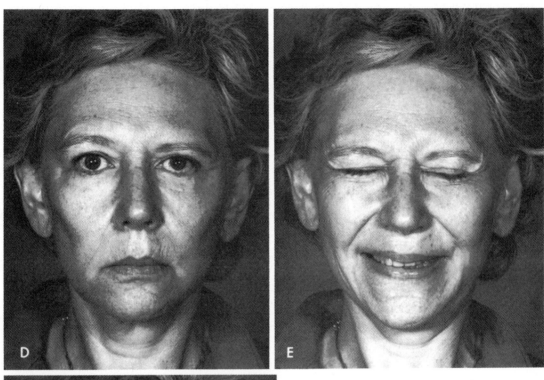

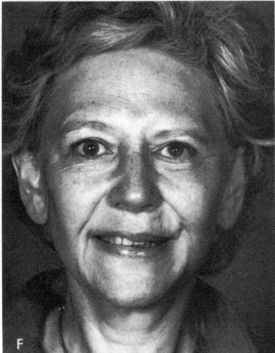

Figure 42–19 *Continued D,* Eight months after nerve repair. Note the improved tone and complete closure of the eyelid *(E). F,* Almost normal return of the upper facial movement can be expected to improve for at least two years after repair. Note the absence of frontalis movement, which returns in only a small percentage of patients. (From Baker, D. C.: Complications of cervicofacial rhytidectomy. Clin. Plast. Surg., *10*:554, 1983.)

ring, fibrosis, and atrophy have complicated the healing process. Of course, there may be compulsory circumstances when delayed nerve grafting is realistic. The decision must be balanced against the irretrievable losses associated with all paralytic processes, as well as the physiologic capacity and potential of the neuromuscular system that is available for rehabilitation.

It must be emphasized that not all patients undergoing radical ablation of the facial nerve are candidates for grafting, because the size of the wound or the quality of the tissue bed may make the procedure unrealistic. These resections usually include the ear, the adjacent skin, the parotid gland, the mandible, the neck, and a portion of the temporal bone.

CHOICE OF THE DONOR GRAFT

The choice of a donor nerve for grafting depends on the size of the recipient nerve and the extent of the functional loss. The most frequently used donor sites are the great auricular, sural, cervical plexus, and lateral femoral cutaneous nerves.

For nerve grafting, the preference is the greater auricular nerve or cervical plexus at the C3 and C4 levels from the ipsilateral side of the neck, unless there is evidence of metastases in the neck from a high-grade malignant tumor (Fig. 42–20) (Conley, 1973). In cases of the latter, the contralateral neck or the sural nerve is used. The cervical plexus is conveniently located in the wound. A single nerve filament or a main trunk with four or five terminal divisions may be obtained. It is ideal to obtain a main trunk that matches the main trunk of the facial nerve in size and also has branches so that the terminal divisions can be accurately approximated without tension. Grafts ranging from 3 to 12 cm have been obtained from the cervical plexus (Fig. 42–21).

When the sural nerve is chosen for autografting, a separate operative site in the lower extremity is necessary. This nerve consists proximally of a few large fascicles, and distally of a few small ones (Hill, Vasconez,

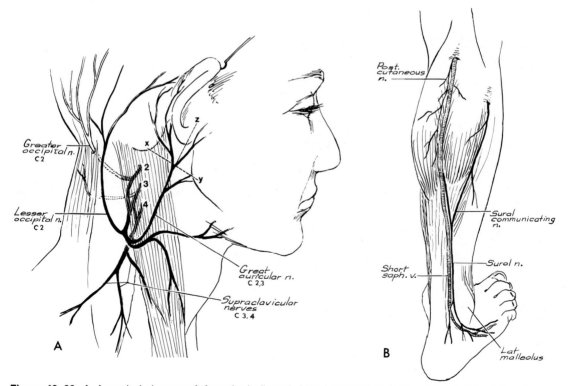

Figure 42–20. *A,* A cervical plexus graft from the ipsilateral side of the neck is preferred (contralateral if nodes are involved). Usually a 9 to 12 cm graft can be obtained with a main trunk and four or five branches of satisfactory physical match. *B,* For crossface nerve grafting, a sural nerve graft 30 to 40 cm in length is obtained. (From Baker, D. C., and Conley, J.: Facial nerve grafting: a thirty year retrospective review. Clin. Plast. Surg., *6:*345, 1979.)

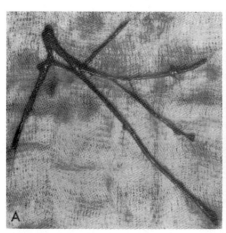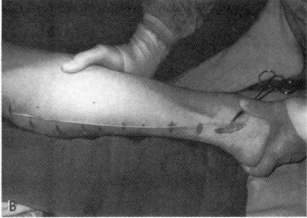

Figure 42–21. *A,* Typical cervical plexus graft. *B,* A sural nerve graft is obtained through small transverse skin incisions. (From Baker, D. C., and Conley, J.: Facial nerve grafting: a thirty year retrospective review. Clin. Plast. Surg., 6:345, 1979.)

and Jurkiewicz, 1978). When multiple or particularly long grafts are needed, as in cross-face nerve grafting, the sural nerve is chosen. Grafts up to 35 cm in length may be obtained, usually composed of two to four fascicles and resulting in minimal functional deficit. However, for ipsilateral facial nerve grafting, the physical match in size is not as satisfactory as that of the cervical plexus, from which four or five terminal branches may also be obtained (Baker, 1985b, 1987a).

SURGICAL TECHNIQUE

It is important that the graft lie in a healthy, well-vascularized recipient area devoid of scar tissue. No attempt should be made to strip the graft of its epineurium and, in preparation of the recipient nerve branches in the face, care should also be taken to maintain the epineurium intact. The anastomosis (see also Chap. 19) is accomplished after placing the nerve graft in position in the pattern that most accurately accommodates the deficiency without tension. If a tumor approaches the stylomastoid foramen or a traumatic neuroma exists at the foramen, it is desirable to remove the tip of the mastoid to isolate normal nerve in the fallopian canal. The facial nerve is usually smaller in size in the mastoid bone than in the parotid gland, and the size differential may be compensated for by obliquely cutting the proximal segment. It is important to control the margins of the proximal nerve stump by frozen section analysis in cases of tumor resection.

The basic techniques of neurorrhaphy have evolved through the early stages of approximation with 6–0 or 7–0 silk sutures to the current level of sophistication in which fascicular repair is accomplished with atraumatic 10–0 nylon sutures using the operating microscope (Fig. 42–22). The early group of cases reported consisted of anastomoses by approximating the main trunk of the facial nerve with four interrupted 6–0 or 7–0 silk sutures placed through the epineurium. The smaller peripheral branches were approximated with a single through and through 7–0 silk suture. Most of these cases were cuffed with a small silicone cylinder. Cases more recently have been repaired by using finer sutures and usually 4 × loupe magnification. An epineural type of repair is favored by the author, although the Millesi (1977a) technique is employed when feasible.

A variety of cylinders have been used to surround the anastomotic site. A soft silicone tube, never exceeding 1 cm in length and nonconstrictive in circumference, is preferred. This was considered to have a dual purpose: to isolate the anastomotic site from heavy exposure to ingrowth of scar tissue, and to keep the cut axons approximated. Studies by Weiss (1944) and Campbell and Luzio (1964) reported encouraging results. However, there are conflicting reports of tubulization causing increased scar formation at the anastomotic site (Millesi, 1977a, 1979). With the newer microsurgical techniques ensuring exact coaptation, there is less invasion by scar tissue and minimal axon aberration, and thus probably less need for cylinders.

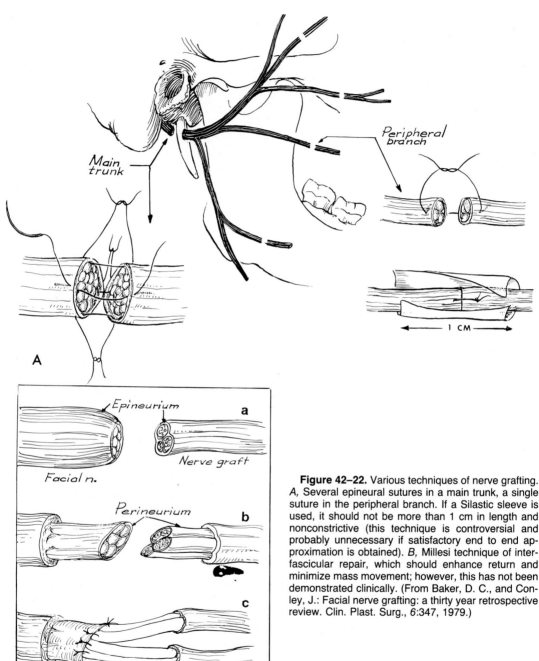

Figure 42–22. Various techniques of nerve grafting. *A,* Several epineural sutures in a main trunk, a single suture in the peripheral branch. If a Silastic sleeve is used, it should not be more than 1 cm in length and nonconstrictive (this technique is controversial and probably unnecessary if satisfactory end to end approximation is obtained). *B,* Millesi technique of interfascicular repair, which should enhance return and minimize mass movement; however, this has not been demonstrated clinically. (From Baker, D. C., and Conley, J.: Facial nerve grafting: a thirty year retrospective review. Clin. Plast. Surg., 6:347, 1979.)

Even the most sophisticated application of grafting techniques consists not only of accurate approximation of the nerve elements, in terms of size and contact, but also approximation of the cut axons in such a way that regrowth has the best opportunity of moving that portion of the face that had previously been under control of the axons in the main trunk of the facial nerve. This goal is realized by positioning the nerve graft and its filaments in such a way to the proximal portion of the facial nerve that the regrowth phenomenon in the anterior portion is utilized to regenerate the lower portion of the face, and the regrowth phenomenon from the posterior portion of the facial nerve to accommodate the upper portion of the face. Although this maneuver does not eliminate dyskinesias or crossed axons, it establishes the most natural conditions for facial movement after regrowth has been accomplished.

Prevention of hematoma is important. Meticulous hemostasis should be obtained and the wound closed without tension on the graft, and the suction drainage should be maintained.

VARIATIONS

Although it is ideal to procure and anastomose a nerve graft of matching size with the four or five principal divisions, this may not be feasible in every case, as in patients with massive tumors of the lower face. The primary terminal division to repair is the zygomatic division, as it is usually the largest and most richly interconnected with the other divisions (Fig. 42–23). If this branch is a minor one, the other dominant division should be selected. The middle third of the face is the area on which to concentrate. However, the more divisions one can supply, the better are the chances for reinnervation (Fig. 42–24). If some of the distal branches cannot be found because of scarring or trauma, a direct muscle implantation may be helpful if the mimetic muscles have survived. If the bifurcation is intact, double grafts can be used, thereby enhancing the result. Nerve grafting can be combined with an immediate masseter muscle transfer to provide some degree of immediate facial movement and to establish a maximal potential for regeneration and myoneurotization.

RESULTS

Baker and Conley (1979a) reported the largest series of facial nerve grafts. Their experience with 170 facial nerve grafts performed over a 30 year period established the efficacy of the technique and proved the high regenerative and adaptive capacities of the facial nerve system. Both the technique of anastomosis and the criteria for selection of patients have evolved and improved considerably. The timing of repair has always been recognized as an important factor, and unquestionably the most ideal situation exists at the time of initial surgery or trauma, when the nerve elements are readily identifiable and scarring is absent. When the surgeon must reenter the wound as a secondary procedure after months or years of paralysis, scar tissue, neuroma formation, and atrophy of the mimetic muscle may hinder the result obtained from nerve grafting.

The follow-up studies ranged from one to 20 years. All patients were evaluated objectively for symmetry at rest and for control, strength, and quality of facial movement (Table 42–3). Good to excellent results were those in which the patient regained facial symmetry in repose, obtained complete closure of the eyelids, and could voluntarily move the corner of the mouth to smile with minimal evidence of synkinesis. Fair results were those in which patients obtained moderate symmetry in repose, partial eyelid closure, and some evidence of mild movement of the commissure. In poor results, patients had little or no symmetry, poor lid closure, and little mimetic muscle action.

Grafts ranging from 3 to 12 cm in length have been used. The time for regeneration depends, among other things, on the length of the graft, the number of scar tissue barriers, the character of the wound, and the duration of the paralysis. The time interval for return of movement in these patients has varied from six to 24 months (Table 42–4). The first signs of regeneration are improvement in facial tone and often a sensation of something moving in the face. Movement usually first appears in the middle third of the face, in the area of the oral commissure. Over a period of months, this extends throughout the middle of the face, including muscles about the mouth, cheek, and orbit. In some patients with long-term facial paral-

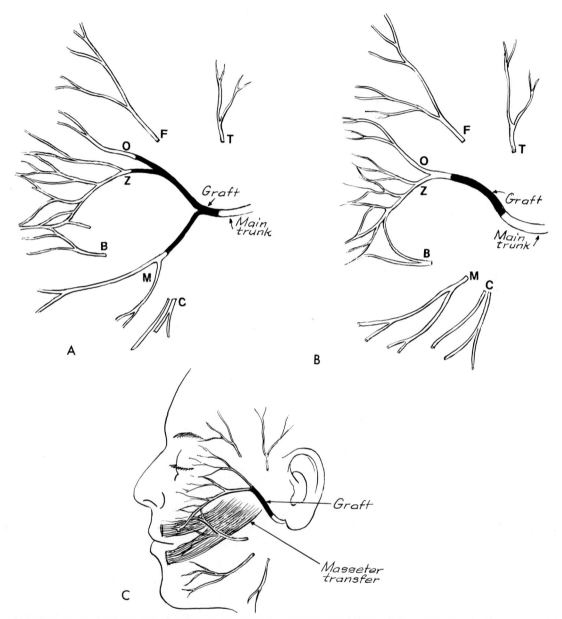

Figure 42–23. Variations in nerve grafting. *A,* A main trunk and three peripheral branches. *B,* A single graft is interposed between the main trunk and the dominant peripheral division (this can be confirmed by electrical testing on the operating table). Satisfactory return of movement could still be anticipated with this single graft because of numerous interconnections with other divisions of the facial nerve. *C,* If a single graft is used, reconstruction should be combined with an immediate masseter muscle transposition. This maneuver immediately rehabilitates the lips and commissure and creates an ideal situation for myoneurotization. (From Baker, D. C., and Conley, J.: Facial nerve grafting: a thirty year retrospective review. Clin. Plast. Surg., *6:*348, 1979.)

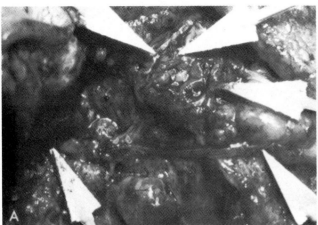

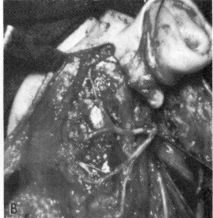

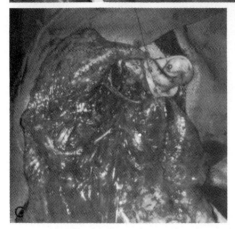

Figure 42–24. *A*, Main trunk and four peripheral branches. The tip of the mastoid was removed in order to resect a neuroma after a traumatic injury. Healthy nerve was confirmed by frozen section examination. *B*, Main trunk and two main divisions. *C*, A single graft to the zygomatic division. (From Baker, D. C., and Conley, J.: Facial nerve grafting: a thirty year retrospective review. Clin. Plast. Surg., *6*:349, 1979.)

ysis (one to two years), improvement may not appear for an interval of one year, and it may be slow and sluggish over the following year (Fig. 42–25). As movements spread throughout the face, the patient is able to close the eyelids and move the middle third of the face on intention. Movement of the face continues to improve for an interval extending over two years. Movement of the forehead and lower lip returns in only approximately 15 per cent of patients. This is most likely explained on the embryologic basis of the separateness of these nerve filaments and their corresponding muscles.

The overriding factor controlling the quality of movement in the cases that are immediately anastomosed is the accuracy of axonal approximation. The latter is rewarded by a rich axonal inflow through the first repaired barrier, followed by a facilitated axonal migration through the second anastomotic barrier into the peripheral segments, end plates, and mimetic muscles.

Although grafting is the only method of restoring emotional expression to the face, complete restitution of facial movement is never obtained (Fig. 42–26). There is always

Table 42–3. Classification of Results

Good	Normal symmetry in repose Complete eyelid closure Voluntary movement of mouth
Fair	Moderate symmetry in repose Partial eyelid closure Mild movement of mouth
Poor	Little or no symmetry in repose Poor eyelid closure Little or no movement of mouth

Table 42–4. Return of Movement

Grafts ranged from 3 to 12 cm
Time interval for return of movement was 6 to 24 months
Facial tone returns first
Movement occurs first in middle third of face
Improvement continues for up to 2 years
Movement of forehead and lower lip returns in only 15 per cent of patients

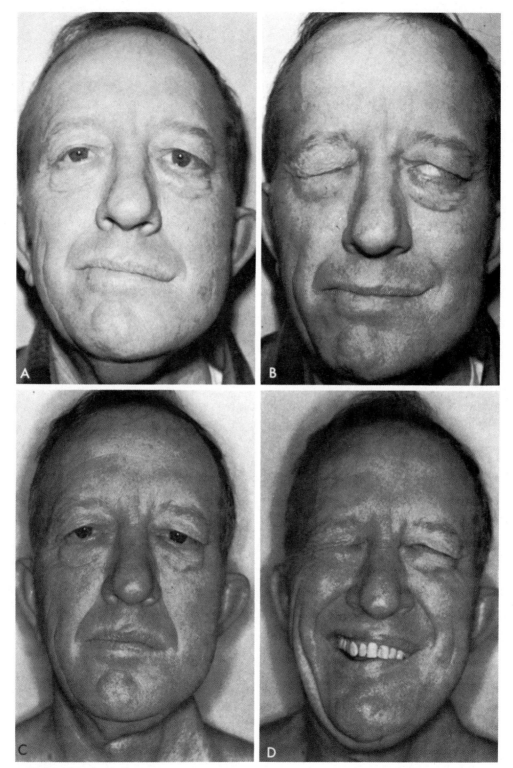

Figure 42–25. A patient with metastatic melanoma from the scalp to the parotid who had undergone radical parotidectomy and immediate facial nerve grafting. *A,* Six months postoperatively, the face is in repose. Tone is beginning to return; the melolabial fold is present. *B,* There is some elevation of the mouth at six months, but poor closure of the eye. *C,* Fourteen months postoperatively the symmetry in repose is satisfactory and tone is excellent. *D,* Satisfactory closure of the eye and strong movement of the face. Movement can be expected to improve for another six months. (From Baker, D. C., and Conley, J.: Facial nerve grafting: a thirty year retrospective review. Clin. Plast. Surg., *6*:351, 1979.)

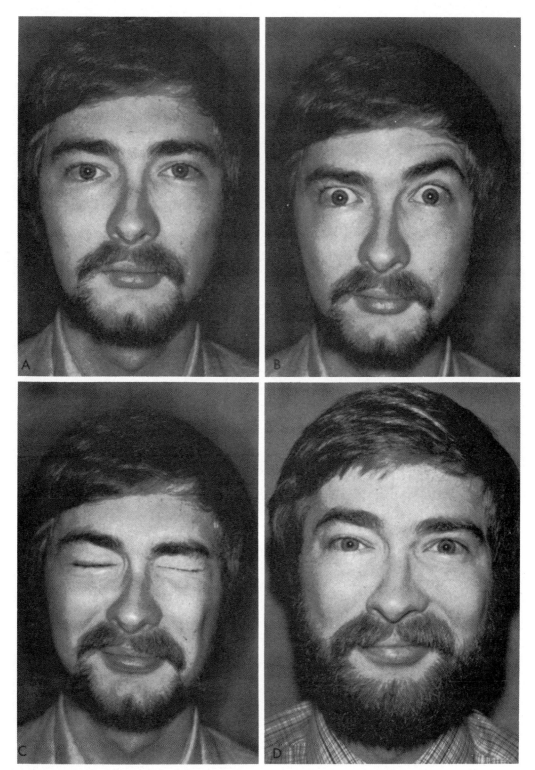

Figure 42–26. *A,* Two years after radical parotidectomy and immediate nerve grafting, facial symmetry in repose is excellent. *B,* Absence of frontalis function. *C,* Closure of eyelids but weakness is still discernible on the grafted side. Note synkinesis with elevation of lip when the eye is closed. *D,* Emotional expression and movement are satisfactory. (From Baker, D. C., and Conley, J.: Facial nerve grafting: a thirty year retrospective review. Clin. Plast. Surg., 6:352, 1979.)

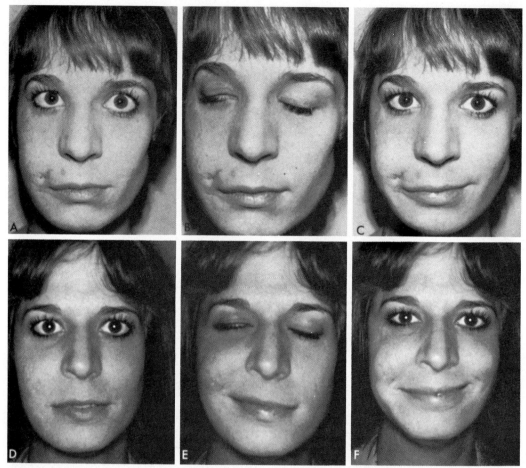

Figure 42–27. This patient underwent a radical parotidectomy for adenoidcystic carcinoma of the parotid. A single nerve graft was placed between the main trunk and the zygomatic division, combined with an immediate masseter muscle transfer. *A,* Two weeks postoperatively the symmetry is good with the face in repose. The right side is completely paralyzed. Note the incision for the muscle transfer. *B,* Two weeks postoperatively the eye is still well protected because of satisfactory facial tone—Bell's phenomenon. *C,* Clenching of the teeth already gives slight movement to the commissure two weeks postoperatively. *D,* Six months postoperatively facial symmetry is excellent. The lip and commissure incisions have softened. *E,* Clenching of the teeth results in satisfactory movement; some tone is returning to the orbicularis oculi. *F,* Symmetry on smiling is already present at six months. Mimetic muscles in the middle third of the face are also functioning, probably from myoneurotization with the masseter muscle as well as from reinnervation by the nerve graft. Movement should continue to improve for another year. (From Baker, D. C., and Conley, J.: Facial nerve grafting: a thirty year retrospective review. Clin. Plast. Surg., 6:354, 1979.)

mass movement, with recognizable dyskinesia and weakness. If most of the axons have been properly directed, the residual mass movement may be refined by concentration and increased awareness of the selective movement of the face. Further improvement may be achieved by exercises in front of a mirror over a period of six to 12 months (Fig. 42–27). Rarely are tics or spasms noted after facial nerve grafting. There is always some deficit in human emotional expression, and although this can be relearned and reoriented by awareness and practice, there will always

be a recognizable deficit when the emotional stimulus is quick and strong (Table 42–5). Movement on intention and command, however, may be almost normal. With consistent training and concentration, approximately 5

Table 42–5. Quality of Movement

Grafting is the only method of restoring emotional expression
Facial movement is never normal
Always some mass movement, dyskinesia
Always some degree of weakness
Always some deficit in emotional expression

Table 42–6. Early Cases (57): 1947 to 1960

High grade malignant cancers:	79 per cent
Low grade malignant cancers:	21 per cent
Preoperative facial paresis:	35 per cent
Good return:	56 per cent
Fair return:	24 per cent
Failures:	20 per cent

per cent of carefully selected patients can attain 80 to 90 per cent function of the facial nerve, although most range between 50 to 70 per cent function.

Early Cases: 1947 to 1960

Fifty-seven cases were reviewed in which complete facial nerve grafting was performed after radical extirpation of the parotid gland (Table 42–6). Seventy-nine per cent were high grade malignant cancers (squamous cell, adenocarcinoma, malignant mixed, mucoepidermoid) and 21 per cent were low grade malignant tumors (acinic cell, mucoepidermoid). Thirty-five per cent of the patients manifested some type and quality of facial nerve paresis preoperatively, resulting either from direct invasion by the tumor or from a previous unsuccessful attempt at tumor extirpation.

Eighty per cent of patients had some type of return of movement to the paralyzed face; 56 per cent of these were classified as having "good" return and 24 per cent as having "fair" return. Twenty per cent were failures, and although 9 per cent demonstrated positive electrical testing in selected muscles, there was no clinical function. In general, electrical nerve and muscle testing usually indicated a more optimistic picture than the patient was able to demonstrate clinically. The failures were associated with the imperfections in anastomotic technique, poor quality of the recipient tissue beds, and poorly selected candidates. Excessively large wounds in which the cheek, a large portion of the mimetic muscles, the mandible, the masticatory muscles, and a portion of the temporal bone were removed were associated with unfavorable results.

Late Cases: 1960 to 1978

Both the technique of anastomosis and the criteria for selection of cases have evolved considerably in the 113 cases reviewed from this period (Table 42–7). Sixty per cent of cases represented nerve grafts after radical ablative procedures for high grade malignant tumors of the parotid, 17 per cent for low grade malignant tumors of the parotid, and 9 per cent for recurrent benign mixed tumors involving the facial nerve. Nerve grafts were employed in 12 patients who suffered trauma from accidents or in whom there were iatrogenic causes, and three patients had resections and grafting for neurilemoma of the facial nerve. The ages of the 113 patients ranged from 12 months to 85 years. Most grafts were performed immediately at the time of the ablative procedure, and no grafts in this series were performed in faces that had been paralyzed longer than two years.

Ninety-five per cent of patients had some type of return of movement to the paralyzed face. Seventy-nine per cent were classified as "good," 16 per cent as "fair," and 5 per cent as "poor." Of interest is that six of ten patients with preoperative facial paralysis and a high grade malignant tumor of the parotid had some return of facial nerve function after ablation and grafting. These findings are directly opposed to those of Lathrop (1963) and Miehlke (1973), who stated that there is never return of function when a preoperative paralysis exists in a high grade malignant tumor of the parotid, and therefore grafting should not be performed. The author agrees with this principle in most cases, but there are certain patients in whom the malignant tumor is situated in the peripheral part of the face or the paralysis is of short duration. The pathologic process can be controlled by frozen section examination taken from the proximal and distal segments of the nerve. In these cases, nerve grafting may be feasible and successful. When the main trunk of the facial nerve is involved, the mastoid tip is removed and the fallopian canal opened to secure the proximal line of resection by frozen section examination.

Table 42–7. Late Cases (113): 1960 to 1978

High grade malignant cancers:	60 per cent
Low grade malignant cancers:	17 per cent
Recurrent mixed tumor:	9 per cent
Trauma or iatrogenic causes:	10 per cent
Neurilemoma of facial nerve:	4 per cent
Good return:	79 per cent
Fair return:	16 per cent
Poor return:	5 per cent

Irradiation and Facial Nerve Grafting

Although Lathrop (1963) reported failure to reinnervate the paralyzed face when postoperative irradiation has been administered, most surgeons (Conley, 1975; Miehlke, 1973) have reported that facial nerve regeneration takes place even in the presence of a therapeutic dose of postoperative irradiation. This has been demonstrated experimentally by McGuirt and McCabe (1977), who performed facial nerve autografts in cats who subsequently received 6000 rads of postoperative irradiation over six weeks. They demonstrated, by clinical appearance and axonal counts, that there was no adverse effect on the return of facial function. Miehlke (1977) irradiated guinea pigs in whom the sciatic nerve was sutured and found the functional results to be the same in the control group and in the irradiated animals, although there was evidence of increased fibrosis at the site of anastomosis in the irradiated group. In general, it is believed that nerve tissue is the most resistant to irradiation.

In the experience of Baker and Conley (1979) with 26 patients who had facial nerve grafts followed by postoperative irradiation, 24 regained some movement of the face. Irradiation was begun two to four weeks after the operation and carried to 6000 rads in six weeks. The quality of movement was considered to be slightly downgraded, but this finding was attributed more to the general effects of irradiation than to a specific effect on the regenerative capacity of the nerve. This effect manifested itself primarily by atrophy and fibrosis of the muscles and subcutaneous tissue. In Miehlke's (1973) review of 56 extratemporal autogenous facial nerve grafts, he found no difference in functional results between those patients who had received full postoperative irradiation and those who had not.

Intracranial Nerve Grafting

Bunnell (1927) repaired a divided facial nerve in the fallopian canal by end to end suture. Several years later he performed the first autotransplant of the nerve in order to bridge an intratemporal defect. Ballance and Duel (1932) did extensive experimental work with nerve grafts to bridge large intratemporal defects in monkeys. In 1931 they performed their new technique on an 8 year old child, and there was successful recovery of facial movement 14 months later. In 1958 Dott successfully used a long nerve graft by an intracranial-extracranial route to bypass the temporal bone.

Today, numerous neurosurgeons and otologists use modern microsurgical techniques to repair or graft the nerve intracranially or perform a bypass operation. If the facial nerve has been interrupted intentionally or damaged inadvertently during removal of posterior or middle fossa tumors, intracranial repair can be accomplished if the proximal nerve stump at the brain stem is identifiable. When anastomoses cannot be accomplished without tension, an intracranial-to-intracranial or an intracranial-to-extracranial graft may be used. The great auricular nerve is adequate to bridge gaps up to 10 cm in length, but the sural nerve is better suited for brain stem extracranial grafts exceeding 12 or more cm in length. Samii (1987) reported 20 patients who underwent reconstruction of the facial nerve in the cerebellopontine angle, 15 of whom had intracranial-intratemporal nerve grafting. A 4 to 5 cm sural nerve graft was placed between the central stump of the facial nerve at the brain stem and the distal end of the facial nerve in a tympanal or mastoidal course. The results were highly encouraging with satisfactory facial movement and symmetry.

Crossface Nerve Grafting (Faciofacial Anastomoses)

Crossface nerve grafting was introduced by Scaramella (1971) in 1970. He presented a case in which the intact buccal ramus on the nonparalyzed side had been sutured to the paralyzed stem of the facial nerve with a sural nerve graft. The patient had gained symmetry and some degree of active movement. The technique was further expanded and developed by Smith (1971), Anderl (1973, 1977a, 1985), Fisch (1974), Freilinger (1975), Ferreira (1987), and Samii (1977). The procedure is based on the principle of crossinnervation from the nonparalyzed side by means of sural nerve grafts that connect the reservoir of healthy peripheral facial nerve fascicles to the corresponding branches of specific muscle groups on the paralyzed side.

The Millesi (1977b) technique of fascicular repair is used, and the lengths of the grafts vary from 6 to 8 cm. Anderl (1985) favored a two-stage procedure, allowing the nerve axons to grow to the opposite side; the neuroma was resected to demonstrate the success of axon regrowth before the graft was sutured to the paralyzed side. Smith (1971) and Samii (1977), on the other hand, repaired both junctures simultaneously. There are no conclusive data showing significant differences in the final result; however, most authors today prefer a two-stage procedure. There is also disagreement as to whether reversal of the nerve graft ensures that all axons entering the tubules on the innervated side present to the opposite end of the graft, or whether nonreversal permits axonal outgrowth and neurotization through nerve branches along the way (Scaramella, 1979).

Although initially there was considerable enthusiasm for this technique, it has taken almost ten years for others to gain sufficient experience with crossface nerve grafting to discover that it has limited applications (except when combined with microneurovascular muscle transfers) and that the overall results are disappointing compared with those from classical procedures (Ba Huy, Monteil, and Rey, 1985).

SURGICAL TECHNIQUE

In the first stage an incision is made lateral to the nasolabial fold on the nonparalyzed side of the face to identify the buccal branches of the facial nerve. A nerve stimulator is used to map the branches supplying the elevators, the upper lip, and the orbicularis oris. A dominant branch of similar cross section to the sural nerve graft is divided, and microsurgical anastomosis performed. Occasionally, the fascicles of the sural nerve may be separated and each fascicle anastomosed to a buccal branch. In cases of early paralyses, if the orbicularis oculi is to be reinnervated, another graft can be anastomosed to a branch of the intact zygomatic or temporal branch. Often a separate incision is required. The long grafts are passed through a subcutaneous tunnel in the upper lip to the paralyzed side and anchored in the dermis near the tragus (Fig. 42–28). A silver clip in proximity to the distal end is helpful in identifying the nerve at the second stage. Sacrifice of facial nerve branches on the normal side does not produce any evidence of significant paralysis, and may even be beneficial in equalizing the two sides.

The second stage is usually performed nine to 12 months later after a positive Tinel's sign has been followed to the distal end of the graft. The neuroma is removed and the graft is sutured to the corresponding branches of the facial nerve on the paralyzed side (or to the nerve of a vascularized muscle).

The concept of crossface nerve grafting is ingenious, and its theoretical advantage is facial reanimation through specific nerve branches to specific mimetic muscle groups. The primary disadvantage, aside from the need for specialized techniques and long operating time, is the period required for return of function. The facial muscles undergo further atrophy during the time needed for axonal growth through the long nerve grafts. Technical difficulties have been encountered with the techniques of Scaramella (1970), Fisch (1979), and Anderl (1977a) in identifying the distal branches of the facial nerve, because of the intimate plexus formation with the trigeminal nerve, which varies considerably and cannot be standardized (Fig. 42–29). Suturing the sensory nerve branches of the infraorbital, buccal, zygomaticofacial, and mental nerves to branches of the facial nerve has been reported (Anderl, 1977a). The greatest disadvantage of this technique, as noted by Samii (1977) and Anderl (1977a), is that only 50 per cent of all nerve fibers of the facial nerve can be used from the normal side, and these are joined to about 50 per cent on the paralyzed side, thereby limiting the amount of axonal input. According to Baker (1987b), the distinct disadvantages include the following:

1. There is surgical intrusion on the normal side of the face with sacrifice of some axonal input, although the resulting deficits are minimal.

2. Highly specialized techniques are required, in addition to a longer operating time (and often two operative stages).

3. There are two suture lines for each nerve graft, increasing the probability of a greater loss of sprouting axons.

4. A longer time is required for reinnervation from the long grafts, during which interval there may be further muscle atrophy.

5. The greatest disadvantage is the reduced axonal input to accomplish a truly powerful reinnervation if one is not to sacri-

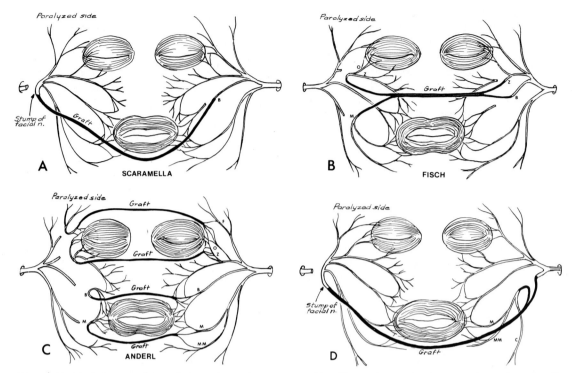

Figure 42–28. *A,* Scaramella's technique of crossface nerve grafting. The graft may also be passed over the upper lip. *B,* Fisch's technique. *C,* Anderl's modifications. In the author's experience the frontal and marginal mandibular functions return in only 15 per cent of patients, even with primary nerve grafting. *D,* The author's preferred technique is to anastomose the entire lower division of the normal side with the main trunk of the paralyzed side. Exposure is easily obtained with standard parotid incisions. The graft may be passed over the upper lip. (From Baker, D. C., and Conley, J.: Facial nerve grafting: a thirty year retrospective review. Clin. Plast. Surg., 6:356, 1979.)

fice too much axonal supply on the normal side.

6. Because of the intimate plexus formation of the trigeminal nerve with the facial nerve, technical difficulties may be encountered in identifying the distal branches of the facial nerve.

7. The results of this method are not free of the mass movements, synkinesis, associated with other methods of rehabilitation.

Samii (1977) reported 10 cases, of whom five showed symmetric position of the face in repose, only one demonstrated satisfactory facial movement, and the others evidenced some degree of movement. Anderl (1977a) reported 15 patients, five of whom demonstrated satisfactory symmetry with some degree of movement. More recently, Anderl (1985) emphasized that if crossface nerve grafting is performed more than six months after paralysis, the results are unacceptable in most cases. In a review of 20 patients by Ba Huy, Monteil, and Rey (1985) only 25 per

cent obtained a satisfactory result with good symmetry during spontaneous and emotional mimics. The authors have since abandoned the technique in favor of the technically easier XII–VII cranial nerve crossovers.

The present consensus among the majority of surgeons operating on patients with facial paralysis is that the crossface nerve graft is only another alternative to the classical procedures of hypoglossal facial nerve crossover and muscle transposition (Baker and Conley, 1982). The alternative proposed by Fisch (1979) and Stennert (1979) of performing an immediate hypoglossal nerve crossover to restore tone and maintain muscular bulk, and then performing a crossface nerve graft for more controlled movement, is gaining in popularity. Further applications consist of reinnervating a free muscle graft (Hakelius, 1979) or combining a crossface nerve graft with masseter and temporalis transfers (Freilinger, 1975) but these have not gained acceptance (Fig. 42–30).

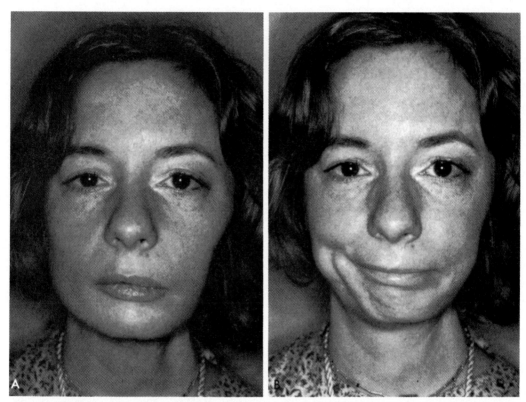

Figure 42–29. This patient underwent radical parotidectomy and temporal bone resection for adenoidcystic carcinoma. The face was immediately rehabilitated with a crossface nerve graft by the technique illustrated in Figure 42–28*D*. *A,* There is fair symmetry with the face in repose 1½ years postoperatively. *B,* Fair movement of the lower and middle face. Results with this technique alone have been disappointing. (From Baker, D. C., and Conley, J.: Facial nerve grafting: a thirty year retrospective review. Clin. Plast. Surg., *6:*357, 1979.)

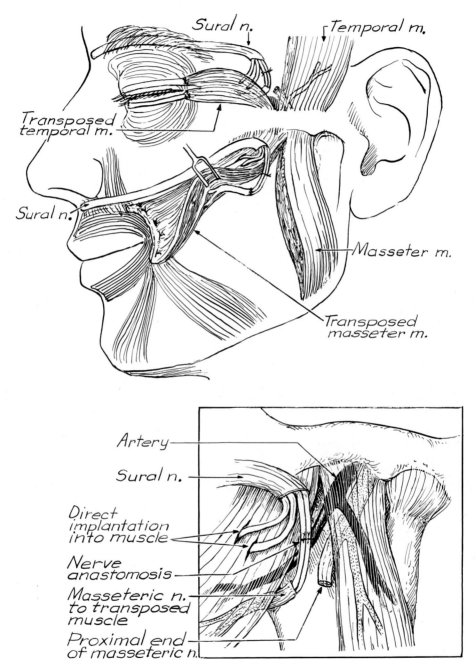

Figure 42–30. Crossface nerve transplantation in combination with temporal and masseter muscle transposition for restoration of the eyelid and oral sphincters, respectively. Sural nerve grafts have previously been inserted across the brow region and upper lip. The inset shows anastomoses of some of the sural nerve fascicles to the nerve of the masseter muscle; the residual fascicles are implanted directly into the transposed muscle.

Nerve Crossovers

When there has been irreversible damage to the facial nerve in its intracranial, intratemporal, or extratemporal portion, direct nerve suture or grafting is not feasible. In these instances, when the mimetic muscles are still functioning adequately, nerve anastomoses from the hypoglossal, spinal accessory, or phrenic nerve have been used for 75 years. However, there has been widespread criticism of these anastomoses because of resultant associated and uncoordinated (mass) movements of the face and because of loss of function of the muscles supplied by the donor nerve. In fact, in one review these techniques were relegated to a category of largely historical interest (Freeman, 1977).

The first description of the hypoglossal-facial nerve anastomosis was by Körte in 1903, who performed it on a patient who had had the temporal bone removed for osteomyelitis. Subsequent reports included those of Sargent (1911–1912), Tavernier and Daum (1961), and Falbe-Hansen and Hermann (1967); and more recently Evans (1974), Hitselberger (1974), Conley (1973), Sterkers (1977), and Stennert (1979). The general consensus among these authors is that it is a satisfactory operation when certain indications and criteria are present.

A review (Conley and Baker, 1979) of 137 cases of hypoglossal-facial nerve crossover established the indications and criteria for the technique and clarified the limitations of its usefulness.

The primary indications for a hypoglossal anastomosis are facial paralyses resulting from
1. Radical resection of the temporal bone.
2. Resection of intracranial tumors.
3. Ear or mastoid surgery.
4. A primary ablative operation for regional cancer, when nerve grafting is not feasible.

The anatomic and physiologic criteria for the use of this anastomosis are
1. An intact peripheral facial nerve from the trunk (distally).
2. An intact mimetic muscle system.
3. An inaccessible locus of the lesion in the central nerve segment, or other reasons why nerve suture or grafting would be preferable.

There are obvious contraindications stemming from the anatomic situation. This technique is usually inapplicable in cases of mild or moderate general paresis (as after a stroke), or regional or segmental facial nerve paralysis. It cannot be used when there is no facial musculature available to respond to reinnervation.

Satisfactory results are usually obtained in paralyses of up to one or two years in duration, and sometimes as late as ten years after loss of facial movement when this is not associated with severe muscular atrophy. When the end stage of muscle fibrosis is present, muscle substitution procedures are essential.

SURGICAL TECHNIQUE

The surgical technique is straightforward and has the advantage of requiring only one anastomosis of nerves that are a satisfactory physical match (Fig. 42–31).

A classic parotid incision is used, with a forward extension below and parallel to the mandible (Fig. 42–32). The main trunk of the facial nerve is identified, dissected free, and divided close to the stylomastoid foramen.

The hypoglossal nerve is easily found immediately below the tendon of the digastric muscle, and it is traced forward toward the tongue where it is divided before it bifurcates deep to the mylohyoid muscle. The proximal end of the hypoglossal nerve is passed beneath the posterior belly of the digastric muscle to join with the distal end of the trunk of the facial nerve.

The cut nerve ends are anastomosed under magnification and without tension, using several epineural sutures of 10–0 nylon. The nerve trunks are usually 2 to 3 mm in diameter, and the use of a four-power loupe magnification has been satisfactory, although the microscope may be employed. Variations of the above have included splitting the hypoglossal nerve to preserve some innervation to the tongue and approximating only the descending branch of the hypoglossal to the facial nerve.

The series of Conley and Baker (1979) was divided into two groups: those who underwent immediate XII–VII crossover (up to two years after paralysis) and those who had delayed XII–VII crossover (over two years) (Tables 42–8, 42–9).

The follow-up studies of these patients ranged from one to 20 years. All patients were evaluated objectively for facial symme-

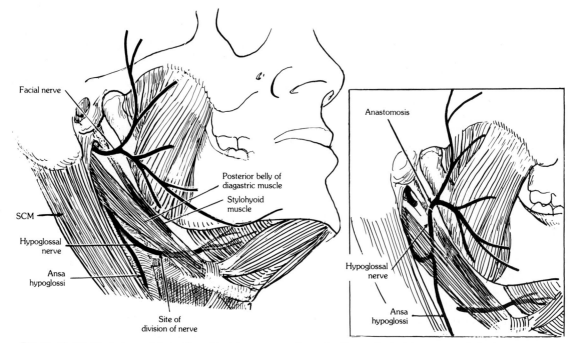

Figure 42–31. Technique of hypoglossal-facial nerve anastomosis. The main facial nerve trunk is divided near the stylomastoid foramen. The hypoglossal nerve is divided just before it dives deep to the mylohyoid muscle. *Inset,* The hypoglossal nerve is passed beneath the posterior belly of the digastric muscle and anastomosed to the main trunk of the facial nerve. Usually the ansa can be maintained intact. The anastomosis must be accomplished without tension. (From Baker, D. C.: Facial reanimation by hypoglossal-facial nerve anastomosis. *In* Brent, B. (Ed.): The Artistry of Reconstructive Surgery. St. Louis, MO, C. V. Mosby Company, 1987, p. 299.)

try at rest and for the control, strength, and quality of facial movement. The degree of tongue atrophy was evaluated in all patients; each was questioned about difficulty in speech and swallowing. Finally, each patient was asked to give a personal assessment of the results of the procedure and any disability resulting from it.

The tone of the facial muscles generally showed signs of recovery in four to six months, with symmetry of the face restored at rest. Movement of that side of the face usually appeared first about the oral commissure, then gradually progressed to the cheek, lips, and orbit during the ensuing 18 months.

Patients must learn to push the tongue against the incisor teeth when they want to smile. With patience, applied concentration, and sustained motivation, some patients can create a habit pattern that simulates normal smiling, and can learn to close the eyes voluntarily (Fig. 42–33).

Much of the movement is, however, basically mass movement associated with eating, chewing, swallowing, and talking. Because these acts are separate from human expression, the results do not include subconscious restoration of the facile expression of the

Table 42–8. Causes of Facial Paralysis in 94 Patients who had Immediate Hypoglossal-Facial Anastomoses

Temporal bone resection	52
Radical parotidectomy	18
Ear resection	10
Temple and mandible resections	8
Acoustic neuroma (less than 1 year)	5
Trauma (less than 1 year)	1
Total	94

Table 42–9. Causes of Facial Paralysis in 43 Patients who had Delayed (More than 2 Years) Hypoglossal-Facial Anastomoses

Postmastoidectomy	11
Acoustic neuroma	11
Bell's palsy (severe)	7
Trauma	5
Tumors	4
Iatrogenic	2
Congenital	2
Spasm	1
Total	43

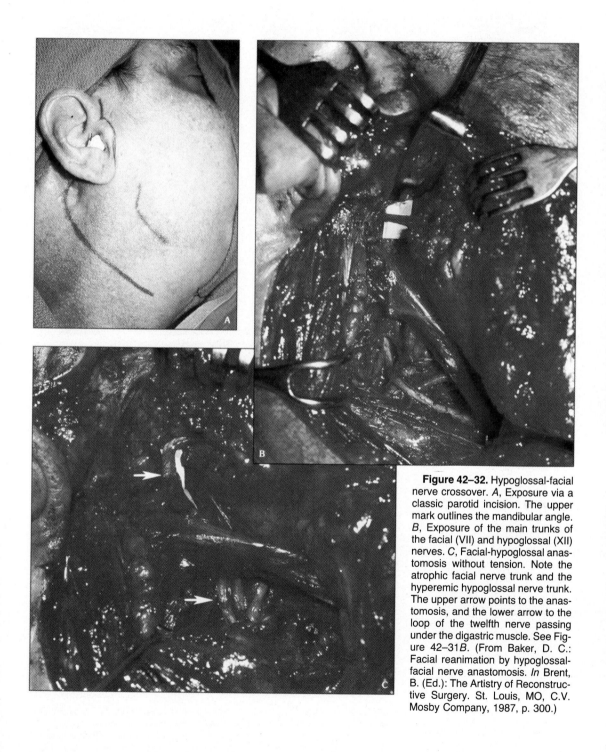

Figure 42–32. Hypoglossal-facial nerve crossover. *A*, Exposure via a classic parotid incision. The upper mark outlines the mandibular angle. *B*, Exposure of the main trunks of the facial (VII) and hypoglossal (XII) nerves. *C*, Facial-hypoglossal anastomosis without tension. Note the atrophic facial nerve trunk and the hyperemic hypoglossal nerve trunk. The upper arrow points to the anastomosis, and the lower arrow to the loop of the twelfth nerve passing under the digastric muscle. See Figure 42–31*B*. (From Baker, D. C.: Facial reanimation by hypoglossal-facial nerve anastomosis. *In* Brent, B. (Ed.): The Artistry of Reconstructive Surgery. St. Louis, MO, C.V. Mosby Company, 1987, p. 300.)

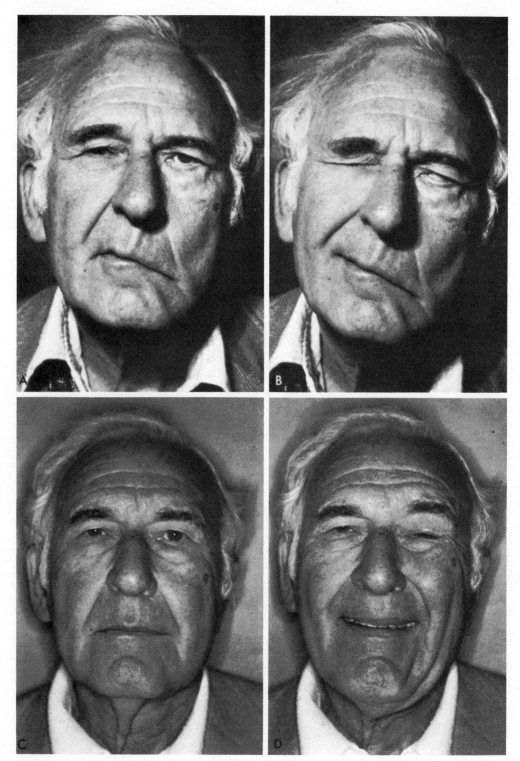

Figure 42–33. Complete paralysis one year after removal of an acoustic neuroma. The facial nerve did not respond to electrical testing. *A*, Preoperative view in repose. *B*, Smiling and closing the eyes preoperatively. *C*, One year after a XII–VII nerve anastomosis, the face is normal in repose. *D*, Excellent movement mimicking a smile. Note the return of the frontal branch. (From Baker, D. C., and Conley, J.: Facial nerve grafting: a thirty year retrospective review. Clin. Plast. Surg., *6*:358, 1979.)

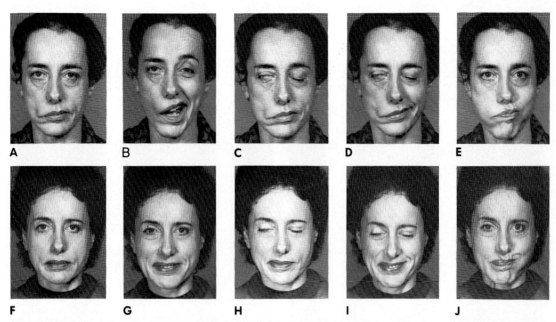

Figure 42–34. Facial reanimation after hypoglossal-facial nerve crossover. Top row, preoperative views; bottom row, postoperative views. *A, F*, Repose. *B, G*, Smiling. *C, H*, Eye closing. *D, I*, Simultaneous eye closing and smiling. *E, J*, Lip pursing. (From Baker, D. C.: Facial reanimation by hypoglossal-facial nerve anastomosis. *In* Brent, B. (Ed.): The Artistry of Reconstructive Surgery. St. Louis, MO, C. V. Mosby Company, 1987, p. 301.)

human emotions. Usually the coincidental movements that occur during speech or swallowing are not a problem, because they are subconscious. The mass movements are usually more dynamic and gross than those seen after autogenous nerve grafting.

Approximately 95 per cent of patients attained satisfactory muscle tone in repose, together with some type and quality of mass movement (Figs. 42–34, 42–35). In 98 per cent of the anastomoses performed immediately, clinical evidence of movement was obtained; in 77 per cent of these the movements were classified as good. In 90 per cent of the delayed anastomoses, movement was obtained, 41 per cent being classified as good.

In some individuals with a "good" return, there was hypertonia, a finding indicating that the neural input from the hypoglossal nerve exceeded that required for natural balance of the face. In these individuals there was an overproduction of facial movements synchronous with physiologic acts relating to the tongue. During eating, talking, or swallowing the face moved excessively in a gross manner.

This type of hyperanimation was conspicuous and could be embarrassing to a sensitive person. However, it did not cause any harm or dysfunction, and those patients who had

the anastomosis as part of an ablative procedure accepted the excessive movement in good grace. On the other hand, a small percentage of those who had had long-standing paralyses were disgruntled, although none would accept the reestablishment of the facial paralysis by having the anastomosis disconnected.

In 22 per cent of the patients there was minimal atrophy of the tongue, in 53 per cent moderate atrophy, and in 25 per cent severe atrophy. In most patients there was residual movement in the paralyzed side of the tongue, and probably the reinnervation crossed the midline from the opposite side (Fig. 42–36). It is well known that patients undergoing a hemiglossectomy can adapt to this condition. Those patients who had the hypoglossal anastomosis as part of a major ablative procedure were much more satisfied than those in the delayed group. There were few complaints in the former group, perhaps owing in part to an overriding concern about the success of the cancer ablation. Only 3 per cent of this group persistently complained about chewing problems, 2 per cent about swallowing difficulties, and 2 per cent about speech problems. Even professionals such as doctors and teachers were able to use their voices with no significant complications.

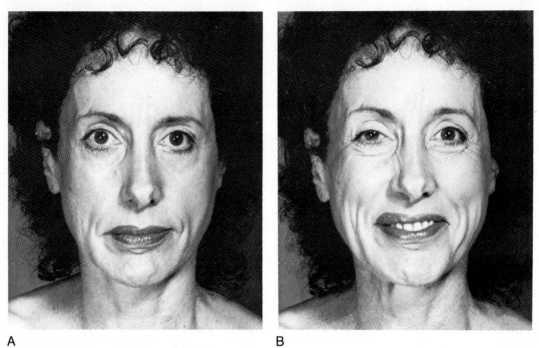

Figure 42–35. Result four years postoperatively (see Fig. 42–34). *A*, Repose. *B*, Smiling. The overall symmetry and appearance have been enhanced by blepharoplasties and neurolysis of the contralateral frontal nerve branch. (From Baker, D. C.: Facial reanimation by hypoglossal-facial nerve anastomosis. *In* Brent, B. (Ed.): The Artistry of Reconstructive Surgery. St. Louis, MO, C. V. Mosby Company, 1987, p. 301.)

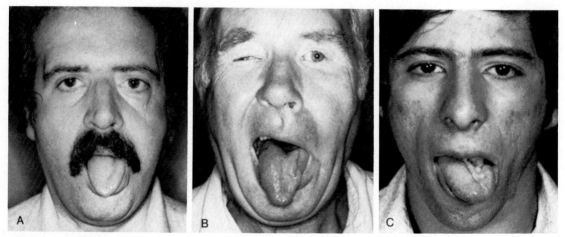

Figure 42–36. Examples of tongue atrophy following XII–VII cranial nerve anastomoses. *A*, Minimal. *B*, Moderate. *C*, Severe. (From Conley, J., and Baker, D. C.: Hypoglossal-facial nerve anastomosis for reinnervation of the paralyzed face. Plast. Reconstr. Surg., *63*:69, 1979.)

In strong contrast to this, individuals with long-standing facial paralysis had a different approach to the problem and responded to the return of movement in a different manner. Preoperatively these patients frequently questioned the advisability of acquiring an additional nerve deficit, particularly when they were already sensitized to a deficiency in chewing and speaking from the facial paralysis. Often, these patients tended to expect much more from the facial rehabilitation than is realistic, and they had an acute sense of guilt concerning their condition. These patients were sometimes negative or suspicious, believing perhaps that the paralysis may not have been necessary and that it had already destroyed a large part of their life style.

All patients with long-standing paralyses complained preoperatively of difficulty in mastication, and 16 per cent complained of this postoperatively. None complained preoperatively about swallowing; 12 per cent complained postoperatively about this. Sixteen per cent complained preoperatively of difficulty with speech; 10 per cent complained postoperatively about this. Thus, a certain number of these patients had improvements of the chewing and speech symptoms associated with their facial paralysis, but swallowing complaints were worse.

OTHER NERVE ANASTOMOSES

Various other nerves have been used for anastomosis to the peripheral part of the trunk of the facial nerve, including the phrenic and the spinal accessory. The hypoglossal nerve is generally the preferred donor nerve.

Phrenic Nerve

When the 11th and 12th cranial nerves have been removed, the phrenic may be a satisfactory alternative, although phrenicofacial anastomoses can result in peculiar resting facial twitches.

Perret (1967) reported relatively normal facial tone in repose after phrenicofacial crossover, although a conspicuous asymmetry occurred with coughing or laughing. These patients usually had difficulty in learning to take a deep breath while smiling.

Production of paralysis of half of the diaphragm would also be contraindicated in any patient with pulmonary disease.

Eleventh Nerve

When the spinal accessory nerve is used, the resulting shoulder drop is obvious and occasionally the shoulder discomfort can be significant. The nerve is a satisfactory physical match to the facial, and generally an almost normal face in repose can be obtained.

Some patients can move the face without moving the shoulder, and move the shoulder without moving the face. This dissociation of movements is the result of a central redirection, requiring intelligence and concentration by the patient; unfortunately, the facial movement cannot be incorporated into a spontaneous emotional response. The greatest disadvantage of the spinal accessory nerve is that it does not accomplish any natural physiologic dynamism or movement in the face (Conley, 1975). The face, therefore, is not active except upon intention or command. It is static during eating, swallowing, and talking; any movement must be produced by conscious direction.

The hypoglossal nerve has the distinct advantage that the face is unconsciously moved during speaking, eating, and swallowing. This creates an exceptional quality of animation on the basis of normal physiologic activity of the tongue in participating in these natural functions. In addition, the patient can voluntarily move the face by intentionally moving the tongue in the oral cavity. Additional control has been accomplished by combining this procedure with a crossface nerve graft. Although the technique is far from ideal and cannot be universally applied, it offers a number of distinct advantages in addition to its high success rate (Baker, 1987b):

1. The surgical technique is direct and uncomplicated, requiring only one suture line.

2. There is greater function, because most facial movements are associated with conscious or unconscious movements of the tongue.

3. There is better balance of the face, as well as the possibility of more rapid facial movements.

4. There is no discomfort from loss of the 12th nerve.

5. There is little functional disability from loss of the 12th nerve.

6. During speech, movement around the mouth is more natural.

7. There is a closer anatomic relationship in the motor zone of the cerebral cortex of the hypoglossal with the facial nerve.

8. A more dynamic functional result is obtained.

The report of Hammerschlag and associates (1987) describing electromyographic rehabilitation after hypoglossal-facial anastomosis is encouraging. Computer technology was used to measure, monitor, and display abnormal electromyographic (EMG) muscle activity, and behavioral techniques were used to reinforce the occurrence of more appropriate motor responses. Thirty-three per cent of patients achieved symmetry and synchrony of function and spontaneity of expression. Synkinetic facial movements associated with use of the tongue were minimal. Fifty-seven per cent of patients accomplished voluntary eye control and lower face function, with only moderate synkinetic movements.

Regional Muscle Transposition

According to Baker and Conley (1979b), when direct nerve suture, autogenous nerve grafting, and nerve crossover are inapplicable in rehabilitation of the paralyzed face, other reconstructive techniques must be used to attempt to supply some type of movement and support. These methods include regional muscle transposition, fascial stripping fixed to a bony point of muscle system, and physical support by synthetic materials. Various techniques of facialplasty and stabilization with dermal flaps have also been used. It can be stated categorically that reactivation of the facial muscles by neural reconstitution or muscle transposition supersedes any type of rehabilitation by suspension or skin stretching except perhaps in very elderly or debilitated patients (Conley and Baker, 1978). These static techniques, however, can be complementary when combined with dynamic reconstruction.

Transposition of regional muscles to rehabilitate the paralyzed face has been employed for almost 75 years. The indications include (1) the absence of mimetic muscles resulting from long-standing atrophy; (2) the need for additional muscle bulk and myoneurotization; and (3) the requirement for a complementary procedure with a nerve graft, nerve crossover, or nerve implantation. Although most of the available muscles in the head and neck have been transposed in whole or in part, by far the most popular muscle transposition techniques are those involving the masseter and temporalis.

The basis of regional muscle transposition is to transfer new muscle innervated by a different cranial nerve, which can furnish pull in various directions and thus accomplish a more normal facial animation. Transposition of a regional muscle presupposes the reeducation of the patient in the use of these voluntary muscles.

The transposition of a dynamic and vital muscle system into a paralyzed face has biologic advantages over other suspension techniques. The living muscle fibers bring with them axons that may have the facility to grow into and support deficient areas in the mimetic muscle system. If the mimetic muscles have atrophied and disappeared, nothing can reverse this situation. However, if there are islands or regions that have survived with paralysis, the introduction of a new dynamic muscle system may be helpful and offers the possibility of myoneurotization.

HISTORY

The use of regional muscle transposition for correction of facial paralysis has been extensively reviewed by Owens (1951) and Conway (1958). Lexer and Eden (1911) performed the first muscle transposition, based on a suggestion of Wrede. They elevated two slips of the anterior half of the masseter muscle from its insertion, and transposed one slip to the upper and the other to the lower lip. To rehabilitate the eye, a slip of temporalis muscle was elevated at its origin, brought forward, and divided, suturing one slip into the upper and the other into the lower lid. As Owens (1951) noted, the results obtained by the use of muscle transposition were fairly satisfactory in some instances, while in others they were questionable. The poor results were undoubtedly due to a disturbance of the neural supply of the transposed muscle, atrophy of the transposed muscle, lack of coordinated movement in the reanimated face, or excessive movement with chewing. However, when the neurovascular supply to the transposed muscle is preserved and when the ideal muscle is chosen for the proper indications, the success rate and patient satisfaction are high.

Some of the poor results reported from use of the Lexer technique of masseter transfer resulted from transection of the nerve supply to the muscle (Fig. 42–37). As noted by de Castro Correia and Zani (1973), if the original drawing of the technique by Lexer and Eden

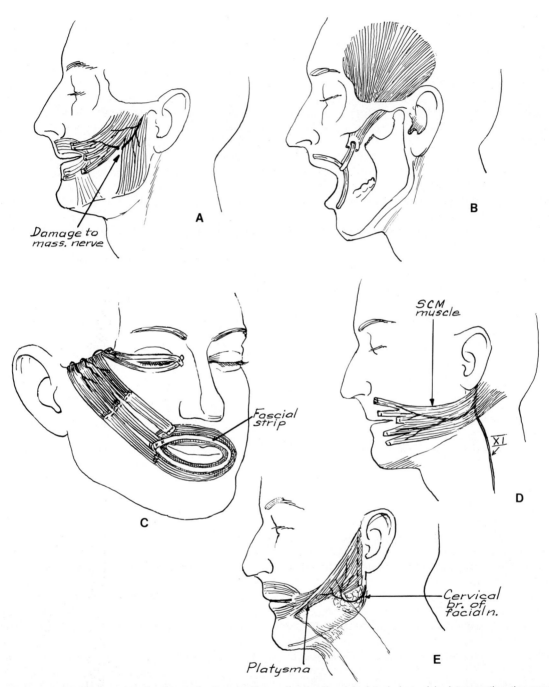

Figure 42–37. Types of regional muscle transpositions. *A*, Lexer's original technique risked transecting the nerve supply to the masseter muscle. *B*, McLaughlin procedure attaching the coronoid process to the circumoral fascia lata suspension. Movement is not at the melolabial crease. *C*, Original technique of temporalis transfer with fascial strips or superficial temporal fascia turned down to obtain length. *D*, Sternocleidomastoid transposition. Movement is more unnatural, in the wrong direction, and muscle is bulky. *E*, Platysma transposition. The muscle is thin and delicate, and does not provide much power; the pull is in the wrong direction. (From Baker, D. C., and Conley, J.: Regional muscle transplantation for rehabilitation of the paralyzed face. Clin. Plast. Surg., 6:318, 1979.)

were to be followed, the nerve to the masseter muscle would be irreversibly damaged in every instance. Modifications of the masseter transposition were made by Jianu (1909), Hastings (1919–1920), and Pickerill (1928). Brunner (1926) was apparently the first to transplant a portion of the masseter muscle by the intraoral approach, thereby eliminating the external incision. Further modifications were made by Owens (1951) and more recently by de Castro Correia and Zani (1973).

Gillies (1934; Gillies and Millard, 1957) popularized the use of the temporalis muscle transfer, and Sheehan (1935) described removal of the zygomatic arch to add length for rotation of the muscle as well as to decrease the deformity associated with the presence of muscle bulk over the zygomatic arch. All these techniques, however, employed strips of fascia as well as temporal muscle to form a sling that was fastened to the upper and lower lips and commissure. This is the basic technique that continues to be employed today, as described by Rubin (1976, 1977), Meyer (1977), and Edgerton, Tuerk, and Fisher (1975). Most surgeons believe that the temporalis muscle is not long enough to reach the mouth or medial canthus without the added fascial attachment. In 1953 Mc-Laughlin described a technique of separating the coronoid process from the mandible, attaching fascial strips to it, and suturing these to the oral commissure for facial movement.

Some of the other regional muscles used in transposition techniques have included the sternocleidomastoid, which was first described by Gomoiu (1913). He sutured the sternal and clavicular insertion into the oral commissure. The disadvantage, however, was that each movement of the head produced a pull on the oral commissure. Schottstaedt, Larsen, and Bost (1955) described a technique for complete mobilization of the sternocleidomastoid muscle by division of its origin and insertion while preserving its neurovascular pedicle. One portion was sutured to the mouth and lips, the other to the parotid and temporal fascia. As noted by Conway (1958), the objections to this procedure are the great muscle bulk and the shortness of the neurovascular pedicle. The one case attempted by Conway (1958) failed because of necrosis of the muscle. Today, this muscle is rarely used because other muscles in the immediate vicinity are more effective.

In order to reanimate the paralyzed eyebrow and forehead, Adams (1946) transposed a flap of frontalis muscle across the midline of the forehead and sutured it to the paralyzed eyebrow. In 1975 Edgerton, Tuerk, and Fisher described a platysma muscle transfer for reanimation of the mouth in Möbius' syndrome. The author has not employed the frontalis or platysma muscle for facial reanimation, and feels that there are several disadvantages associated with these muscles: (1) the direction of muscle pull is incorrect to obtain the reanimation desired; (2) both muscles are thin and delicate, with a fine neurovascular supply that could easily be damaged; and (3) both muscles lack the strength required to accomplish adequate facial movement, as compared with that of the masseter and temporalis.

The use of an innervated trapezius flap to accomplish movement in the paralyzed face has been described by Ryan, Waterhouse, and Davies (1988). Because of the bulk of the muscle flap, it is best employed where soft tissue reconstruction, in addition to facial reanimation, is required, such as after extensive facial tumor resections.

MASSETER MUSCLE TRANSPOSITION

The surgical anatomy and location of the masseter muscle make it ideal for transposition to rehabilitate the upper lip, oral commissure, and lower lip (Figs. 42–38, 42–39). The muscle is short, thick, and rectangular in shape and originates on the inferior surface of the zygomatic complex. Its insertion is into the lateral aspect of the ascending ramus of the mandible, and the tendinous attachments interdigitate into the periosteum and bone. The muscle fibers run obliquely and posteriorly from the zygomatic complex to the angle of the mandible. Its physiologic function is to close the mandible against the maxilla in the act of biting, chewing, and grinding.

The neurovascular supply has been studied by de Castro Correia and Zani (1973), who noted that the muscle receives innervation and blood supply from the masseteric nerve and artery, which arise from the mandibular nerve and internal maxillary artery in the infratemporal fossa. The neurovascular bundle passes through the coronoid notch of the mandible and runs obliquely forward and diagonally downward across the rectangle of

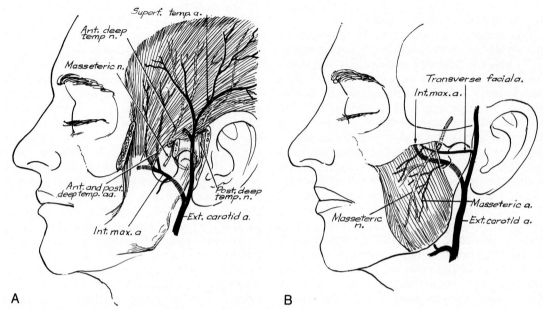

Figure 42–38. *A,* Neurovascular supply of the temporalis muscle. *B,* Neurovascular supply of the masseter muscle; note the oblique direction of the nerve. (From Baker, D. C., and Conley, J.: Regional muscle transplantation for rehabilitation of the paralyzed face. Clin. Plast. Surg., 6:320, 1979.)

Figure 42–39. *A,* It is recommended to transfer the entire masseter muscle. The incision need be only several centimeters to avoid damage to the nerve. *B,* The anterior portion of the muscle is sutured to the orbicularis oris and to the dermis anterior to the melolabial fold. The posterior portion of the muscle is sutured to the lower lip and commissure. (From Baker, D. C., and Conley, J.: Regional muscle transplantation for rehabilitation of the paralyzed face. Clin. Plast. Surg., 6:321, 1979.)

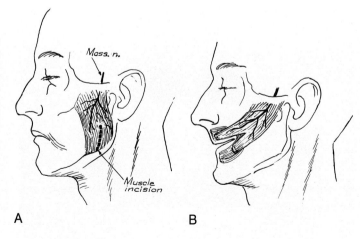

the muscle, becoming more superficial as it passes inferiorly. de Castro Correia and Zani (1973) recommended that separation of the muscle should be performed at the junction of the anterior two-thirds with the posterior one-third. The height of the incision should not be more than 3.5 cm. A safer technique is to transpose the entire muscle.

The masseter muscle may be approached intraorally or externally. When total paralysis is present, the circumauricular approach provides the optimal exposure to the entire muscle belly, and the incision usually is cosmetically acceptable. A preauricular incision is made with a submandibular extension, and the cheek flap is elevated to expose the entire masseter muscle. The tendinous insertion of the muscle is incised on the lowermost portion of the horizontal ramus, preserving the tendinous fibers because they provide a strong attachment for suturing. All the muscle is elevated from the mandibular ramus up to the glenoid notch. Care is taken not to disturb the nerve or blood supply entering the muscle at the level of the coronoid notch. If further mobilization is required, the anterior portion of the muscle may be freed from the ascending portion of the mandible.

The lateral cheek is undermined to create a tunnel for the muscle. The tunnel is intentionally extended through the mimetic muscles of the cheek, commissure, and lips. As the tunnel approaches the lips, it develops a superior and inferior extension similar to the shape of a "Y." One of the tunnels leads into the upper lip and the other toward the commissure and lower lip (Fig. 42–39).

Skin incisions approximately 1 cm long are made medial to the melolabial fold in the upper lip and medial to the angular incision at the commissure and lower lip. They are connected to the tunnel in the cheek, and extended medially over the orbicularis oris muscle (Figs. 42–40, 42–41).

The method of cutting the muscle is extremely important. At the inferior portion of the muscle, some attempt should be made to separate the superficial from the deep bundle. The inferior portion of the muscle is cut in the center, creating two distal bundles. It is important that the muscle be back cut no more than a third in order to protect the neurovascular supply in the distal segments.

The masseter muscle is transposed into the tunnels. If it is too short, it may be lengthened by the partial release of its tendinous origin from the zygomatic complex. The lips and commissure are pulled laterally. There should always be overcorrection of the lip by pulling it in a posterior direction with appropriate hooks or small retractors. The masseter muscle is delivered through the skin incision in the lip and fixed to the orbicularis oris muscle with nonabsorbable sutures in each segment. It should also be sutured to the deep layer of the dermis and fixed in a tunnel in the lip with a pull-out suture (Fig. 42–41).

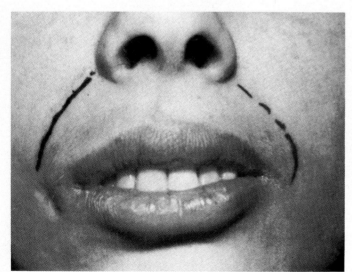

Figure 42–40. The important preoperative marking of the melolabial fold, which must be recreated by the muscle pull. The muscle must be sutured to the dermis anterior to the fold. (From Baker, D. C., and Conley, J.: Regional muscle transplantation for rehabilitation of the paralyzed face. Clin. Plast. Surg., 6:321, 1979.)

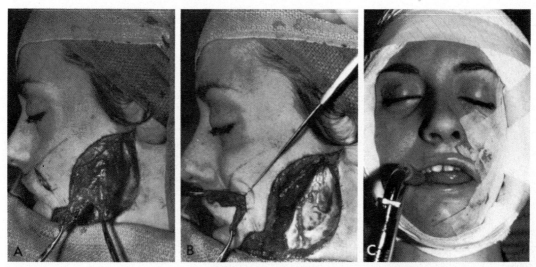

Figure 42–41. *A,* The entire masseter muscle is elevated and divided. *B,* Transposition to the upper lip, melolabial fold, lower lip, and commissure. Overcorrection is essential. *C,* A suture tied over a bolus maintains the muscle in position over the upper lip and orbicularis oris. Steri-Strips and a bulky head dressing help to immobilize the area. Tube feeding is often employed for several days postoperatively to maintain the face and mouth at rest. (From Baker, D. C., and Conley, J.: Regional muscle transplantation for rehabilitation of the paralyzed face. Clin. Plast. Surg., 6:322, 1979.)

Meticulous hemostasis is obtained and the wound drained with Hemovac catheters. Incisions are closed with absorbable subcuticular sutures and 6–0 nylon cutaneous sutures. The face is immobilized and supported with large Steri-Strips for a period of two weeks. The patient is fed with a nasogastric tube for six days to ensure immobilization of the muscle and suture lines. A liquid diet is maintained for two weeks, and chewing is gradually resumed and increased as the patient is taught to practice control of facial movements in front of a mirror.

Intraoral Approach

Transfer of the anterior portion of the masseter muscle has been found to have value in segmental paresis about the upper lip and commissure. When there is weakness of this particular region about the mouth, it is not necessary to expose the entire parotid gland and masseter muscle by the classical lateral approach. Under these circumstances, an incision is made along the lateral horizontal ramus intraorally and extended into the posterior buccal and retromolar areas. The periosteum of the mandible is elevated along with the anterior portion of the masseter muscle. This section of the masseter muscle is split vertically with right-angled scissors. The split should be less than half the length of

the muscle and should be directed slightly posteriorly. A tunnel is made through the same intraoral incision, directed toward the commissure and upper lip. The muscle is fixed in an overcorrected position with 4–0 silk sutures.

There are two disadvantages to this approach. Bleeding within the belly of the muscle is difficult to control because of inaccessibility, and there can be injury to some of the adjacent residual branches of the facial nerve. The intraoral approach is somewhat awkward and is not recommended except for limited segmental transpositions.

Indications

All or portions of the masseter muscle may be considered for transfer in congenital paralyses of the face associated with Möbius' syndrome and in long-standing facial paralysis in which there has been degeneration of the mimetic muscles (Fig. 42–42). The muscle is primarily suited to the rehabilitation of the mouth and lips. If the eye requires rehabilitation, masseter transfer must be combined with a temporalis transfer or other techniques.

One of the most advantageous uses of masseter transposition is as an integral part of the primary ablative operation in the treatment of high grade malignant tumors of the

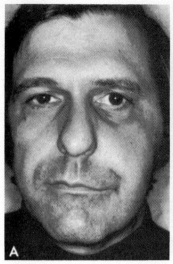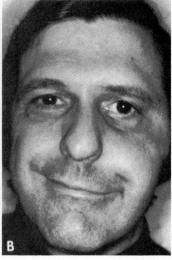

Figure 42–42. *A,* The face is in repose three months after masseter transfer. *B,* Elevation of the upper lip and commissure with clenching of teeth. Movement will improve for another one to two years. (From Baker, D. C., and Conley, J.: Regional muscle transplantation for rehabilitation of the paralyzed face. Clin. Plast. Surg., *6*:322, 1979.)

parotid gland that result in facial paralysis (Fig. 42–43), especially in infirm patients over 60 years of age. Transfer of this muscle rehabilitates the face in a more expeditious manner than facial nerve grafting. This technique shortens the period of rehabilitation. The patient experiences a quicker return of movement and is in satisfactory condition for postoperative irradiation (Fig. 42–44).

The masseter muscle may also be used in conjunction with free autogenous facial nerve grafting when there is a contraindication to nerve grafting in the lower third of the face because of extensive tumor ablation in this region. Under these circumstances, a single large nerve graft may be anastomosed to the principal upper (zygomatic) division of the facial nerve. The masseter transposition to the lower third of the face reactivates the lower third and the nerve graft supplies additional movement to the middle and upper thirds of the face (see Fig. 42–23*C*).

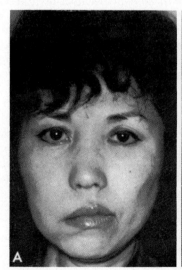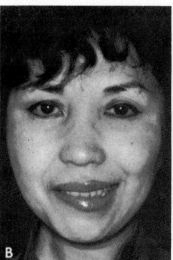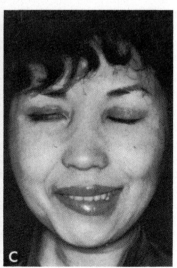

Figure 42–43. *A,* Patient who had a radical parotidectomy including facial nerve resection. Rehabilitation was only with immediate masseter muscle transposition interdigitated with the mimetic muscles. The face is in repose two years postoperatively. *B,* Clenching of teeth demonstrates satisfactory movement of the lower and middle third of the face. Significant myoneurotization with the mimetic muscles has occurred. *C,* Almost complete closure of the eye. (From Baker, D. C., and Conley, J.: Regional muscle transplantation for rehabilitation of the paralyzed face. Clin. Plast. Surg., *6*:323, 1979.)

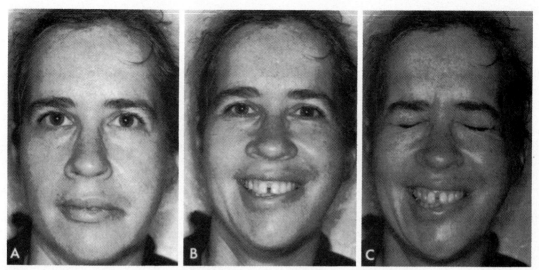

Figure 42–44. *A,* Patient who had total parotidectomy and sacrifice of the *entire* lower division of the facial nerve for a malignant tumor. An immediate masseter muscle transfer was performed to rehabilitate the lips and commissure. The face is in repose two months postoperatively. *B,* Patient is clenching teeth and also using the upper division of the VII nerve. *C,* Eye closure is excellent and facial symmetry is satisfactory except for weakness of the lower lip depressors. (From Baker, D. C., and Conley, J.: Regional muscle transplantation for rehabilitation of the paralyzed face. Clin. Plast. Surg., *6:*324, 1979.)

TEMPORALIS MUSCLE TRANSPOSITION

The temporalis muscle has enjoyed more popularity in facial rehabilitation than has the masseter, because it has the ability to rehabilitate the paralyzed eye and achieve greater excursion of mouth movement. The surgical anatomy of the temporalis muscle was reviewed by Rubin (1977) and Holmes and Marshall (1979). The muscle is fan-shaped, being thin peripherally and thicker centrally. The deep origin of the muscle fibers interdigitate into the periosteum and temporal bone over the entire fossa, from the inferior temporal line above to the infratemporal crest below. The superficial origin of the muscle is from the temporalis fascia, which originates from the superior temporal line of the skull. The muscle inserts on the entire coronoid process and a portion of the ascending ramus of the mandible.

The blood supply is from the anterior and deep temporal arteries and veins, which are tributaries of the internal maxillary system. They enter the infratemporal fossa beneath the zygoma and lateral to the external pterygoid muscle, predominantly on the anterior medial portion of the muscle, to spread out through the muscle superiorly.

The nerve supply is from the anterior and posterior deep temporal nerves, which are branches of the mandibular division of the trigeminal. Their origin is deeper and more posterior than the vascular supply, and they enter the muscle in proximity with the vessels.

Both the concept and technique of temporalis muscle transposition have undergone considerable modification during the past 50 years. Almost all the procedures devised for transposition of the temporalis muscle have been concerned not only with muscle placement but also with some type of maneuver to increase muscle length. The techniques of lengthening have included suturing fascia lata to the end of the muscle (Gillies, 1934), folding and advancing the temporal fascia on the muscle, and, most recently, using free muscle grafts attached to the temporalis transfer (Millesi, 1979). These lengthening concepts are based on the assumption that the muscle is not long enough to reach the medial canthus and mouth. In the author's experience (Baker and Conley, 1979), however, in over 100 temporalis transfers it has been noted that, by following the temporal ridge and taking the full body of the muscle with several centimeters of pericranium, the medial canthus, upper lip, and oral commissure can be reached without much difficulty.

This technique has the following advantages:

1. Elimination of a nonvascularized unit (fascia) that carries the risk of necrosis, breakage, atrophy, slippage, and stretching.

2. Direct insertion of the muscle into the area to be reanimated.

3. Augmentation of an atrophic face in long-standing paralysis.

4. If some functioning mimetic muscle remains in the face, the ability to interdigitate the temporalis muscle with these fibers, thus enhancing the possibility of myoneurotization.

The temporal muscle is exposed through a crescent-shaped, cruciate, or "T" type of incision in the temple, and the entire muscle, with 2 cm of pericranium about its peripheral margin, is elevated for transposition (Fig. 42–45). Two anterior segments are back cut to be adapted about the upper and lower eyelids. Appropriate tunnels are made in both lids in a subcutaneous plane. The levator muscle is protected, and the tunnels communicate in the region of the medial canthus. The two anterior strips of temporal muscle with the pericranium are pulled into the tunnels with lead sutures and sutured to the medial canthal ligament. Sufficient tension is maintained so that the upper lid overlaps the lower lid by several millimeters.

The lateral cheek is undermined and tunnels are made to the upper lip, commissure, and lower lip. If the temporal muscle is exceptionally thick and bulky, the zygomatic arch can be removed to reduce the bulk at this level. This maneuver adds approximately 2 cm to the length of the muscle. If the muscle is not bulky, it is draped over the arch. The muscle is back cut in two sections, using the anterior section for the orbit and the posterior section for the cheek, face, and lips. The

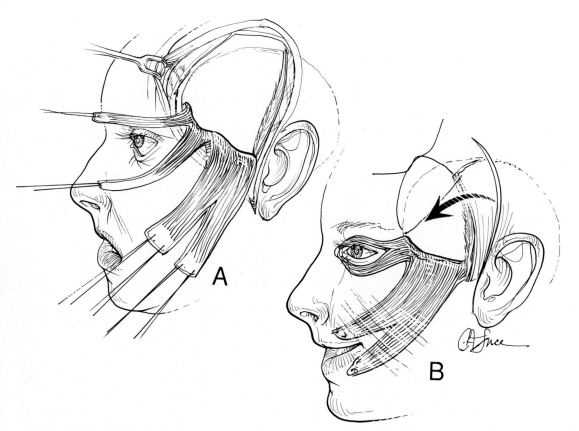

Figure 42–45. Technique of temporalis transposition. *A,* Preauricular incision with extension into the scalp. The entire muscle is elevated and four or five incisions are made for the slips to be inserted. *B,* Muscle slips are transposed to the upper and lower eyelids, upper lip and melolabial fold, lower lip, and commissure. Overcorrection is essential. The muscle should be sutured medial to the melolabial fold and interdigitated with the orbicularis oris muscle in the upper lip.

posterior section is tailored with minimal back cutting to accommodate the prepared tunnels in the cheek and lips. Back cutting should be restricted because of the danger of transecting nerves and small blood vessels to the distal segment of the muscle. The muscle strips are pulled through the tunnels and sutured into the dermis of the skin. It is important to attach the muscle medially to the melolabial fold so that this natural crease is recreated by the muscle pull. If there are mimetic muscles remaining in the face, an attempt should be made to interdigitate the transposed temporalis fibers into them. This is often possible over the orbicularis oris, since there is frequently crossinnervation from the normal side (Nishimura, Morimoto, and Yanagihara, 1977).

In the melolabial fold the crease may be deepened to recreate contour by transposing a deepithelized skin flap based on the line of the future nasolabial fold, as described by Clodius (1976). This flap may also serve as an anchoring point for the transposed muscle to imitate the movement of the quadratus labii superioris and levator anguli oris (Fig. 42–46). To imitate the action of the zygomaticus major, a muscle strip should be sutured to the angle of the mouth.

Overcorrection and exaggeration of the nasolabial fold and corner of the mouth are essential. The overcorrection resolves spontaneously within a few weeks. After meticulous hemostasis, the wounds are drained and closed as in the masseter transfer. The face is supported by large Steri-Strips, and the postoperative care is the same as that after masseter transfer.

After temporalis transposition there may be considerable depression in the region of the temple donor area. This may be camouflaged by hair styling, or eliminated at the time of the primary operation by the insertion of a silicone rubber block. There is always some bulging of the muscle over the zygoma, but when the muscle is excessively thick the zygoma may be removed. This maneuver, however, eliminates the fulcrum action of the zygomatic arch, and the muscle passes straight down instead of going up and down. Most patients have a slight web at the inner canthal region where the muscle is sutured to the medial canthal tendon, although this is not usually a significant deformity (Fig. 42–47).

Indications

Temporalis muscle transposition can be used to advantage in complete facial paralysis with atrophy of the mimetic muscles, sagging and hollowness of the face, and drooping of the oral commissure. Rubin (1976, 1977) used it extensively in facial rehabilitation for Möbius' syndrome. In these instances it provides support, movement, and augmentation. The temporalis muscle is also helpful in protecting the eye.

Temporalis transfer is rarely used as the rehabilitative technique with a primary ablative operation causing facial paralysis. When the other preferred methods are not feasible, such as in a massive tumor resection, primary rehabilitation with the temporalis muscle may offer some advantage. In most instances, however, the temporal muscle has

Figure 42–46. Muscle slips are sutured to the dermis medial to the melolabial fold and also interdigitated with the orbicularis oris muscle. (From Baker, D. C., and Conley, J.: Regional muscle transplantation for rehabilitation of the paralyzed face. Clin. Plast. Surg., 6:327, 1979.)

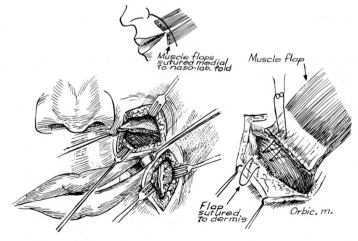

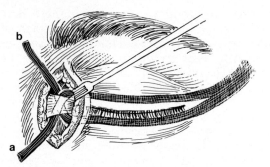

Figure 42–47. Slips are sutured to the medial canthus with nonabsorbable suture. Extreme care must be taken to minimize the size of tunnels in the eyelids and to prevent drifting of the muscle (occasionally a suture placed in the midportion of the lid maintains the position). Tension should be sufficient to overlap the lower lid by the upper lid by several millimeters. The overcorrection rapidly corrects itself. (From Baker, D. C., and Conley, J.: Regional muscle transplantation for rehabilitation of the paralyzed face. Clin. Plast. Surg., 6:327, 1979.)

been used as a secondary procedure in postoperative or long-standing facial paralysis.

RESULTS OF TEMPORALIS AND MASSETER MUSCLE TRANSPOSITION

In all cases one should expect some degree of minimal movement of the face several weeks after surgery. The movement is always associated with voluntary action of the masticatory muscles initiated by clenching of the teeth. Failure to attain movement in the face may result from excessive back cutting and interference with the neurovascular supply, with resultant muscle atrophy and fibrosis. Improper suture of the muscle to the dermis may result in slippage or breakage; the latter may also represent improper postoperative immobilization or early movement of the face. If fascial strips are used to lengthen the muscle, they may atrophy, slip, or stretch.

The greatest observed movement involves the region about the lips and cheek. If significant myoneurotization occurs (frequently, when a masseter muscle transfer is used for immediate rehabilitation of the face in an ablative procedure), the movement gradually extends, over an interval of one to two years, to include all the muscles of the lower and middle thirds of the face. This may include satisfactory movement of the lower eyelid, cheek, upper lip, commissure, and lower lip (Fig. 42–48). The movement is always intentional and not associated with emotion. Many patients, however, can train themselves to imitate an emotional reaction. The strength of the movement is usually satisfactory, although the tone of the muscles on that side of the face may be poor. In the temporalis transfer, eyelid closure is usually adequate.

Because the impulse for muscle movement in temporalis and masseter transfers originates from the trigeminal nerve, facial movement is produced upon chewing, clenching the teeth (Fig. 42–49), and moving the mandible. A few patients may complain of excessive movement while eating. These are obvious limitations and disadvantages, and they have stimulated the search for other means to reinnervate these muscles (Fig. 42–50). One can perform a facial nerve graft from the proximal segment of the ipsilateral facial nerve, if it is intact, and implant it into the transposed muscle, or anastomose it to the masseteric or temporal nerves at the foramen ovale. Crossface nerve grafts with muscle implantation have also been performed (Anderl, 1977a, 1985), as have crossface nerve grafts to the masseteric nerve at the foramen ovale (Freilinger, 1975). The results of these procedures have not been sufficiently evaluated to justify their routine use.

The basic advantage of masseter and temporalis transfer is the introduction of a large volume of living and dynamic muscle into the face. Additional advantages include the simplicity of the technique, the support provided, enhancement of the possibility of myoneurotization, and no loss of other significant function. In many instances, facial movement improves for approximately two years, and the long-term effect suggests some degree of rehabilitation of the facial muscles.

Free Muscle Grafts

In 1971 Thompson reported the successful transplantation of free autogenous muscle grafts in humans, and in 1974 he established its clinical application in the treatment of unilateral facial paralysis. According to Thompson, the success of this procedure depends on three factors: (1) the muscle selected for transplantation must be denervated 14 days before transplantation; (2) a full length of muscle fiber must be preserved; and (3) the denervated muscle must be placed in direct contact with normal, fully innervated, and vascularized skeletal muscle at the recipient

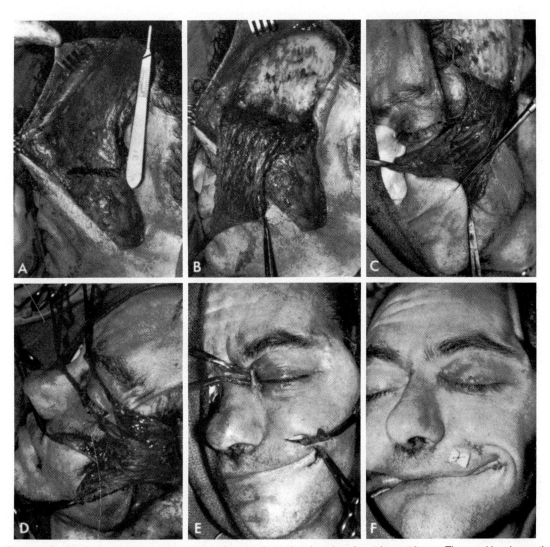

Figure 42–48. *A,* The length of the temporalis muscle and epicranium is at least 10 cm. The marking is on the zygomatic arch. *B,* The entire temporalis muscle is transposed, and it easily reaches the lower lip and commissure without the need for fascial strips or temporalis fascia. *C,* The transposed muscle also easily reaches the medial canthus. *D,* The divided slips are in place. The lowermost muscle slip reaches the commissure with overcorrection. *E,* The slips are passed through tunnels and are ready for suturing. *F,* Note the overcorrection, the recreation of the melolabial fold, and the bolus maintaining the muscle over the orbicularis oris muscle. (From Baker, D. C., and Conley, J.: Regional muscle transplantation for rehabilitation of the paralyzed face. Clin. Plast. Surg., *6:*328, 1979.)

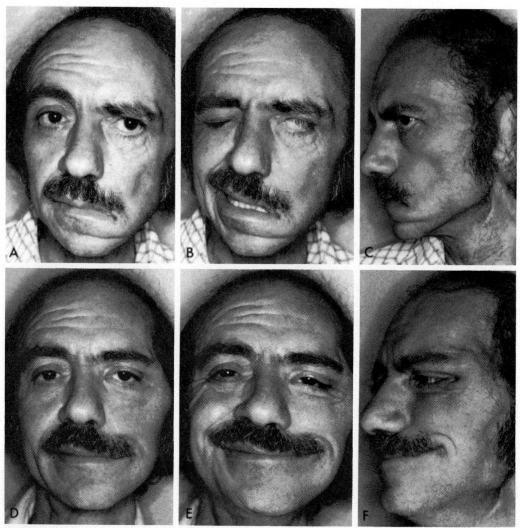

Figure 42–49. The patient (see Fig. 42–48) had a temporal bone resection for squamous cell carcinoma of the ear. Immediate facial rehabilitation was by a crossface nerve graft. *A*, The result two years postoperatively is shown. The face is in repose. *B*, Smiling and closing the eye. *C*, Note ectropion, sagging of the face, and atrophy of the facial tissues. *D*, Results are shown three months after temporalis muscle transposition. The face is in repose. *E*, Mimicking a smile by clenching the teeth. *F*, Note the augmentation of the face by the transposed muscle. The bulge over the zygoma could be corrected by insertion of a Silastic implant in the temporal region or by removal of the zygomatic arch. (From Baker, D. C., and Conley, J.: Regional muscle transplantation for rehabilitation of the paralyzed face. Clin. Plast. Surg., *6*:329, 1979.)

Figure 42–50. *A,* Patient with Möbius' syndrome with the face in repose. *B,* The patient is attempting to smile. *C,* One year after bilateral temporalis muscle transfer, fullness of the malar areas and accentuation of the epicanthal folds are seen. *D,* Satisfactory movement of the mouth and cheeks is achieved by clenching the teeth. In females, the depression in the temporal donor site is easily camouflaged by the hair style. (From Baker, D. C., and Conley, J.: Regional muscle transplantation for rehabilitation of the paralyzed face. Clin. Plast. Surg., *6*:330, 1979.)

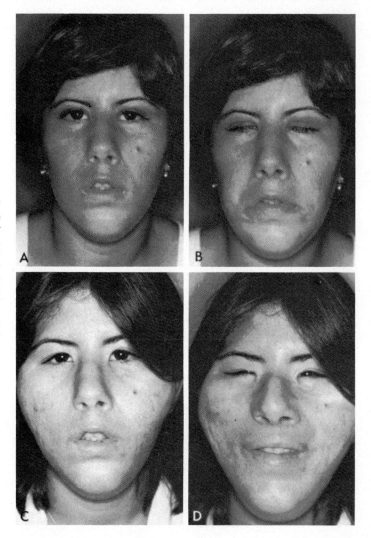

site before neurotization can occur. Thus, a minimum of two operations is required, with an interval of 14 days between them. The technique consists of placing denervated muscle in contact with normal muscle on the nonparalyzed side of the face. The transplanted muscle tendon is then sutured to the appropriate area to obtain movement (e.g., the zygomatic arch for the oral sphincter and the lateral canthal tendon for the eye sphincter).

Thompson (1971) reported that of 54 patients treated for oral sphincter reconstruction, 90 per cent had good results and 10 per cent showed satisfactory improvement. Seventeen per cent of the patients required another surgical procedure to tighten the tendon sling. In the reconstruction of the paralyzed eyelids of 62 patients, 48 per cent showed good results and 45 per cent satisfactory results. Secondary operations to adjust tension or perform tenolysis were required in 22 per cent of the patients. The advantage of this technique is that movement is controlled by the normal side of the face.

In spite of the reports of success by Thompson (1971) and Hakelius (1979), considerable skepticism exists about the reproducibility of free muscle grafting for reconstructive surgery. The attempt by Mayou and associates (1981) to reproduce Thompson's experiments in dogs proved unsuccessful, and it is still uncertain which factors are responsible for the survival of free muscle grafts. In addition to this uncertainty and reports that grafts have become fibrotic, other disadvantages include the multiple surgical stages required, the high incidence of reoperation, and the intrusion on the nonparalyzed side of the face.

With the present high success rates of microneurovascular muscle transfer, the technique of free muscle grafting has little or no place in facial paralysis reconstruction.

Nerve-Muscle Pedicle Techniques

From previous work involving reinnervation of paralyzed vocal cords, Tucker (1979) extended the nerve-muscle pedicle technique to the treatment of facial paralysis. The technique involves transplanting an intact motor nerve with an attached small block of donor muscle from the point of nerve entry, after which the pedicle is sutured to the muscle to

be reinnervated. If most motor end plates are preserved, the pedicle is prevented from degenerating, and reinnervation of the recipient muscle takes place within two to eight weeks (as demonstrated by experimental work in rabbits). The ansa hypoglossi nerve is used with muscle pedicles from the anterior belly of the omohyoid, the sternohyoideus, and the sternothyroideus. The pedicles have sufficient length to be implanted in the levator anguli oris and the orbicularis oris, but they cannot reach the eye. For reconstruction of the orbicularis oculi, Tucker (1979) recommended a temporalis muscle pedicle. Minimal clinical experience has been amassed on this technique; in theory, however, it could rehabilitate the face without loss of function, perhaps doing so in a shorter time than some other present techniques.

The technique can be applied only to the perioral musculature, and it has yet to capture the interest of surgeons.

Microneurovascular Muscle Transfers

The most recent contribution to reanimation of the paralyzed face is the microneurovascular muscle transfer, combined with crossface nerve graft, ipsilateral nerve graft, or split hypoglossal anastomoses. The technique provides new, vascularized muscle to the face that can produce pull in various directions and accomplish more normal facial animation. The indications for its use are similar to those for regional muscle transfer; the advantage over the latter technique is that the transferred muscle can be reinnervated by a crossface nerve graft, thereby enhancing control of voluntary facial movement. In spite of the success of and enthusiasm for this technique, its limitations must be kept in mind and the indications for its use should be clear. At present, it is merely another alternative in the surgeon's armamentarium of facial reanimation procedures.

Harii, Ohmori, and Torii (1976) were the first to report a successful microvascular transfer of the gracilis muscle to provide elevation of the oral commissure. In the first case, performed in 1973, the motor nerve to the temporalis muscle was employed. In subsequent cases a crossface nerve graft was anastomosed to the transferred muscle at a second stage. Harii's report of 18 cases (1979) demonstrated encouraging results. Two of the major drawbacks were the excessive bulk of the transferred muscle and the excessive movement. In 1980 O'Brien, Franklin, and Morrison reported favorable results.

Tolhurst and Bos (1982) reported seven cases in which the extensor digitorum brevis muscle was used, with only two satisfactory results. The experience of Harii and O'Brien using this as a donor muscle was similarly disappointing, and most surgeons no longer employ it for facial paralysis reconstruction. Terzis and Manktelow (1982) recommended the pectoralis minor muscle for facial reanimation, and this report was followed by Harrison (1985), who used the same donor muscle in ten patients with five excellent results, three good results, and two failures. The advantages of this muscle are its small, flat configuration, the minimal functional loss, and an acceptable donor scar. Buncke (1983) reported the successful use of the serratus anterior muscle for facial reanimation. More recent reports by Manktelow (1987), O'Brien and Morrison (1987), and Harii (1988) appear to favor the gracilis as the donor muscle of choice.

The ideal donor muscle should provide the following:

1. Excursion equal to that of the normal side of the face.

2. A reliable vascular and nerve pattern of similar size to that of the recipient.

3. No functional deficit from removal of the muscle.

4. Location of a donor site sufficiently distant from the face to allow for two operating teams to work simultaneously.

Numerous muscles have been used for transplantation to the face (Terzis, 1987). The most commonly used at present are listed below.

Gracilis muscle has a predictable and adequate neurovascular pedicle, with adequate bulk but excessive length (Hamilton, Terzis, and Carraway, 1987). Because various portions are supplied by different fascicles, the muscle can be split longitudinally and cut transversely to produce the required size of muscle needed for transfer. The initial reports of Harii (Harii, Ohmori, and Torii, 1976; Harii, 1979) described the use of the entire gracilis muscle, with resultant facial bulk and distortion. With the refinements of Manktelow (1987), a single fascicle supplying the anterior third of the muscle can be taken to provide the desired length and bulk.

Pectoralis minor muscle has adequate weight but excessive length; its flat shape facilitates insertion into the face. However, as Manktelow (1985) pointed out, the neurovascular pedicle is complex and variable, and its motor supply may present significant problems in reinnervation. In addition, the proximity on the upper chest makes simultaneous two-team dissection difficult. Nevertheless, Terzis (1987) has been encouraged with the results of using this muscle in facial reanimation.

Latissimus dorsi muscle and *serratus muscle* have a predictable neurovascular pedicle and longitudinal intramuscular pattern. The latissimus dorsi can be segmentally separated like the gracilis in order to reduce its bulk. The nerve to the serratus is short (Hamilton, 1987) and usually the lower four segments are utilized; it also requires segmental separation to reduce its bulkiness.

Rectus abdominis muscle is bulky and long but can be transferred. It has a long, predictable vascular supply and a laterally based segmental nerve supply.

Platysma muscle is a thin facial muscle supplied by the facial artery and the cervical branch of the facial nerve. Because of its weight and thinness, Terzis (1987) used it in reconstructing the orbicularis oculi.

All the aforementioned muscles leave minimal or no functional deficit when sacrificed. As operative techniques have been refined, the emphasis has shifted toward harvesting well-innervated pieces of muscle that have the correct functional length to replace the appropriate facial muscles. There are numerous muscles with a predictable neurovascular supply from which such pieces of muscle may be taken.

SURGICAL TECHNIQUE

The operative procedure is usually divided into two stages unless the ipsilateral facial nerve can be used or the hypoglossal is split and anastomosed. The first stage consists of a classical crossface nerve graft. If muscle transfer is to reanimate both the eye and mouth, two crossface nerve grafts are required. Tinel's sign is followed, and approximately nine to 12 months later the vascularized muscle is transferred and its neural element anastomosed to the distal end of the crossface nerve graft.

For the second stage the two-team approach is best, one to prepare the facial nerve graft and recipient vessels (usually the superficial temporal or facial), while the other harvests and prepares the donor muscle on its neurovascular pedicle. It is important to carry out fascicular nerve stimulation of the donor muscle to determine which portion of the muscle each fascicle supplies. For example, the anterior one-third of the gracilis is usually utilized (Fig. 42–51).

According to Manktelow (1985), the zygomaticus major is the single facial muscle most nearly producing a normal smile. It is approximately 5 cm in length and produces a maximal shortening of 1.5 to 2 cm in the normal face. With preoperative observation the excursion of the oral commissure and shape of the patient's smile can be recorded, and an attempt should be made to simulate the normal side with the transferred muscle. The muscle should usually run from the oral commissure to the body of the zygoma along the normal course of the zygomaticus major (Fig. 42–52). A functioning muscle length of 5 to 6 cm is generally required.

The transferred muscle is sutured into the commissure and can be interdigitated with any remaining facial muscles in the upper and lower lip, nasolabial fold, and alar base. The site of the muscle's origin depends on the direction of pull desired, usually between the zygomatic arch and tragus.

The correct tension at which the muscle should be inserted has not yet been fully demonstrated. Manktelow (1987) placed the muscle in sufficient tension so that under anesthesia it is tight enough to place the paralyzed oral commissure in balance with the normal side. Microvascular anastomoses of artery and vein and fascicular nerve repair are completed. Overlying skin closure should avoid tension on the vascular anastomoses, and drains should be kept distant to the latter.

RESULTS

The reports of Harrison (1985); Harii, Ohmori, and Torii (1976); Harii (1979);

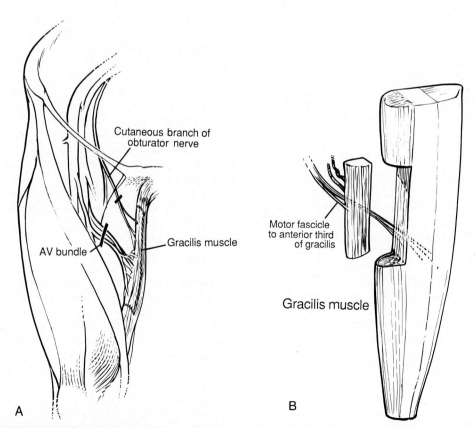

Figure 42–51. Gracilis microneurovascular transfer. *A,* Overview of the muscle with the cutaneous branch of the obturator nerve and the arteriovenous bundle, which are divided. *B,* The three longitudinal fascicular motor territories. The anterior territory containing the dominant neurovascular pedicle has been harvested. (*A* and *B* from Manktelow, R. T.: Free muscle transplantation for facial paralysis. Clin. Plast. Surg., *11:*218, 1984.)

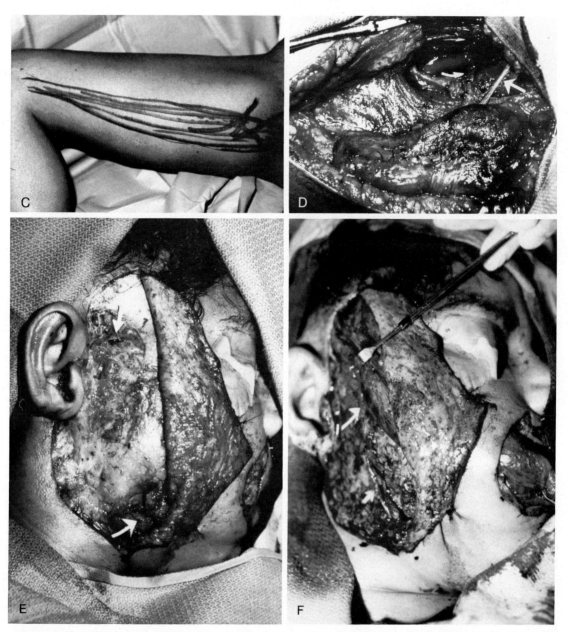

Figure 42–51 *Continued C*, Outline of the gracilis muscle and neurovascular pedicle. *D*, The gracilis muscle flap dissected with the nerve and vascular pedicles isolated *(arrows)*. *E*, Recipient facial vessels and the distal end of the crossface nerve graft *(arrows)*. *F*, The muscle flap transferred to the face. The anastomoses of facial vessels and crossface nerve graft completed.

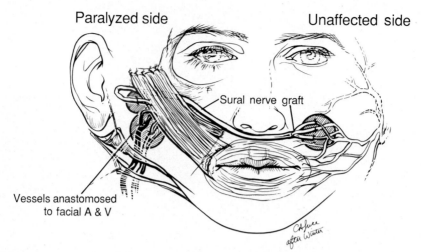

Paralyzed side   Unaffected side

Sural nerve graft

Vessels anastomosed
to facial A & V

Figure 42–52. Microneurovascular transfer of the gracilis muscle on the paralyzed side. The muscle is sutured to the zygomatic arch and the sural nerve graft is anastomosed to the motor nerve to the gracilis muscle. The gracilis arteriovenous bundle is sutured to the respective facial artery and vein. The other end of the gracilis muscle is sutured into the oral commissure, orbicularis oris, and nasolabial fold.

O'Brien and Morrison (1987); and Manktelow (1987) have all been encouraging, with a majority of good to excellent results (Fig. 42–53). In 35 out of 40 of the patients of O'Brien and Morrison adequate symmetry was obtained at rest and reasonably active lifting of the angle of the mouth and cheek. In addition, 19 patients obtained independent movements of the face in spite of the fact that both sides of the face were supplied by the same facial nerve. No satisfactory explanation has been determined for this phenomenon.

It is important to emphasize that movement of the face after microneurovascular muscle transfer is never normal. As pointed out by Rayment, Poole, and Rushworth (1987), it is simplistic to use one reinnervated muscle along one vector to reanimate the oral commissure and upper lip—an area that normally has ten muscles acting on it along different vectors. Patients do learn to produce a definitive smile, but the ability to produce the involuntary, spontaneous "flash" smile rarely returns. Therefore, during speech some asymmetry of the face is usually evident. It is also difficult to obtain independent movements in the eye and mouth (Manktelow, 1987).

Rayment, Poole, and Rushworth (1987) analyzed the problem of poor symmetry of synergistic facial movement in patients who have had successful reinnervation of transplanted muscle. They explained that the ad-

equacy of reinnervation of muscle is directly related to the numbers of axons that manage to cross the sural nerve graft to the muscle: different ratios of axons to muscle fibers exist for different muscles. Normal facial muscles have approximately 25 muscle fibers innervated by one axon (Feinstein, 1955), while gracilis and pectoralis minor muscles have 150 to 200 muscle fibers to each axon. Muscles with a smaller ratio of muscle fibers to axons, such as the facial muscles are capable of producing a wide variety of finely tuned movements (Rayment, Poole, and Rushworth, 1987). The facial muscles have been described as "intelligent," while the gracilis and pectoralis minor muscles are "stupid" (Terzis, 1988).

Crossface nerve grafting, even with the most meticulous technique, has demonstrated that only 20 to 50 per cent of axons cross the nerve graft (Harrison, 1985). The different muscle fiber to axon ratio would explain the limited success of crossface nerve grafting alone, as opposed to combining it with a microvascular muscle transfer (muscles requiring fewer axons to reinnervate a larger number of muscle fibers).

INDICATIONS

Microneurovascular muscle transfer is another alternative in facial paralysis reconstruction. Some of the best candidates for this

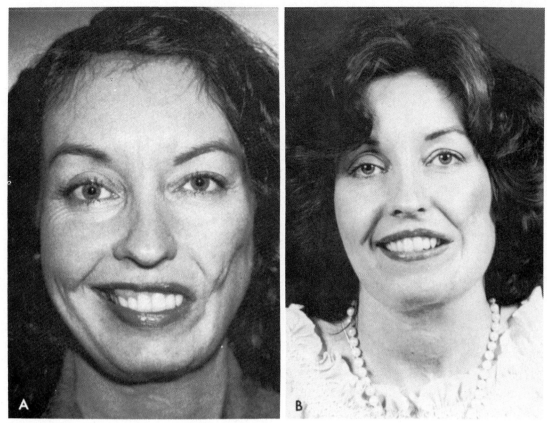

Figure 42–53. *A*, Preoperative appearance, smiling, showing inability to elevate the corner of the mouth and a soft tissue defect in the left cheek. *B*, Postoperative appearance, smiling. (From Manktelow, R. T.: Free muscle transplantation for facial paralysis. Clin. Plast. Surg., *11*:219, 1984.)

technique are patients with a regional paralysis, especially involving the elevators of the lip. Others are patients in whom the ipsilateral facial nerve is intact, as after trauma or extensive facial tumor resections where the facial muscles are ablated. Younger patients with congenital paralysis or those who have had intracranial tumor resection are also well suited for this technique. Older or infirmed patients with facial paralysis more often prefer a simpler, pragmatic approach to facial reanimation such as regional muscle transfers.

The main advantage of the technique is that facial movement is provided and controlled by the contralateral facial nerve, providing for better symmetry and perhaps a more definitive smile. Many disadvantages, however, remain: (1) there are at least two operative stages with prolonged surgical time; (2) there are two donor site scars; (3) there is usually a lapse of two years before return of facial movement; (4) complete eyelid closure, forehead movement, oral sphincter, and depressor lip function are almost never restored; (5) the technique is not free of synkinesis; and (6) there is a deficit of involuntary emotional expression common to most other rehabilitative techniques.

Static and Ancillary Techniques

All the previous procedures for facial reanimation used nerve and muscle or a combination of the two to provide for a dynamic reconstruction of the paralyzed face. At present these techniques are well accepted and easily accomplished with a high degree of success and minimal risk. Consequently there is rarely any place for the static methods of reconstruction that were popular several decades ago.

FASCIAL TRANSPLANTS

According to Freeman (1977), the use of autogenous fascia for blepharoptosis was initiated by Payr and applied to the treatment of facial paralysis by Stein (1913). However, it was Blair's advocacy (1926) of the suspension of paralyzed facial muscles by fascia lata bands that popularized the method. The technique (Fig. 42–54) varies considerably with the individual problem, but a modified fascial sling has proved of value as a method of primary treatment in older adults, and as an adjunct method while waiting for the functional results of nerve crossings, grafts, or nerve end approximations. It is also used in association with muscle transplants and the resection of contralateral muscles, and may be helpful in prolonging the effects of skin excisions, face lifts, and blepharoplasties.

DERMAL TRANSPLANTS

Strips of dermis of a width and length comparable with that of strips of fascia inserted in the same manner have a tendency to stretch (Freeman, 1977). Dermis and lyophilized fascia are more liable to stimulate fibrous proliferation than autogenous fascia, because they fragment and disintegrate early. Postoperative subcutaneous infections are higher with dermal implants than with fascia, because saprophytic infection carried into the repaired field is manifest many days or weeks after the operation rather than in the usual 12 to 36 hours after surgery (Pick, 1949).

INORGANIC (ALLOPLAST) IMPLANTS

Static methods to relieve distortion employ the suspension of paralyzed facial muscles by various materials, varying from wire and silk to stainless steel and tantalum. There are advocates for the use of nonreactive plastic tapes of polyethylene, Teflon, or Silastic with or without either Marlex or Dacron mesh reinforcement (Fig. 42–55). Clinical experience has led to a distrust of inorganic material placed in a position of suspension or tension in superficial locations (Freeman,

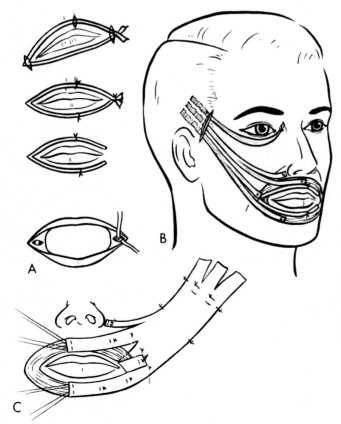

Figure 42–54. Fascia lata suspension. *A,* Placement of a circumoral fascial strip. Inserted via extraoral or buccal incisions, the loops are tightened on the unaffected side to elevate the paralyzed angle of the mouth. The knotted attachment at the unaffected commissure is excised after five weeks. The lowermost sketch shows the oral incisions for insertion of the circumoral band of fascia after it has been threaded through and knotted, before the suturing. *B,* The fascial sling to the lower lid is secured at the nasal periosteum. The lateral end is attached to the temporal fascia. The fascial band is attached through a temporal incision to the orbicularis oris. The three tails for attachment at both insertions are shortened for clarity. *C,* The typical fashioning of a fascial ribbon for adequate support using three tails for insertion: one for each lip well past the midline and another folded around the dissected orbicularis oris muscle. The similarly tailed lateral end is woven into the temporal fascia or tacked securely to the adjacent periosteum.

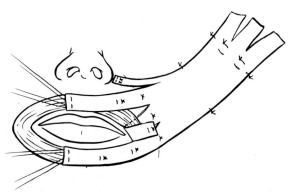

Figure 42–55. Method of attachment of the fascia lata or Marlex mesh by nonabsorbable mattress sutures at the pterygomandibular raphé (rather than at the mandible). The central slip of the anterior end is wrapped securely around the orbicularis oris muscle at the oral commissure. The inferior and superior slips are secured temporarily by pull-out mattress sutures to the undersurface of the dermis. (The optional small strip to the ala is secured firmly.) Insertion can also be made to the mandible.

1977). The reviews of Bäckdahl and D'Alessio (1958) and Conway (1958) should be consulted before inorganic (alloplast) materials are used for facial suspension.

Selective Neurectomy

Selective sectioning of the intact facial nerve in order to accomplish a more balanced face has been practiced for over 100 years (Freeman, 1977). It is best carefully to evaluate the degree of antagonist muscle pull and distortion and to map the nerves to be sectioned.

UPPER FACIAL PARALYSIS

The degree and permanency of the paralysis may be established by electrical testing of the facial nerve and recording of the chronaxial levels. If these levels remain high for more than six months, there will most likely be no return of movement to the brow.

If the paralysis persists, the frontal muscles atrophy, with a resultant ptosis of the brow. Any improvement at this stage involves an equalization of the movement of the forehead by a selective cutting of the corresponding nerve on the opposite side. This may be carried out through the temporal incision used in the face lift, with identification of the responsible nerve by electrical testing. At this anatomic level there are frequently two or three filaments requiring division (as determined by electrical stimulation). They should be sectioned step by step, until the brow is paretic. Even with this approach to nerve section, equalization of movement of the brow does not result in every case (Baker, 1984). Occasionally, after the operation the paralysis of the normal side may not be as much as desired, and a "second look" may be necessary. According to Baker and Conley (1979) in equalizing the brow one should always attempt to save the filament that goes to the corrugator muscles, to the eyebrow, and to the orbicularis muscles, because this retains an active and lively expression about the eyebrows. Not uncommonly, however, patients with a paralysis of the frontal branch prefer to have a smooth, immobile forehead with minimal frown lines.

MIDDLE FACIAL PARALYSIS

If the paresis is recognized postoperatively, it is reasonable to wait because almost all middle facial paralyses recover considerably during a period of months, owing to collateral budding from the network that these nerves share with each other. The result may be complicated, however, by a slight motor tic. If a persistent or troublesome tic or spasm of the face develops, consideration may be given to a selective division of the particular nerve filament causing it. This is accomplished by exposing the particular branch, electrical testing, and a neurotomy. The weakness that develops in the muscle systems supplied by this nerve is marked in the beginning, but over six months there is considerable return of movement via the network pathways. Unfortunately, in some instances when the balance becomes restored there may be a reappearance of the tic, but usually not as marked as it was originally.

LOWER FACIAL PARALYSIS

A persistent paralysis of the marginal mandibular branch may be handled by division of the opposite mandibular branch after an interval of one year. A neurectomy at this level places the lower lip in relative balance. Again, this may be difficult to accomplish permanently, because of variations in the network connections of the distal branches of the facial nerve. A combination of this procedure with a selected myectomy, accomplished through a mucosal incision (Rubin, 1977), gives more assurance of permanent symmetry.

Selective Myectomy

Freeman (1977) outlined the various techniques for selective myectomy of the facial muscles to accomplish better balance in repose and during facial expression.

The muscles most frequently causing distortion during speech, emotion, and associated actions are the quadratus labii superioris, the depressor labii inferioris, and the zygomaticus. A study of the muscle or muscle groups responsible for the distortion permits these to be isolated and sectioned and varying amounts of muscle tissue to be resected. This procedure can be helpful in segmental paralysis not amenable to surgical neurorrhaphy or grafting. Alleviation of the spastic, antagonistic muscles on the nonpalsied side has aided symmetry during action, both voluntary and emotional.

To correct excessive upward deviation of the opposite side of the face during a smile, the zygomaticus muscle is outlined at the angle of the mouth. The fibers, which spread up and out and become deeper superiorly, are isolated under the subcutaneous tissue and retracted for a distance of approximately 2 cm from the relatively diffuse origin of the muscle to its insertion into the orbicularis oris. Careful dissection exposes the tiny nerves that enter the muscle from the undersurface. It is a simple procedure to remove a segment 1 to 2 cm in length, depending on the age of the patient (Freeman, 1977).

Deviation of the philtrum to the contralateral side and the upward pull of the cheek can be lessened by resecting a segment of the quadratus labii superioris muscle, as well as a short segment of the orbicularis oris in this area.

Abnormal depression of the lip during labial speech, simulating a sneer, can be alleviated by isolating the quadratus labii inferioris through the mucosa and removing a segment of the muscle. The muscle outline is marked during forceful speech. The lip is everted, the mucosa incised, the muscle isolated and sectioned, and the mucosa closed.

An intraoral approach is also adequate for resection of the depressor muscles. After everting the lip, a mucosal flap is elevated, and the quadratus muscle, together with the triangularis and the associated segments of the orbicularis oris, is outlined. The muscles, isolated from the skin and mucosa, are clipped and ligated, and resected.

The incision to expose the zygomaticus or the quadratus labii superioris (the levators) is placed in the nasolabial fold. The stouter and thickened muscles are outlined, and after careful dissection a 2 cm segment of muscle is removed.

Elevation and spasm of the contralateral forehead and eyebrow can be adjusted by myectomy. Through an incision of 2 cm or less at the upper median border of the eyebrow, the corrugator and procerus muscles are exposed, isolated, and resected. Since the procerus, frontalis, orbicularis oculi, and corrugator muscles act synergistically, a small median segment of the conjoint muscle of the first three muscles, which covers the corrugator muscle, is removed.

Face Lifts, Brow Lifts, and Excision of Redundant Skin and Mucosa

Removal of redundant skin and mucosa (Fig. 42–56), either by direct excision or the

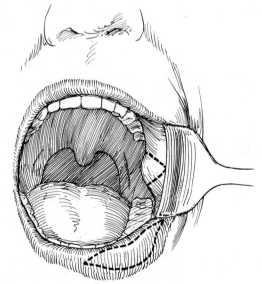

Figure 42–56. Excision of the redundant and hypertrophied buccal and labial mucosa affords access to the underlying musculature for repair of the diastasis. (From Freeman, B. S.: Late reconstruction of the lax oral sphincter in facial paralysis. Plast. Reconstr. Surg., *51*:144, 1973. Copyright ©1973. The Williams & Wilkins Company, Baltimore.)

various rhytidectomy techniques outlined in Chapter 43, may also be useful in balancing the paralyzed face and accomplishing a more esthetically pleasing result. Most often a combination of the foregoing techniques yields the maximal result.

TREATMENT OF THE PARALYZED EYELID

Facial paralysis affecting the orbicularis oculi muscle results in an inability to close the eyelids, a condition referred to as lagophthalmos (from the Greek word *lagos* meaning hare, an animal that sleeps with its eyes open). Because of the loss of orbicularis muscle tone, gravity pulls the atonic lower lid into a sagging position (ectropion). When the lower lid margin and lacrimal punctum are no longer in apposition with the globe, normal tear flow and the lacrimal drainage system are disturbed. Constant exposure of the cornea results in evaporation of the tear film, dryness of the cornea, and exposure keratitis. This condition may progress to infection, corneal ulceration, and eventual blindness. Fortunately, because of Bell's phenomenon, the eyeball rotates upward and the cornea comes to lie under the upper lid, helping to protect it from trauma and desiccation. However, in patients with a totally paralyzed orbicularis oculi this is usually insufficient to protect the eye.

Management of Lagophthalmos

NONSURGICAL METHODS

These methods are directed at providing comfort and protecting the cornea from trauma and drying. Numerous artificial tears and eye ointments (Jelks, Smith, and Bosniak, 1979) are available to keep the eye moist. Lid taping at night may also prevent corneal exposure during sleep. Other measures include occlusive moisture chambers, soft contact lenses and scleral shells (Goren and Clemis, 1973), and temporary lid suturing. These methods are most helpful in patients with acute facial paralysis in whom recovery of orbicularis oculi function is expected. However, if recovery does not occur or is incomplete, numerous surgical procedures are available to improve eyelid closure.

SURGICAL METHODS

It must be remembered that the ocular complications of orbicularis oculi paralysis follow a progressive course. It is therefore necessary to individualize procedures according to the degree of deformity and dysfunction. Furthermore, before dynamic lid procedures such as the application of lid weights, magnets, springs, or silicone strips can be attempted, it is necessary to repair any lid abnormalities, including paralytic ectropion. A protective program of ocular lubrication must also be well established.

Tarsorrhaphy

For many years lateral tarsorrhaphy was the accepted method for treating lagophthalmos in facial paralysis. The McLaughlin procedure (1953) is preferred because it preserves the lashes to camouflage the lateral lid adhesion. The disadvantages of tarsorrhaphy, however, are the narrowing of the lid aperture, a downward displacement of the lateral canthus, and difficulty in separating the lids without considerable residual deformity. The last-named may be a significant problem if the patient has return of orbicularis oculi function and the tarsorrhaphy is no longer needed. At present, horizontal lid shortening and medial and lateral canthoplasties are more popular in correcting ectropion and alleviating lagophthalmos.

Canthoplasties

Laxity of the lower lid or ectropion may be the prominent features of patients with facial paralysis. A standard wedge excision to obtain a horizontal shortening of the lower lid is often satisfactory in mild cases of lid laxity. However, with marked lower lid laxity, lateral canthoplasties that support the lower lid from the lateral orbital rim are the best reconstructive methods (Fig. 42–57). Edgerton and Wolfort (1969) were the first to describe a technique for support of the lower eyelids in patients with facial paralysis. Their technique employs a dermal flap secured to the lateral orbital rim. In 1978 Montandon modified this technique by incorporating a portion of the upper and lower eyelid margins with the dermal flap. There is also an occasional need for a medial canthoplasty in patients with facial paralysis (Fig. 42–58).

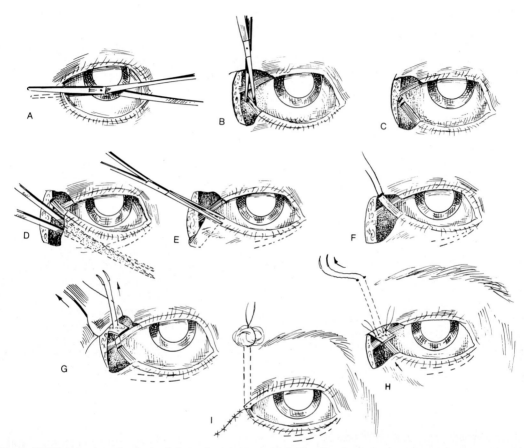

Figure 42–57. Lateral canthoplasty. *A,* Lateral canthotomy. *B, C,* The lateral canthal tendon is exposed and the lower limb of the tendon is divided at the orbital rim. *D,* Scissors undermine the skin of the lower lid and also cut retracting bands that connect the orbital rim to the tarsus of the lower lid. *E,* The desired position of the new lateral canthal angle is determined along the lower lid margin by placing upward and lateral traction on the lower lid. The lid margin is excised to this point. The dotted lines show the planned excision of excess orbicularis oculi muscle, cilia, and skin, leaving a long lower lid tarsal tongue. *F,* The lower lid tarsal tongue has a double-armed 4–0 silk suture passed through it. With this suture, the lower lid is elevated anterior and superior to the superior limb of the lateral canthal tendon (which is still attached to the lateral orbital rim). *G,* A laterally based flap of periosteum is developed from the orbital rim superior and lateral to the upper lid contribution to the lateral canthal tendon. The 4–0 silk suture is passed through the base of this flap. *H,* The suture is passed along a subcutaneous track to emerge superior to the lateral brow level. This suture is tied over a cotton bolster after adjusting the desired elevation and tightening of the lower lid. Two 4–0 Dexon sutures are used to reinforce the tarsal tongue–periosteal flap attachment. *I,* The final result shows slight overcorrection with the lateral lower lid elevated. The tendon can also be secured to a hole in the orbital rim. (From Jelks, G. W., Smith, B., and Bosniak, S.: The evaluation and management of the eye in facial palsy. Clin. Plast. Surg., *6:*411, 1979.)

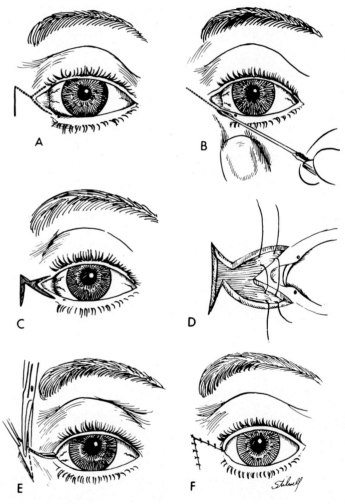

Figure 42–58. Medial canthoplasty, which places the everted punctum against the globe and tightens a moderately sagging lower lid. *A*, The outline of the incisions. *B*, A probe is placed in the canaliculus in order to avoid severing this structure. *C*, After completion of the incisions. *D*, The edges of the medial canthus are sutured by means of inverting sutures. *E*, Traction is placed on the skin flap, and excess skin is removed. *F*, The skin incision is sutured. (From Kazanjian and Converse.)

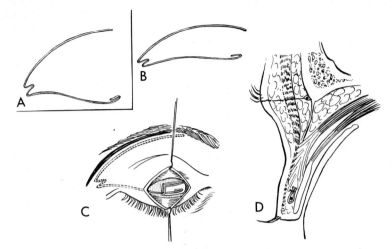

Figure 42–59. The palpebral spring in the treatment of paralysis of the eyelid (technique of Morel-Fatio). *A, B,* Stainless steel wire formed in the shape of a "W." *C,* Dacron felt covering over the doubled lower end. Note the incisions. *D,* Cross-sectional view.

The Morel-Fatio Spring (Morel-Fatio and Lalardrie, 1964) is a stainless steel wire formed into a figure "W," which is inserted into the upper lid to provide synchronous closure of the eye with levator relaxation (Fig. 42–59). At best, the results can be excellent, but a high rate of spring extrusion has decreased the popularity of this technique.

Morel-Fatio (1976) reported his results in 72 cases: 27 secondary operations were required; 11 complications occurred (five springs broke; two springs were extruded; infection occurred in four cases); and in five cases the spring was deliberately removed. In Guy's (1969) experience, using a slightly different technique, of a series of 24 patients, six springs were removed, eight required minor adjustments, and 18 were still functioning after three years.

Lid Magnets

Mühlbauer, Segeth, and Viessmann (1973) implanted two miniaturized, siliconized curved magnets beneath the orbicularis muscle near the upper and lower eyelid margins. The tarsal plates prevent erosion of the rods into the conjunctival sacs. The magnetic force employed in the open-eye position for the double-magnet system was 200 to 300 m p, and this corresponds to the absent muscle tone of the orbicularis muscle, thus preventing upper lid retraction, corneal irritation, and epiphora. Normal lid opening is maintained by the intact levator mechanism.

Initially the lid magnets are taped to the lid margins to determine the ideal magnet force. When this is established, the lid magnets are implanted under local anesthesia. The results with lid magnets can be excellent (Mühlbauer, 1977), but unfortunately the extrusion rate is unacceptably high.

Silicone Sling (Arion Prosthesis)

In 1972 Arion described a method of placing a silicone band in the lids inducing just enough tension to allow the lids to close with levator relaxation. The procedure has been modified by Wood-Smith (1973), as shown in Figure 42–60. Because silicone is a material that does not wear well, it is subject to stress, relaxation, and breakage. For this reason, there has not been much support for this technique.

Upper Lid Loading

A technique of accentuation of gravity by a weight (Fig. 42–61) in the lid was described by Sheehan (1927). He initially recommended the use of stainless steel mesh in the upper lid. According to Freeman (1979) tantalum, which is malleable, became available during World War II. It is nonreactive, can be readily fashioned during the operation, and has proved to be useful. The upper lid weight is increased by implanting a tantalum strip of 0.75 gm. Nonetheless, the various implants of gold seem to provide a better color match for white patients and have been commercially prepared (Jobe, 1974).

To assess the required load, a series of weights are taped to the eyelid until normal closure is obtained. This weight is then in-

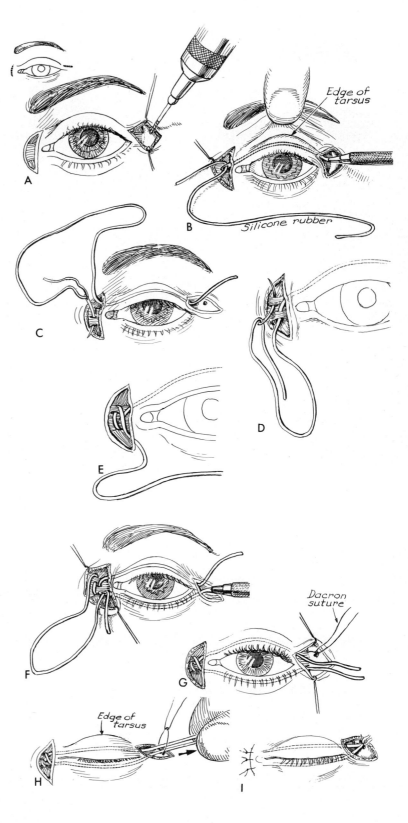

Figure 42–60. Construction of an orbicularis sphincter by a circumorbital Silastic string—technique of Arion (courtesy of Dr. D. Wood-Smith). A fine Silastic band is threaded around the lids. The band is sutured to the medial canthal tendon and secured to the lateral orbital rim by a Dacron suture passed through a drill hole. The technique is performed under local anesthesia, because the cooperation of the patient in adjusting tension is essential. The small vertical incision over the medial canthal tendon and the small horizontal incision over the lateral orbital rim are closed with fine nylon sutures. Note the special instrument used to pass the Silastic string through the upper and lower eyelids. (From Kazanjian and Converse, 1974.)

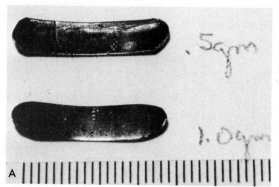 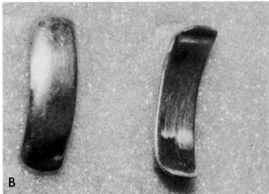

Figure 42–61. Upper lid implants. *A,* Implants hand-fashioned in the operating room out of tantalum. *B,* Gold implants weighing approximately 1.0 gm. The former can be altered; the latter cannot be changed.

serted into the upper lid. Complications of this technique include insufficient loading, infection, and extrusion. The weight may also be visible in the upper lid, appearing as a lump.

Other Procedures

Temporalis muscle transfers (Fig. 42–62) and nerve grafting have already been reviewed. Jelks, Smith, and Bosniak (1979) made an extensive review of the various procedures to reconstruct the paralyzed eye. Table 42–10 summarizes the alternative approaches.

CHOICE OF CORRECTIVE PROCEDURE

The choice of corrective procedure is dependent on a detailed analysis of the etiology, the degree of paralysis, the patient's age, and the overall prognosis. No single method can routinely offer the efficacy of a multiple technique approach modified to suit the end desired and progressively achieved over a period of time (Freeman, 1975, 1979).

There are few procedures proposed for the alleviation of facial paralysis that have not been of some value in selected cases. None, however, with the possible exception of an early nerve repair or graft, is suitable for all

Table 42–10. Surgical Procedures for Orbicularis Oculi Palsy According to Expected Duration and Severity of Lagophthalmos

Severity of Lagophthalmos	Expected Duration		
	Six Months	*Two Years*	*More Than Two Years*
Mild (70 to 90 per cent lid closure)	Nonsurgical	1,2,3 (4,5,6,7)*	1,2,3 (4,5,6,7)*
Moderate (30 to 70 per cent lid closure)	2,3	1,2,3,† (4,5,6,7)*	2,3† (4,5,6,7,8)*
Severe (less than 30 per cent lid closure)	2,3† (4,5,6,7)*	2,3† (4,5,6,7)*	2,3† (4,5,6,7,8)*

*To further protect the cornea and to restore dynamic eyelid function.
†Horizontal lid shortening is usually required.
1, lateral tarsorrhaphy; 2, medial canthoplasty; 3, lateral canthoplasty; 4, lid weights; 5, lid magnets; 6, palpebral spring; 7, silicone encircling band; 8, temporal muscle transfer.
After Jelks, G. W., Smith, B., and Bosniak, S.: The evaluation and management of the eye in facial palsy. Clin. Plast. Surg., 6:397, 1979.

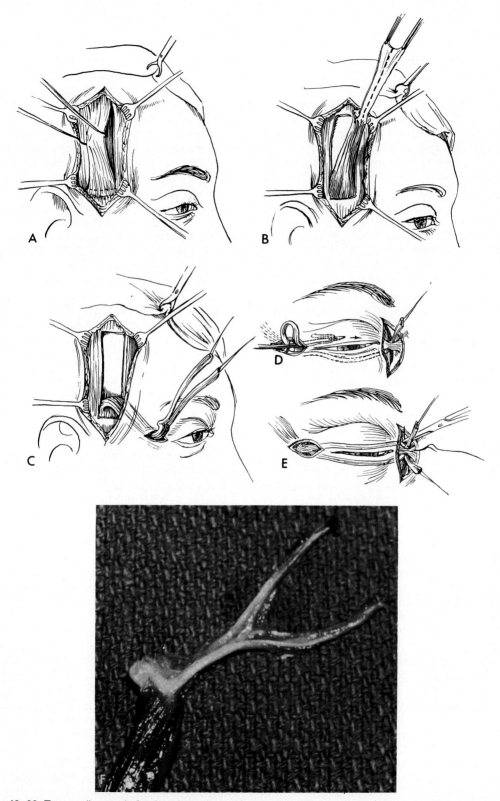

Figure 42–62. Temporalis muscle-fascia unit used as a circumorbital sling and motor unit. *A* to *E*, Gillies technique as modified by Andersen (1961). *F* shows a segment of temporalis muscle and its attachment to the temporal fascia. (This attachment may be tenuous and should be reinforced with Dacron sutures.)

patients. The selection of the procedure or procedures to be applied to the individual patient is based on an analysis of the deformity, a knowledge of the usual results by that surgeon, and the requirements and physical condition of the patient.

To perform a two-stage microneurovascular muscle transfer in an elderly patient who has had a cerebrovascular accident is inappropriate when there are numerous simple and highly successful techniques to improve that patient's appearance. For the teenager with a congenital facial paralysis, on the other hand, the microneurovascular technique may provide the best opportunity for natural facial movement. All the techniques previously described have certain limitations as well as requirements for their use. In virtually every case of facial paralysis there are several alternative methods of reconstruction, each with advantages and disadvantages, higher or lower success rates, longer or shorter operating times. It is essential that the surgeon evaluate and present the various methods and alternatives to each patient who desires rehabilitation of the paralyzed face.

Limitations of Facial Paralysis Reconstruction

Conley and Baker (1983) reviewed some of the misconceptions, limitations, and myths of rehabilitation of the paralyzed face.

The ideal is to reestablish complete facial movement that automatically exhibits the complete spectrum of human expression. This degree of perfection is unrealistic, and most patients and surgeons are satisfied with results that are less optimal than these ideals. The poignancy of facial paralysis, the vast number of techniques that have been described to ameliorate it, and the methods of reporting these results have created hopes and beliefs that are, in many instances, totally unrealistic.

The most common myth that has developed is the presumption that a variety of operations can restore involuntary facial movement. Three basic operations (free ipsilateral facial nerve grafting, hypoglossal nerve crossover, and regional masticatory muscle transfer) improve the stigmata of facial paralysis in most instances, but do not restore the capability for spontaneous emotional expression. There are many ingenious variations of these fundamental techniques: crossface anastomosis, muscle transplants with neurovascular microsurgical techniques, myotomies and myectomies, and Z-plasties. However, none of these operations restores natural emotional expression.

One of the most appealing arguments for using the proximal segment of either the ipsilateral or the contralateral facial nerve in a free nerve grafting technique has been the statement by some operating surgeons that they intend to restore involuntary facial expression (Anderl, 1977a,b; Ben-Hur, 1977; Fisch, 1979). This myth should not be propagated. No one has ever found or described the involuntary neural pathways to the face (Brodal, 1965; Goss, 1973; Carpenter, 1978). Pure involuntary facial movement is associated with human emotion, which has its primary reservoir in the frontal lobes, but its essence and mechanism of production and transit are unknown. It has been assumed by many surgeons that involuntary emotional communication is through the facial nerve, but this has never been substantiated. Indeed, emotional expression may be beyond the concept of a mere physical tract. It certainly has never been totally restored by any surgical technique that attempts to rehabilitate the face.

The movement that does return, however, regardless of the technique used, is always weaker than that of the normal side, and is associated with depletion of the number of axons and nuclei and certain central neural connections on the affected side. The movement that returns is generally gross, not regionalized or refined, has a conglomerate mass quality, and is associated with dyskinesia (Stennert, 1979). When the patient responds to pure emotion, it is essentially the normal side of the face that moves. The persistence of this imbalance and this discrepancy in natural human emotional response are, indeed, the hallmarks of facial paralysis.

The movement that the patient can produce in the rehabilitated face is intentional. The muscular contraction is a disciplined act within the realm of consciousness and awareness. Many of these patients can simulate a smile and other human expressions by practice, training, and adaptation. All photographs, however, that are taken of the rehabilitated paralyzed face depict precisely this smile, which is an intentional performance that patients demonstrate before the camera.

Motion pictures taken when patients intentionally move the face and when they spontaneously move it as an emotional response are the most accurate method of assessing the results of surgical rehabilitation. Even though the results, in some instances, are far better than had been hoped for, the myth of restoring spontaneous emotional expression should be dispelled.

The question of specific fascicular grafting in the main trunk of the facial nerve on the basis of topography has stimulated the hope of reducing mass movement and dyskinesia (May, 1977a; Crumley, 1980). No specific report on humans has supported this proposition, however. Indeed, there is not complete agreement on the regional topography of the facial nerve in the temporal bone (Miehlke, 1958; Harris, 1968; May, 1973; Kempe, 1980). All animal experiments and studies indicate that in the temporal bone portion of the nerve, the motor axons are not regionalized but are diffusely scattered in all portions of the nerve, even though separate fascicles are readily identifiable (Sunderland, 1953; Thomander, Aldskogius, and Grant, 1981; Gacek and Radpour, 1982).

Surgery and disease affecting the facial nerve in the temporal bone support diffusion of axons by causing a general, rather than a regional, weakness in the movement of the face. Certain pathologic conditions affecting the main trunk of the nerve outside the temporal bone may cause a regional weakness first. This may progress or remain localized, depending on the cause. Involvement of a peripheral division of the nerve affects only one region. It is therefore unrealistic to propose that restoration of regional and individual facial movement can be accomplished by fascicular facial nerve grafting within the temporal bone. The randomized position of the axons in the main trunk always predisposes to a misdirection of the regenerating axons, with the physiologic consequences of weakness, mass movement, and dyskinesia (Young, Wray, and Weeks, 1981).

These misconceptions are a derivative of surgical hopefulness and have created a false attitude toward what is real and what can be accomplished in rehabilitation of the paralyzed face. It is never possible to restore natural, spontaneous expression, complete motor power, and perfect synchronous movement by any operation. However, the patient can use the movement that does return to the mimetic muscles or a transferred muscle to imitate emotional expression. This is attained by patient awareness, practice, and adaptation.

REFERENCES

Adams, W.: The use of the masseter, temporalis, and frontalis muscles in the correction of facial paralysis. Plast. Reconstr. Surg., *1*:216, 1946.

Anderl, H.: Reconstruction of the face through cross-face nerve transplantation in facial paralysis. Chir. Plast. (Berl.), *2*:17, 1973.

Anderl, H.: Reconstruction of the face through cross-face nerve transplantation in facial paralysis. *In* Converse, J. M. (Ed.): Reconstructive Plastic Surgery. 2nd Ed. Philadelphia, W. B. Saunders Company, 1977a, p. 1848.

Anderl, H. (Moderator): Rehabilitation of the face by VIIth nerve substitution (panel discussion no. 6). *In* Fisch, U. (Ed.): Facial Nerve Surgery. Birmingham, AL, Aesculapius Publishing Company, 1977b.

Anderl, H.: Cross face grafting in facial palsy. *In* Portmann, M. (Ed.): Facial Nerve. New York, Masson, 1985.

Arion, H. G.: Dynamic closure of the lids in paralysis of the orbicularis muscle. Int. Surg., *57*:48, 1972.

Bäckdahl, M., and D'Alessio, E.: Experience with static reconstruction in cases of facial paralysis. Plast. Reconstr. Surg., *21*:211, 1958.

Ba Huy, P. T., Monteil, J. P., and Rey, A.: Results of twenty cases of trans facio-facial anastomosis as compared with those of XII–VII anastomoses. *In* Portmann, M. (Ed.): Facial Nerve. New York, Masson, 1985.

Baker, D. C.: Anatomy and injuries of the facial nerve in cervicofacial rhytidectomy. *In* Kaye, B. L., and Gradinger, G. P. (Eds.): Symposium on Problems and Complications in Aesthetic Plastic Surgery of the Face. St. Louis, C. V. Mosby Company, 1984.

Baker, D. C.: Hypoglossal-facial nerve anastomosis, indications and limitations. *In* Portmann, M. (Ed.): Facial Nerve. New York, Masson, 1985a.

Baker, D. C.: Reanimation of the paralyzed face: nerve crossover, cross-face nerve grafting, and muscle transfers. *In* Chretien, P. B., Johns, M. E., Shedd, D. P., Strong, E. W., and Ward, P. H. (Eds.): Head and Neck Cancer. Philadelphia, B. C. Decker, 1985b.

Baker, D. C.: Facial paralysis. *In* Smith, B., Nesi, F., DellaRocca, R., and Lisman, R. (Eds.): Ophthalmic Plastic and Reconstructive Surgery. St. Louis, C. V. Mosby Company, 1987a.

Baker, D. C.: Hypoglossal-facial nerve anastomoses. *In* Brent, B. (Ed.): The Artistry of Reconstructive Surgery. St. Louis, C. V. Mosby Company, 1987b.

Baker, D. C., and Conley, J.: Facial nerve grafting: a thirty year retrospective review. Clin. Plast. Surg., *6*:343, 1979a.

Baker, D. C., and Conley, J.: Regional muscle transposition for rehabilitation of the paralyzed face. Clin. Plast. Surg., *6*:317, 1979b.

Baker, D. C., and Conley, J.: Avoiding facial nerve injuries in rhytidectomy. Anatomical variations and pitfalls. Plast. Reconstr. Surg., *64*:781, 1979c.

Baker, D. C., and Conley, J.: Reanimation of facial

paralysis. *In* English, G. M. (Ed.): Otolaryngology. Philadelphia, J. B. Lippincott Company, 1982.

Ballance, C.: Results obtained in some experiments in which the facial and recurrent laryngeal nerves were anastomosed with other nerves. Br. Med. J., *2*:349, 1924.

Ballance, C., and Duel, A. B.: The operative treatment of facial palsy by the introduction of nerve grafts into the fallopian canal and by other intratemporal methods. Arch. Otolaryngol., *15*:1, 1932.

Bell, C.: On the nerves, giving an account of some experiments on their structure and functions, which leads to a new arrangement of the system. Trans. R. Soc. Lond. (Phil.), *3*:398, 1821.

Ben-Hur, N.: Primary nerve suturing of severed motor nerves in facial trauma. *In* Rubin, L. R. (Ed.): Reanimation of the Paralyzed Face. St. Louis, C. V. Mosby Company, 1977.

Blair, V. P.: Notes on the operative correction of facial palsy. South. Med. J., *19*:116, 1926.

Brodal, A.: The Cranial Nerves: Anatomy and Anatomico-Clinical Correlations. 2nd Ed. London, Blackwell Scientific Publications, 1965.

Brunner, H.: Surgical treatment of facial paralysis. Ztschr. Hals Nasen Ohrenheilkd., *15*:379, 1926.

Buncke, H.: Serratus anterior free muscle grafts for facial paralysis. Presented at the American Association for Plastic Surgery annual meeting, 1983.

Bunnell, S.: Suture of the facial nerve within the temporal bone with a report of the first successful case. Surg. Gynecol. Obstet., *45*:7, 1927.

Bunnell, S.: Surgical repair of the facial nerve. Arch. Otolaryngol., *25*:235, 1937.

Campbell, J. B., and Luzio, J.: Facial nerve repair: new surgical techniques. Trans. Am. Acad. Ophthalmol. Otolaryngol., *68*:1068, 1964.

Carpenter, M. B.: Core Text of Neuroanatomy. 2nd Ed. Baltimore, Williams & Wilkins Company, 1978.

Clodius, L.: Selective neurectomies to achieve symmetry in partial and complete facial paralysis. Br. J. Plast. Surg., *29*:43, 1976.

Conley, J. J.: Facial nerve grafting in treatment of parotid gland tumors. Arch. Surg., *70*:359, 1955.

Conley, J. J.: Facial rehabilitation following radical parotid gland surgery. Arch. Otolaryngol., *66*:58, 1957.

Conley, J. J.: Facial nerve grafting. Arch. Otolaryngol., *73*:322, 1961.

Conley, J. J.: Techniques of extratemporal facial nerve surgery. *In* Miehlke, A. (Ed.): Surgery of the Facial Nerve. 2nd Ed. Philadelphia, W. B. Saunders Company, 1973.

Conley, J. J.: Salivary Glands and the Facial Nerve. Stuttgart, Georg Thieme Verlag, 1975.

Conley, J., and Baker, D. C.: The surgical treatment of extratemporal facial paralysis: an overview. Head Neck Surg., *1*:12, 1978.

Conley, J., and Baker, D. C.: Hypoglossal-facial nerve anastomosis for reinnervation of the paralyzed face. Plast. Reconstr. Surg., *63*:63, 1979.

Conley, J., and Baker, D. C.: Myths and misconceptions in the rehabilitation of facial paralysis. Plast. Reconstr. Surg., *71*:538, 1983.

Conley, J., Baker, D. C., and Selfe, R. W.: Paralysis of the mandibular branch of the facial nerve. Plast. Reconstr. Surg., *70*:569, 1982.

Conway, H.: Muscle plastic operations for facial paralysis. Ann. Surg., *147*:541, 1958.

Crumley, R. L.: Spatial anatomy of facial nerve fibers—a preliminary report. Laryngoscope, *90*:274, 1980.

Crumley, R. L.: Muscle evaluation of facial reanimation surgery. *In* Portmann, M. (Ed.): Facial Nerve. New York, Masson, 1985.

Davis, R. A., Anson, B. J., Budinger, J. M., and Kurth, L. E.: Surgical anatomy of the facial nerve and parotid gland based upon a study of 350 cervicofacial halves. Surg. Gynecol. Obstet., *102*:385, 1956.

de Castro Correia, P., and Zani, R.: Masseter muscle rotation in the treatment of inferior facial paralysis. Plast. Reconstr. Surg., *52*:370, 1973.

Dingman, R. O., and Grabb, W. C.: Surgical anatomy of the mandibular ramus of the facial nerve based on the dissection of 100 facial halves. Plast. Reconstr. Surg., *29*:266, 1962.

Dott, N. M.: Facial paralysis—restitution by extrapetrous nerve graft. Proc. R. Soc. Med. Lond., *51*:900, 1958.

Drobnik: Über die Behandlung der Kinderlämung mit Funktionstheilung und Funktionsübertragung der Muskeln. Dtsch. Z. Chir., *43*:473, 1896.

Edgerton, M. T., Tuerk, D. B., and Fisher, J. C.: Surgical treatment of Moebius syndrome by platysma and temporalis muscle transfers. Plast. Reconstr. Surg., *55*:305, 1975.

Edgerton, M. T., and Wolfort, F. G.: The dermal-flap canthal lift for lower eyelid support. Plast. Reconstr. Surg., *43*:42, 1969.

Ellenbogen, R.: Pseudo-paralysis of the mandibular branch of the facial nerve after platysmal face-lift operation. Plast. Reconstr. Surg., *63*:364, 1979.

Erlacher, P.: Direct and muscular neurotization of paralyzed muscles. Experimental research. Am. J. Orthop. Surg., *13*:22, 1915.

Esslen, E.: Electrodiagnosis of facial palsy. *In* Miehlke, A. (Ed.): Surgery of the Facial Nerve. Munich, Urban & Schwarzenberg, 1973.

Esslen, E.: *In* Fisch, U. (Ed.): Facial Nerve Surgery. Birmingham, AL, Aesculapius Publishing Company, 1977.

Evans, D.: Hypoglossal-facial anastomosis in the treatment of facial palsy. Br. J. Plast. Surg., *27*:251, 1974.

Falbe-Hansen, J., and Hermann, S.: Hypoglosso-facial anastomosis. Acta Neurol. Scand., *43*:472, 1967.

Ferreira, M. C.: Cross-facial nerve grafting. *In* Terzis, J. K. (Ed.): Microreconstruction of Nerve Injuries. Philadelphia, W. B. Saunders Company, 1987, p. 601.

Fisch, U.: Facial nerve grafting. Otolaryngol. Clin. North Am., 7:517, 1974.

Fisch, U.: Current surgical treatment of intratemporal facial palsy. Clin. Plast. Surg., *6*:377, 1979.

Freeman, B. S.: Comparative long-term results following reconstruction of the palsied face. Presented at the Sixth International Congress of Plastic and Reconstructive Surgery, Paris, August 25, 1975.

Freeman, B. S.: Facial palsy. *In* Converse J. M. (Ed.): Reconstructive Plastic Surgery. 2nd Ed. Philadelphia, W. B. Saunders Company, 1977, p. 1774.

Freeman, B. S.: Review of long-term results in supportive treatment of facial paralysis. Plast. Reconstr. Surg., *63*:214, 1979.

Freilinger, G.: A new technique to correct facial paralysis. Plast. Reconstr. Surg., *56*:44, 1975.

Gacek, R. R., and Radpour, S.: Fiber orientation of the facial nerve: an experimental study in the cat. Laryngoscope, *92*:547, 1982.

Gillies, H. D.: Experience with fascia lata grafts in the operative treatment of facial paralysis. Proc. R. Soc. Med., *27*:1372, 1934.

Gillies, H. D., and Millard, D. R., Jr.: The Principles and the Art of Plastic Surgery. Boston, Little, Brown & Company, 1957.

Gomoiu, V.: La methode myoplastique dans le traitement de la paralysie faciale. Lyon Chir., *9*:5, 1913.

Goren, S. B., and Clemis, J. D.: Care of the eye in facial paralysis. Arch. Otolaryngol., *97*:227, 1973.

Goren, S. B., and Shoch, D.: The use of the flush-fitting scleral contact shell after surgical intervention on acoustic neuroma. Trans. Am. Ophthalmol. Surg., *68*:277, 1970.

Goss, C. M. (Ed.): Gray's Anatomy. 29th Ed. Philadelphia, Lea & Febiger, 1973.

Guy, C. L.: The palpebral spring for paralysis of the upper eyelid in facial nerve paralysis. Presented at the American Society of Plastic and Reconstructive Surgeons, St. Louis, 1969.

Hakelius, L.: Free muscle grafting. Clin. Plast. Surg., *6*:301, 1979.

Hamilton, S. G., Terzis, J. K., and Carraway, J. T.: Surgical anatomy of the facial musculature and muscle transplantation. *In* Terzis, J. K. (Ed.): Microreconstruction of Nerve Injuries. Philadelphia, W. B. Saunders Company, 1987, p. 571.

Hammerschlag, P. E., Brudny, J., Cusumano, R., and Cohen, N. L.: Hypoglossal-facial nerve anastomosis and electromyographic feedback rehabilitation. Laryngoscope, *97*:705, 1987.

Harii, K.: Microneurovascular free muscle transplantation for reanimation of facial paralysis. Clin. Plast. Surg., *6*:361, 1979.

Harii, K.: Personal communication, 1988.

Harii, K., Ohmori, K., and Torii, S.: Free gracilis muscle transplantation with microneurovascular anastomoses for the treatment of facial paralysis. Plast. Reconstr. Surg., *57*:133, 1976.

Harris, W. D.: Topography of the facial nerve. Arch. Otolaryngol., *88*:264, 1968.

Harrison, D. H.: The pectoralis minor vascularized muscle graft for the treatment of unilateral facial palsy. Plast. Reconstr. Surg., *75*:206, 1985.

Hastings, S.: Transplantation of anterior half of masseter muscle for facial paralysis. Proc. R. Soc. Med., *13*:64, 1919–1920.

Hill, H. L., Vasconez, L. O., and Jurkiewicz, M. J.: Method for obtaining a sural nerve graft. Plast. Reconstr. Surg., *61*:177, 1978.

Hitselberger, W. E.: Hypoglossal-facial anastomosis. Otolaryngol. Clin. North Am., 7:545, 1974.

Holmes, A. D., and Marshall, K. A.: Use of the temporalis muscle flap in blanking out orbits. Plast. Reconstr. Surg., *63*:336, 1979.

Huber, E.: Evaluation of Facial Musculature and Facial Expression. Baltimore, Johns Hopkins University Press, 1931.

Hueston, J. T., and Cuthbertson, R. A.: Duchenne de Boulogne and facial expression. Ann. Plast. Surg., *1*:411, 1978.

Hughes, G. B.: Electroneurography: objective prognostic assessment of facial paralysis. Am. J. Otol., *4*:73, 1982.

Jelks, G. W., Smith, B., and Bosniak, S.: The evaluation and management of the eye in facial palsy. Clin. Plast. Surg., *6*:397, 1979.

Jianu, A.: The surgical treatment of facial paralysis. Deutsche Ztschr. Chir., *102*:377, 1909.

Jobe, R. P.: A technique for lid loading in the management of lagophthalmos of facial palsy. Plast. Reconstr. Surg., *53*:29, 1974.

Kempe, L. G.: Topical organization of the distal portion of the facial nerve. J. Neurosurg., *52*:671, 1980.

Körte, W.: Ein Fall von Nervenpfropfung des Nervus facialis auf den Nervus hypoglossus. Dtsch. Med. Wochenschr., *17*:293, 1903.

Lathrop, F. D.: Affections of the facial nerve. J.A.M.A., *152*:19, 1953.

Lathrop, F. D.: Surgical repair of facial nerve: technique. Surg. Clin. North Am., *36*:583, 1956.

Lathrop, F. D.: Management of the facial nerve during operations on the parotid gland. Ann. Otol., *72*:780, 1963.

Lathrop, F. D.: Facial nerve grafting. Trans. Am. Acad. Ophthalmol. Otolaryngol., *68*:1060, 1964.

Lexer, E., and Eden, R.: Über die chirurgische Behandlung der peripheren Facialislähmung. Beitr. Klin. Chir., *73*:116, 1911.

Manktelow, R.: Free muscle transplantation for facial paralysis. Clin. Plast. Surg., *11*:215, 1984.

Manktelow, R. T.: Discussion of the pectoralis minor vascularized muscle graft for the treatment of unilateral facial palsy by Douglas H. Harrison. Plast. Reconstr. Surg., *75*:214, 1985.

Manktelow, R. T.: Free muscle transplantation for facial paralysis. *In* Terzis, J. K. (Ed.): Microreconstruction of Nerve Injuries. Philadelphia, W. B. Saunders Company, 1987, p. 607.

Martin, H., and Helsper, J. T.: Spontaneous return of function following surgical section or excision of the seventh cranial nerve in the surgery of parotid tumors. Ann. Surg., *146*:715, 1957.

May, M.: Anatomy of the facial nerve (spatial orientation of fibers in the temporal bone). Laryngoscope, *83*:1311, 1973.

May, M.: Anatomy of cross-section of facial nerve in the temporal bone: clinical application. *In* Fisch, U. (Ed.): Facial Nerve Surgery. Birmingham, AL, Aesculapius Publishing Company, 1977a.

May, M.: Factors influencing regeneration and quality of recovery after facial nerve lesions (panel discussion no. 1). *In* Fisch, U. (Ed.): Facial Nerve Surgery. Birmingham, AL, Aesculapius Publishing Company, 1977b.

May, M.: Facial paralysis: differential diagnosis and indications for surgical therapy. Clin. Plast. Surg., *6*:275, 1979.

May, M.: The Facial Nerve. New York, Thieme Medical Publishers, 1986.

Mayou, B. J., Watson, J. S., Harrison, D. H., and Parry, C. B.: Free microvascular and microneural transfer of the extensor digitorum brevis muscle for the treatment of unilateral facial palsy. Br. J. Plast. Surg., *34*:362, 1981.

McGuirt, W. F., and McCabe, B. F.: Effect of radiation therapy on facial nerve cable autografts. Laryngoscope, *87*:415, 1977.

McLaughlin, C. R.: Surgical support in permanent facial paralysis. Plast. Reconstr. Surg., *11*:302, 1953.

Meyer, R.: New concepts in rehabilitation of long-standing facial paralysis (panel discussion no. 7). *In* Fisch, U. (Ed.): Facial Nerve Surgery. Birmingham, AL, Aesculapius Publishing Company, 1977.

Miehlke, A.: Uber die Topographie des Faserverlaufes in Facialisstamm. Arch. Ohren Nas. Kehlk., *171*:340, 1958.

Miehlke, A.: Surgery of the Facial Nerve. 2nd Ed. Philadelphia, W. B. Saunders Company, 1973.

Miehlke, A.: Factors influencing results in extratemporal

facial nerve repair (panel discussion no. 5). *In* Fisch, U. (Ed.): Facial Nerve Surgery. Birmingham, AL, Aesculapius Publishing Company, 1977.

Miehlke, A., Stennert, E., and Chilla, R.: New aspects in facial nerve surgery. Clin. Plast. Surg., *6*:451, 1979.

Miller, T. A., Korn, H. N., Wheeler, E. S., and Eldrige, L.: Can one muscle reinnervate another? Plast. Reconstr. Surg., *61*:50, 1978.

Millesi, H.: Technique of free nerve grafting in the face. *In* Rubin, L. R. (Ed.): Reanimation of the Paralyzed Face. St. Louis, C. V. Mosby Company, 1977a.

Millesi, H.: Facial nerve suture. *In* Fisch, U. (Ed.): Facial Nerve Surgery. Birmingham, AL, Aesculapius Publishing Company, 1977b.

Millesi, H.: Nerve suture and grafting to restore the extratemporal facial nerve. Clin. Plast. Surg., *6*:333, 1979.

Millesi, H., Berger, A., and Meisal, G.: Experimentelle Untersuchungen zur Heilung durchtrennter Nerven. Chir. Plast. (Berl.), *1*:174, 1972.

Mitz, V., and Peyronie, M.: The superficial musculoaponeurotic system (SMAS) in the parotid and cheek area. Plast. Reconstr. Surg., *58*:80, 1976.

Montandon, D. A.: A modification of the dermal-flap canthal lift for correction of the paralyzed lower lid. Plast. Reconstr. Surg., *61*:555, 1978.

Morel-Fatio, D., and Lalardrie, J. P.: Palliative surgical treatment of facial paralysis. The palpebral spring. Plast. Reconstr. Surg., *33*:446, 1964.

Morel-Fatio, D.: The palpebral spring (round table discussion). *In* Marchac, D., and Hueston, J. T. (Eds.): Transactions of the Sixth International Congress of Plastic and Reconstructive Surgery. Paris, Masson, 1976.

Mühlbauer, W. D.: Five years' experience with lid magnet implantation for paretic lagophthalmos. Klin. Monatsbl. Augenheilkd., *171*:938, 1977.

Mühlbauer, W. D., Segeth, H., and Viessmann, H.: Restoration of lid function in facial palsy with permanent magnets. Chir. Plast. (Berl.), *1*:295, 1973.

Nishimura, H., Morimoto, M., and Yanagihara, N.: Contralateral innervation of the facial nerve. *In* Fisch, U. (Ed.): Facial Nerve Surgery. Birmingham, AL, Aesculapius Publishing Company, 1977.

O'Brien, B. M., Franklin, J. D., and Morrison, W. A.: Cross-facial nerve grafts and microneurovascular free muscle transfer for long-established facial palsy. Br. J. Plast. Surg., *33*:202, 1980.

O'Brien, B. M., and Morrison, W.: Facial palsy. *In* Reconstructive Microsurgery. London, Churchill Livingstone, 1987.

Owens, N.: The surgical treatment of facial paralysis. Plast. Reconstr. Surg., *7*:61, 1951.

Pansky, B., and House, E. L.: Review of Gross Anatomy. New York, Macmillan Company, 1964.

Perret, G.: Results of phrenicofacial nerve anastomosis for facial paralysis. Arch. Surg., *94*:505, 1967.

Pick, J. F.: The Surgery of Repair. Vol. 2. Philadelphia, J. B. Lippincott Company, 1949, p. 617.

Pickerill, P.: Facial paralysis, palatal repair, and some other plastic operations. Med. J. Aust., *1*:543, 1928.

Rayment, R., Poole, M. D., and Rushworth, G.: Cross-facial nerve transplants: why are spontaneous smiles not restored? Br. J. Plast. Surg., *40*:592, 1987.

Romanes, G. J. (Ed.): Cunningham's Textbook of Anatomy. 10th Ed. London, Oxford University Press, 1964.

Rubin, L. R.: The anatomy of a smile: its importance in the treatment of facial paralysis. Plast. Reconstr. Surg., *53*:384, 1974.

Rubin, L. R.: The Moebius syndrome: bilateral facial diplegia. Clin. Plast. Surg., *3*:625, 1976.

Rubin, L. R.: Reanimation of the Paralyzed Face. St. Louis, C. V. Mosby Company, 1977.

Ryan, R. M., Waterhouse, N., and Davies, D. M.: The innervated trapezius flap in facial paralysis. Br. J. Plast. Surg., *41*:344, 1988.

Sade, J.: Facial nerve reconstruction and its prognosis. Ann. Otol. Rhinol. Laryngol., *84*:695, 1975.

Samii, M.: Rehabilitation of the face by VIIth nerve substitution (panel discussion no. 6). *In* Fisch, U. (Ed.): Facial Nerve Surgery. Birmingham, AL, Aesculapius Publishing Company, 1977.

Samii, M.: Facial nerve grafting in acoustic neurinoma. *In* Terzis, J. K. (Ed.): Microreconstruction of Nerve Injuries. Philadelphia, W. B. Saunders Company, 1987, p. 651.

Sargent, P.: Four cases of facial paralysis treated by hypoglossal-facial anastomosis. Proc. R. Soc. Med., *5*:69, 1911–1912.

Scaramella, L. F.: Preliminary report on facial nerve anastomosis. Read before the Second International Symposium on Facial Nerve Surgery, Osaka, Japan, 1970.

Scaramella, L. F.: On the repair of the injured facial nerve. Ear Nose Throat J., *58*:127, 1979.

Schottstaedt, E. K., Larsen, L. G., and Bost, T. C.: Complete muscle transposition. J. Bone Joint Surg., *37A*:897, 1955.

Seddon, H. J.: Three types of nerve injury. Brain, *66*:238, 1943.

Sheehan, J. E.: Plastic Surgery of the Orbit. New York, Macmillan Company, 1927.

Sheehan, J. E.: The muscle nerve graft. Surg. Clin. North Am., *15*:471, 1935.

Smith, J. W.: A new technique of facial reanimation. *In* Hueston, J. T. (Ed.): Transactions of the Fifth International Congress of Plastic and Reconstructive Surgery. Melbourne, Butterworths, 1971.

Stein, A. E.: Die kosmetische Korrektur der Fazialislaehmung durch freie Faszienplastic. Münch. Med. Wochenschr., *60*:1370, 1913.

Stennert, E.: I. Hypoglossal facial anastomosis: its significance for modern facial surgery. II. Combined approach in extratemporal facial nerve reconstruction. Clin. Plast. Surg., *6*:471, 1979.

Sterkers, J. M.: Rehabilitation of the face by VIIth nerve substitution. *In* Fisch, U. (Ed.): Facial Nerve Surgery. Birmingham, AL, Aesculapius Publishing Company, 1977.

Sunderland, S.: Mass movements after facial nerve injury. *In* Fisch, U. (Ed.): Facial Nerve Surgery. Birmingham, AL, Aesculapius Publishing Company, 1977.

Sunderland, S., and Cossar, D. F.: The structure of the facial nerve. Anat. Rec., *116*:147, 1953.

Szal, G. J., and Miller, T.: Surgical repair of facial nerve branches. Arch. Otolaryngol., *101*:160, 1975.

Tavernier, J. B., and Daum, S.: Hypoglossal-facial anastomosis as a treatment for peripheral facial paralysis. Neurochirurgie, *7*:173, 1961.

Terzis, J.: Microreconstruction of Nerve Injuries. Philadelphia, W. B. Saunders Company, 1987.

Terzis, J.: Personal communication, 1988.

Terzis, J., and Manktelow, R.: Personal communication, 1982.

Thomander, L., Aldskogius, H., and Grant, G.: Motor fiber organization in the intratemporal portion of the cat and rat facial nerve studied with the horse-radish peroxidase technique. Acta Universitatis Upsaliensis. Abstr. of Uppsala Dissert. Fac. Med., No. 404, iii, 1–24, 1981.

Thompson, N.: Autogenous free grafts of skeletal muscle. A preliminary experimental and clinical study. Plast. Reconstr. Surg., *48*:11, 1971.

Thompson, N.: A review of autogenous skeletal muscle grafts and their clinical applications. Clin. Plast. Surg., *1*:349, 1974.

Tolhurst, D. E., and Bos, K. E.: Free revascularized muscle grafts and facial palsy. Plast. Reconstr. Surg., *69*:760, 1982.

Tucker, H. M.: Restoration of selective facial nerve function by the nerve-muscle pedicle technique. Clin. Plast. Surg., *6*:293, 1979.

Weiss, P.: The technology of nerve regeneration: a review. Sutureless tubulation and related methods of nerve repair. J. Neurosurg., *1*:400, 1944.

Wood-Smith, D.: Encircling Silastic band for paralysis of the orbicularis oculi muscle. Presented at the Society of Ophthalmic Plastic Surgeons, Dallas, TX, September 16, 1973.

Wrede, L.: Die Operationen am Nervus facialis, chirurgisches Operationenslehre. Band I. Leipzig, J. A. von Verlag, 1933.

Young, L., Wray, R. C., and Weeks, P. M.: A randomized prospective comparison of fascicular and epineural digital nerve repairs. Plast. Reconstr. Surg., *68*:89, 1981.

43

Thomas D. Rees
Sherrell J. Aston
Charles H. M. Thorne

Blepharoplasty and Facialplasty
Including Forehead-Brow Lift

BLEPHAROPLASTY

Blepharoplasty has become one of the most common esthetic procedures performed today. It is a highly gratifying operation for both surgeon and patient alike. The results can be significant and often predictable. Blepharoplasty for the purpose of improving one's appearance can be indicated at almost any age, but is most commonly performed in middle age. Blepharoplasty in the younger age group is usually indicated in patients with a familial genetic predisposition to eyelid deformities, especially bulging of excessive periorbital fat. This deformity is commonly known as "herniated orbital fat," although there is considerable question as to whether the fat actually herniates through the orbital septum, or is simply displacing a somewhat attenuated septum forward.

Another reason to perform blepharoplasty in patients of a relatively early age is to correct a condition known as *blepharochalasis*. Blepharochalasis is characterized by a true excess of skin, orbicularis muscle, and occasionally fat. In severe deformities the condition can interfere with upward fields of vision. For insurance compensation it must be demonstrated that there is interference with the visual fields, or that at least 3 mm of iris is covered (Fig. 43–1). In fact, blepharoplasty of the upper eyelids was first performed to correct this condition. The term "blepharochalasis" was coined by Fuchs (1896) from two Greek words used to designate relaxation of the eyelids; however, the term is technically inappropriate since excess skin may be present without actual interference with vision, especially in younger patients. The upper eyelid problem is com-

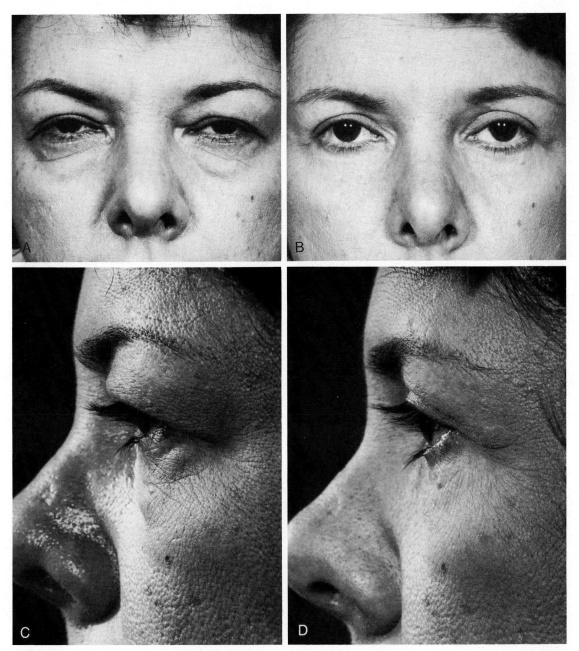

Figure 43–1. Blepharochalasis. *A, C,* Interference with superior fields of vision from true blepharochalasis. Visual loss was confirmed by visual field examination and documented with photographs showing that the upper lids obscured more than 3 mm of the iris. *B, D,* The postoperative result.

pounded by aging, because the brows tend to descend and progressive relaxation of all the tissues of both the upper and lower lids occurs, leading to the formation of a larger and larger fold on the upper eyelids. Progressive "senile" sagging or frank ectropion of the lower eyelids can result from natural aging changes in the lower lids.

With the aging process there is progressive loss of elasticity not only of the skin, but also of the tarsus, the muscle, and the orbital septum. There is also a build-up of periorbital fat over the years so that it becomes redundant and tends to bulge through an attenuated orbital septum. These progressive anatomic changes, associated with brow ptosis, result in the familiar changes seen in the eyes of the older patient. If atrophy of the levator aponeurosis also occurs, this structure becomes attenuated, and ptosis of the upper lids can result. Many of the changes are partially or completely correctable by esthetic blepharoplasty. Various technical variations in the procedure may be required to meet the challenge and to correct the specific morphologic problems. In addition to genetic make-up and the aging process, there are other factors that influence the structure of the eyelids and contribute to the deformity of "baggy eyelids." Perhaps chief among these are recurrent bouts of edema of the lids, which may result from normal fluid accumulation associated with the premenstrual period; idiopathic edema (not uncommon in women); allergies; heart disease; renal disease; hormonal imbalances; overindulgence in alcohol; thyroid dysfunctions (both hyperthyroid and hypothyroid states); and more obscure factors. Recurrent idiopathic edema of the lids and the malar eminences constitutes a difficult problem to overcome. Blepharoplasty may worsen the deformity in certain instances and, especially in the presence of malar edema, patients should be made aware that the proposed surgery *will not* correct the problem. Some of the early descriptions by Dupuytren (1839) of the "baggy eyelid syndrome" and by Sichel (1844) of the condition in young patients very likely represented the result of recurrent edema in young women, as well as the belief that congenital weakness of the orbital septum was the principal cause. Panneton (1936) described the baggy eyelid deformity in members of the same family for several generations.

The eyes are first to register the telltale signs of aging, and therefore are frequently the reference point that brings a patient to a plastic surgeon for consultation. Blepharoplasty is often indicated before a full face lift and is often performed several years prior to a face lift. In this regard, it should be mentioned that blepharoplasty does not eliminate the small wrinkles of the eyelid skin, especially those lateral to the lateral canthus in the temporal skin, the "crow's feet." This fact also should be made clear to the patient.

Hyperpigmentation of the lower lids is often seen in patients with darker skin, usually descendants of inhabitants of the Mediterranean area, or is the result of extensive lentigines. The pigmented lesions generally are not improved by blepharoplasty, but they may appear somewhat lighter if the bulges are removed, thereby eliminating the shadows. Deep chemical peel (chemabrasion) is often helpful in such patients.

Blepharoplasty of two or all four eyelids can be performed for two basic reasons: (1) to correct a functional problem such as diminution of visual field, ptosis, or involutional changes of the lower lids (senile ectropion); or (2) to improve the patient's appearance. The design of the operation must vary according to the individual problem presented by each patient. In the patient in the third or fourth decade of life, simple removal of the excessive fat may be all that is required. A small stab wound (made transconjunctivally or transcutaneously) may be sufficient, whereas in the older patient a satisfactory correction often requires excision of excess skin, orbicularis muscle, and fat, as well as possible tightening of the levator expansion, raising of the brows, and a horizontal shortening of the lower lid by tarsal resection, lateral canthoplasty, or both. The plastic surgeon should be versed in all the technical variations and should know when and how to apply them.

ANATOMY AND MORPHOLOGY

A detailed description of the anatomy of the orbital region including the eyelids is presented in Chapter 34. There are, however, certain technical highlights, unique to the eyelids, that can spell the difference between success or a result that falls short of expectations. In some instances there results a problem that could have been avoided by preoperative recognition of the specific role of the anatomic features present.

Much depends on the quality of the eyelid skin. The skin of the eyelids is very thin in some individuals, and in everyone there is a difference in thickness at the orbital margin where the skin of the eyelids joins the skin of the cheek at the border of the maxilla (Fig. 43–2). It is along this interface that chronic recurrent edema can result in a band of subcutaneous scar tissue that blepharoplasty not only fails to remove, but can exacerbate. Many changes in the eyelid skin occur with aging. Dehydration of the skin with loss of the elastic fibers and collagen, dermal thinning, and acanthosis are seen with advancing age. These changes account for many of the visible changes, such as wrinkling, that are so distressing to many patients. Surgery is only partially helpful for such wrinkling, and chemabrasion may be required as a secondary procedure (Fig. 43–3). Telangiectasis, keratoses, syringomas, and other benign as well as malignant skin lesions, especially basal cell carcinoma, are common in the eyelid skin. Such lesions should be identified before surgery since in many instances they can be treated concomitantly with blepharoplasty.

Some lesions cannot be adequately treated but should be noted and discussed with the patient. An example is multiple syringomas, which are particularly distressing to the patient and surgeon alike. Since they are cosmetically disfiguring, the treatment is difficult, and the results usually are disappointing.

The periorbital fat is usually the culprit in the young patient with bulging eyelids. Castañares (1951, 1977) classified the collection of periorbital fat into specific compartments of both upper and lower eyelids. The compartments are separated by thin fibrous septa and by the inferior oblique muscle. This concept of compartmentalization of the periorbital fat is generally accepted as useful clinically, but it was challenged by Hugo and Stone (1974). They injected 54 orbits in 27 cadavers with Evans blue dye. Dissection showed generalized diffusion of the dye throughout the orbit, leading these authors to believe that there is no true compartmentalization. The concept of compartmentalization is of practical use to the operating surgeon. The fat accumulations differ in character in both the upper and lower lids (Fig. 43–4). The middle compartment of the upper and lower lids is typical "butter-col-

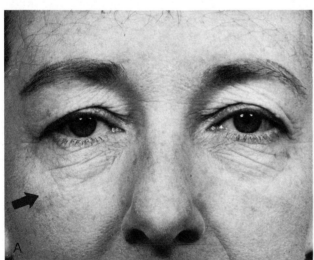
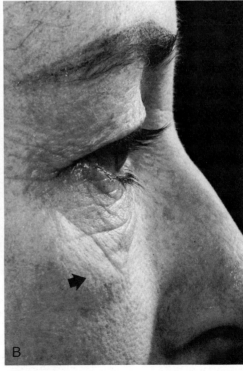

Figure 43–2. *A, B,* Arrow indicates the so-called "malar pouch," not infrequently found in women. Treatment is unsatisfactory. Severe problems require excision (see Fig. 43–11). (From Rees, T. D., and Wood-Smith, D.: Cosmetic Facial Surgery. Philadelphia, W. B. Saunders Company, 1973.)

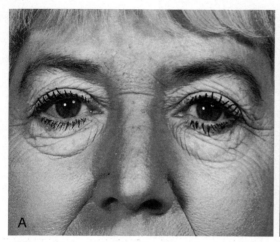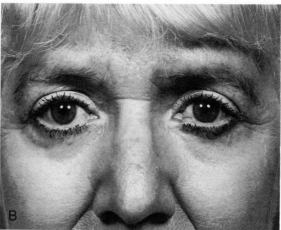

Figure 43–3. *A,* Preoperative view of a patient who underwent blepharoplasty and chemical peeling for marked palpebral bags and rhytidosis of eyelid skin. Such wrinkling cannot be eliminated by surgery alone and requires subsequent peeling. *B,* Final result. (From Rees, T. D., and Wood-Smith, D.: Cosmetic Facial Surgery. Philadelphia, W. B. Saunders Company, 1973.)

ored" yellow fat, while the fat of the remaining compartments is pale, almost white in color, and interlaced with a fine fibrous network of septa. The relationships of the fat to the orbital rims are of prime importance and are discussed in the following section on examination. A prominent orbital rim and over-reduction of the fat can result in "pseudoenophthalmos." The periorbital fat is, for the most part, found beneath the orbital septum in both the upper and lower lids. The exception to this is a sausage-shaped cylinder of yellow fat found in the upper eyelids in some Oriental persons. It is this fat pad, along with the disinsertion of the levator expansion from the skin, that results in an absence of the supratarsal fold in many non-Caucasians.

In recent years, more attention has been focused on the role of the orbicularis muscle in blepharoplasty. It has been recognized by many that this muscle, especially in middle-aged and older individuals, is redundant and therefore requires judicious resection during surgery. Many surgeons (including the author) routinely resect a strip of muscle comparable in size with the skin strip from the upper lids, and remove a similar strip of skin and muscle from the lower lids. Removal of a muscle strip from the upper eyelids has increased the ability to achieve a clean supratarsal crease and has eliminated the necessity for levator fixation into the skin, at least in most Caucasian patients.

The orbicularis muscle can be hypertrophied in a portion of the lid. An unsightly bulge commonly seen along the horizontal width of the lower lid often results from this type of hypertrophy (Fig. 43–5). Excision of such hypertrophic segments may be required (Rees, 1980). Furnas (1978) aptly described ptotic folds of orbicularis muscle of the lower lids as "festoons" of muscle (Fig. 43–6). His description of this deformity began a new era in surgical treatment of muscle deformities that had previously been ignored. Such muscle "festoons" are approached directly during the surgical procedure.

The orbital septum is frequently thinned out and attenuated. Whether this condition is developmental or is the result of continuous pressure from the bulging fat is unknown. Involutional changes occur in the septum with advancing age, along with the changes described in the skin, muscle, and fat. The problem seems to be of little practical significance in blepharoplasty since removal of the offending fat bulges appears to correct any visible weakness attributable to the orbital septum. Recently, tightening or "reefing" of the orbital septum has been used as the chief method of correcting baggy eyelids without the excision of either fat, skin, or muscle in many patients except those in the senile category. The results are intriguing, and further study and experience will dictate the validity of such a technique.

The actual size and shape of the globe are of considerable importance in blepharoplasty and should be carefully evaluated preoperatively. In some patients one or both globes

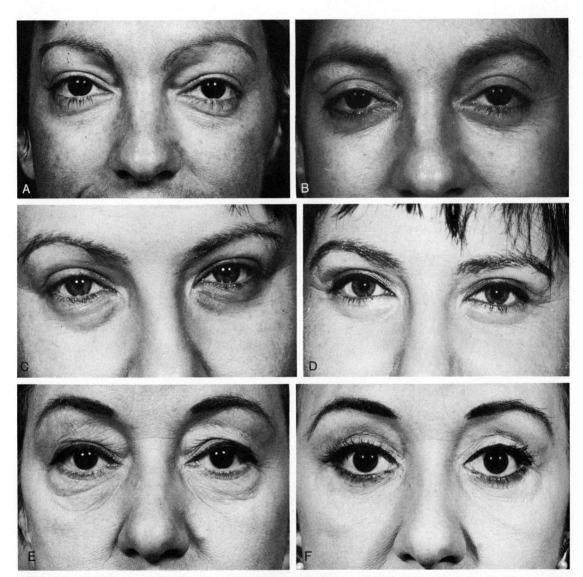

Figure 43–4. A 30 year old female with familial fat bags of the lower eyelids. *A,* Preoperative view. *B,* After correction with the skin-muscle flap technique. *C, D,* Pre- and postoperative views of a 38 year old female with typical perioribtal fat excess of the upper and lower eyelids. Corrected with upper and lower blepharoplasty (skin-muscle flap). *E, F,* Pre- and postoperative views of a 55 year old female with advanced palpebral bags of skin, muscle, and fat excess. Corrected by the skin-muscle flap blepharoplasty shown in Figs. 43–14 to 43–17.

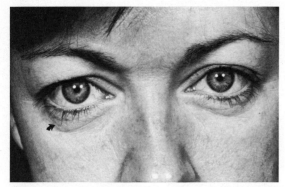

Figure 43–5. An example of a hypertrophic muscle roll extending horizontally along the lower lid. The deformity is accentuated by animation. The surgical correction is illustrated in Figs. 43–20 and 43–21.

may be larger than normal, as the result of either genetic inheritance or myopia, the so-called high myopic eye. Exophthalmos can also project the globes forward so that they appear to be larger. If such departures from the normal anatomy are not heeded, the surgical result can be severely impaired and the likelihood of scleral show or frank ectropion is markedly increased. Such increase in size or change in shape of the globe becomes of clinical significance during surgery, since the lower eyelid often is stretched around the inferior border of the globe. The lid is, in fact,

displaced inferiorly and, like a bowstring, stretched around the eyeball. If such a condition is unrecognized, postoperative scleral show or even ectropion can result from simple conservative blepharoplasty with minimal skin, fat, and muscle excision as a natural result of the wound contracture. The bowstringing is increased, and the show of white sclera likewise increased. In selected patients, horizontal tightening of the lid by wedge resection or tarsal suspension can be useful in preventing untoward results.

CLASSIFICATION

Castañares (1951, 1977) proposed a classification of eyelid deformities that is useful to the surgeon.

Blepharochalasis is a condition characterized by loss of tone and relaxation of the lid skin, particularly the skin of the upper lids (see Fig. 43–1). A redundant fold of skin and often muscle hanging like a curtain from the upper eyelid is the result. It is this type of deformity that can interfere with upward field of vision.

Dermochalasis is often confused with blepharochalasis. It is also the condition of an excess fold of skin of the upper eyelid. The

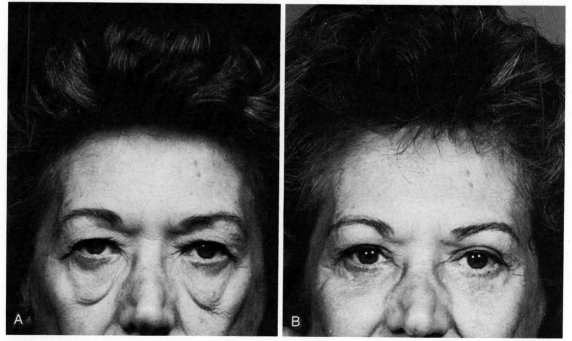

Figure 43–6. *A,* Example of a patient with "festoons" of orbicularis muscle (Furnas, 1978). *B,* Postoperative view (see Figs. 43–18 and 43–19.)

skin is thin and hangs over the ciliary margin. The fold of skin does not contain fat, and while the orbicularis may or may not be included, it is not a feature of the deformity. Dermochalasis usually occurs from middle age onward and is probably a normal consequence of the aging process. The condition was most likely first described by Sichel in 1844.

Hypertrophy of the orbicularis oculis muscle is often manifest as a ridge of bulging muscle running horizontally along the lower lid just below the ciliary margin. The "festoons" of muscle (Furnas, 1978) also represent hypertrophy of muscle and should probably be included in this category.

Herniated orbital fat is most likely a misnomer since it is doubtful whether the excess periorbital fat actually herniates through the orbital septum, but it is more accurately characterized as a pseudoherniation against an attenuated orbital septum. It is this condition that occurs first in the young patient. In the older patient, pseudoherniation of the fat is only one component of the overall problem.

Ptosis of the eyebrows is a contributing factor in many patients in addition to hooding of the upper lids. Planning operative correction may require consideration of the eyebrow correction as well as a blepharoplasty. A forehead and brow lift via a coronal incision may be necessary.

The senile lid may be characterized by a combination of all the above features plus other changes that are characteristic of degenerative changes of the lid structures, such as idiopathic attenuation of the levator aponeurosis resulting in *ptosis,* and loss of substance of the tarsus of the lower lids in combination with elastic tissue atrophy, which results in lower lid sag or ectropion.

PREOPERATIVE EVALUATION

The purpose of the preoperative consultation is to evaluate the patient from an ophthalmologic as well as an overall systemic point of view in order to prevent untoward results and complications and to ensure a satisfactory result. A complete history and physical examination are necessary to achieve this goal. Some systemic conditions can directly affect the eyes as well as the eyelids, and these can often be elicited in the history and physical examination. In the older age group, it is often advisable to obtain a complete work-up before surgery from the patient's family doctor or internist. A history of eye disease may or may not require a consultation with an ophthalmologist, depending on the severity of the problem. Needless to say, if any doubt exists, a consultation is in order.

Prevention of complications is an important aspect of esthetic blepharoplasty. Prevention begins long before the actual surgical procedure and starts with the first consultation.

An adequate examination of the eye, orbit, and adnexa is mandatory. A superficial examination of the eyelids does not suffice. The examination should include a visual acuity evaluation. A small portable Snellen chart is convenient and can be used by a trained nurse or assistant. Each eye should be tested separately. Examination of the mobility of the extraocular muscles is important to determine whether there is paresis or paralysis of one or more of these structures, because these could lead to serious or potentially serious postoperative complications. Paralysis of the superior rectus muscle, with an absent Bell's phenomenon, coupled with the usual temporary tethering of the upper eyelid (lagophthalmos) that occurs immediately after surgery, could lead to desiccation of the cornea with eventual ulceration. Simple observation of the eyes in all fields of gaze can often elicit lagophthalmos, ptosis or pseudoptosis, and scleral show, both above and below the pupil. Scleral show above the pupil is most often caused by spasm of Müller's muscle, a suspicious sign of hyperthyroidism (Fig. 43–7). Acquired ptosis, especially in middle age and beyond, should be investigated. The most common cause is idiopathic attenuation of the levator aponeurosis. Unexplained ptosis is an indication for additional diagnostic studies to rule out myasthenia gravis and other related neuromuscular diseases.

It is important to note the presence or absence and frequency of the blinking phenomenon. The nonblinking patient is more subject to corneal problems after surgery, especially as there is also a diminuation in tear production. The nonblinking, staring patient should also be considered as having significant emotional or psychiatric problems.

The symmetry and actual size of the eyes are important to note. Varying degrees of asymmetry are common. Significant asym-

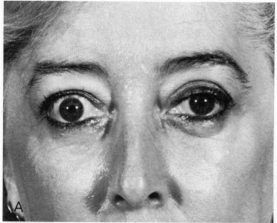

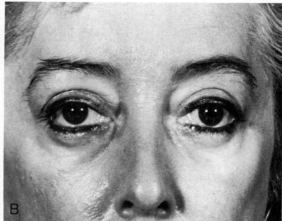

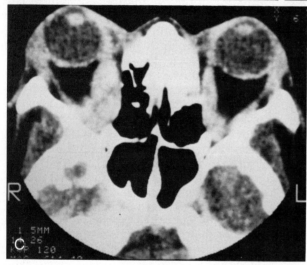

Figure 43–7. *A,* A patient with bilateral exophthalmos (more severe on the right) and spasm of Müller's muscle, with lid retraction and scleral show above the iris. *B,* Postoperative result after resection of Müller's muscle, fascial grafts to the levator and lid release following medical control of the hyperthyroidism. *C,* Typical CT scan appearance of Graves' ophthalmopathy showing marked enlargement of the extraocular muscles (the medial and lateral recti) due to edema. The CT scan findings are pathognomonic. (From Lisman, R., Rees, T. D., Baker, D., and Smith, B.: Experience with tarsal suspension as a factor in lower lid blepharoplasty. Plast. Reconstr. Surg., *79:*897, 1987.)

metry may be masked by folds of skin, muscle, and large fat pockets. Patients who have significant asymmetry are often surprisingly unaware of the condition. It is not uncommon for such patients to first notice the natural asymmetry of their face and especially of their eyes *after* surgery. Asymmetry should be pointed out and discussed before surgery to avoid misunderstanding. It is important to notice differences in the size and shape of the eyeballs. The unilaterally enlarged eyeball of the patient with high myopia (Fig. 43–8) can lead to scleral show and even ectropion after simple blepharoplasty. Lateral tarsal suspension may be indicated in such patients as an integral part of the blepharoplasty procedure (see Fig. 43–25). Fat and skin removal in the protruding eyeball of high myopia must be exceedingly conservative. Slight unilateral or bilateral bulging of the globes is not always an indication of a pathologic condition: it may

be and, in fact, usually is familial. However, familial or not, even slight exophthalmos can become a problem of scleral show or ectropion unless care is taken to minimize the excisional surgery. Factors that contribute to scleral show along with the bulging eye include a hypoplastic maxilla, the absence of a strongly defined orbital rim, and shallow orbits. All these features except shallow orbits can be determined by simple physical examination. Shallow orbits as well as high unilateral myopia are identified by CT scan (Fig. 43–9).

Scleral show, either unilateral or bilateral, in the presence of a bulging eye and levator spasm is strong presumptive evidence of Graves' ophthalmopathy (see Fig. 43–7). Failure to recognize this problem can result in exacerbation of the physical findings postoperatively. Scleral show may be noted in minimal cases for the first time after blepharo-

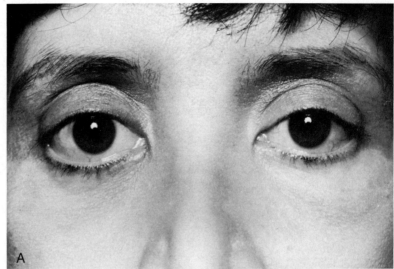

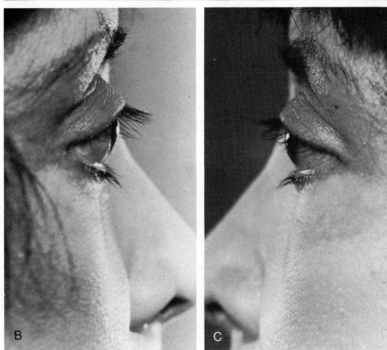

Figure 43–8. *A*, Frontal view of a patient with a unilateral high myopic eye. Note how much larger the right eye is than the left. Both globes seem larger than the normal and both have scleral show. Blepharoplasty in such a patient is hazardous, and lateral tarsal suspension is indicated (see Fig. 43–25). *B, C*, Note the marked bulging of the right eye. The left eye is mildly proptotic. (From Lisman, R., Rees, T. D., Baker, D., and Smith, B.: Experience with tarsal suspension as a factor in lower lid blepharopasty. Plast. Reconstr. Surg., *79*:897, 1987.)

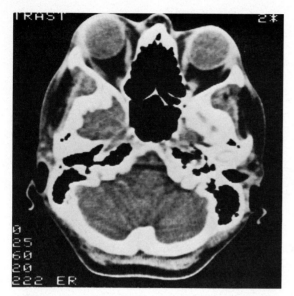

Figure 43–9. Typical CT axial scan of a patient with unilateral high myopia. Note the forward projection of the enlarged right globe. (From Lisman, R., Rees, T. D., Baker, D., and Smith, B.: Experience with tarsa suspension as a factor in lower lid blepharoplasty. Plast. Reconstr. Surg., 79:897, 1987.)

plasty, or existing scleral show may be considerably aggravated. Fifteen to 20 per cent of patients with Graves' disease are euthyroid, and exophthalmos or scleral show may precede chemical changes by many months. Thyroid disease can also result in other physical signs involving the orbital structures. Localized signs include edema of the lids and extraocular muscles. Early in the course of Graves' ophthalmopathy, the extraocular muscles may become considerably enlarged because of accumulation of edema in the orbital structures, especially the extraocular muscles. Enlargement of these muscles on sagittal CT scan (see Fig. 43–7C) is almost pathognomonic of the hyperthyroid state (Lisman and associates, 1987). Hypothyroidism also can result in localized or generalized edema of the orbit that is manifest primarily as baggy eyelids. Blepharoplasty in the myxedematous lid can be disastrous, or at the very least ineffective. Marked edema, scleral show, levator spasm, or protrusion of one or both globes should arouse suspicion of thyroid disease. When any of these signs or symptoms are present, the thyroid status of the patient should be scrutinized.

The patient who presents for blepharoplasty later in life, without previous surgical intervention, should be examined for involutional changes that predispose the lower lids in such patients to sagging or frank ectropion. A general loss of elasticity and tone of the lid tissues is a natural consequence of the aging process. The structures of concern to the surgeon planning a blepharoplasty are the levator aponeurosis, the tarsus, the orbicularis oculis muscle, and the skin. The tarsus shrinks with age and fails to provide the needed "batten" support to the lower eyelid. All the structures sag, resulting in a pre-ectropion environment that can readily produce ectropion after surgery. In the senile or presenile lid the tone of the lid can be grossly assessed by the "snap-back" test (Fig. 43–10) (Rees and Tabbal, 1981). The lower lid is held between the examiner's index finger and thumb, drawn away from the globe, and allowed to snap back. Lids that do not readily snap back against the globe, and especially those that slowly sink back into position, are certainly suspect as being predisposed to postoperative ectropion. In such hypotonic lids, horizontal lid shortening by tarsal suspension should be strongly considered as part of the blepharoplasty procedure (see Fig. 43–25). This maneuver strengthens the lower lid sling and helps to avoid bowstringing the weakened lower lid around the eyeball.

The medial portion of the lower lid should also be evaluated for deformities or weakness.

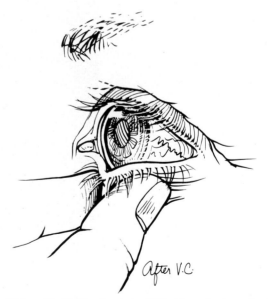

after V.C.

Figure 43–10. The "snap-back" test is a simple method of detecting involutional changes of the lower lid. Hypotonia is indicated by a sluggish return of the lid to the globe.

The punctum is the entrance to the lacrimal outflow apparatus. If the punctum faces vertically, just out of the lacrimal lake, and the medial lid is lax, significant punctal eversion or ectropion of the medial portion of the lower lid can occur as a result of the surgical procedure. The punctum must be tight and properly positioned to drain the lacrimal lake. The tone of the medial canthal tendon should also be noted.

The presence or absence of a tear film should be noted. A history of dry eyes with recurrent irritation or corneal ulceration is an important signal that the patient has a potential or existing dry eye syndrome. The expected scar tethering after blepharoplasty results in a certain amount of lagophthalmos, which can have serious consequences in such patients, often converting a potential problem into a real one. The problem of the dry eye syndrome and its relationship to blepharoplasty was reviewed by Rees (1975) and Rees and Jelks (1981). Deficient tear production can be caused by cigarette smoking, menopause, thyroid dysfunction, aging, drug intake (antihistamines), and other factors. A tearing deficiency may be difficult to diagnose accurately. Serial examinations may be required at different times, since the flow of tears may vary considerably from day to day and even hour to hour. Schirmer's test is the simplest clinical test available, although the clinical application of the results in terms of blepharoplasty may be open to question (Rees and LaTrenta, 1988). It is wise to perform Schirmer's test on all patients over 40 years of age, which is a purely arbitrary age limit. The results are recorded as the number of millimeters of tear wetting that occurs within 5 minutes on a strip of Whatman's No. 41 filter paper, 5 mm wide and 35 mm long. The test is best performed in a semidarkened room after anesthetizing the conjunctival sac with a topical anesthetic. Normal wetting is between 15 and 30 mm. Less than 10 mm of wetting is considered a reduction of both basic and reflex secretion. The difficulty with such a test lies in the large number of borderline results that are seen, which make it difficult to decide whether or not a blepharoplasty could convert a symptomless patient into one with irritative symptoms. Obviously, a patient who tolerates hard contact lenses can easily endure the added stresses of blepharoplasty incisions and subsequent scarring. Patients with dry eyes, however, can tolerate soft lenses, so that it is still advisable to test patients with soft lenses. Should the surgeon elect to proceed with cosmetic blepharoplasty after marginal (or low) Schirmer's test results, caution and conservatism should be exercised both in the degree of surgery and particularly in regard to the amount of tissue excised. The upper eyelids must be especially protected since coverage of the cornea, and therefore lubrication, is primarily dependent on upper lid mobility. A marginal or low Schirmer's test result is an indication for a preoperative ophthalmologic consultation, including a slit lamp examination.

Patches of edema along the malar eminences lying below the eyelid skin proper should be noted, since these will not be eliminated by surgery, and can, in fact, be exacerbated (see Fig. 43–2). The surgeon should identify the "cheek pouches" to the patient in a mirror or photograph so that their separateness from the eyelid bags is understood. The patient thus has a clear understanding before surgery that the cheek defects will not be eliminated. The natural edema after blepharoplasty can increase the swelling along the malar rims for a short period. The cause of the malar pouches is not known, but they seem to result from repeated bouts of localized edema, eventually causing a small patch of subcutaneous scar tissue. The cycle of edema-scar-edema is repeated each time the scar tissue volume is increased, so that eventually the defect is permanent. The localized areas of edema are most often seen in women and are often related to premenstrual edema. In other patients with systemic disease in which edema is a feature, such as chronic renal disease, allergy, and cirrhosis, malar bags may also be present. There is no satisfactory treatment for the condition except in severe cases in which direct excision may be required (Fig. 43–11).

Hypertrophy of eyelid tissue can result from various localized lesions such as lymphangioma, hemangioma, neurofibromatosis, lipomatosis, reactions from foreign body injections such as paraffin or silicone, and conditions that cause a localized low-grade inflammatory response.

The measurement of intraocular tension and the slit lamp examination appear to be unnecessary as a routine part of the work-up in each blepharoplasty candidate. If the history or physical examination arouses suspicion that there is a pathologic condition of

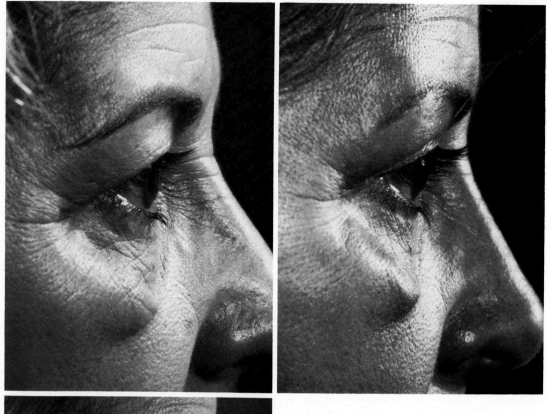

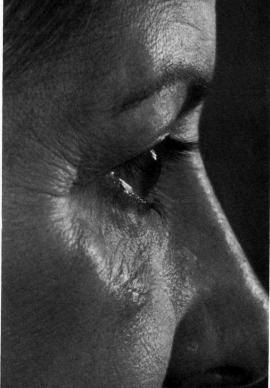

Figure 43–11. Malar "pouches" often are not related to blepharoplasty and certainly are not corrected by the operation. Such malar swellings are often the result of a localized collection of edema, which may be exacerbated by the operation. This patient required a secondary direct surgical excision of the malar pouch to achieve a reasonable correction. A permanent external scar must be accepted, but is a reasonable trade-off for the deformity. *A,* Preoperative view. *B,* After blepharoplasty. The malar swelling has been worsened by the procedure. *C,* The final result after direct excision of an ellipse of skin and subcutaneous tissue. (From Rees, T. D.: Aesthetic Plastic Surgery. Philadelphia, W. B. Saunders Company, 1980, p. 569.)

the eyes or adnexa, consultation with an ophthalmologist, preferably one who is surgically oriented, should be sought. Any question of muscular imbalance, protruding eye (high myopic), or reduced tear production is an indication for more intensive ophthalmologic work-up, often including tomography and CT scans.

Excessive wrinkling of the eyelids, especially on animation of the face, imposes a limitation on the postoperative result. Some patients complain of fine wrinkling or animated wrinkling as their chief concern. Blepharoplasty only partially improves wrinkling and patients should be advised of this limitation. Fine rhytides of the skin are often the result of prolonged solar exposure. Such wrinkling may require chemabrasion for further improvement after blepharoplasty (see Fig. 43–3) or, in some instances, as the primary procedure. Generalized wrinkling of the lids on smiling or grimacing must be differentiated from the localized "muscle roll" (Rees, 1980), which can be eliminated by direct excision. The experimental use of botulism toxin to reduce the neuromuscular activity has been extended to certain patients with severe wrinkling of the skin and muscle of the eyelid region, especially those cases exacerbated by animation. To date, the results are moderately encouraging in severe cases, but they seem to be temporary in nature, lasting only a few months, at which time further injections of the toxin are required. Only long-term follow-up will provide accurate evaluation of this technique.

Prolapse of the lacrimal gland should be noted so that a lateral bulge of the upper lid is not confused with protruding fat. The prolapsed gland presents as a bulging mass in the lateral upper lid region, and can readily be identified by everting the upper lid. With the lid retracted, the gland can be seen in the temporal corner of the orbit (Fig. 43–12B). Prolapse of the gland often occurs in "crowded" orbits, with a smaller volume and

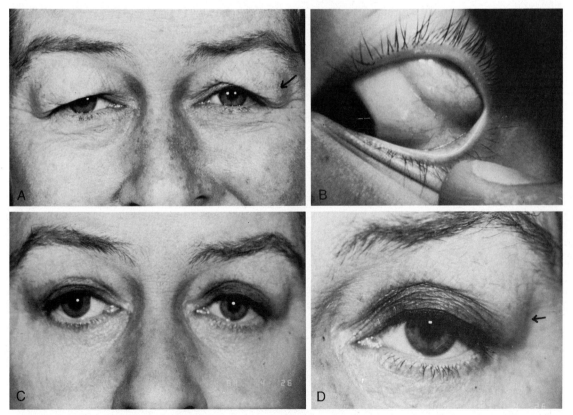

Figure 43–12. *A*, A patient with marked hooding of the upper lids. The hoods are camouflaging protruding masses in the upper lids *(arrow)*, which are ptotic and enlarged lacrimal glands. *B*, Displaced lacrimal glands as well as herniated orbital fat can present subconjunctivally in the temporal aspect of the orbit with the lid retracted. *C, D*, Postoperative views after upper blepharoplasty and partial resection of the lacrimal glands. Note that the gland remnant still bulges slightly in the lateral orbit *(arrow)*. Partial resection of the lacrimal gland requires careful preoperative evaluation of the tearing mechanism.

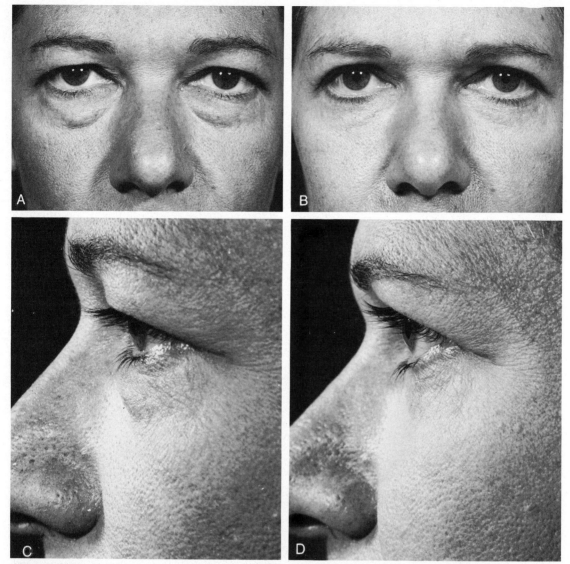

Figure 43–13. *A, C,* Preoperative views of a 40 year old female with palpebral bags and a marked brow ptosis. Brow ptosis in a relatively young woman is often familial; it is the rule in men. *B, D,* Blepharoplasty corrects the bags, but not the brow ptosis. Such ptosis can only be improved by a brow-forehead lift via a transcoronal approach.

a shallow superior bony rim. It is of little significance except as a cosmetic problem. Provided there is no tearing deficiency, a portion of the gland can safely be resected at surgery to provide more room. Attempts to elevate the gland higher in the orbit with fascial strips and fixation sutures are generally disappointing. Preoperative recognition of the problem is important as a point of information for the patient.

Ptosis of the brow requires study and thought. Brow ptosis occurs with advancing age, at a younger age in some than in others. It can be the result of hereditary factors often related to a low superior orbital rim. In marked ptosis, simple blepharoplasty may not suffice, since it is virtually impossible in such patients to eliminate the folds of skin and/or muscle of the upper lids without also elevating the brows or deepening the sulcus (Fig. 43–13). A bicoronal forehead lift is indicated in such patients to achieve the optimal result. Direct elevation of the brows, removing a segmental ellipse of skin from the forehead just above the eyebrow hairline, has been disappointing; however, it can be considered in older patients with significant horizontal wrinkling of the forehead skin (so that the resulting scar will be camouflaged) or in men who have male pattern baldness in which a coronal incision would be contraindicated. The coronal forehead lift is described later in the chapter. It can be done in conjunction with four-lid blepharoplasty, but the upper eyelid excision must be conservative in the combined procedures. It is wise not to premark the eyelid skin in such patients *before* the forehead lift, otherwise a shortage of skin can easily result.

SURGICAL TECHNIQUE

Anesthesia

Blepharoplasty can be performed under general or local anesthesia. Except in patients in whom a ptosis correction is planned along with the esthetic blepharoplasty, it is unnecessary to elicit facial motion during the operation provided the surgeon pays attention to certain technical details to ensure proper lid positioning before and during skin and muscle excision. The technical details are described later in this chapter. Ptosis correction and perhaps tarsal suspension procedures are considered by some surgeons to require eyelid motion, so that local anesthesia is indicated.

Skin Marking

The design of the incisions should take into account the different morphologic factors that constitute the composite deformity. Eyelid markings should vary to account for even slight differences in the architecture of the soft tissues, as well as the configuration of the bony vault. In a four-lid blepharoplasty the upper eyelid is marked first. The inferior marking of the rough ellipse is located at varying distances from the ciliary border according to the natural supratarsal fold (Fig. 43–14). The fold, formed by an insertion of fibers from the levator expansion into the dermis, is located at different distances from one individual to another, varying from approximately 7 mm to over 12 mm. There is no uniform distance to locate the line. In patients with "deep-set eyes," i.e., high bony arches and enlarged intraorbital space, the supratarsal fold is apt to be much higher than in those with a smaller or more shallow

orbit. Examination of the patient, except in some Oriental individuals in whom the fold may be completely absent, will identify the line. The line is drawn from the medial aspect of the eyelid along the supratarsal line to the lateral canthus, where it is angled somewhat in a cephalad direction. The amount of resection is judged with the aid of the Green forceps (Fig. 43–14C), the lateral extension angled cephalically to minimize the possibility of placing the final scar in too low a position and too close to the incision of the lower lid. When the incisions are placed too close to each other, a small web contracture can result. The excisional design of the upper lid includes both skin and muscle in almost all patients now treated by the author, a change in technique of recent years.

The incisional marking along the lower lid is begun at the medial extent of the ciliary margin and carried laterally in the first small natural crease, usually approximately 2 to 3 mm below the lash margin (Fig. 43–15). Marking the incision any closer to the lid margin is unnecessary and can be troublesome, especially if a secondary procedure is performed. In the older patient with increased lid laxity or senile ectropion, the lower lid incision should be made even farther below the ciliary margin to obviate scar contracture, which can accentuate the tendency for the lid to evert. In such instances it is made 3 mm or even more below the ciliary margin. At the lateral canthus the lower marking follows a natural skin crease, which is readily identified as a laugh line. This line often runs almost directly horizontally or angles slightly in a caudal direction. It is unnecessary to angle the lateral extent of the incision sharply in a caudal direction, as indicated in many reports.

It is important not to transgress the thin skin of the medial upper lid and extend the incision line onto the thicker skin of the nose, otherwise a hypertrophic contracted scar is likely to result. A pseudoepicanthus is then obvious and is exceedingly difficult to eradicate even by interdigitating flaps.

Upper Eyelids

The area to be incised is injected with local solution containing a 1:100,000 solution of epinephrine whether or not local or general anesthesia is used. The incisions are made

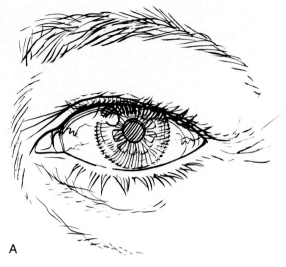

A

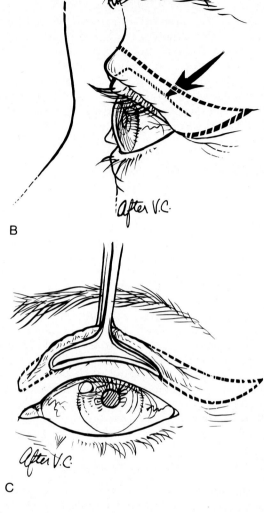

B

Figure 43–14. *A*, Typical example of aging eyelids. The natural supratarsal groove is covered by the excess fold of skin (and muscle). *B*, The supratarsal fold *(arrow)* lies beneath the skin hood approximately 7 to 14 mm from the ciliary margin. The supratarsal crease should be identified preoperatively in each patient. Note that the lateral extension of the excision is directed in a slightly cephalic direction in a natural expression line. *C*, The Green forceps aid in determining the amount of resection.

C

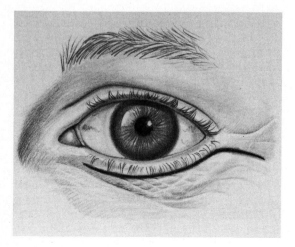

Figure 43–15. The incision in the lower lid is located in the first natural line below the ciliary margin, usually approximated 2 to 3 mm below. It extends laterally in a line of expression and is only slightly angled downward.

with a No. 15 blade or a permanent diamond knife, and the ellipse of skin and muscle is excised (Fig. 43–16*A*). For the learning surgeon it is recommended that the skin be excised first, followed by the muscle. Care is taken during the muscle excision not to injure the levator expansion that lies below. Hemostasis is obtained by electrocoagulation with a pinpoint cautery. The orbital septum is opened and the medial and horizontal (longitudinal) fat pads are identified, dissected free from the orbital septum, clamped, and excised (Fig. 43–16*B*). The fat pedicles are coagulated. Technical variations in this basic procedure, such as ptosis repair, tarsal fixation, partial resection of the lacrimal gland, or sculpting of the supraorbital bony rim, can be performed through the above exposure. Ptosis repair is described in Chapter 34. The reconstruction of a supratarsal fold in Oriental patients is described in Chapter 44. Lassus (1979) emphasized recontouring the supraorbital rim with sharp osteotomes or high speed drills. This technique, in carefully selected patients with a low positioning of the bony rims, results in a higher arch, and consequently a higher position of the brows. Contouring of the orbital rims can also be accomplished by a coronal approach; however, direct surgical alteration of the bone architecture requires experience and should not be performed casually. The reader is referred to the publications of Flowers (1976). Tarsal fixation as a routine step in upper lid blepharoplasty is unnecessary in most Caucasian patients. The routine excision of a strip of muscle (Fig. 43–16*C*) has resulted in a more clearly defined supratarsal fold and has obviated the need for tarsal fixation to achieve a sharp crease, except in reconstruction of the Oriental eyelid.

The upper lid is sutured with a subdermal running suture of 5–0 nylon and interrupted 6–0 nylon (Fig. 43–16*D, E*). The orbital septum is not sutured.

Lower Eyelids

Until recently, correction of the lower lid implied only excision of redundant periorbital fat and skin. Only occasionally was orbicularis muscle intentionally removed. It has been recognized that in most instances there is also a redundancy of muscle, often in proportion to the skin excess (Rees and Tabbal, 1981). This concept has provided renewed impetus to the skin-muscle flap technique of lower lid blepharoplasty as championed by McIndoe and Beare (Beare, 1967), Rees and Dupuis (1969), and Rees and Wood-Smith (1973).

The incisions are marked as described above. If conditions dictate, provision is made in the initial planning for horizontal shortening of the lower lid by V-excision (McKinney, 1977; Rees, 1983) or lateral tarsal suspension (Smith, 1969; Lisman and associates, 1987). The technical variations are discussed in more detail later in this chapter.

The tissues are infiltrated with the local solution. A skin-muscle flap is elevated by first making a small incision in the lateral aspect of the incisional line with a No. 15 blade, then completing the incision medially with a small, sharp, straight scissors. Scissors are preferred since more exact control is afforded the surgeon. The incision is carried through both skin and muscle, care being taken to preserve a strip of pretarsal muscle on the anterior surface of the tarsal plate. These fibers are thought to provide important support and to protect normal lid function. The flap is then dissected. Gentle upward traction is provided with skin hooks. Small scissors facilitate the dissection, which is relatively bloodless compared with the subcutaneous dissection of a skin flap. A ready plane lies between the orbicularis muscle and the underlying orbital septum. The dissection is extended caudally for varying distances according to the particular anatomic configuration of the patient. Usually the dissection extends at least to the infraorbital rim, and in patients with marked palpebral bags or muscle "festoons" the dissection is carried further on the anterior surface of the zygoma just above the periosteum. In severe deformities, wide detachment of the soft tissues may be required; in minimal deformities, the dissection is much more limited (Fig. 43–17*A*).

Slight pressure on the eyeball readily identifies the major fat compartments of the lower lids. Often there is obvious attenuation of the orbital septum, and the fat is seen to bulge through. In most patients the medial and middle compartments predominate in the deformity, and the lateral compartment is the least noticeable; however, when the major component of the deformity is excess periorbital fat, all three compartments can contribute equally to the deformity. At this point in

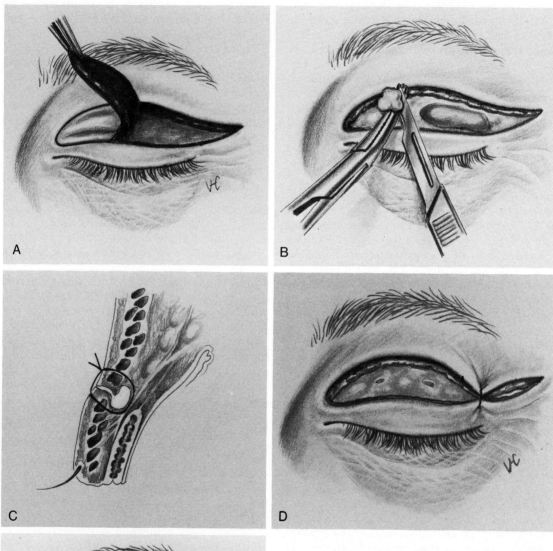

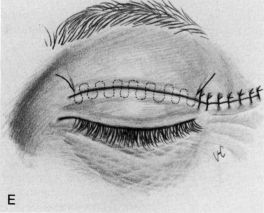

Figure 43–16. *A,* The excess eyelid is resected, including the orbicularis muscle, which is redundant in almost all cases. *B,* The medial and longitudinal periorbital fat excess is located and excised after the orbital septum is opened. *C,* Removal of a strip of muscle ensures the formation of a defined supratarsal crease. The two edges of the wound adhere to the underlying structures, creating a crease. Routine levator fixation in Caucasians is unnecessary. *D,* The first suture is a reference point and is placed approximately at the lateral canthus. *E,* The lid is sutured with intradermal and simple interrupted sutures.

the procedure, scrupulous attention to hemostasis is important to minimize ecchymosis and reduce hematoma formation. Bleeding points are cauterized with the finest tipped jeweler's forceps and electrocautery. The fat compartments can be infiltrated with local solution to minimize the pain of traction and cauterization; however, deep injections should be performed with caution to avoid penetrating a vessel and initiating a retrobulbar hematoma. For the same reason, deep injections of the orbit are not recommended during blepharoplasty. The danger of penetrating a vessel deep in the retrobulbar space is great and the consequence of such vessel injury can be a retrobulbar hematoma.

The orbital septum is opened. The extent of the incision is a matter of personal preference. Some surgeons prefer to open the septum widely for full exposure; however, in most cases the fat can be retrieved through small stab wounds made directly through the septum overlying the pockets. The redundant fat should be teased from the wound, clamped with a hemostat, and excised (Fig. 43–17B). The stump should be thoroughly coagulated to avoid bleeding after retraction of the stump behind the orbital septum. The fat should be excised with caution, especially in patients with prominent infraorbital bony rims. It is difficult for the learning surgeon to "guesstimate" the amount of fat for removal; only experience and careful evaluation of the anatomy in each patient will dictate the amount. Patients with a prominent inferior orbital rim and relative enophthalmos or "deep-set" eyes must be approached with caution since even minimal overexcision can result in enophthalmos. If the fat excision seems excessive at this point in the procedure, the surgeon should not hesitate to return small amounts of fat as free grafts. The exact fate of such grafts is unknown, but as a practical matter they seem to result in a space-filling effect either by survival as fat or by resolution as fibrous tissue.

During removal of fat, the location of the inferior oblique muscle should be appreciated by the surgeon. The muscle lies astraddle the medial and middle fat compartment, and care should be taken not to injure it by either incision or cautery during the fat removal. It is often helpful, especially for teaching purposes, to identify the muscle visually. Injury to the inferior oblique muscle can result in temporary or permanent diplopia. The lateral fat compartments must be carefully identified since its role in the deformity varies considerably from one individual to another. Its volume is often incompletely reduced, and therefore a secondary procedure may be required. After all redundant fat has been removed, it is wise to take a second look at all fat remnants to check for bleeding points and to remove any excess. The fat pedicles are carefully tucked behind the orbital septum.

The excision of excess skin and muscle is begun by carefully draping the skin-muscle flap over the lid wound in a cephalic direction (Fig. 43–17C, D). The flap is simply teased over the superior wound edge without applying traction to the flap in any way. The lid should be in a neutral position, and this maneuver is facilitated by slight pressure on the globe to elevate the lid in a cephalic direction. It is also important to determine that the lid is in no way "tethered." Complete freedom of the lid should be ensured with forceps. There is no need to exert traction on the flap in a lateral direction, a maneuver often described in the past. The flap is simply draped over the wound margin.

With the flap so located, a vertical cut is made with a small, sharp, straight scissors through the entire thickness of the skin and muscle at the level of the lateral canthus, progressing carefully, 1 mm at a time, until the obvious excess to be excised is determined (Fig. 43–17E). A 6–0 suture is placed precisely at this point. The redundant skin and muscle are excised throughout the length of the lower lid with straight scissors. The line of excision is directed medially at first, and then laterally (Fig. 43–17F, G). During excision, it is helpful to maintain slight pressure on the globe so that the lid is kept in a neutral position.

Individual differences in anatomy should be met with variations in technique for each patient. Patients with marked excess of muscle (the "festoons" of Furnas, 1978) require more extensive dissection to isolate the muscle from the skin as a separate layer. Various maneuvers can be designed to excise excess muscle separately from the skin or to tighten, bolster, or otherwise support the lid by fashioning a sling of the orbicularis muscle, reefing it laterally, excising a lateral triangle, or fixing the muscle flap to the periosteum of the orbit (Figs. 43–18, 43–19). Isolated horizontal muscle rolls can be excised or imbricated (Figs. 43–20, 43–21).

Text continued on page 2345

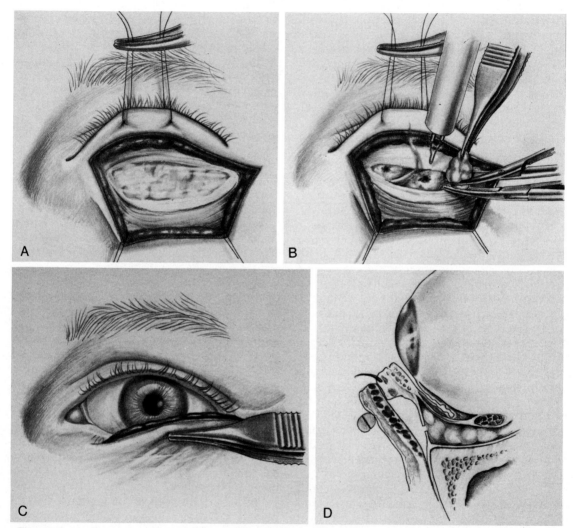

Figure 43–17. Skin-muscle flap technique. *A*, The skin-muscle flap of the lower lid has been completely developed. The medial, middle, and lateral fat compartments can be seen beneath the attenuated orbital septum. *B*, The orbital septum is incised, the excess fat from each compartment is clamped and resected, and the base is coagulated. *C*, The skin-muscle flap is gently draped over the superior wound edge without traction. The lid should be in the neutral position. *D*, Sagittal view. It is important to redrape the skin-muscle flap into the defect. Tenting must be avoided. Note the presence of the pretarsal orbicularis muscle fibers.

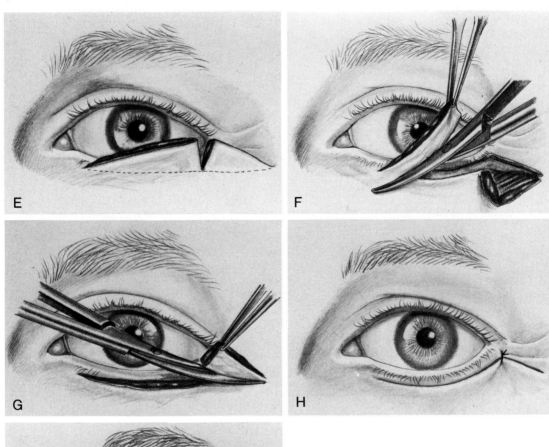

Figure 43–17 *Continued E*, A vertical cut is made at the lateral canthus. *F*, The excess skin and muscle are excised along the length of the lid. Care is taken to maintain the lower lid in a neutral position. *G*, The lateral full-thickness skin and muscle wedge are excised. *H*, A key suture is placed at the lateral canthus. *I*, Suturing is completed.

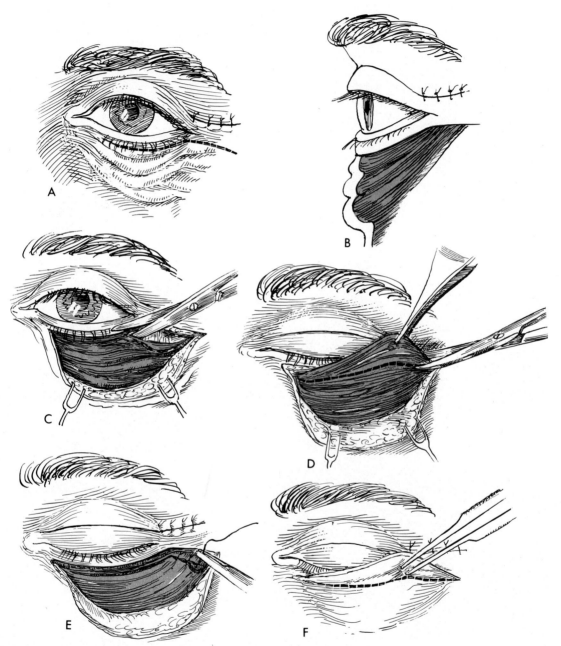

Figure 43–18. Surgical correction of muscle excess (Furnas). *A,* The deformity and the location of the incision. *B,* Lateral view of the deformity. *C,* The skin has been extensively undermined and the muscle is incised separately. *D,* The muscle is pulled gently in a cephalolateral direction to take up the slack. The excess is excised. *E,* The muscle is sutured laterally to soft tissue or preferably to periosteum. The muscle acts as a hammock support. *F,* The redundant skin is excised in the manner described previously (Furnas, 1978). (From Rees, T. D.: Aesthetic Plastic Surgery. Philadelphia, W. B. Saunders Company, 1980, p. 502.)

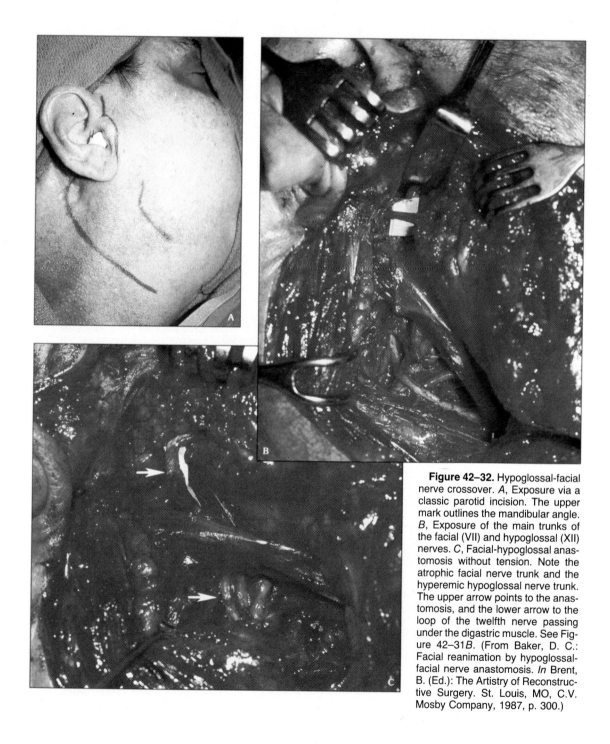

Figure 42–32. Hypoglossal-facial nerve crossover. *A*, Exposure via a classic parotid incision. The upper mark outlines the mandibular angle. *B*, Exposure of the main trunks of the facial (VII) and hypoglossal (XII) nerves. *C*, Facial-hypoglossal anastomosis without tension. Note the atrophic facial nerve trunk and the hyperemic hypoglossal nerve trunk. The upper arrow points to the anastomosis, and the lower arrow to the loop of the twelfth nerve passing under the digastric muscle. See Figure 42–31*B*. (From Baker, D. C.: Facial reanimation by hypoglossal-facial nerve anastomosis. *In* Brent, B. (Ed.): The Artistry of Reconstructive Surgery. St. Louis, MO, C.V. Mosby Company, 1987, p. 300.)

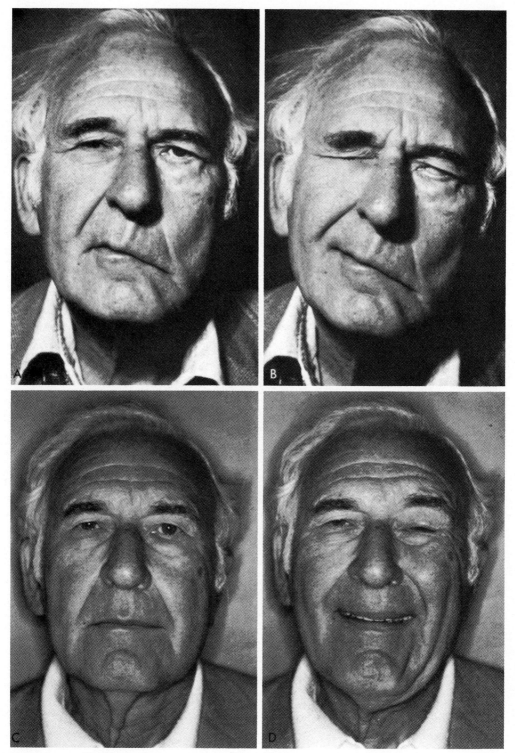

Figure 42–33. Complete paralysis one year after removal of an acoustic neuroma. The facial nerve did not respond to electrical testing. *A,* Preoperative view in repose. *B,* Smiling and closing the eyes preoperatively. *C,* One year after a XII–VII nerve anastomosis, the face is normal in repose. *D,* Excellent movement mimicking a smile. Note the return of the frontal branch. (From Baker, D. C., and Conley, J.: Facial nerve grafting: a thirty year retrospective review. Clin. Plast. Surg., *6:*358, 1979.)

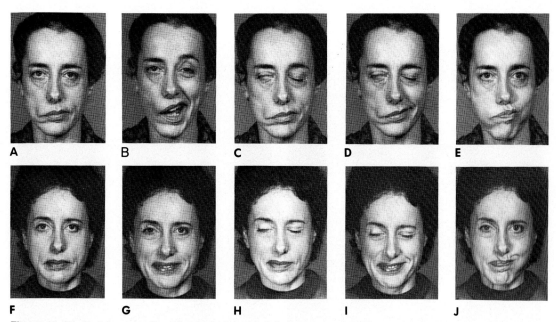

Figure 42–34. Facial reanimation after hypoglossal-facial nerve crossover. Top row, preoperative views; bottom row, postoperative views. *A, F,* Repose. *B, G,* Smiling. *C, H,* Eye closing. *D, I,* Simultaneous eye closing and smiling. *E, J,* Lip pursing. (From Baker, D. C.: Facial reanimation by hypoglossal-facial nerve anastomosis. *In* Brent, B. (Ed.): The Artistry of Reconstructive Surgery. St. Louis, MO, C. V. Mosby Company, 1987, p. 301.)

human emotions. Usually the coincidental movements that occur during speech or swallowing are not a problem, because they are subconscious. The mass movements are usually more dynamic and gross than those seen after autogenous nerve grafting.

Approximately 95 per cent of patients attained satisfactory muscle tone in repose, together with some type and quality of mass movement (Figs. 42–34, 42–35). In 98 per cent of the anastomoses performed immediately, clinical evidence of movement was obtained; in 77 per cent of these the movements were classified as good. In 90 per cent of the delayed anastomoses, movement was obtained, 41 per cent being classified as good.

In some individuals with a "good" return, there was hypertonia, a finding indicating that the neural input from the hypoglossal nerve exceeded that required for natural balance of the face. In these individuals there was an overproduction of facial movements synchronous with physiologic acts relating to the tongue. During eating, talking, or swallowing the face moved excessively in a gross manner.

This type of hyperanimation was conspicuous and could be embarrassing to a sensitive person. However, it did not cause any harm or dysfunction, and those patients who had

the anastomosis as part of an ablative procedure accepted the excessive movement in good grace. On the other hand, a small percentage of those who had had long-standing paralyses were disgruntled, although none would accept the reestablishment of the facial paralysis by having the anastomosis disconnected.

In 22 per cent of the patients there was minimal atrophy of the tongue, in 53 per cent moderate atrophy, and in 25 per cent severe atrophy. In most patients there was residual movement in the paralyzed side of the tongue, and probably the reinnervation crossed the midline from the opposite side (Fig. 42–36). It is well known that patients undergoing a hemiglossectomy can adapt to this condition. Those patients who had the hypoglossal anastomosis as part of a major ablative procedure were much more satisfied than those in the delayed group. There were few complaints in the former group, perhaps owing in part to an overriding concern about the success of the cancer ablation. Only 3 per cent of this group persistently complained about chewing problems, 2 per cent about swallowing difficulties, and 2 per cent about speech problems. Even professionals such as doctors and teachers were able to use their voices with no significant complications.

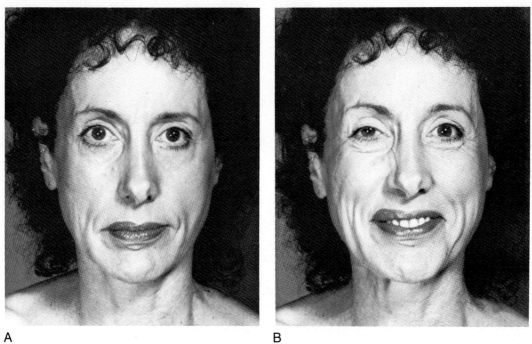

A   B

Figure 42–35. Result four years postoperatively (see Fig. 42–34). *A*, Repose. *B*, Smiling. The overall symmetry and appearance have been enhanced by blepharoplasties and neurolysis of the contralateral frontal nerve branch. (From Baker, D. C.: Facial reanimation by hypoglossal-facial nerve anastomosis. *In* Brent, B. (Ed.): The Artistry of Reconstructive Surgery. St. Louis, MO, C. V. Mosby Company, 1987, p. 301.)

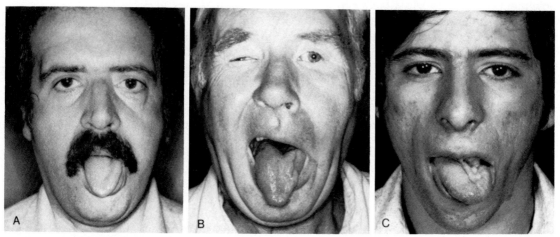

Figure 42–36. Examples of tongue atrophy following XII–VII cranial nerve anastomoses. *A*, Minimal. *B*, Moderate. *C*, Severe. (From Conley, J., and Baker, D. C.: Hypoglossal-facial nerve anastomosis for reinnervation of the paralyzed face. Plast. Reconstr. Surg., *63*:69, 1979.)

In strong contrast to this, individuals with long-standing facial paralysis had a different approach to the problem and responded to the return of movement in a different manner. Preoperatively these patients frequently questioned the advisability of acquiring an additional nerve deficit, particularly when they were already sensitized to a deficiency in chewing and speaking from the facial paralysis. Often, these patients tended to expect much more from the facial rehabilitation than is realistic, and they had an acute sense of guilt concerning their condition. These patients were sometimes negative or suspicious, believing perhaps that the paralysis may not have been necessary and that it had already destroyed a large part of their life style.

All patients with long-standing paralyses complained preoperatively of difficulty in mastication, and 16 per cent complained of this postoperatively. None complained preoperatively about swallowing; 12 per cent complained postoperatively about this. Sixteen per cent complained preoperatively of difficulty with speech; 10 per cent complained postoperatively about this. Thus, a certain number of these patients had improvements of the chewing and speech symptoms associated with their facial paralysis, but swallowing complaints were worse.

OTHER NERVE ANASTOMOSES

Various other nerves have been used for anastomosis to the peripheral part of the trunk of the facial nerve, including the phrenic and the spinal accessory. The hypoglossal nerve is generally the preferred donor nerve.

Phrenic Nerve

When the 11th and 12th cranial nerves have been removed, the phrenic may be a satisfactory alternative, although phrenicofacial anastomoses can result in peculiar resting facial twitches.

Perret (1967) reported relatively normal facial tone in repose after phrenicofacial crossover, although a conspicuous asymmetry occurred with coughing or laughing. These patients usually had difficulty in learning to take a deep breath while smiling.

Production of paralysis of half of the diaphragm would also be contraindicated in any patient with pulmonary disease.

Eleventh Nerve

When the spinal accessory nerve is used, the resulting shoulder drop is obvious and occasionally the shoulder discomfort can be significant. The nerve is a satisfactory physical match to the facial, and generally an almost normal face in repose can be obtained.

Some patients can move the face without moving the shoulder, and move the shoulder without moving the face. This dissociation of movements is the result of a central redirection, requiring intelligence and concentration by the patient; unfortunately, the facial movement cannot be incorporated into a spontaneous emotional response. The greatest disadvantage of the spinal accessory nerve is that it does not accomplish any natural physiologic dynamism or movement in the face (Conley, 1975). The face, therefore, is not active except upon intention or command. It is static during eating, swallowing, and talking; any movement must be produced by conscious direction.

The hypoglossal nerve has the distinct advantage that the face is unconsciously moved during speaking, eating, and swallowing. This creates an exceptional quality of animation on the basis of normal physiologic activity of the tongue in participating in these natural functions. In addition, the patient can voluntarily move the face by intentionally moving the tongue in the oral cavity. Additional control has been accomplished by combining this procedure with a crossface nerve graft. Although the technique is far from ideal and cannot be universally applied, it offers a number of distinct advantages in addition to its high success rate (Baker, 1987b):

1. The surgical technique is direct and uncomplicated, requiring only one suture line.

2. There is greater function, because most facial movements are associated with conscious or unconscious movements of the tongue.

3. There is better balance of the face, as well as the possibility of more rapid facial movements.

4. There is no discomfort from loss of the 12th nerve.

5. There is little functional disability from loss of the 12th nerve.

6. During speech, movement around the mouth is more natural.

7. There is a closer anatomic relationship in the motor zone of the cerebral cortex of the hypoglossal with the facial nerve.

8. A more dynamic functional result is obtained.

The report of Hammerschlag and associates (1987) describing electromyographic rehabilitation after hypoglossal-facial anastomosis is encouraging. Computer technology was used to measure, monitor, and display abnormal electromyographic (EMG) muscle activity, and behavioral techniques were used to reinforce the occurrence of more appropriate motor responses. Thirty-three per cent of patients achieved symmetry and synchrony of function and spontaneity of expression. Synkinetic facial movements associated with use of the tongue were minimal. Fifty-seven per cent of patients accomplished voluntary eye control and lower face function, with only moderate synkinetic movements.

Regional Muscle Transposition

According to Baker and Conley (1979b), when direct nerve suture, autogenous nerve grafting, and nerve crossover are inapplicable in rehabilitation of the paralyzed face, other reconstructive techniques must be used to attempt to supply some type of movement and support. These methods include regional muscle transposition, fascial stripping fixed to a bony point of muscle system, and physical support by synthetic materials. Various techniques of facialplasty and stabilization with dermal flaps have also been used. It can be stated categorically that reactivation of the facial muscles by neural reconstitution or muscle transposition supersedes any type of rehabilitation by suspension or skin stretching except perhaps in very elderly or debilitated patients (Conley and Baker, 1978). These static techniques, however, can be complementary when combined with dynamic reconstruction.

Transposition of regional muscles to rehabilitate the paralyzed face has been employed for almost 75 years. The indications include (1) the absence of mimetic muscles resulting from long-standing atrophy; (2) the need for additional muscle bulk and myoneurotization; and (3) the requirement for a complementary procedure with a nerve graft, nerve crossover, or nerve implantation. Although most of the available muscles in the head and neck have been transposed in whole or in part, by far the most popular muscle transposition techniques are those involving the masseter and temporalis.

The basis of regional muscle transposition is to transfer new muscle innervated by a different cranial nerve, which can furnish pull in various directions and thus accomplish a more normal facial animation. Transposition of a regional muscle presupposes the reeducation of the patient in the use of these voluntary muscles.

The transposition of a dynamic and vital muscle system into a paralyzed face has biologic advantages over other suspension techniques. The living muscle fibers bring with them axons that may have the facility to grow into and support deficient areas in the mimetic muscle system. If the mimetic muscles have atrophied and disappeared, nothing can reverse this situation. However, if there are islands or regions that have survived with paralysis, the introduction of a new dynamic muscle system may be helpful and offers the possibility of myoneurotization.

HISTORY

The use of regional muscle transposition for correction of facial paralysis has been extensively reviewed by Owens (1951) and Conway (1958). Lexer and Eden (1911) performed the first muscle transposition, based on a suggestion of Wrede. They elevated two slips of the anterior half of the masseter muscle from its insertion, and transposed one slip to the upper and the other to the lower lip. To rehabilitate the eye, a slip of temporalis muscle was elevated at its origin, brought forward, and divided, suturing one slip into the upper and the other into the lower lid. As Owens (1951) noted, the results obtained by the use of muscle transposition were fairly satisfactory in some instances, while in others they were questionable. The poor results were undoubtedly due to a disturbance of the neural supply of the transposed muscle, atrophy of the transposed muscle, lack of coordinated movement in the reanimated face, or excessive movement with chewing. However, when the neurovascular supply to the transposed muscle is preserved and when the ideal muscle is chosen for the proper indications, the success rate and patient satisfaction are high.

Some of the poor results reported from use of the Lexer technique of masseter transfer resulted from transection of the nerve supply to the muscle (Fig. 42–37). As noted by de Castro Correia and Zani (1973), if the original drawing of the technique by Lexer and Eden

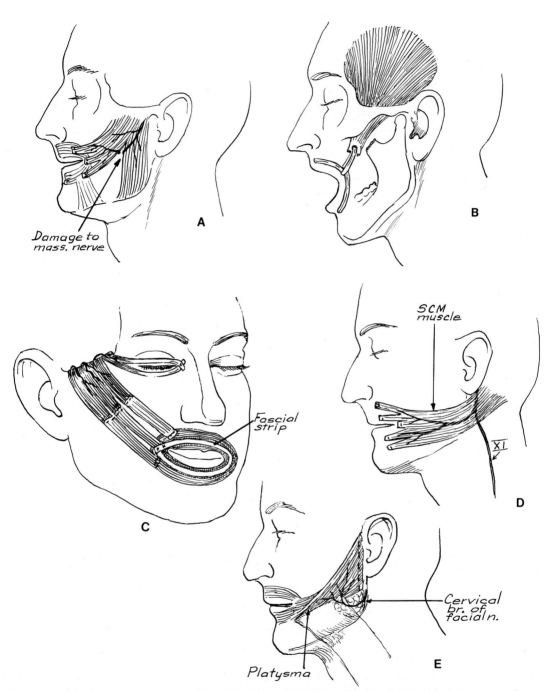

Figure 42–37. Types of regional muscle transpositions. *A*, Lexer's original technique risked transecting the nerve supply to the masseter muscle. *B*, McLaughlin procedure attaching the coronoid process to the circumoral fascia lata suspension. Movement is not at the melolabial crease. *C*, Original technique of temporalis transfer with fascial strips or superficial temporal fascia turned down to obtain length. *D*, Sternocleidomastoid transposition. Movement is more unnatural, in the wrong direction, and muscle is bulky. *E*, Platysma transposition. The muscle is thin and delicate, and does not provide much power; the pull is in the wrong direction. (From Baker, D. C., and Conley, J.: Regional muscle transplantation for rehabilitation of the paralyzed face. Clin. Plast. Surg., 6:318, 1979.)

were to be followed, the nerve to the masseter muscle would be irreversibly damaged in every instance. Modifications of the masseter transposition were made by Jianu (1909), Hastings (1919–1920), and Pickerill (1928). Brunner (1926) was apparently the first to transplant a portion of the masseter muscle by the intraoral approach, thereby eliminating the external incision. Further modifications were made by Owens (1951) and more recently by de Castro Correia and Zani (1973).

Gillies (1934; Gillies and Millard, 1957) popularized the use of the temporalis muscle transfer, and Sheehan (1935) described removal of the zygomatic arch to add length for rotation of the muscle as well as to decrease the deformity associated with the presence of muscle bulk over the zygomatic arch. All these techniques, however, employed strips of fascia as well as temporal muscle to form a sling that was fastened to the upper and lower lips and commissure. This is the basic technique that continues to be employed today, as described by Rubin (1976, 1977), Meyer (1977), and Edgerton, Tuerk, and Fisher (1975). Most surgeons believe that the temporalis muscle is not long enough to reach the mouth or medial canthus without the added fascial attachment. In 1953 McLaughlin described a technique of separating the coronoid process from the mandible, attaching fascial strips to it, and suturing these to the oral commissure for facial movement.

Some of the other regional muscles used in transposition techniques have included the sternocleidomastoid, which was first described by Gomoiu (1913). He sutured the sternal and clavicular insertion into the oral commissure. The disadvantage, however, was that each movement of the head produced a pull on the oral commissure. Schottstaedt, Larsen, and Bost (1955) described a technique for complete mobilization of the sternocleidomastoid muscle by division of its origin and insertion while preserving its neurovascular pedicle. One portion was sutured to the mouth and lips, the other to the parotid and temporal fascia. As noted by Conway (1958), the objections to this procedure are the great muscle bulk and the shortness of the neurovascular pedicle. The one case attempted by Conway (1958) failed because of necrosis of the muscle. Today, this muscle is rarely used because other muscles in the immediate vicinity are more effective.

In order to reanimate the paralyzed eyebrow and forehead, Adams (1946) transposed a flap of frontalis muscle across the midline of the forehead and sutured it to the paralyzed eyebrow. In 1975 Edgerton, Tuerk, and Fisher described a platysma muscle transfer for reanimation of the mouth in Möbius' syndrome. The author has not employed the frontalis or platysma muscle for facial reanimation, and feels that there are several disadvantages associated with these muscles: (1) the direction of muscle pull is incorrect to obtain the reanimation desired; (2) both muscles are thin and delicate, with a fine neurovascular supply that could easily be damaged; and (3) both muscles lack the strength required to accomplish adequate facial movement, as compared with that of the masseter and temporalis.

The use of an innervated trapezius flap to accomplish movement in the paralyzed face has been described by Ryan, Waterhouse, and Davies (1988). Because of the bulk of the muscle flap, it is best employed where soft tissue reconstruction, in addition to facial reanimation, is required, such as after extensive facial tumor resections.

MASSETER MUSCLE TRANSPOSITION

The surgical anatomy and location of the masseter muscle make it ideal for transposition to rehabilitate the upper lip, oral commissure, and lower lip (Figs. 42–38, 42–39). The muscle is short, thick, and rectangular in shape and originates on the inferior surface of the zygomatic complex. Its insertion is into the lateral aspect of the ascending ramus of the mandible, and the tendinous attachments interdigitate into the periosteum and bone. The muscle fibers run obliquely and posteriorly from the zygomatic complex to the angle of the mandible. Its physiologic function is to close the mandible against the maxilla in the act of biting, chewing, and grinding.

The neurovascular supply has been studied by de Castro Correia and Zani (1973), who noted that the muscle receives innervation and blood supply from the masseteric nerve and artery, which arise from the mandibular nerve and internal maxillary artery in the infratemporal fossa. The neurovascular bundle passes through the coronoid notch of the mandible and runs obliquely forward and diagonally downward across the rectangle of

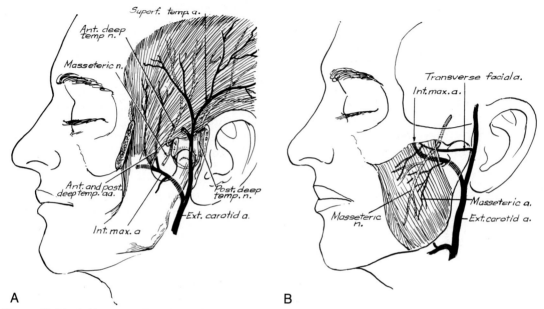

Figure 42–38. *A*, Neurovascular supply of the temporalis muscle. *B*, Neurovascular supply of the masseter muscle; note the oblique direction of the nerve. (From Baker, D. C., and Conley, J.: Regional muscle transplantation for rehabilitation of the paralyzed face. Clin. Plast. Surg., *6*:320, 1979.)

Figure 42–39. *A*, It is recommended to transfer the entire masseter muscle. The incision need be only several centimeters to avoid damage to the nerve. *B*, The anterior portion of the muscle is sutured to the orbicularis oris and to the dermis anterior to the melolabial fold. The posterior portion of the muscle is sutured to the lower lip and commissure. (From Baker, D. C., and Conley, J.: Regional muscle transplantation for rehabilitation of the paralyzed face. Clin. Plast. Surg., *6*:321, 1979.)

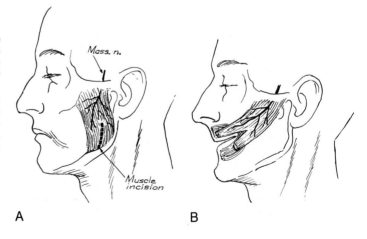

the muscle, becoming more superficial as it passes inferiorly. de Castro Correia and Zani (1973) recommended that separation of the muscle should be performed at the junction of the anterior two-thirds with the posterior one-third. The height of the incision should not be more than 3.5 cm. A safer technique is to transpose the entire muscle.

The masseter muscle may be approached intraorally or externally. When total paralysis is present, the circumauricular approach provides the optimal exposure to the entire muscle belly, and the incision usually is cosmetically acceptable. A preauricular incision is made with a submandibular extension, and the cheek flap is elevated to expose the entire masseter muscle. The tendinous insertion of the muscle is incised on the lowermost portion of the horizontal ramus, preserving the tendinous fibers because they provide a strong attachment for suturing. All the muscle is elevated from the mandibular ramus up to the glenoid notch. Care is taken not to disturb the nerve or blood supply entering the muscle at the level of the coronoid notch. If further mobilization is required, the anterior portion of the muscle may be freed from the ascending portion of the mandible.

The lateral cheek is undermined to create a tunnel for the muscle. The tunnel is intentionally extended through the mimetic muscles of the cheek, commissure, and lips. As the tunnel approaches the lips, it develops a superior and inferior extension similar to the shape of a "Y." One of the tunnels leads into the upper lip and the other toward the commissure and lower lip (Fig. 42–39).

Skin incisions approximately 1 cm long are made medial to the melolabial fold in the upper lip and medial to the angular incision at the commissure and lower lip. They are connected to the tunnel in the cheek, and extended medially over the orbicularis oris muscle (Figs. 42–40, 42–41).

The method of cutting the muscle is extremely important. At the inferior portion of the muscle, some attempt should be made to separate the superficial from the deep bundle. The inferior portion of the muscle is cut in the center, creating two distal bundles. It is important that the muscle be back cut no more than a third in order to protect the neurovascular supply in the distal segments.

The masseter muscle is transposed into the tunnels. If it is too short, it may be lengthened by the partial release of its tendinous origin from the zygomatic complex. The lips and commissure are pulled laterally. There should always be overcorrection of the lip by pulling it in a posterior direction with appropriate hooks or small retractors. The masseter muscle is delivered through the skin incision in the lip and fixed to the orbicularis oris muscle with nonabsorbable sutures in each segment. It should also be sutured to the deep layer of the dermis and fixed in a tunnel in the lip with a pull-out suture (Fig. 42–41).

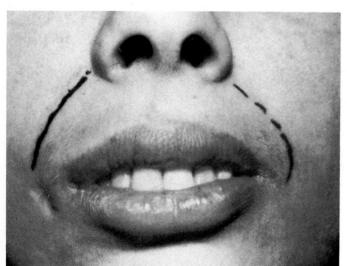

Figure 42–40. The important preoperative marking of the melolabial fold, which must be recreated by the muscle pull. The muscle must be sutured to the dermis anterior to the fold. (From Baker, D. C., and Conley, J.: Regional muscle transplantation for rehabilitation of the paralyzed face. Clin. Plast. Surg., 6:321, 1979.)

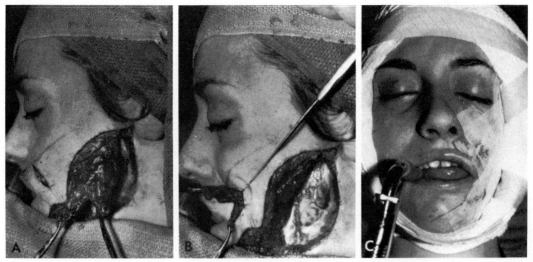

Figure 42–41. *A*, The entire masseter muscle is elevated and divided. *B*, Transposition to the upper lip, melolabial fold, lower lip, and commissure. Overcorrection is essential. *C*, A suture tied over a bolus maintains the muscle in position over the upper lip and orbicularis oris. Steri-Strips and a bulky head dressing help to immobilize the area. Tube feeding is often employed for several days postoperatively to maintain the face and mouth at rest. (From Baker, D. C., and Conley, J.: Regional muscle transplantation for rehabilitation of the paralyzed face. Clin. Plast. Surg., *6:*322, 1979.)

Meticulous hemostasis is obtained and the wound drained with Hemovac catheters. Incisions are closed with absorbable subcuticular sutures and 6–0 nylon cutaneous sutures. The face is immobilized and supported with large Steri-Strips for a period of two weeks. The patient is fed with a nasogastric tube for six days to ensure immobilization of the muscle and suture lines. A liquid diet is maintained for two weeks, and chewing is gradually resumed and increased as the patient is taught to practice control of facial movements in front of a mirror.

Intraoral Approach

Transfer of the anterior portion of the masseter muscle has been found to have value in segmental paresis about the upper lip and commissure. When there is weakness of this particular region about the mouth, it is not necessary to expose the entire parotid gland and masseter muscle by the classical lateral approach. Under these circumstances, an incision is made along the lateral horizontal ramus intraorally and extended into the posterior buccal and retromolar areas. The periosteum of the mandible is elevated along with the anterior portion of the masseter muscle. This section of the masseter muscle is split vertically with right-angled scissors. The split should be less than half the length of

the muscle and should be directed slightly posteriorly. A tunnel is made through the same intraoral incision, directed toward the commissure and upper lip. The muscle is fixed in an overcorrected position with 4–0 silk sutures.

There are two disadvantages to this approach. Bleeding within the belly of the muscle is difficult to control because of inaccessibility, and there can be injury to some of the adjacent residual branches of the facial nerve. The intraoral approach is somewhat awkward and is not recommended except for limited segmental transpositions.

Indications

All or portions of the masseter muscle may be considered for transfer in congenital paralyses of the face associated with Möbius' syndrome and in long-standing facial paralysis in which there has been degeneration of the mimetic muscles (Fig. 42–42). The muscle is primarily suited to the rehabilitation of the mouth and lips. If the eye requires rehabilitation, masseter transfer must be combined with a temporalis transfer or other techniques.

One of the most advantageous uses of masseter transposition is as an integral part of the primary ablative operation in the treatment of high grade malignant tumors of the

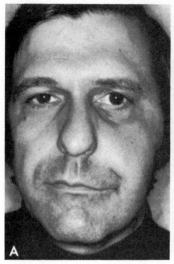
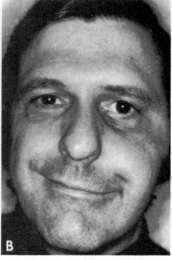

Figure 42–42. *A*, The face is in repose three months after masseter transfer. *B*, Elevation of the upper lip and commissure with clenching of teeth. Movement will improve for another one to two years. (From Baker, D. C., and Conley, J.: Regional muscle transplantation for rehabilitation of the paralyzed face. Clin. Plast. Surg., *6*:322, 1979.)

parotid gland that result in facial paralysis (Fig. 42–43), especially in infirm patients over 60 years of age. Transfer of this muscle rehabilitates the face in a more expeditious manner than facial nerve grafting. This technique shortens the period of rehabilitation. The patient experiences a quicker return of movement and is in satisfactory condition for postoperative irradiation (Fig. 42–44).

The masseter muscle may also be used in conjunction with free autogenous facial nerve grafting when there is a contraindication to nerve grafting in the lower third of the face because of extensive tumor ablation in this region. Under these circumstances, a single large nerve graft may be anastomosed to the principal upper (zygomatic) division of the facial nerve. The masseter transposition to the lower third of the face reactivates the lower third and the nerve graft supplies additional movement to the middle and upper thirds of the face (see Fig. 42–23*C*).

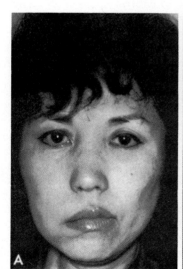
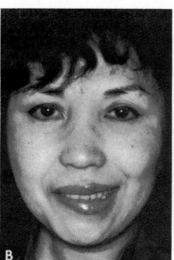
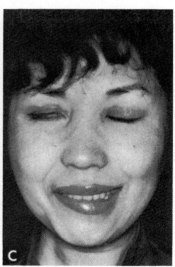

Figure 42–43. *A*, Patient who had a radical parotidectomy including facial nerve resection. Rehabilitation was only with immediate masseter muscle transposition interdigitated with the mimetic muscles. The face is in repose two years postoperatively. *B*, Clenching of teeth demonstrates satisfactory movement of the lower and middle third of the face. Significant myoneurotization with the mimetic muscles has occurred. *C*, Almost complete closure of the eye. (From Baker, D. C., and Conley, J.: Regional muscle transplantation for rehabilitation of the paralyzed face. Clin. Plast. Surg., *6*:323, 1979.)

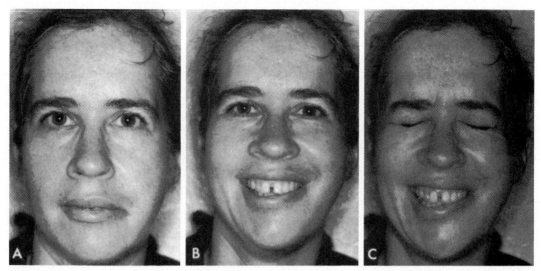

Figure 42–44. *A,* Patient who had total parotidectomy and sacrifice of the *entire* lower division of the facial nerve for a malignant tumor. An immediate masseter muscle transfer was performed to rehabilitate the lips and commissure. The face is in repose two months postoperatively. *B,* Patient is clenching teeth and also using the upper division of the VII nerve. *C,* Eye closure is excellent and facial symmetry is satisfactory except for weakness of the lower lip depressors. (From Baker, D. C., and Conley, J.: Regional muscle transplantation for rehabilitation of the paralyzed face. Clin. Plast. Surg., *6:*324, 1979.)

TEMPORALIS MUSCLE TRANSPOSITION

The temporalis muscle has enjoyed more popularity in facial rehabilitation than has the masseter, because it has the ability to rehabilitate the paralyzed eye and achieve greater excursion of mouth movement. The surgical anatomy of the temporalis muscle was reviewed by Rubin (1977) and Holmes and Marshall (1979). The muscle is fan-shaped, being thin peripherally and thicker centrally. The deep origin of the muscle fibers interdigitate into the periosteum and temporal bone over the entire fossa, from the inferior temporal line above to the infratemporal crest below. The superficial origin of the muscle is from the temporalis fascia, which originates from the superior temporal line of the skull. The muscle inserts on the entire coronoid process and a portion of the ascending ramus of the mandible.

The blood supply is from the anterior and deep temporal arteries and veins, which are tributaries of the internal maxillary system. They enter the infratemporal fossa beneath the zygoma and lateral to the external pterygoid muscle, predominantly on the anterior medial portion of the muscle, to spread out through the muscle superiorly.

The nerve supply is from the anterior and posterior deep temporal nerves, which are branches of the mandibular division of the trigeminal. Their origin is deeper and more posterior than the vascular supply, and they enter the muscle in proximity with the vessels.

Both the concept and technique of temporalis muscle transposition have undergone considerable modification during the past 50 years. Almost all the procedures devised for transposition of the temporalis muscle have been concerned not only with muscle placement but also with some type of maneuver to increase muscle length. The techniques of lengthening have included suturing fascia lata to the end of the muscle (Gillies, 1934), folding and advancing the temporal fascia on the muscle, and, most recently, using free muscle grafts attached to the temporalis transfer (Millesi, 1979). These lengthening concepts are based on the assumption that the muscle is not long enough to reach the medial canthus and mouth. In the author's experience (Baker and Conley, 1979), however, in over 100 temporalis transfers it has been noted that, by following the temporal ridge and taking the full body of the muscle with several centimeters of pericranium, the medial canthus, upper lip, and oral commissure can be reached without much difficulty.

This technique has the following advantages:

1. Elimination of a nonvascularized unit (fascia) that carries the risk of necrosis, breakage, atrophy, slippage, and stretching.

2. Direct insertion of the muscle into the area to be reanimated.

3. Augmentation of an atrophic face in long-standing paralysis.

4. If some functioning mimetic muscle remains in the face, the ability to interdigitate the temporalis muscle with these fibers, thus enhancing the possibility of myoneurotization.

The temporal muscle is exposed through a crescent-shaped, cruciate, or "T" type of incision in the temple, and the entire muscle, with 2 cm of pericranium about its peripheral margin, is elevated for transposition (Fig. 42–45). Two anterior segments are back cut to be adapted about the upper and lower eyelids. Appropriate tunnels are made in both lids in a subcutaneous plane. The levator muscle is protected, and the tunnels communicate in the region of the medial canthus. The two anterior strips of temporal muscle with the pericranium are pulled into the tunnels with lead sutures and sutured to the medial canthal ligament. Sufficient tension is maintained so that the upper lid overlaps the lower lid by several millimeters.

The lateral cheek is undermined and tunnels are made to the upper lip, commissure, and lower lip. If the temporal muscle is exceptionally thick and bulky, the zygomatic arch can be removed to reduce the bulk at this level. This maneuver adds approximately 2 cm to the length of the muscle. If the muscle is not bulky, it is draped over the arch. The muscle is back cut in two sections, using the anterior section for the orbit and the posterior section for the cheek, face, and lips. The

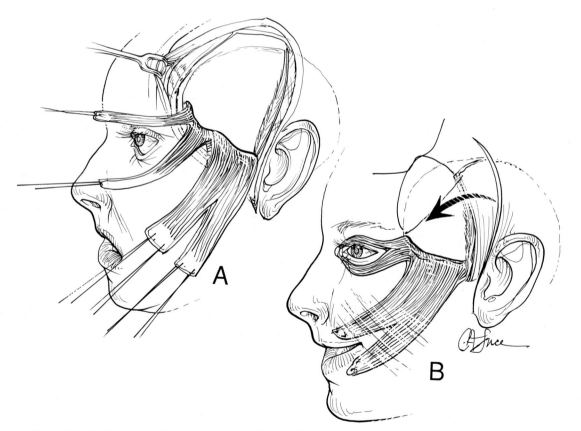

Figure 42–45. Technique of temporalis transposition. *A,* Preauricular incision with extension into the scalp. The entire muscle is elevated and four or five incisions are made for the slips to be inserted. *B,* Muscle slips are transposed to the upper and lower eyelids, upper lip and melolabial fold, lower lip, and commissure. Overcorrection is essential. The muscle should be sutured medial to the melolabial fold and interdigitated with the orbicularis oris muscle in the upper lip.

posterior section is tailored with minimal back cutting to accommodate the prepared tunnels in the cheek and lips. Back cutting should be restricted because of the danger of transecting nerves and small blood vessels to the distal segment of the muscle. The muscle strips are pulled through the tunnels and sutured into the dermis of the skin. It is important to attach the muscle medially to the melolabial fold so that this natural crease is recreated by the muscle pull. If there are mimetic muscles remaining in the face, an attempt should be made to interdigitate the transposed temporalis fibers into them. This is often possible over the orbicularis oris, since there is frequently crossinnervation from the normal side (Nishimura, Morimoto, and Yanagihara, 1977).

In the melolabial fold the crease may be deepened to recreate contour by transposing a deepithelized skin flap based on the line of the future nasolabial fold, as described by Clodius (1976). This flap may also serve as an anchoring point for the transposed muscle to imitate the movement of the quadratus labii superioris and levator anguli oris (Fig. 42–46). To imitate the action of the zygomaticus major, a muscle strip should be sutured to the angle of the mouth.

Overcorrection and exaggeration of the nasolabial fold and corner of the mouth are essential. The overcorrection resolves spontaneously within a few weeks. After meticulous hemostasis, the wounds are drained and closed as in the masseter transfer. The face is supported by large Steri-Strips, and the postoperative care is the same as that after masseter transfer.

After temporalis transposition there may be considerable depression in the region of the temple donor area. This may be camouflaged by hair styling, or eliminated at the time of the primary operation by the insertion of a silicone rubber block. There is always some bulging of the muscle over the zygoma, but when the muscle is excessively thick the zygoma may be removed. This maneuver, however, eliminates the fulcrum action of the zygomatic arch, and the muscle passes straight down instead of going up and down. Most patients have a slight web at the inner canthal region where the muscle is sutured to the medial canthal tendon, although this is not usually a significant deformity (Fig. 42–47).

Indications

Temporalis muscle transposition can be used to advantage in complete facial paralysis with atrophy of the mimetic muscles, sagging and hollowness of the face, and drooping of the oral commissure. Rubin (1976, 1977) used it extensively in facial rehabilitation for Möbius' syndrome. In these instances it provides support, movement, and augmentation. The temporalis muscle is also helpful in protecting the eye.

Temporalis transfer is rarely used as the rehabilitative technique with a primary ablative operation causing facial paralysis. When the other preferred methods are not feasible, such as in a massive tumor resection, primary rehabilitation with the temporalis muscle may offer some advantage. In most instances, however, the temporal muscle has

Figure 42–46. Muscle slips are sutured to the dermis medial to the melolabial fold and also interdigitated with the orbicularis oris muscle. (From Baker, D. C., and Conley, J.: Regional muscle transplantation for rehabilitation of the paralyzed face. Clin. Plast. Surg., 6:327, 1979.)

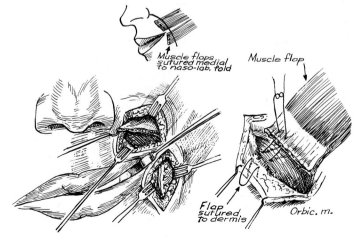

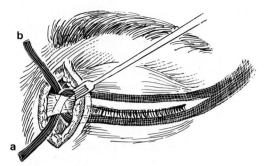

Figure 42–47. Slips are sutured to the medial canthus with nonabsorbable suture. Extreme care must be taken to minimize the size of tunnels in the eyelids and to prevent drifting of the muscle (occasionally a suture placed in the midportion of the lid maintains the position). Tension should be sufficient to overlap the lower lid by the upper lid by several millimeters. The overcorrection rapidly corrects itself. (From Baker, D. C., and Conley, J.: Regional muscle transplantation for rehabilitation of the paralyzed face. Clin. Plast. Surg., 6:327, 1979.)

been used as a secondary procedure in postoperative or long-standing facial paralysis.

RESULTS OF TEMPORALIS AND MASSETER MUSCLE TRANSPOSITION

In all cases one should expect some degree of minimal movement of the face several weeks after surgery. The movement is always associated with voluntary action of the masticatory muscles initiated by clenching of the teeth. Failure to attain movement in the face may result from excessive back cutting and interference with the neurovascular supply, with resultant muscle atrophy and fibrosis. Improper suture of the muscle to the dermis may result in slippage or breakage; the latter may also represent improper postoperative immobilization or early movement of the face. If fascial strips are used to lengthen the muscle, they may atrophy, slip, or stretch.

The greatest observed movement involves the region about the lips and cheek. If significant myoneurotization occurs (frequently, when a masseter muscle transfer is used for immediate rehabilitation of the face in an ablative procedure), the movement gradually extends, over an interval of one to two years, to include all the muscles of the lower and middle thirds of the face. This may include satisfactory movement of the lower eyelid, cheek, upper lip, commissure, and lower lip (Fig. 42–48). The movement is always intentional and not associated with emotion. Many patients, however, can train themselves to imitate an emotional reaction. The strength of the movement is usually satisfactory, although the tone of the muscles on that side of the face may be poor. In the temporalis transfer, eyelid closure is usually adequate.

Because the impulse for muscle movement in temporalis and masseter transfers originates from the trigeminal nerve, facial movement is produced upon chewing, clenching the teeth (Fig. 42–49), and moving the mandible. A few patients may complain of excessive movement while eating. These are obvious limitations and disadvantages, and they have stimulated the search for other means to reinnervate these muscles (Fig. 42–50). One can perform a facial nerve graft from the proximal segment of the ipsilateral facial nerve, if it is intact, and implant it into the transposed muscle, or anastomose it to the masseteric or temporal nerves at the foramen ovale. Crossface nerve grafts with muscle implantation have also been performed (Anderl, 1977a, 1985), as have crossface nerve grafts to the masseteric nerve at the foramen ovale (Freilinger, 1975). The results of these procedures have not been sufficiently evaluated to justify their routine use.

The basic advantage of masseter and temporalis transfer is the introduction of a large volume of living and dynamic muscle into the face. Additional advantages include the simplicity of the technique, the support provided, enhancement of the possibility of myoneurotization, and no loss of other significant function. In many instances, facial movement improves for approximately two years, and the long-term effect suggests some degree of rehabilitation of the facial muscles.

Free Muscle Grafts

In 1971 Thompson reported the successful transplantation of free autogenous muscle grafts in humans, and in 1974 he established its clinical application in the treatment of unilateral facial paralysis. According to Thompson, the success of this procedure depends on three factors: (1) the muscle selected for transplantation must be denervated 14 days before transplantation; (2) a full length of muscle fiber must be preserved; and (3) the denervated muscle must be placed in direct contact with normal, fully innervated, and vascularized skeletal muscle at the recipient

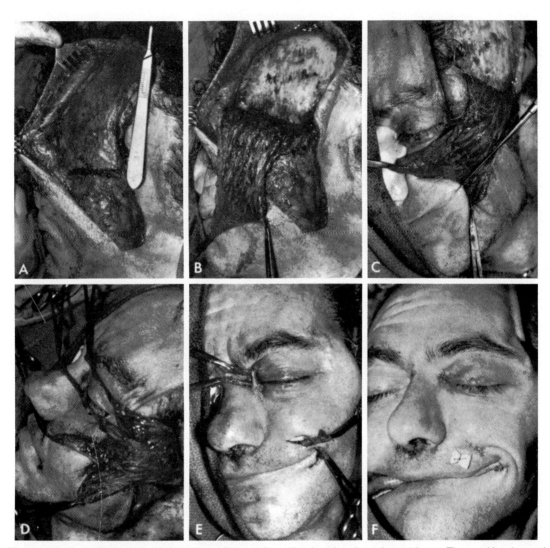

Figure 42–48. *A,* The length of the temporalis muscle and epicranium is at least 10 cm. The marking is on the zygomatic arch. *B,* The entire temporalis muscle is transposed, and it easily reaches the lower lip and commissure without the need for fascial strips or temporalis fascia. *C,* The transposed muscle also easily reaches the medial canthus. *D,* The divided slips are in place. The lowermost muscle slip reaches the commissure with overcorrection. *E,* The slips are passed through tunnels and are ready for suturing. *F,* Note the overcorrection, the recreation of the melolabial fold, and the bolus maintaining the muscle over the orbicularis oris muscle. (From Baker, D. C., and Conley, J.: Regional muscle transplantation for rehabilitation of the paralyzed face. Clin. Plast. Surg., *6:*328, 1979.)

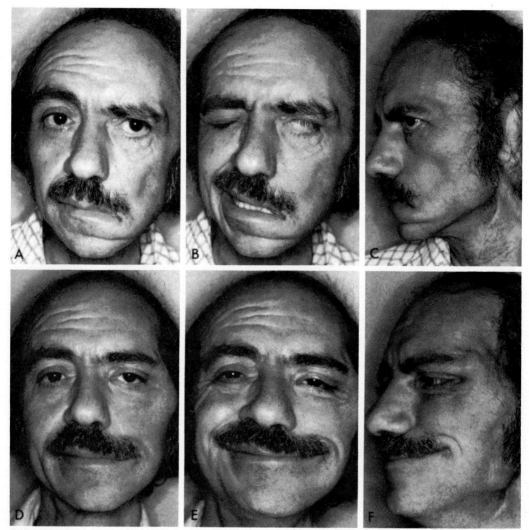

Figure 42–49. The patient (see Fig. 42–48) had a temporal bone resection for squamous cell carcinoma of the ear. Immediate facial rehabilitation was by a crossface nerve graft. *A,* The result two years postoperatively is shown. The face is in repose. *B,* Smiling and closing the eye. *C,* Note ectropion, sagging of the face, and atrophy of the facial tissues. *D,* Results are shown three months after temporalis muscle transposition. The face is in repose. *E,* Mimicking a smile by clenching the teeth. *F,* Note the augmentation of the face by the transposed muscle. The bulge over the zygoma could be corrected by insertion of a Silastic implant in the temporal region or by removal of the zygomatic arch. (From Baker, D. C., and Conley, J.: Regional muscle transplantation for rehabilitation of the paralyzed face. Clin. Plast. Surg., *6:*329, 1979.)

Figure 42–50. *A*, Patient with Möbius' syndrome with the face in repose. *B*, The patient is attempting to smile. *C*, One year after bilateral temporalis muscle transfer, fullness of the malar areas and accentuation of the epicanthal folds are seen. *D*, Satisfactory movement of the mouth and cheeks is achieved by clenching the teeth. In females, the depression in the temporal donor site is easily camouflaged by the hair style. (From Baker, D. C., and Conley, J.: Regional muscle transplantation for rehabilitation of the paralyzed face. Clin. Plast. Surg., *6*:330, 1979.)

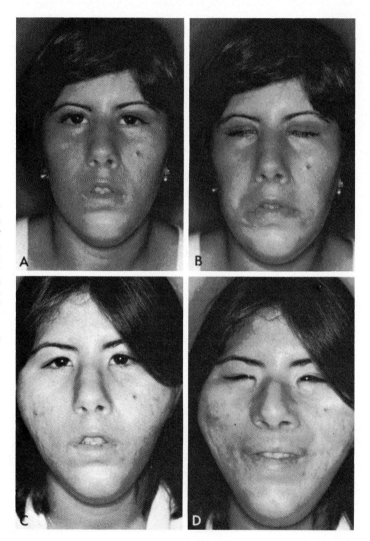

site before neurotization can occur. Thus, a minimum of two operations is required, with an interval of 14 days between them. The technique consists of placing denervated muscle in contact with normal muscle on the nonparalyzed side of the face. The transplanted muscle tendon is then sutured to the appropriate area to obtain movement (e.g., the zygomatic arch for the oral sphincter and the lateral canthal tendon for the eye sphincter).

Thompson (1971) reported that of 54 patients treated for oral sphincter reconstruction, 90 per cent had good results and 10 per cent showed satisfactory improvement. Seventeen per cent of the patients required another surgical procedure to tighten the tendon sling. In the reconstruction of the paralyzed eyelids of 62 patients, 48 per cent showed good results and 45 per cent satisfactory results. Secondary operations to adjust tension or perform tenolysis were required in 22 per cent of the patients. The advantage of this technique is that movement is controlled by the normal side of the face.

In spite of the reports of success by Thompson (1971) and Hakelius (1979), considerable skepticism exists about the reproducibility of free muscle grafting for reconstructive surgery. The attempt by Mayou and associates (1981) to reproduce Thompson's experiments in dogs proved unsuccessful, and it is still uncertain which factors are responsible for the survival of free muscle grafts. In addition to this uncertainty and reports that grafts have become fibrotic, other disadvantages include the multiple surgical stages required, the high incidence of reoperation, and the intrusion on the nonparalyzed side of the face.

With the present high success rates of microneurovascular muscle transfer, the technique of free muscle grafting has little or no place in facial paralysis reconstruction.

Nerve-Muscle Pedicle Techniques

From previous work involving reinnervation of paralyzed vocal cords, Tucker (1979) extended the nerve-muscle pedicle technique to the treatment of facial paralysis. The technique involves transplanting an intact motor nerve with an attached small block of donor muscle from the point of nerve entry, after which the pedicle is sutured to the muscle to

be reinnervated. If most motor end plates are preserved, the pedicle is prevented from degenerating, and reinnervation of the recipient muscle takes place within two to eight weeks (as demonstrated by experimental work in rabbits). The ansa hypoglossi nerve is used with muscle pedicles from the anterior belly of the omohyoid, the sternohyoideus, and the sternothyroideus. The pedicles have sufficient length to be implanted in the levator anguli oris and the orbicularis oris, but they cannot reach the eye. For reconstruction of the orbicularis oculi, Tucker (1979) recommended a temporalis muscle pedicle. Minimal clinical experience has been amassed on this technique; in theory, however, it could rehabilitate the face without loss of function, perhaps doing so in a shorter time than some other present techniques.

The technique can be applied only to the perioral musculature, and it has yet to capture the interest of surgeons.

Microneurovascular Muscle Transfers

The most recent contribution to reanimation of the paralyzed face is the microneurovascular muscle transfer, combined with crossface nerve graft, ipsilateral nerve graft, or split hypoglossal anastomoses. The technique provides new, vascularized muscle to the face that can produce pull in various directions and accomplish more normal facial animation. The indications for its use are similar to those for regional muscle transfer; the advantage over the latter technique is that the transferred muscle can be reinnervated by a crossface nerve graft, thereby enhancing control of voluntary facial movement. In spite of the success of and enthusiasm for this technique, its limitations must be kept in mind and the indications for its use should be clear. At present, it is merely another alternative in the surgeon's armamentarium of facial reanimation procedures.

Harii, Ohmori, and Torii (1976) were the first to report a successful microvascular transfer of the gracilis muscle to provide elevation of the oral commissure. In the first case, performed in 1973, the motor nerve to the temporalis muscle was employed. In subsequent cases a crossface nerve graft was anastomosed to the transferred muscle at a second stage. Harii's report of 18 cases (1979) demonstrated encouraging results. Two of the major drawbacks were the excessive bulk of the transferred muscle and the excessive movement. In 1980 O'Brien, Franklin, and Morrison reported favorable results.

Tolhurst and Bos (1982) reported seven cases in which the extensor digitorum brevis muscle was used, with only two satisfactory results. The experience of Harii and O'Brien using this as a donor muscle was similarly disappointing, and most surgeons no longer employ it for facial paralysis reconstruction.

Terzis and Manktelow (1982) recommended the pectoralis minor muscle for facial reanimation, and this report was followed by Harrison (1985), who used the same donor muscle in ten patients with five excellent results, three good results, and two failures. The advantages of this muscle are its small, flat configuration, the minimal functional loss, and an acceptable donor scar. Buncke (1983) reported the successful use of the serratus anterior muscle for facial reanimation. More recent reports by Manktelow (1987), O'Brien and Morrison (1987), and Harii (1988) appear to favor the gracilis as the donor muscle of choice.

The ideal donor muscle should provide the following:

1. Excursion equal to that of the normal side of the face.

2. A reliable vascular and nerve pattern of similar size to that of the recipient.

3. No functional deficit from removal of the muscle.

4. Location of a donor site sufficiently distant from the face to allow for two operating teams to work simultaneously.

Numerous muscles have been used for transplantation to the face (Terzis, 1987). The most commonly used at present are listed below.

Gracilis muscle has a predictable and adequate neurovascular pedicle, with adequate bulk but excessive length (Hamilton, Terzis, and Carraway, 1987). Because various portions are supplied by different fascicles, the muscle can be split longitudinally and cut transversely to produce the required size of muscle needed for transfer. The initial reports of Harii (Harii, Ohmori, and Torii, 1976; Harii, 1979) described the use of the entire gracilis muscle, with resultant facial bulk and distortion. With the refinements of Manktelow (1987), a single fascicle supplying the anterior third of the muscle can be taken to provide the desired length and bulk.

Pectoralis minor muscle has adequate weight but excessive length; its flat shape facilitates insertion into the face. However, as Manktelow (1985) pointed out, the neurovascular pedicle is complex and variable, and its motor supply may present significant problems in reinnervation. In addition, the proximity on the upper chest makes simultaneous two-team dissection difficult. Nevertheless, Terzis (1987) has been encouraged with the results of using this muscle in facial reanimation.

Latissimus dorsi muscle and *serratus muscle* have a predictable neurovascular pedicle and longitudinal intramuscular pattern. The latissimus dorsi can be segmentally separated like the gracilis in order to reduce its bulk. The nerve to the serratus is short (Hamilton, 1987) and usually the lower four segments are utilized; it also requires segmental separation to reduce its bulkiness.

Rectus abdominis muscle is bulky and long but can be transferred. It has a long, predictable vascular supply and a laterally based segmental nerve supply.

Platysma muscle is a thin facial muscle supplied by the facial artery and the cervical branch of the facial nerve. Because of its weight and thinness, Terzis (1987) used it in reconstructing the orbicularis oculi.

All the aforementioned muscles leave minimal or no functional deficit when sacrificed. As operative techniques have been refined, the emphasis has shifted toward harvesting well-innervated pieces of muscle that have the correct functional length to replace the appropriate facial muscles. There are numerous muscles with a predictable neurovascular supply from which such pieces of muscle may be taken.

SURGICAL TECHNIQUE

The operative procedure is usually divided into two stages unless the ipsilateral facial nerve can be used or the hypoglossal is split and anastomosed. The first stage consists of a classical crossface nerve graft. If muscle transfer is to reanimate both the eye and mouth, two crossface nerve grafts are required. Tinel's sign is followed, and approximately nine to 12 months later the vascularized muscle is transferred and its neural element anastomosed to the distal end of the crossface nerve graft.

For the second stage the two-team approach is best, one to prepare the facial nerve graft and recipient vessels (usually the superficial temporal or facial), while the other harvests and prepares the donor muscle on its neurovascular pedicle. It is important to carry out fascicular nerve stimulation of the donor muscle to determine which portion of the muscle each fascicle supplies. For example, the anterior one-third of the gracilis is usually utilized (Fig. 42–51).

According to Manktelow (1985), the zygomaticus major is the single facial muscle most nearly producing a normal smile. It is approximately 5 cm in length and produces a maximal shortening of 1.5 to 2 cm in the normal face. With preoperative observation the excursion of the oral commissure and shape of the patient's smile can be recorded, and an attempt should be made to simulate the normal side with the transferred muscle. The muscle should usually run from the oral commissure to the body of the zygoma along the normal course of the zygomaticus major (Fig. 42–52). A functioning muscle length of 5 to 6 cm is generally required.

The transferred muscle is sutured into the commissure and can be interdigitated with any remaining facial muscles in the upper and lower lip, nasolabial fold, and alar base. The site of the muscle's origin depends on the direction of pull desired, usually between the zygomatic arch and tragus.

The correct tension at which the muscle should be inserted has not yet been fully demonstrated. Manktelow (1987) placed the muscle in sufficient tension so that under anesthesia it is tight enough to place the paralyzed oral commissure in balance with the normal side. Microvascular anastomoses of artery and vein and fascicular nerve repair are completed. Overlying skin closure should avoid tension on the vascular anastomoses, and drains should be kept distant to the latter.

RESULTS

The reports of Harrison (1985); Harii, Ohmori, and Torii (1976); Harii (1979);

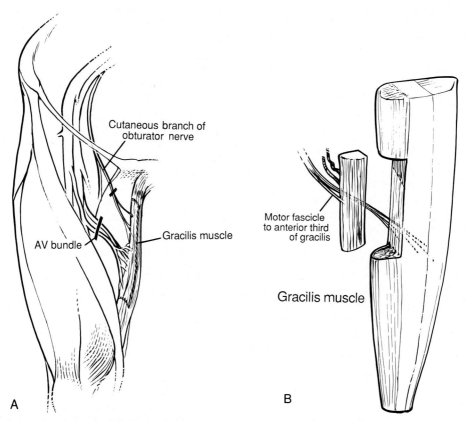

Figure 42–51. Gracilis microneurovascular transfer. *A,* Overview of the muscle with the cutaneous branch of the obturator nerve and the arteriovenous bundle, which are divided. *B,* The three longitudinal fascicular motor territories. The anterior territory containing the dominant neurovascular pedicle has been harvested. (*A* and *B* from Manktelow, R. T.: Free muscle transplantation for facial paralysis. Clin. Plast. Surg., *11:*218, 1984.)

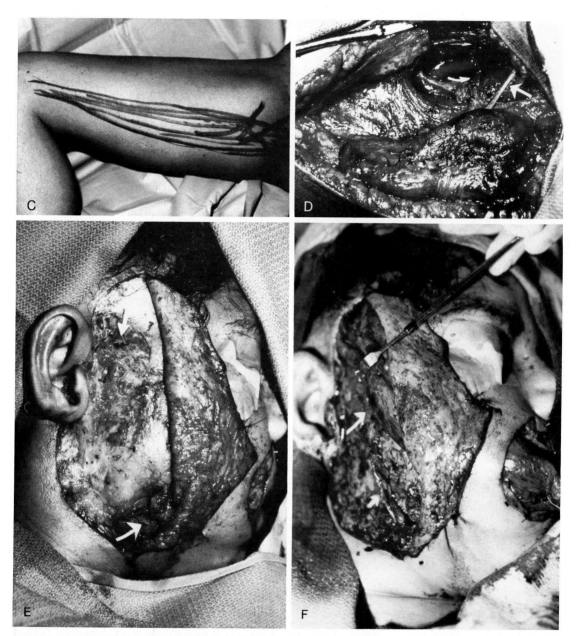

Figure 42–51 *Continued C*, Outline of the gracilis muscle and neurovascular pedicle. *D*, The gracilis muscle flap dissected with the nerve and vascular pedicles isolated *(arrows)*. *E*, Recipient facial vessels and the distal end of the crossface nerve graft *(arrows)*. *F*, The muscle flap transferred to the face. The anastomoses of facial vessels and crossface nerve graft completed.

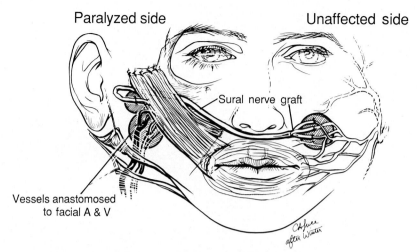

Paralyzed side   Unaffected side

Sural nerve graft

Vessels anastomosed
to facial A & V

Figure 42–52. Microneurovascular transfer of the gracilis muscle on the paralyzed side. The muscle is sutured to the zygomatic arch and the sural nerve graft is anastomosed to the motor nerve to the gracilis muscle. The gracilis arteriovenous bundle is sutured to the respective facial artery and vein. The other end of the gracilis muscle is sutured into the oral commissure, orbicularis oris, and nasolabial fold.

O'Brien and Morrison (1987); and Manktelow (1987) have all been encouraging, with a majority of good to excellent results (Fig. 42–53). In 35 out of 40 of the patients of O'Brien and Morrison adequate symmetry was obtained at rest and reasonably active lifting of the angle of the mouth and cheek. In addition, 19 patients obtained independent movements of the face in spite of the fact that both sides of the face were supplied by the same facial nerve. No satisfactory explanation has been determined for this phenomenon.

It is important to emphasize that movement of the face after microneurovascular muscle transfer is never normal. As pointed out by Rayment, Poole, and Rushworth (1987), it is simplistic to use one reinnervated muscle along one vector to reanimate the oral commissure and upper lip—an area that normally has ten muscles acting on it along different vectors. Patients do learn to produce a definitive smile, but the ability to produce the involuntary, spontaneous "flash" smile rarely returns. Therefore, during speech some asymmetry of the face is usually evident. It is also difficult to obtain independent movements in the eye and mouth (Manktelow, 1987).

Rayment, Poole, and Rushworth (1987) analyzed the problem of poor symmetry of synergistic facial movement in patients who have had successful reinnervation of transplanted muscle. They explained that the ad-

equacy of reinnervation of muscle is directly related to the numbers of axons that manage to cross the sural nerve graft to the muscle: different ratios of axons to muscle fibers exist for different muscles. Normal facial muscles have approximately 25 muscle fibers innervated by one axon (Feinstein, 1955), while gracilis and pectoralis minor muscles have 150 to 200 muscle fibers to each axon. Muscles with a smaller ratio of muscle fibers to axons, such as the facial muscles are capable of producing a wide variety of finely tuned movements (Rayment, Poole, and Rushworth, 1987). The facial muscles have been described as "intelligent," while the gracilis and pectoralis minor muscles are "stupid" (Terzis, 1988).

Crossface nerve grafting, even with the most meticulous technique, has demonstrated that only 20 to 50 per cent of axons cross the nerve graft (Harrison, 1985). The different muscle fiber to axon ratio would explain the limited success of crossface nerve grafting alone, as opposed to combining it with a microvascular muscle transfer (muscles requiring fewer axons to reinnervate a larger number of muscle fibers).

INDICATIONS

Microneurovascular muscle transfer is another alternative in facial paralysis reconstruction. Some of the best candidates for this

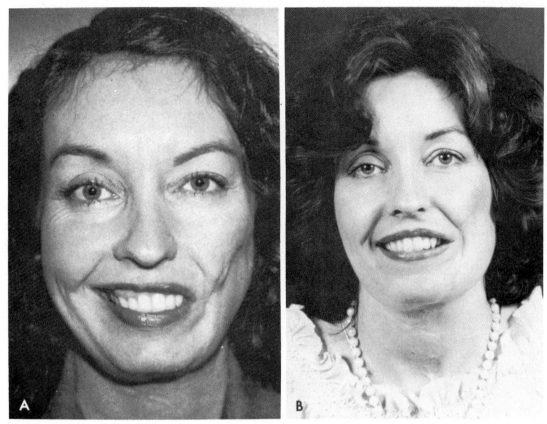

Figure 42–53. *A,* Preoperative appearance, smiling, showing inability to elevate the corner of the mouth and a soft tissue defect in the left cheek. *B,* Postoperative appearance, smiling. (From Manktelow, R. T.: Free muscle transplantation for facial paralysis. Clin. Plast. Surg., *11*:219, 1984.)

technique are patients with a regional paralysis, especially involving the elevators of the lip. Others are patients in whom the ipsilateral facial nerve is intact, as after trauma or extensive facial tumor resections where the facial muscles are ablated. Younger patients with congenital paralysis or those who have had intracranial tumor resection are also well suited for this technique. Older or infirmed patients with facial paralysis more often prefer a simpler, pragmatic approach to facial reanimation such as regional muscle transfers.

The main advantage of the technique is that facial movement is provided and controlled by the contralateral facial nerve, providing for better symmetry and perhaps a more definitive smile. Many disadvantages, however, remain: (1) there are at least two operative stages with prolonged surgical time; (2) there are two donor site scars; (3) there is usually a lapse of two years before

return of facial movement; (4) complete eyelid closure, forehead movement, oral sphincter, and depressor lip function are almost never restored; (5) the technique is not free of synkinesis; and (6) there is a deficit of involuntary emotional expression common to most other rehabilitative techniques.

Static and Ancillary Techniques

All the previous procedures for facial reanimation used nerve and muscle or a combination of the two to provide for a dynamic reconstruction of the paralyzed face. At present these techniques are well accepted and easily accomplished with a high degree of success and minimal risk. Consequently there is rarely any place for the static methods of reconstruction that were popular several decades ago.

FASCIAL TRANSPLANTS

According to Freeman (1977), the use of autogenous fascia for blepharoptosis was initiated by Payr and applied to the treatment of facial paralysis by Stein (1913). However, it was Blair's advocacy (1926) of the suspension of paralyzed facial muscles by fascia lata bands that popularized the method. The technique (Fig. 42–54) varies considerably with the individual problem, but a modified fascial sling has proved of value as a method of primary treatment in older adults, and as an adjunct method while waiting for the functional results of nerve crossings, grafts, or nerve end approximations. It is also used in association with muscle transplants and the resection of contralateral muscles, and may be helpful in prolonging the effects of skin excisions, face lifts, and blepharoplasties.

DERMAL TRANSPLANTS

Strips of dermis of a width and length comparable with that of strips of fascia inserted in the same manner have a tendency to stretch (Freeman, 1977). Dermis and lyophilized fascia are more liable to stimulate fibrous proliferation than autogenous fascia, because they fragment and disintegrate early. Postoperative subcutaneous infections are higher with dermal implants than with fascia, because saprophytic infection carried into the repaired field is manifest many days or weeks after the operation rather than in the usual 12 to 36 hours after surgery (Pick, 1949).

INORGANIC (ALLOPLAST) IMPLANTS

Static methods to relieve distortion employ the suspension of paralyzed facial muscles by various materials, varying from wire and silk to stainless steel and tantalum. There are advocates for the use of nonreactive plastic tapes of polyethylene, Teflon, or Silastic with or without either Marlex or Dacron mesh reinforcement (Fig. 42–55). Clinical experience has led to a distrust of inorganic material placed in a position of suspension or tension in superficial locations (Freeman,

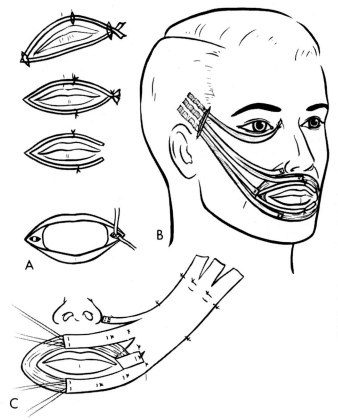

Figure 42–54. Fascia lata suspension. *A*, Placement of a circumoral fascial strip. Inserted via extraoral or buccal incisions, the loops are tightened on the unaffected side to elevate the paralyzed angle of the mouth. The knotted attachment at the unaffected commissure is excised after five weeks. The lowermost sketch shows the oral incisions for insertion of the circumoral band of fascia after it has been threaded through and knotted, before the suturing. *B*, The fascial sling to the lower lid is secured at the nasal periosteum. The lateral end is attached to the temporal fascia. The fascial band is attached through a temporal incision to the orbicularis oris. The three tails for attachment at both insertions are shortened for clarity. *C*, The typical fashioning of a fascial ribbon for adequate support using three tails for insertion: one for each lip well past the midline and another folded around the dissected orbicularis oris muscle. The similarly tailed lateral end is woven into the temporal fascia or tacked securely to the adjacent periosteum.

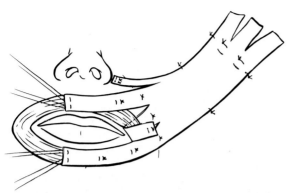

Figure 42–55. Method of attachment of the fascia lata or Marlex mesh by nonabsorbable mattress sutures at the pterygomandibular raphé (rather than at the mandible). The central slip of the anterior end is wrapped securely around the orbicularis oris muscle at the oral commissure. The inferior and superior slips are secured temporarily by pull-out mattress sutures to the undersurface of the dermis. (The optional small strip to the ala is secured firmly.) Insertion can also be made to the mandible.

1977). The reviews of Bäckdahl and D'Alessio (1958) and Conway (1958) should be consulted before inorganic (alloplast) materials are used for facial suspension.

Selective Neurectomy

Selective sectioning of the intact facial nerve in order to accomplish a more balanced face has been practiced for over 100 years (Freeman, 1977). It is best carefully to evaluate the degree of antagonist muscle pull and distortion and to map the nerves to be sectioned.

UPPER FACIAL PARALYSIS

The degree and permanency of the paralysis may be established by electrical testing of the facial nerve and recording of the chronaxial levels. If these levels remain high for more than six months, there will most likely be no return of movement to the brow.

If the paralysis persists, the frontal muscles atrophy, with a resultant ptosis of the brow. Any improvement at this stage involves an equalization of the movement of the forehead by a selective cutting of the corresponding nerve on the opposite side. This may be carried out through the temporal incision used in the face lift, with identification of the responsible nerve by electrical testing. At this anatomic level there are frequently two or

three filaments requiring division (as determined by electrical stimulation). They should be sectioned step by step, until the brow is paretic. Even with this approach to nerve section, equalization of movement of the brow does not result in every case (Baker, 1984). Occasionally, after the operation the paralysis of the normal side may not be as much as desired, and a "second look" may be necessary. According to Baker and Conley (1979) in equalizing the brow one should always attempt to save the filament that goes to the corrugator muscles, to the eyebrow, and to the orbicularis muscles, because this retains an active and lively expression about the eyebrows. Not uncommonly, however, patients with a paralysis of the frontal branch prefer to have a smooth, immobile forehead with minimal frown lines.

MIDDLE FACIAL PARALYSIS

If the paresis is recognized postoperatively, it is reasonable to wait because almost all middle facial paralyses recover considerably during a period of months, owing to collateral budding from the network that these nerves share with each other. The result may be complicated, however, by a slight motor tic. If a persistent or troublesome tic or spasm of the face develops, consideration may be given to a selective division of the particular nerve filament causing it. This is accomplished by exposing the particular branch, electrical testing, and a neurotomy. The weakness that develops in the muscle systems supplied by this nerve is marked in the beginning, but over six months there is considerable return of movement via the network pathways. Unfortunately, in some instances when the balance becomes restored there may be a reappearance of the tic, but usually not as marked as it was originally.

LOWER FACIAL PARALYSIS

A persistent paralysis of the marginal mandibular branch may be handled by division of the opposite mandibular branch after an interval of one year. A neurectomy at this level places the lower lip in relative balance. Again, this may be difficult to accomplish permanently, because of variations in the network connections of the distal branches of the facial nerve. A combination of this procedure with a selected myectomy, accomplished through a mucosal incision (Rubin, 1977), gives more assurance of permanent symmetry.

Selective Myectomy

Freeman (1977) outlined the various techniques for selective myectomy of the facial muscles to accomplish better balance in repose and during facial expression.

The muscles most frequently causing distortion during speech, emotion, and associated actions are the quadratus labii superioris, the depressor labii inferioris, and the zygomaticus. A study of the muscle or muscle groups responsible for the distortion permits these to be isolated and sectioned and varying amounts of muscle tissue to be resected. This procedure can be helpful in segmental paralysis not amenable to surgical neurorrhaphy or grafting. Alleviation of the spastic, antagonistic muscles on the nonpalsied side has aided symmetry during action, both voluntary and emotional.

To correct excessive upward deviation of the opposite side of the face during a smile, the zygomaticus muscle is outlined at the angle of the mouth. The fibers, which spread up and out and become deeper superiorly, are isolated under the subcutaneous tissue and retracted for a distance of approximately 2 cm from the relatively diffuse origin of the muscle to its insertion into the orbicularis oris. Careful dissection exposes the tiny nerves that enter the muscle from the undersurface. It is a simple procedure to remove a segment 1 to 2 cm in length, depending on the age of the patient (Freeman, 1977).

Deviation of the philtrum to the contralateral side and the upward pull of the cheek can be lessened by resecting a segment of the quadratus labii superioris muscle, as well as a short segment of the orbicularis oris in this area.

Abnormal depression of the lip during labial speech, simulating a sneer, can be alleviated by isolating the quadratus labii inferioris through the mucosa and removing a segment of the muscle. The muscle outline is marked during forceful speech. The lip is everted, the mucosa incised, the muscle isolated and sectioned, and the mucosa closed.

An intraoral approach is also adequate for resection of the depressor muscles. After everting the lip, a mucosal flap is elevated,

and the quadratus muscle, together with the triangularis and the associated segments of the orbicularis oris, is outlined. The muscles, isolated from the skin and mucosa, are clipped and ligated, and resected.

The incision to expose the zygomaticus or the quadratus labii superioris (the levators) is placed in the nasolabial fold. The stouter and thickened muscles are outlined, and after careful dissection a 2 cm segment of muscle is removed.

Elevation and spasm of the contralateral forehead and eyebrow can be adjusted by myectomy. Through an incision of 2 cm or less at the upper median border of the eyebrow, the corrugator and procerus muscles are exposed, isolated, and resected. Since the procerus, frontalis, orbicularis oculi, and corrugator muscles act synergistically, a small median segment of the conjoint muscle of the first three muscles, which covers the corrugator muscle, is removed.

Face Lifts, Brow Lifts, and Excision of Redundant Skin and Mucosa

Removal of redundant skin and mucosa (Fig. 42–56), either by direct excision or the

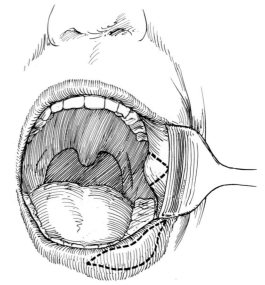

Figure 42–56. Excision of the redundant and hypertrophied buccal and labial mucosa affords access to the underlying musculature for repair of the diastasis. (From Freeman, B. S.: Late reconstruction of the lax oral sphincter in facial paralysis. Plast. Reconstr. Surg., *51*:144, 1973. Copyright ©1973. The Williams & Wilkins Company, Baltimore.)

various rhytidectomy techniques outlined in Chapter 43, may also be useful in balancing the paralyzed face and accomplishing a more esthetically pleasing result. Most often a combination of the foregoing techniques yields the maximal result.

TREATMENT OF THE PARALYZED EYELID

Facial paralysis affecting the orbicularis oculi muscle results in an inability to close the eyelids, a condition referred to as lagophthalmos (from the Greek word *lagos* meaning hare, an animal that sleeps with its eyes open). Because of the loss of orbicularis muscle tone, gravity pulls the atonic lower lid into a sagging position (ectropion). When the lower lid margin and lacrimal punctum are no longer in apposition with the globe, normal tear flow and the lacrimal drainage system are disturbed. Constant exposure of the cornea results in evaporation of the tear film, dryness of the cornea, and exposure keratitis. This condition may progress to infection, corneal ulceration, and eventual blindness. Fortunately, because of Bell's phenomenon, the eyeball rotates upward and the cornea comes to lie under the upper lid, helping to protect it from trauma and desiccation. However, in patients with a totally paralyzed orbicularis oculi this is usually insufficient to protect the eye.

Management of Lagophthalmos

NONSURGICAL METHODS

These methods are directed at providing comfort and protecting the cornea from trauma and drying. Numerous artificial tears and eye ointments (Jelks, Smith, and Bosniak, 1979) are available to keep the eye moist. Lid taping at night may also prevent corneal exposure during sleep. Other measures include occlusive moisture chambers, soft contact lenses and scleral shells (Goren and Clemis, 1973), and temporary lid suturing. These methods are most helpful in patients with acute facial paralysis in whom recovery of orbicularis oculi function is expected. However, if recovery does not occur or is incomplete, numerous surgical procedures are available to improve eyelid closure.

SURGICAL METHODS

It must be remembered that the ocular complications of orbicularis oculi paralysis follow a progressive course. It is therefore necessary to individualize procedures according to the degree of deformity and dysfunction. Furthermore, before dynamic lid procedures such as the application of lid weights, magnets, springs, or silicone strips can be attempted, it is necessary to repair any lid abnormalities, including paralytic ectropion. A protective program of ocular lubrication must also be well established.

Tarsorrhaphy

For many years lateral tarsorrhaphy was the accepted method for treating lagophthalmos in facial paralysis. The McLaughlin procedure (1953) is preferred because it preserves the lashes to camouflage the lateral lid adhesion. The disadvantages of tarsorrhaphy, however, are the narrowing of the lid aperture, a downward displacement of the lateral canthus, and difficulty in separating the lids without considerable residual deformity. The last-named may be a significant problem if the patient has return of orbicularis oculi function and the tarsorrhaphy is no longer needed. At present, horizontal lid shortening and medial and lateral canthoplasties are more popular in correcting ectropion and alleviating lagophthalmos.

Canthoplasties

Laxity of the lower lid or ectropion may be the prominent features of patients with facial paralysis. A standard wedge excision to obtain a horizontal shortening of the lower lid is often satisfactory in mild cases of lid laxity. However, with marked lower lid laxity, lateral canthoplasties that support the lower lid from the lateral orbital rim are the best reconstructive methods (Fig. 42–57). Edgerton and Wolfort (1969) were the first to describe a technique for support of the lower eyelids in patients with facial paralysis. Their technique employs a dermal flap secured to the lateral orbital rim. In 1978 Montandon modified this technique by incorporating a portion of the upper and lower eyelid margins with the dermal flap. There is also an occasional need for a medial canthoplasty in patients with facial paralysis (Fig. 42–58).

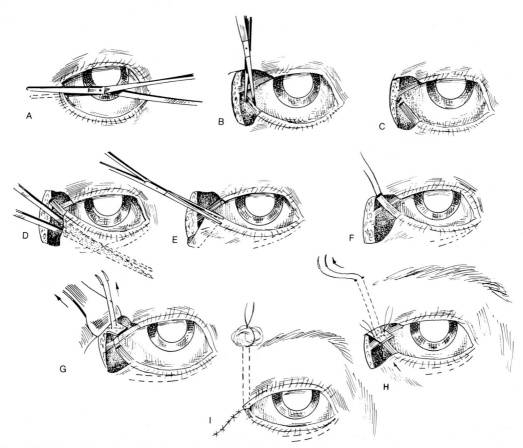

Figure 42–57. Lateral canthoplasty. *A,* Lateral canthotomy. *B, C,* The lateral canthal tendon is exposed and the lower limb of the tendon is divided at the orbital rim. *D,* Scissors undermine the skin of the lower lid and also cut retracting bands that connect the orbital rim to the tarsus of the lower lid. *E,* The desired position of the new lateral canthal angle is determined along the lower lid margin by placing upward and lateral traction on the lower lid. The lid margin is excised to this point. The dotted lines show the planned excision of excess orbicularis oculi muscle, cilia, and skin, leaving a long lower lid tarsal tongue. *F,* The lower lid tarsal tongue has a double-armed 4–0 silk suture passed through it. With this suture, the lower lid is elevated anterior and superior to the superior limb of the lateral canthal tendon (which is still attached to the lateral orbital rim). *G,* A laterally based flap of periosteum is developed from the orbital rim superior and lateral to the upper lid contribution to the lateral canthal tendon. The 4–0 silk suture is passed through the base of this flap. *H,* The suture is passed along a subcutaneous track to emerge superior to the lateral brow level. This suture is tied over a cotton bolster after adjusting the desired elevation and tightening of the lower lid. Two 4–0 Dexon sutures are used to reinforce the tarsal tongue–periosteal flap attachment. *I,* The final result shows slight overcorrection with the lateral lower lid elevated. The tendon can also be secured to a hole in the orbital rim. (From Jelks, G. W., Smith, B., and Bosniak, S.: The evaluation and management of the eye in facial palsy. Clin. Plast. Surg., 6:411, 1979.)

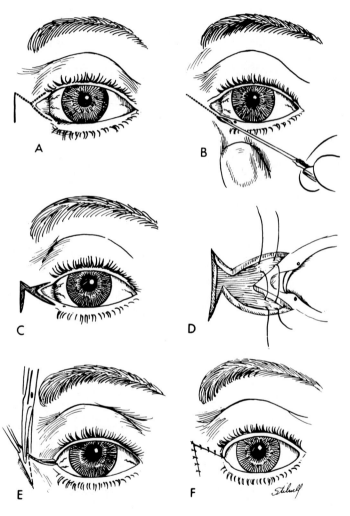

Figure 42–58. Medial canthoplasty, which places the everted punctum against the globe and tightens a moderately sagging lower lid. *A*, The outline of the incisions. *B*, A probe is placed in the canaliculus in order to avoid severing this structure. *C*, After completion of the incisions. *D*, The edges of the medial canthus are sutured by means of inverting sutures. *E*, Traction is placed on the skin flap, and excess skin is removed. *F*, The skin incision is sutured. (From Kazanjian and Converse.)

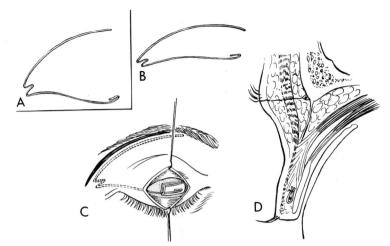

Figure 42–59. The palpebral spring in the treatment of paralysis of the eyelid (technique of Morel-Fatio). *A, B,* Stainless steel wire formed in the shape of a "W." *C,* Dacron felt covering over the doubled lower end. Note the incisions. *D,* Cross-sectional view.

The Morel-Fatio Spring (Morel-Fatio and Lalardrie, 1964) is a stainless steel wire formed into a figure "W," which is inserted into the upper lid to provide synchronous closure of the eye with levator relaxation (Fig. 42–59). At best, the results can be excellent, but a high rate of spring extrusion has decreased the popularity of this technique.

Morel-Fatio (1976) reported his results in 72 cases: 27 secondary operations were required; 11 complications occurred (five springs broke; two springs were extruded; infection occurred in four cases); and in five cases the spring was deliberately removed. In Guy's (1969) experience, using a slightly different technique, of a series of 24 patients, six springs were removed, eight required minor adjustments, and 18 were still functioning after three years.

Lid Magnets

Mühlbauer, Segeth, and Viessmann (1973) implanted two miniaturized, siliconized curved magnets beneath the orbicularis muscle near the upper and lower eyelid margins. The tarsal plates prevent erosion of the rods into the conjunctival sacs. The magnetic force employed in the open-eye position for the double-magnet system was 200 to 300 m p, and this corresponds to the absent muscle tone of the orbicularis muscle, thus preventing upper lid retraction, corneal irritation, and epiphora. Normal lid opening is maintained by the intact levator mechanism.

Initially the lid magnets are taped to the lid margins to determine the ideal magnet force. When this is established, the lid magnets are implanted under local anesthesia. The results with lid magnets can be excellent (Mühlbauer, 1977), but unfortunately the extrusion rate is unacceptably high.

Silicone Sling (Arion Prosthesis)

In 1972 Arion described a method of placing a silicone band in the lids inducing just enough tension to allow the lids to close with levator relaxation. The procedure has been modified by Wood-Smith (1973), as shown in Figure 42–60. Because silicone is a material that does not wear well, it is subject to stress, relaxation, and breakage. For this reason, there has not been much support for this technique.

Upper Lid Loading

A technique of accentuation of gravity by a weight (Fig. 42–61) in the lid was described by Sheehan (1927). He initially recommended the use of stainless steel mesh in the upper lid. According to Freeman (1979) tantalum, which is malleable, became available during World War II. It is nonreactive, can be readily fashioned during the operation, and has proved to be useful. The upper lid weight is increased by implanting a tantalum strip of 0.75 gm. Nonetheless, the various implants of gold seem to provide a better color match for white patients and have been commercially prepared (Jobe, 1974).

To assess the required load, a series of weights are taped to the eyelid until normal closure is obtained. This weight is then insor labii inferioris and the depressor anguli oris muscles. Thus, loss of function of the platysma muscle may cause a transient weakness in the depressor function of the lateral lower lip. However, loss of platysma function does not produce a permanent deficit in lower lip depression (Ellenbogen, 1979).

Two anatomic studies have directed specific attention to the anterior platysma muscle anatomy. Vistnes and Souther (1979) in 21 surgical and 14 cadaver specimens noted (1) platysma fiber decussation across the midline from the level of the hyoid to the border of the mandible in 61 per cent and (2) free medial platysma borders from the mandible to clavicles in 39 per cent. Cardoso de Castro (1980) in a study of 50 cadaver specimens divided the findings into three groups: (1) 1 to 2 cm of decussated fibers just below the mandibular border in 75 per cent, (2) decussation of fibers from the level of the thyroid cartilage up to the mandible in 15 per cent, and (3) free medial borders in 10 per cent (Fig. 43–46).

The important facts regarding the medial platysma anatomy can be summarized as follows: (1) the medial borders of the right and left platysma muscles are separated below the level of the hyoid bone in most patients; (2) the medial borders frequently produce vertical bands that patients wish to have eliminated; (3) above the level of the hyoid bone, some platysma fibers decussate from each side across the midline in 60 to 90 per cent of patients, although in some individuals the decussation involves only a few fibers; (4) a group of patients have undecussated medial platysma borders extending from the clavicles to the mandible; and (5) other variations of the medial platysma borders may be seen.

When muscle fiber decussation is absent or when high fusion occurs near the mentum (Vistnes and Souther, 1979; Cardoso de Castro, 1980), the medial borders of each muscle may form bilateral vertical platysma bands, sometimes referred to as the "turkey gobbler" deformity. In some patients, medial platysma fibers decussate across the midline above the

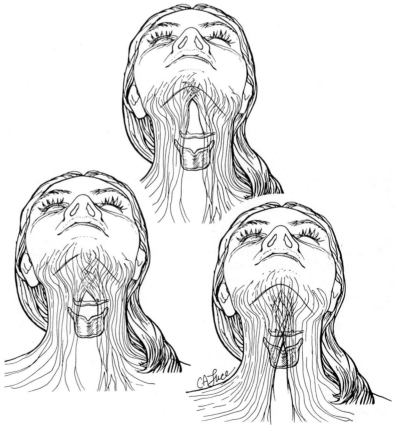

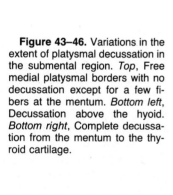

Figure 43–46. Variations in the extent of platysmal decussation in the submental region. *Top,* Free medial platysmal borders with no decussation except for a few fibers at the mentum. *Bottom left,* Decussation above the hyoid. *Bottom right,* Complete decussation from the mentum to the thyroid cartilage.

level of the hyoid, but platysma bands are nonetheless formed and lie lateral to the decussated fibers. In other words, the clinical presentation in these patients does not necessarily correlate with the actual anatomy seen during surgery.

SMAS ANATOMY

Mitz and Peyronie (1976) described in detail the anatomy of the superficial musculoaponeurotic system (SMAS) of the face. The SMAS is a layer of superficial fascia of the face most easily defined over the parotid gland and cheek area. The SMAS system is in continuity with the frontoparietal fascia and galea superiorly, and extends inferiorly where it is in continuity with the platysma muscle along the jawline and in the upper neck (see Fig. 43–45). According to the dissections of Mitz and Peyronie (1976), the SMAS overlies and is distinct from the parotid fascia.

The SMAS is attached to the dermis of the overlying skin by numerous fibrous septa that separate the subcutaneous tissue into many small fat lobules and establish multiple connections between the skin and underlying SMAS. The fascia is dense in the pretragal area and particularly over the parotid gland, but becomes thinner anterior to the border of the parotid gland. Anterior to the masseter muscle the SMAS separates the septated subcutaneous fat from the buccal fat pad of Bichat.

Only sensory nerves are located between the dermis and the SMAS; all motor nerves are deep to the SMAS and provide innervation via the deep surface of the respective facial muscles. Anterior to the parotid gland the SMAS becomes thin, and because the facial nerve branches lie immediately beneath this fragile layer, surgical dissection is difficult and dangerous in this region.

In the temporozygomatic area the SMAS is just superficial to the zygomatic arch. Since the frontal branch of the facial nerve lies deep to the SMAS, it is easily injured in this region.

Whether the SMAS inserts into the nasolabial fold or the nasolabial crease has been a subject of debate. Mitz and Peyronie (1976) stated that the SMAS appears to insert into the nasolabial fold. Webster and associates (1982), Owsley (1985), and Pensler, Ward, and Parry (1985) concluded that the SMAS

actually inserts into the nasolabial crease. Clinically the latter observation appears to be more accurate, as traction on the SMAS and facial animation deepen the fixed crease and increase the size of the mobile nasolabial fold.

Jost and Levet (1984) reported a study of animal and human dissections and concluded that the SMAS was actually a fibrous remnant of the primitive platysma muscle. In contrast to the finding of Mitz and Peyronie (1976), these authors believe that the SMAS forms the external surface of the parotid capsule, and therefore it is impossible to separate the SMAS from the parotid fascia. In practical terms one can accept either the description of Mitz and Peyronie (1976) or that of Jost and Levet (1984), because once it is dissected, traction on the SMAS is functionally the same. Lateral dissection and cephaloposterior traction on the SMAS produces a "pull" across the cheek and jawline. If correction of the patient's deformities has required extensive subcutaneous undermining, lifting of the SMAS changes the underlying foundation over which the skin is redraped. If the deformity is less severe and there is less skin undermining, lifting of the SMAS also elevates the skin via the intact connections into the dermis. As the SMAS is in continuity with the platysma, the SMAS and platysma are dissected in continuity and advanced as a single flap. Rotation and advancement of this additional layer formed by the SMAS-platysma lifts and contours the cheeks, jawline, and neck.

PLATYSMA TECHNIQUES

Surgical alteration of the platysma muscle can be performed at its lateral border, medial border, or both (Figs. 43–47, 43–48). The most frequently used lateral platysma modifications are (1) elevation and advancement of the lateral borders of the platysma without cutting the muscle, (2) partial-width (L-shaped platysma) flaps, and (3) full-width platysma muscle flaps. The surgeon can employ the following medial platysma modifications: (1) midline suturing of the platysma borders, (2) wedge resection of the anterior platysma borders, and (3) vertical resection of the redundant medial platysma bands. Regardless of which platysma techniques are chosen, complete SMAS-platysma dissection and advancement are performed.

Figure 43–47. Variations in platysma surgery. *A*, Cephaloposterior advancement of the SMAS-platysma flap without cutting the platysma laterally and without midline alteration. *B*, Rotation of the SMAS-platysma flap with a partial cut across the lateral platysma. *C*, Rotation of the SMAS-platysma flap with a partial lateral cut, plication of the medial platysma borders, and excision of a midline wedge to interrupt the continuity of the bands. *D*, SMAS-platysma flap, full-width platysma transection, and midline plication. Note that full-width transection extends from a level 6 cm below the mandibular angle to the thyroid cartilage. In addition the cut muscle edges are contoured under direct vision to avoid irregularities in the neck.

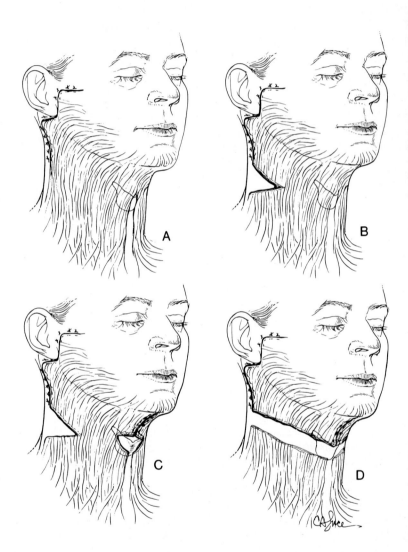

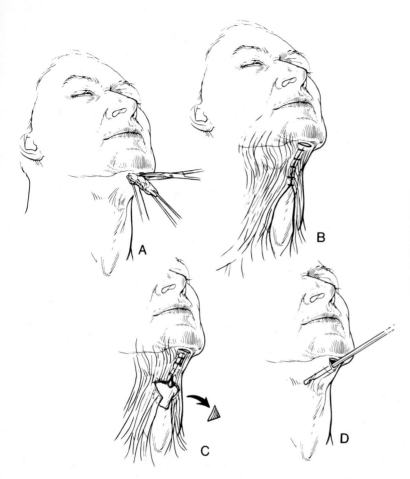

Figure 43–48. Variations in submental surgery. *A*, Fat removed from the submental region under direct vision. *B*, Midline plication of the platysma after submental defatting. *C*, Midline plication and excision of a muscle wedge after submental defatting. *D*, Defatting of the submental region using suction assisted lipectomy.

Full-Width Transection of Platysma

Full-width platysma transection (Fig. 43–47*D*) helps in obtaining the best possible result for patients when it is desirable to produce the maximal discrepancy in size between the mandible and the neck. This technique, like other new surgical procedures that require evaluation over the long term, was overused during the early stages of platysma surgery. There are, however, definite indications for its use. It is critical that the platysma be divided at least 6 cm below the mandibular border and that the cut edges of the muscle be beveled to yield a smooth contour.

Obtuse Cervicomental Angle. Patients with an obtuse cervicomental angle were previously considered by most plastic surgeons to be poor candidates for a rhytidoplasty (Fig. 43–49). Conventional face lifting procedures and submental lipectomy did little to correct the anatomic deformity of these patients and

sometimes resulted in other deformities. Submental lipectomy and submental skin excision may increase the obtuse angle deformity or cause a midline submental depression by removal of fat from the region between the medial borders of the platysma muscles. As there is a relative deficiency of skin on the anterior surface of the obtusely angled neck, excision of skin in the submental area exaggerates the deformity. Patients with an obtuse cervicomental angle are among those receiving the greatest benefit from full-width platysma division. Frequently these deformities have been present from childhood and can be dramatically improved.

Patients with an obtuse cervicomental angle can be divided into two categories: (1) those who have a true obtuse cervicomental angle and (2) those with a pseudo-obtuse cervicomental angle. In both groups, patients have a platysma veil across the anterolateral surfaces of the neck from the mandible to the clavicles, submental and submandibular fat

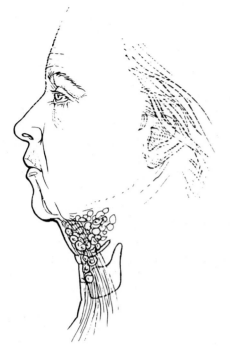

Figure 43–49. A true obtuse cervicomental angle with a low hyoid bone.

deposits, possible subplatysma fat deposits, and often microgenia. The difference between the two categories lies in the position of the hyoid bone relative to the chin.

The normal position for the hyoid bone is at the level of the third cervical vertebra. When it is lower, a true obtuse cervicomental angle exists. Patients with a pseudo-obtuse cervicomental angle have normal hyoid positions but appear to have obtuse cervicomental angles because of the platysmal veil over the anterior neck. Fat deposits may contribute to the deformity but are not the cause. In fact, fat deposits are often relatively small. Correction of both obtuse angle categories requires appropriate excision of fat, midline muscle stabilization, and full-width platysma muscle division. Interrupting the platysma veil is of major importance in deepening the cervicomental angle and defining the jawline.

The main difference in correcting the two categories of obtuse cervicomental angles relates to the level of platysma transection and midline suturing. When the hyoid bone is low, the platysma is transected just below the upper level of the thyroid cartilage so that the transected muscle retracts above the thyroid notch, allowing the thyroid cartilage to be visible on the anterior surface of the neck.

The prominence of the thyroid cartilage suggests a deeper cervicomental angle than is actually present. When the hyoid bone is in a normal position, better neck and jawline contouring is obtained by suturing the medial platysma borders together so as to cover the upper one-half to three-fourths of the thyroid cartilage. This creates a longer, straighter neck with a deepened cervicomental angle. When microgenia is a component of the deformity, a silicone chin implant dramatically improves the surgical result.

Narrow Mandible, Thick Necks, Fat Faces. Full-width platysma division is also used when it is desirable to decrease the apparent size of the neck relative to the cheeks and jawline (e.g., a narrow mandible in combination with a thick neck). Patients with a reduced transverse (bigonial) distance between the mandibular rami often present with a blending of the cheeks, jawline, and neck when seen on profile. Platysma transection helps to define the mandibular border and separates the neck and cheeks as specific anatomic areas. Some women have thick, masculine necks. Full-width platysma division produces more of a discrepancy between the jawline and neck, a result that is desirable because it makes the neck smaller as the platysmal veil is interrupted.

In patients with fat faces and necks in profile, the cheek, jawline, and neck often blend with little or no distinction between the anatomic areas, an appearance similar to that described for patients with narrow mandibles. Appropriate selective fat resection and resculpturing can often provide better definition and a more pleasing contour. For most of these patients, correction is usually obtained by lower facial, submental, and submandibular lipectomies; medial platysma suturing; full-width platysma transection; and cephaloposterior SMAS-platysma flap rotation.

Some patients with fat deposits in the submental and submandibular areas have a very thin, attenuated platysma muscle that need not be transected to contour the neck. These patients can usually be recognized preoperatively by a hanging fat waddle and distinct depressions in the neck at the anterior borders of the sternocleidomastoid muscles. For such patients, partial-width platysma flaps or cephaloposterior advancement of the uninterrupted lateral platysma border, midline platysma suturing, and anterior wedge resection yield a superior result.

The most difficult area for fat excision is the lower face extending across the mandibular border anterior to the submaxillary gland. Exposure through both submental and face lift incisions facilitates fat removal from this area. Suction assisted lipectomy under direct vision is of significant benefit in removing fat from this area.

The transition between the defatted platysma and the remaining cheek fat must be a gradual one, otherwise a line of demarcation will be obvious through the skin. Similarly, the junction between the defatted and nondefatted neck will be obvious unless it is smoothed by beveling and feathering of the fat. The platysma just below the mandibular border should not be completely defatted, nor should final jawline contouring be attempted until the SMAS-platysma flap has been sutured into its final position (Fig. 43–50). Otherwise, the defatted platysma lying just below the mandibular border will be rotated to lie along the mandible or higher, giving the lateral lower face a flat or depressed appearance. In addition, overresection of midline fat results in a concavity that is almost impossible to correct. The necessity for subplatysma fat excision is best determined after the platysma flaps have been sutured into the final lateral position, so that the cervical sling is tight and makes the anterior fat bulge more obvious.

The relative concavity on the anterior neck produced by fat resection takes up a large percentage of the apparent excess skin as it is redraped on the neck. Submental skin excision is rarely, if ever, necessary even in older patients when the neck is defatted in conjunction with a cervicofacial rhytidectomy.

Singer (1984) reported excellent results in young patients from extensive submandibular defatting and midline platysma alteration. A submental incision is made to provide exposure of the anterior platysma, which is modified as indicated. Suction assisted lipectomy has made this an even more favorable procedure, as the fat removal is done with minimal bleeding through small, stab incisions.

Partial-Width Platysma Flaps

Partial-width platysma L-shaped flaps help to define the posterior jawline and mandibular angles (see Fig. 43–47B, C). The break in continuity of the lateral platysma, the cephaloposterior platysma-SMAS rotation, and the redraping of the platysma beneath the posterior mandible produces a relative concavity anterior to the sternocleidomastoid muscle. The optimal results with lateral partial platysma division are achieved in patients with poorly defined posterior jawlines and moderately thin necks. In these patients, a full-width platysma division would produce an overoperated appearance of the neck.

When the mandibular angles are prominent and the neck shows depressions below the mandibular angles anterior to the sternocleidomastoid muscle, even partial transection of the platysma may cause a depression that is too deep at the angles of the mandible. Elevation and cephaloposterior advancement of the lateral platysma muscle border without transection prevents this problem (see Fig. 43–47A).

Slight and Moderate Platysma Laxity. Slight and moderate platysma muscle laxity associated with a well-developed mandible can be improved by SMAS-platysma flap advancement. If the lateral jawline needs defining, partial lateral platysma division enhances the contour. Suturing of the medial platysma borders is not needed when there is only slight laxity of the platysma. Moderate laxity may require midline platysma suturing to eliminate platysma laxity. Patients with slight or moderate laxity may require excision of localized fat deposits and, when indicated, small anterior muscle excisions may contribute to the final result. Although SMAS-platysma surgery may be eliminated

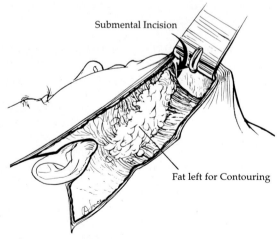

Submental Incision

Fat left for Contouring

Figure 43–50. Fat is intentionally left on the mandibular border for contouring to be done after the SMAS-platysma flap rotation.

in patients with slight to moderate platysma laxity, it is the opinion of the authors that the incidence of recurrent platysma laxity is lessened and the jawline contour improved for a longer period if SMAS-platysma tightening procedures are performed.

Midline Approximation of Platysma

The goals of midline platysma approximation (see Fig. 43–48C) are (1) elimination of free medial platysma borders or bands, (2) reduction of skin laxity, (3) stabilization of the cervical muscle sling, and (4) deepening of the cervical angle. Suture approximation of the medial platysma borders before the creation of platysma flaps laterally stabilizes the midline, producing a secure sling effect when the platysma flaps are advanced in a cephaloposterior direction. If the skin of the neck has not been adequately undermined, skin puckering occurs in the neck when the medial platysma borders are sutured. Midline platysma suturing is not indicated if (1) there is slight platysma laxity, (2) platysma bands are absent, and (3) there is a relatively normal cervicomental angle.

Vertical Platysma Bands. Vertical platysma bands are one of the most frequent complaints of patients requesting cervicofacialplasty, and frequently recur in the early postoperative period after conventional face lifting techniques.

Vertical bands on the anterior neck usually represent the free medial margins of the platysma muscle. Voluntary platysma contraction with the neck extended demonstrates the underlying platysma muscle and helps to define the full extent of the platysma bands. It is true that patients with a large number of decussated fibers in the midline do not usually have vertical bands, but it is not infrequent to find, at the time of surgery, platysmal bands lateral to the midline even though there is evidence of decussation of some medial platysma fibers. Regardless of the presence or absence of platysmal decussation, platysma bands are best eliminated by dealing directly with the bands, even if this requires suturing the medial platysma bands over the decussated fibers or excising the medial decussated fibers to eliminate bulk.

Advancement of Lateral SMAS-Platysma

In patients with slight platysma laxity, cephaloposterior advancement of the lateral

platysma and SMAS without partial muscle transection (see Fig. 43–47A) is a satisfactory technique for young face lift patients and patients with thin necks in whom partial muscle transection may give an "operated" look. This is similar to Skoog's (1974) technique, but as performed by the authors the subcutaneous dissection is much greater than that advocated by Skoog.

OPERATIVE TECHNIQUE OF SMAS-PLATYSMA CERVICOFACIALPLASTY

A wide cervicofacial skin flap dissection is performed as discussed above for the classic face lift operation. If indicated, a submental skin incision is made first. The anterior cervical area is undermined in the subcutaneous plane. Lateral to medial facial flap dissection establishes continuity with the anterior cervical flap dissection so that the face and neck are completely dissected and the anterior and lateral neck is completely exposed. Any excess fat is removed from the surface of the platysma muscle, care being taken to leave the fat along the mandibular border (and a distance of 2 cm below). Final fat resection and jawline contouring is done after the platysma-SMAS flap has been rotated and sutured into its final position. The medial platysma borders are sutured or resected as indicated by the anatomy of the individual patient.

SMAS-platysma flap dissection is performed as follows (Fig. 43–51). The lateral border of the platysma muscle is located at a point 5 cm below the angle of the mandible, by vacuuming the muscle with a suction cannula under direct vision. The border of the platysma muscle is grasped with tissue forceps and pulled laterally. This maneuver

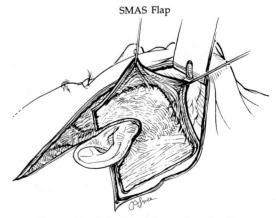

SMAS Flap

Figure 43–51. SMAS-platysma flap elevation.

places tension on the platysma muscle, making it easier to pass the scissor tips between the anterior border of the sternocleidomastoid muscle and the posterior surface of the platysma muscle. The scissor blades pass just superficial to the external jugular vein and the great auricular nerve. This establishes the lateral border of the platysma muscle at approximately 5 cm below the angle of the mandible. The lateral platysma border is dissected inferiorly for another 3 to 4 cm. Attention is directed to the SMAS dissection.

SMAS dissection is begun with a 4 cm transverse incision through the SMAS at the level of the inferior border of the zygomatic arch (Fig. 43–51). An attempt is made to divide only the SMAS, sparing the parotid fascia. A vertical incision is made approximately 0.5 cm anterior to the tragus and extended from the level of the transverse SMAS incision, passing inferiorly and posteriorly to the mandibular angle to connect with the previously defined lateral margin of the platysma muscle. The lateral borders of the SMAS and platysma are thus dissected in continuity. The SMAS is elevated from the parotid fascia by scalpel dissection. The SMAS dissection extends at least to the anterior border of the parotid gland and is usually carried anteriorly onto the surface of the masseter muscle. Occasionally, when the SMAS is thin, the SMAS and parotid fascia are dissected together. Dissection deep to the parotid fascia has not resulted in complications; however, there generally is more bleeding if the parotid fascia is violated. Buccal and marginal mandibular nerve branches are frequently seen lying on the masseter muscle deep to the thin areolar layer anterior to the parotid gland. Platysma undermining is carried anteriorly to the same extent as SMAS dissection.

When the desired dissection of the SMAS-platysma flap is completed in a medial direction, the lateral platysma muscle can be altered as indicated by the specific anatomy of the patient (partial transection, full-width transection, or no transection) (Fig. 43–52). The dissected SMAS-platysma border is grasped with an Allis clamp at the level of the transverse SMAS cut, and with a second clamp 5 cm below the angle of the mandible. Cephaloposterior rotation of the flap produces tension on the platysma muscle and lifts the jawline and lower one-third of the face. The SMAS-platysma flap can be secured in the lifted position without altering the platysma muscle further. When platysma division (partial or full width) is indicated, the scissor tips are used to cut the muscle fibers under direct vision. Any muscle transection begins at least 6 cm below the angle of the mandible and transverses the neck on a line parallel to the border of the mandible. The platysma-SMAS flap is rotated in a cephaloposterior direction, the excess SMAS-platysma is excised (Fig. 43–53), and the flap is sutured into final position by using buried horizontal mattress sutures of 4–0 white Mersilene.

The first horizontal mattress suture secures the lateral platysma border to the sternocleidomastoid muscle fascia. A triangle of redundant rotated SMAS is excised at the level of the zygomatic arch, and the resultant transverse incision is sutured with two or three buried figure-of-eight sutures to fix the SMAS flap into position. Several buried horizontal mattress sutures complete the fixation of the lateral SMAS-platysma to the upper sternocleidomastoid fascia. The lateral edge of the flap is thinned with scissors or a suction cannula in order to blend it into the underlying tissue and eliminate a visible or palpable ridge. The upper and lower edges of the platysma caused by the platysma transection are also feathered into the underlying fascia. It is at this point that final contouring of the residual fat is performed by using either scissors or a suction cannula under direct vision (Fig. 43–54).

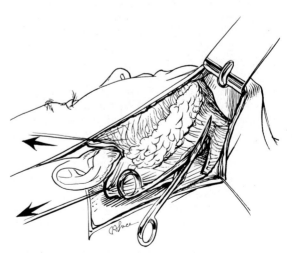

Figure 43–52. A partial cut in the lateral platysma is made while tension is maintained on the SMAS-platysma flap.

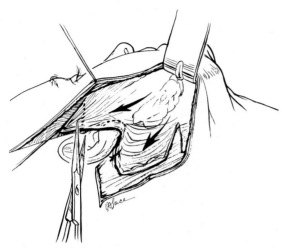

Figure 43–53. Redraping and trimming of the SMAS flap.

OPERATIVE TECHNIQUE OF SUBMENTAL LIPECTOMY

In patients who require submental lipectomy or surgery on the medial borders of the platysma muscle, the cervicofacialplasty is begun with a submental incision. The incision is made in the submental crease in males when an incision may produce a scar that bears no hair. In females the incision is made slightly anterior to the crease to help to offset, rather than deepen, the submental crease. The neck is hyperextended in order to tighten the anterior neck skin, facilitating scissor dissection of the flap. It is critical to leave a layer of subcutaneous fat 2 to 3 mm in thickness on the undersurface of the anterior neck skin. The remaining fat is resected down to

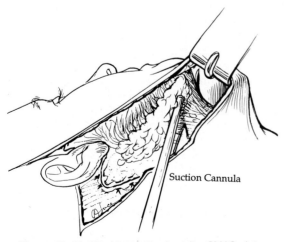

Suction Cannula

Figure 43–54. Final fat contouring after SMAS-platysma flap advancement.

the surface of the platysma muscle. Medial subplatysmal fat is resected if there is a subplatysmal bulge, but care is taken not to cause a depression in the midline by excessive fat resection. Fat removal laterally must be graduated if the lipectomy is being performed as an isolated procedure. Suction assisted lipectomy facilitates fat removal and contouring. When performed as part of a cervicofacialplasty with in-continuity dissection of cervical and facial flaps, the fat on the surface of the platysma is resected or suctioned from a lateral to a medial direction (after rotation and fixation of the SMAS-platysma) to join the defatted submental area. The defatting extends inferiorly as far as necessary to obtain the desired neck contour. Any fat remaining on the surface of the platysma near the mandibular border may be accentuated by platysma transection, which decreases the circumference of the neck below the transected muscle edge.

Secondary surgery designed to correct residual fat deposits usually requires complete undermining of the facial flaps and reopening of the submental incision to provide the same exposure required for the primary operation. Suction assisted lipectomy can be used in secondary procedures for isolated fat removal when further skin redraping is not needed.

Frequently, the patient presenting with facial aging suffers from ptosis of the soft tissue of the chin or a "witch's chin" deformity. The correction of the cleft between the drooping chin and cervical region requires soft tissue to fill the defect. No single method has consistently succeeded in correcting this problem, including external triangular or elliptic excisions and internal shifting of the medial raphé. Peterson's (1982) experience with local dermal-fat and platysma flaps was of improvement in his hands. For the chin with adequate vertical height and projection, anterior advancement and anchoring to the mentum of a posteriorly based elliptic dermis-fat flap is advised (Peterson, 1982). If the chin lacks vertical height and anterior projection, distributing the drooping chin by posterior advancement of an anteriorly based dermis-fat flap to the underlying platysma with augmentation mentoplasty has been suggested.

ANCILLARY PROCEDURES

Chin Implant. Some degree of microgenia is a frequently seen deformity in patients requesting facialplasty. A silicone chin implant can provide considerable improvement in skeletal proportions. Standard stock sizes can also be carved to the appropriate size and shape. A small implant is all that is usually needed. It is better to be conservative in this body image changing procedure. The submental approach for placing a chin implant has the advantage that the implant can be sutured to the inferior border of the mandible, thus securing the implant position. Inserting the implant at the end of the facialplasty just before applying the dressing reduces the risk of inadvertent movement of the implant during surgery.

Cheek Implants. The midface of some patients may be partially recontoured by augmenting a depressed malar region with a prosthesis (Hinderer, 1975). This can be accomplished by an intraoral, subciliary, or face lift approach. The intraoral approach is preferred (see Chap. 33).

A 2 to 3 cm incision is made in the upper buccal mucosa perpendicular to the upper first premolar and extended through the periosteum of the maxilla. A subperiosteal pocket is made only sufficiently large to accommodate the implant. Dissection in this region is relatively easy but must be done with caution. Direct vision or palpation of the infraorbital foramen and nerve is necessary.

Excluding the possibility of an infection, there are three main problems associated with cheek implants: (1) difficulty in obtaining symmetric placement, (2) difficulty in maintaining the implant in the exact position desired, and (3) the appearance of "something under the skin" after a fibrous capsule has occurred. The ideal cheek implant has not yet been developed and the above complications are sufficiently frequent for the procedure to be reserved for severe deformities.

Buccal Fat Pad Excision. This maneuver may further enhance the angularity of the zygomatic prominence and reduce the fullness of the cheeks in both old and young patients. The buccal fat pad can be removed through either an intraoral or a face lift incision. The intraoral incision begins at the first premolar and extends posteriorly for 2 cm, leaving a generous cuff of cheek mucosa parallel to the upper buccal sulcus. The fibers of the buccinator are separated by blunt dissection. Scissors are introduced in the direction of the temporomandibular joint to expose the well-defined yellow buccal fat pad (Bi-

chat) within its thin capsule. Gentle traction with forceps draws the fat into the oral cavity. Small vessels in the pedicle are clamped and electrocoagulated before the fat pad is excised. The pocket is packed with a wet sponge, which is removed after five minutes. The oral mucosa is approximated with absorbable sutures. There usually is moderate trismus, which spontaneously disappears in a few days.

An alternative method is to remove the buccal fat pad under direct vision beneath the facial skin flap. A fingertip is placed anterior to the masseter into the buccal fat pad space to identify the exact location. Tissue forceps are used to grasp the SMAS just over the fat pad and retract it gently toward the ear. Blunt-tipped scissors are advanced into the fat pad space between the buccal branches of the facial nerve and the tips are spread. The light yellow fat pad is seen, grasped with the forceps, and easily delivered. The base of the fat pad containing one or two small vessels is electrocoagulated and the fat removed.

DRESSING

At the end of the face lift procedure, a large-tooth comb is used to remove loose hair and dried blood. The face and hair are washed gently with benzalkonium chloride, and all hair tangles and snarls are removed. Flat cotton strips soaked in mineral oil are placed over the incisions and along the jawline. Gauze sponges are placed over the cheeks, and an elastic net dressing is placed over the head and opened in the front to expose the face and eyes. The dressing serves to cushion the skin flaps, helps to eliminate dead space beneath the flaps, absorbs drainage, and reminds the patient that there has been a surgical procedure. It is *not* a pressure dressing and it should be noted that an excessively tight dressing (1) is extremely uncomfortable, (2) does nothing to prevent hematoma formation, and (3) causes increased swelling by occluding venous and lymphatic outflow.

Selected case studies are illustrated in Figures 43–55 to 43–61.

Secondary Facialplasty

It is impossible to predict when a secondary face lift will be required, whether the primary

Text continued on page 2392

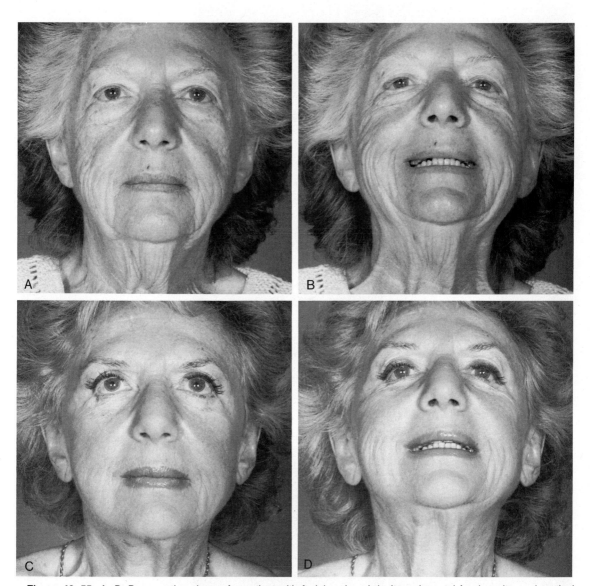

Figure 43–55. *A, B,* Preoperative views of a patient with facial and neck laxity, submental fat deposits, and vertical platysma bands extending from the anterior border of the mandible to the clavicles. *C, D,* Vertical platysma bands persist 13 months after facialplasty, submental lipectomy, partial lateral platysma division, and rotation of lateral platysma-SMAS flaps. Midline platysma suturing and anterior wedge resection of platysma muscle would have eliminated the vertical platysma bands.

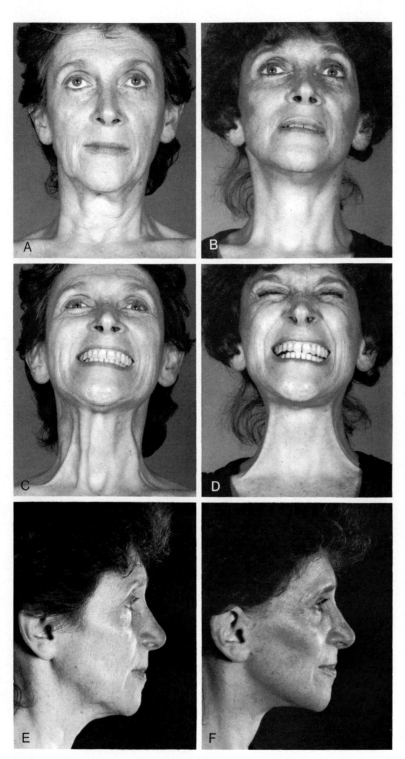

Figure 43–56. *A, C, E,* Preoperative views of a patient with facial and neck laxity, midline vertical platysma bands, and poor delineation of the posterior mandibular border. *B, D, F,* Elimination of the midline vertical platysma bands, deepening of the cervicomental angle, and posterior mandibular contouring by midline platysma suturing, anterior platysma wedge resection, partial lateral platysma division, and rotation of platysma-SMAS flaps. Animation photographs confirm the elimination of the midline platysma bands but the retained continuity of the midplatysma muscle.

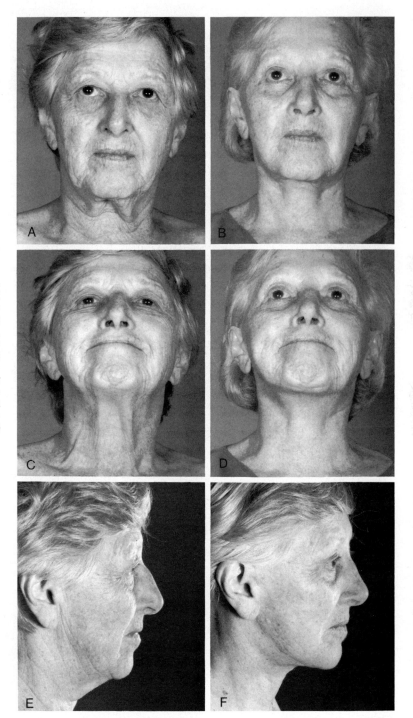

Figure 43–57. *A, C, E,* Preoperative views of a patient with facial and neck laxity, midline vertical platysma bands and lack of definition of the entire mandibular border. *B, D, F,* Elimination of the vertical platysma bands, deepending of the cervicomental angle, and contouring of the entire mandibular border by midline platysma suturing, full-width transection of the platysma muscle, and rotation of the platysma-SMAS flaps. The patient also underwent an eyelidplasty.

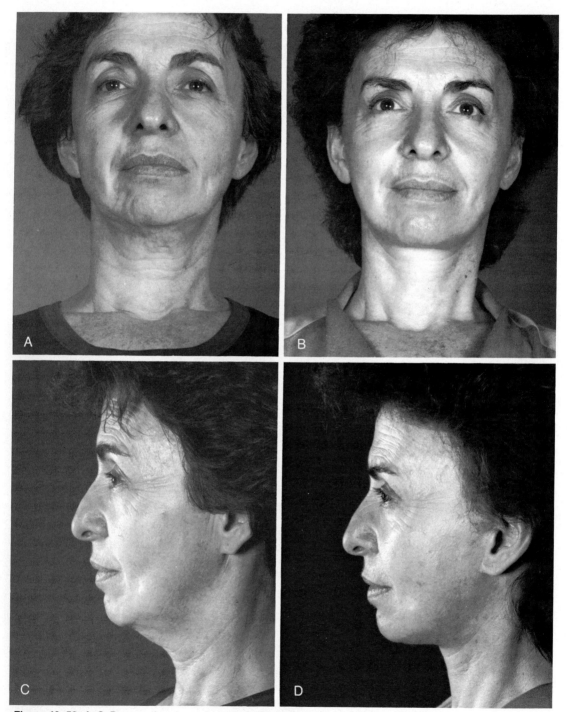

Figure 43–58. *A, C,* Preoperative views of a patient with facial and neck laxity, small submental and submandibular fat deposits, and lack of jawline definition. *B, D,* Correction of facial and neck laxity by wide subcutaneous undermining, submental and submandibular lipectomy, partial lateral platysma division, and rotation of lateral platysma-SMAS flaps without midline platysma sutures.

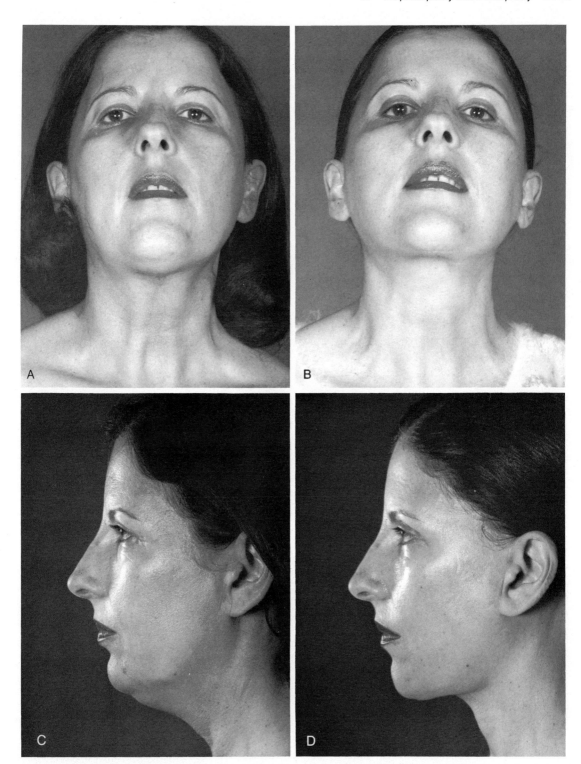

Figure 43–59. *A, C,* Preoperative views of a patient with a pseudo-obtuse cervicomental angle with small submental and submandibular fat deposits. Note the flatness at the angles of the mandible and the ptotic submandibular glands. *B, D,* Deepening of the cervicomental angle and jawline contouring by submental and submandibular lipectomy, midline suturing of the platysma muscle, and full-width platysma transection. Midline platysma approximation covered the upper one-half of the thyroid cartilage.

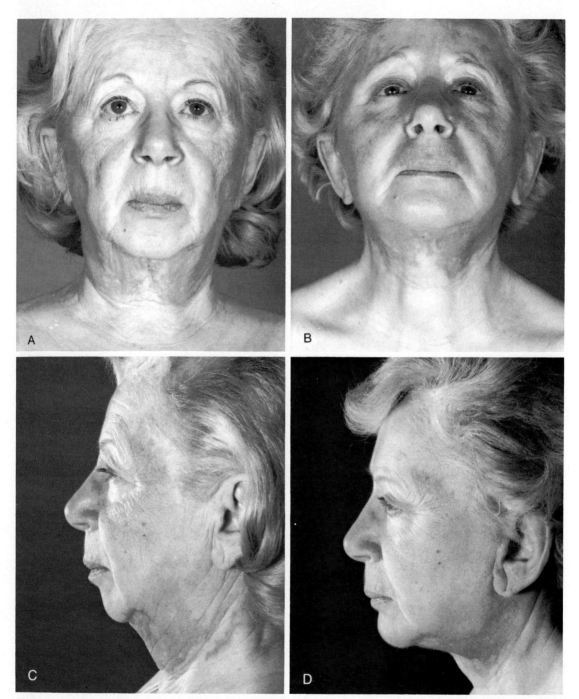

Figure 43–60. *A, C*, Preoperative views of a patient with facial and neck laxity, an obtuse cervicomental angle, inferiorly positioned hyoid bone, and microgenia. There is no distinction between the cheeks, jawline, and neck. *B, D*, Jawline contouring separating the cheeks from the neck, correction of the obtuse cervicomental angle and microgenia by submental and submandibular lipectomies, midline platysma suturing, full-width platysma transection, lateral rotation of platysma-SMAS flaps, and insertion of a Silastic chin implant. The platysma was transected at the upper margin of the thyroid cartilage.

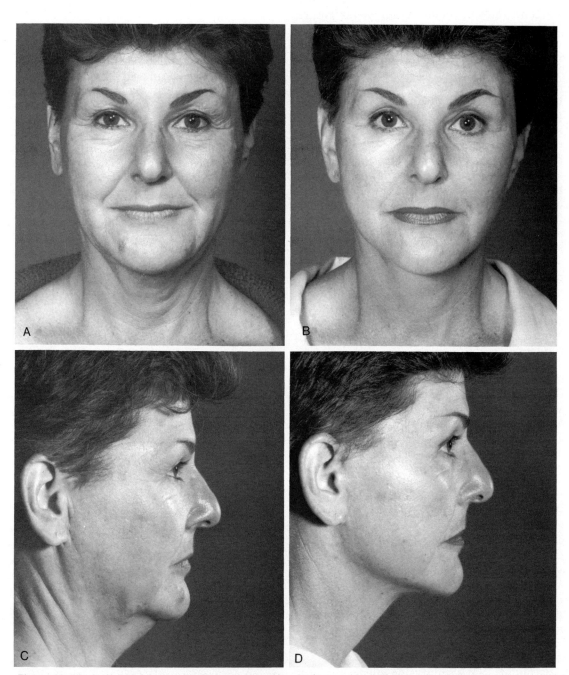

Figure 43–61. *A, C,* Preoperative views of a patient with a fat face and neck, facial and neck laxity, heavy nasolabial folds, an obtuse cervicomental angle, and lack of jawline definition. *B, D,* Improvement in the nasolabial folds, deepening of the cervicomental angle, and contouring of the mandibular border by suction lipectomy across the cheeks, wide facial and cervical skin undermining, submental and submandibular lipectomies, midline platysma suturing, full-width platysma transection, and rotation of lateral platysma-SMAS flaps.

operation was a subcutaneous procedure or an SMAS-platysma procedure. The benefit of the operation is permanent in that the skin, fat, and muscle removed can never return. However, the aging process continues, and between five and ten years later the patient may wish to undergo the procedure again. Younger patients, in whom the degenerative process of aging has not destroyed the elasticity of the skin, usually enjoy a longer period before a secondary procedure is desired. The aims of secondary face lifting are (1) to relift the face and neck, (2) to remove the primary surgical scars, and (3) to preserve a maximal amount of temporal and sideburn hair. This last goal frequently requires variations from the primary face lift incisions. Most often a transverse cut made under a sideburn helps to preserve the temporal and sideburn hair.

Secondary flap dissection is usually technically easier than the primary dissection, unless there was a hematoma at the time of the primary lift. There is generally less intraoperative bleeding during a secondary procedure and postoperative hematomas are less common.

The amount of skin excised at a secondary (or tertiary or quaternary) lift is much less than at a primary facialplasty. For this reason, one should never preexcise any skin in a secondary face lift. The skin is undermined, a small amount is resected, and the remainder is redistributed to a more cephaloposterior position. As in primary facialplasty, skin tension should be moderate at the "key" sutures above and behind the ear and there should be no tension in the preauricular region. The benefit of face lifting comes from undermining and flap rotation, not skin tension. As the skin ages and the degenerative aging process continues, repeated face lifting with *excess* tension causes the skin to look stretched and masklike. The great popularity of face lifting began approximately 20 years ago. Consequently, an ever-increasing number of patients are now requesting secondary, tertiary, and quaternary face lifts.

Secondary SMAS-platysma surgery is performed as indicated according to the anatomy. If midline platysma suturing was performed at a primary face lift, lateral SMAS-platysma work alone may accomplish the desired result. Secondary SMAS-platysma dissection requires considerable care and attention, because tissue planes, and possibly the location

of facial nerve branches, may be distorted by previous surgery.

Male Facialplasty

In the past decade the social and psychologic barriers against male face lifts have been broken. Most plastic surgeons have noted a definite change in the type of man seeking esthetic surgery. Previously, face lifting was an operation for men in the "spotlight." Today, business executives, doctors, lawyers, stockbrokers, cab drivers, and athletes want to look "well" and physically fit. Baker and Gordon (1969) described two categories of male face lift candidates: (1) well-adjusted, married businessmen in their early 50's; and (2) esthetic surgery—oriented single men in their late 40's or early 50's, many of whom have had cosmetic surgical procedures before the time of their face lift. These two categories were also described by Baker and associates (1977).

Cervicofacial rhytidectomy for males differs from the same operation in females. In general, the following characteristics hold true for male face lifting: (1) the skin is thicker and more rubbery than female skin; (2) fibrous connections between the SMAS and the overlying dermis are more numerous and more tenacious, making the dissection considerably more difficult; (3) there is more intraoperative and postoperative bleeding than in females, the incidence of hematomas being twice as high; (4) postoperative edema in the skin and subcutaneous tissue persists longer than in females; (5) the platysma muscle and SMAS are usually thicker than in females; (6) during surgery, male patients are usually less cooperative than females and require more premedication, anesthesia, and surgical time; and (7) the result is often less dramatic.

SURGICAL INCISIONS

A point of controversy among plastic surgeons regarding male face lifts has been the location of the surgical incisions. Incisions are more difficult to camouflage in most men because of their relatively short haircuts. Also, the beard and sideburns must be dealt with appropriately.

Many surgeons have advocated preserving the area of hairless skin or at least a portion of it between the tragus of the ear and the sideburn. Incisions designed to leave a large strip of non–hair-bearing skin in the preauricular area may eliminate the sideburn when the flap is pulled back and excess skin is resected. Other surgeons have advocated an incision extending horizontally at the level of the temporal hairline and connecting with the lateral extension of the blepharoplasty incision. For most patients these incisions are unnecessary and undesirable. Most male patients prefer incisions that can be well camouflaged within their hair and that do not distort the hairline. The loss of beardless skin in the preauricular area is less of a handicap if the sideburns are preserved. Care must be taken to prevent making a "stair step" in the hairline in the mastoid area. Such an irregularity can be quite obvious with a short hairstyle, but it may be unavoidable in extreme cases of redundant skin. By moving the face lift flaps in the cephaloposterior direction, the facial beard is also displaced behind the ear. Patients should be advised beforehand that they will have to shave in this area. In most male patients, incisions should not vary a great deal from those used in females. The incision begins in the temporal hair and extends caudally in the natural preauricular skin crease, passing anterior to the tragus and curving under the earlobe. A small footplate of beardless skin is left just behind the earlobe to avoid bringing the beard into this area. The incision continues posteriorly behind the ear and lies in the postauricular sulcus. The upper limit of the postauricular incision is at least as high as the point at which the ear covers the posterior hairline. The posterior incision extends horizontally into the mastoid scalp and must be long enough to accommodate redraping of all excess skin.

A large percentage of male patients, just like females, require a submental incision for lipectomy or surgery on the medial borders of the platysma muscle. In males it is especially important to place the incision in the submental skin crease as opposed to a position lower on the neck. If there is more than a very thin beard, a scar lower on the neck will be obvious owing to the lack of beard growth in the scar.

Skin flap undermining should extend superiorly across the malar prominences and medially to the nasolabial folds, as indicated by the individual deformity. Undermining of the cervical skin flaps across the midline, giving complete continuity of flap dissection, is usually necessary. Submental skin excision is almost never necessary in male or female patients because (1) extensive undermining permits cephaloposterior skin advancement and resection laterally and (2) some apparent excess skin is used to fill the space created by cervical fat excision and platysma muscle tightening. However, submental skin excision is more often needed in males than in females because of the rubbery skin texture and excess in the former. If the incision is maintained in the submental skin crease, the scar will be relatively inconspicuous. When there is marked redundant skin on the anterior surface of the neck, some surgeons have advocated H-type incisions, W-plasties, and Z-plasties (Johnson and Hadley, 1964; Adamson, Horton, and Crawford, 1964; Morel-Fatio, 1964; Conley, 1968; Cronin and Biggs, 1971; Cannon and Pantazelos, 1971; Gurdin and Carlin, 1972). Scars produced by these incisions are almost always unsightly and are rarely, if ever, indicated.

Complications

Every surgical procedure has associated complications. Those occurring after facialplasty may be of minor significance, such as temporary hair loss in the temporal area, or of major significance, such as slough of a large area of preauricular skin (Table 43–2). In addition, patients vary considerably in their ability to deal with complications. One patient may be frantic over a 1 cm postauricular skin slough, while another may demonstrate only minimal anxiety while awaiting a marginal mandibular paresis to subside. When complications occur, the surgeon must acknowledge them (to himself and the patient), take appropriate measures to remedy the problem, and be available to see the patient and discuss the situation as often as necessary.

HEMATOMAS

Hematomas, the most frequent complication after rhytidectomy, vary from a large collection of blood that threatens skin flap survival to small collections that are only obvious when facial edema subsides. Most expanding hematomas occur during the first

Table 43–2. Complications After Face Lift

Author (Year)	No. of Pts	% Hematomas	No. of Pts	% Facial Nerve Palsies	No. of Pts	% Skin Sloughs	No. of Pts	% Hair Loss
Subcutaneous Without SMAS								
Baker and Gordon, 1967	300	0.3	300	0.6	300	0	—	—
Conway, 1970	325	6.5	325	0.6	325	0.3	325	0
Pitanguy et al., 1971	1600	5.5	—	—	—	—	—	
Mcgregor and Greenberg, 1972	527	8.1	527	2.6	527	3.0	527	2.8
McDowell, 1972	105	2.9	105	2.0	105	0.9	105	0
Stark, 1972	100	3.0	—	—	—	—	—	—
Webster, 1972	221	0.9	—	—	—	—	—	—
Gleason, 1973	102	1.0	102	0.9	102	2.9	—	—
Morgan, 1973	40	2.5	—	—	—	—	—	—
Pitanguy et al., 1973	52	7.7	52	0	52	0	52	1.9
Rees et al., 1973	806	2.9	—	—	—	—	—	—
Barker, 1974	151	1.3	—	—	—	—	—	—
Stark, 1977	500	2.6	500	0.4	500	0.2	500	0.2
Leist et al., 1977	324	5.9	324	0.9	324	0.9	324	3.0
Baker et al., 1977	1500	3.1	1500	0.5	1500	1.1	—	–
Thompson and Ashley, 1978	922	4.8	922	0.6	922	14.2	—	—
Baker, 1983	9460	3.3	6119	0.9	—	—	—	—
Cohen and Webster, 1983	149	0	149	2.0	149	0	149	1.3
	Total	3.5%	Total	1%	Total	2.1%	Total	1.3%
With SMAS								
Lemmon and Hamra, 1980	577	0.8	577	1.7	577	0.8	577	0.5
Hugo, 1980	82	2.4	82	2.4	82	2.4	82	0
Matsunaga, 1981	427	0.2	427	0	427	0.2	427	0.2
Owsley, 1983	460	1.3	460	2.8	460	0	435	2.3
Lemmon, 1983	1449	0.5	1449	4.6	1449	0	—	—
	Total	1%	Total	2.2%	Total	0.7%	Total	0.9%

Compiled from tables in Barton, F. Jr.: The aging face/rhytidectomy. Select Read Plast Surg, 4, No. 20, 1987.

10 to 12 hours postoperatively. The usual scenario is that the patient becomes apprehensive and restless and experiences pain isolated to one side of the face or neck. Pain is extremely unusual after an uncomplicated face lift and is a sign of a hematoma until it is proved otherwise. Likewise, unilateral facial fullness, swelling of the lips, ecchymosis of the buccal mucosa, and excessive periorbital edema and ecchymosis are signs of a hematoma until this is proved not to be the case.

If the above signs and symptoms are present, the dressing should be removed immediately to permit accurate examination. Analgesics should not be given to alleviate pain until the patient is examined. In addition to causing skin flap ischemia, a large bilateral expanding hematoma under tight skin flaps has the potential to cause respiratory compromise, which could be made worse by sedatives and analgesics.

The etiology of hematomas is multifactorial (Pitanguy, Cansancao, and Daher, 1971; McDowell, 1972; Stark, 1972; Webster, 1972; Rees, Lee, and Coburn, 1973). Most often there is little correlation between the amount of intraoperative bleeding and postoperative hematoma formation; the patient in whom hemostasis was easily achieved intraoperatively is just as likely to bleed postoperatively as the patient who required additional operating time to obtain hemostasis.

Most anti-inflammatory agents (vitamin E, aspirin, and aspirin-containing products such as Alka-Seltzer, Anacin, Bufferin, Darvon Compound, Empirin, Excedrin, and Midol) interfere with platelet aggregation and should not be taken for 12 to 14 days preoperatively and seven to eight days postoperatively. Likewise, any other drugs (such as clofibrate, dipyridamole, and sulfinpyrazone) with anticoagulating properties are discontinued for a sufficient preoperative period for all pharmacologic properties to be eliminated.

Rees and Aston (1978) and Baker (1983)

reviewed and discussed possible causes of hematoma following rhytidectomy. Rees, Lee, and Coburn (1973), in a retrospective study of 23 hematomas in 806 rhytidectomy patients, noted an association with blood pressure elevation in the immediate postoperative period and the development of hematomas at that time. Transient increases in blood pressure and hematoma formation are also associated with (1) upper respiratory infection with coughing, (2) vomiting or wretching, and (3) episodes of hyperkinesia.

Stark (1972, 1977) suggested general anesthesia with controlled hypotension to help prevent hematoma formation. However, Rees, Lee, and Coburn (1973) reported that general anesthesia was used in 20 of 23 rhytidectomy patients who developed hematomas and, in addition, 12 of the 20 had controlled hypotension with systolic pressures of 60 to 80 mm Hg during surgery. These findings are explainable if not predictable. Both the low perfusion pressure and the vasoconstriction caused by the hemostatic solution prevent bleeding intraoperatively, but after the blood pressure returns to normal in the postoperative period, uncoagulated vessels may begin bleeding. Berner, Morain, and Noe (1976) evaluated 202 rhytidectomy patients and found that, in general, during the first two postoperative hours, blood pressure recordings did not deviate significantly from the preoperative levels. In the succeeding three hours, when postoperative and intraoperative medications lost their effect, there was considerable blood pressure elevation. The authors suggested that chlorpromazine (Thorazine) be used in the early postoperative course to reduce the "reactive hypertension" associated with hematoma formation. Straith, Raju, and Hipps (1977) evaluated 500 consecutive rhytidectomy patients and found that patients with blood pressures above 150/100 mm Hg on admission developed hematomas 2.6 times more often than normotensive patients.

The reported incidence of major hematomas (expanding, large hematomas) requiring surgical evacuation ranges from 0.9 per cent (Webster, 1972) to 8 per cent (McDowell, 1972). Baker and associates (1977) compiled statistics on 7700 rhytidectomy patients, 4 to 5 per cent of whom were male, and found the average incidence of major hematomas to be 3.7 per cent.

The incidence of hematomas in males is more than twice that in females. Pitanguy and associates (1973) reported a series specifically dealing with males and noted hematomas in 7.7 per cent. In the series of Baker and associates (1977) of 130 male face lifts, the incidence of hematomas requiring operative evacuation was 8.7 per cent.

The question why hematomas in males should necessarily be higher than in females has not been answered definitively. The male skin is thicker and more sebaceous than the female facial skin, and the blood vessels are larger. The vascular supply around the hair follicles in the male beard may represent a significant difference between males and females.

The treatment of expanding hematomas is always surgical. When a large hematoma is present, there is usually tension on the skin flaps with some degree of circulatory compromise. Sutures should be removed to relieve tension on the skin flaps while making preparations for surgery. The patient's anxiety and discomfort usually make general anesthesia preferable for hematoma evacuation. After the patient has been sterilely prepared, all sutures are removed; the facial flaps are elevated for visualization and the hematoma is completely evacuated. A fiberoptic retractor provides a valuable light source for this procedure. After removal of large blood clots, vigorous irrigation of sterile saline washes away clinging small clots and aids in visualization of any bleeding vessels. A single bleeding vessel is rarely detected.

Small hematomas of 2 to 20 ml, which are not usually visible until edema begins to subside, occur in approximately 10 to 15 per cent of patients. Initially, a small area of firmness is palpable, followed by ecchymosis in the overlying skin, and, depending on the amount of hematoma present, the skin surface may become irregular. Between the seventh and tenth day small hematomas liquefy, making it possible to express most of the blood by fingertip manipulation through a small stab incision. A No. 11 knife blade placed tangentially through the skin gives access to the blood, and the scar heals extremely well. A small Silastic cannula (butterfly intravenous tubing) inserted in the stab wound can be manipulated to remove the blood without the skin trauma caused by finger manipulation. Small hematomas can occasionally be aspirated by using a 5 ml syringe and a 15 or 16 gauge needle. Either technique must be repeated on two to four successive days in order to remove as much blood as possible.

Hematomas not detected and evacuated during the period of clot liquefication result in skin firmness, irregularity, and discoloration that may persist for several weeks to months. On occasion, the hemosiderin deposits in the skin result in permanent discoloration. Most patients need psychologic support. Warm compresses and gentle daily massage by the patient may be helpful by making the patient an active participant in the healing process. Small intralesional injections of dilute steroids are occasionally helpful. Large-dose steroid injection will produce subcutaneous fat atrophy and a depression when the hematoma has resolved.

SKIN SLOUGH

All skin sloughs are caused by vascular compromise of the involved tissue. A full-thickness skin slough in a visible area of the face and neck is a devastating complication that results in some degree of permanent scarring. A superficial slough of the epidermis usually heals with little or no residual scar. The postauricular and mastoid areas are the sites most frequently involved, probably because the skin is thinnest in this area and it is farthest from the pedicle of the cervicofacial skin flap. Fortunately, small sloughs in this area are concealed by the ear and hair.

Major skin sloughs can be caused by (1) undiagnosed hematoma, (2) a skin flap that is too thin or is damaged by scissors or scalpel during flap dissection, (3) skin flap injury due to retractor or digital trauma during flap elevation or deep layer procedures, (4) excessive tension on closure, or (5) thermal injury due to electrocoagulation or a light source burn from movie or television filming. All facial skin sloughs, even when in a highly visible area, are treated by careful observation, *not surgical intervention.*

The devitalized skin develops a thick, black eschar. The eschar should be left in place and progressively trimmed around the edges as epithelization occurs and the edges of the eschar separate. It may take three to four weeks for the eschar to separate completely. Any evidence of infection beneath the eschar requires immediate debridement.

The areas of skin slough epithelize and contract dramatically. The resultant scar is usually better than would be anticipated from the initial wound appearance. Sloughs behind the ear may extend below the earlobe and continue along the mandibular border. Preauricular sloughs contract most. Skin grafting usually is not indicated because there would be a remaining scar patch. Depending on the size of the sloughed area, scar excision and advancement of the facial skin may provide improvement when sufficient time has elapsed for skin laxity to return.

There is no question that cigarette smoking increases the risk of skin slough. Rees, Liverett, and Guy (1984) demonstrated a risk of skin slough 12 times greater in smokers than in nonsmokers. Skin flap experiments in animals have supported this conclusion (Lawrence and associates, 1984; Kaufman and associates, 1984; Rees, Liverett, and Guy, 1984; Craig and Rees, 1985; Nolan and associates, 1985). Webster and associates (1986) recommended conservative undermining in patients who smoke. It is the opinion of the authors of this chapter, however, that abstinence from smoking for at least two weeks preoperatively, although not reducing the risk to the level of nonsmokers, is preferable to operating on a patient who has not given up smoking and compromising the surgical procedure.

NERVE INJURY

Transient numbness or hypoesthesia of the lower two-thirds of the ear, the preauricular area, and the cheeks occurs for the first two to six weeks postoperatively as a result of the interruption of small sensory nerves during surgery, and is unavoidable.

The most common nerve injured during facialplasty is the great auricular nerve. Injury to the great auricular nerve can produce a permanent loss of sensation or paresthesias over the lower portion of the ear and the immediate preauricular and postauricular areas. Injury to this nerve occurs when the dissection is too deep, piercing the fascia over the middle portion of the sternocleidomastoid muscle. McKinney and Katrana (1980) studied the course of the great auricular nerve and found that, with the head turned 45 degrees toward the contralateral side, the nerve consistently crosses the midportion of the sternocleidomastoid muscle at a level 6.5 cm below the caudal edge of the bony external auditory canal. The great auricular nerve then courses cephalad just beneath the

SMAS, 0.5 cm posterior and parallel to the external jugular vein. McKinney and Gottlieb (1985) suggested that the safest place to incise the SMAS-platysma during a face lift procedure is at a point immediately anterior to the sternocleidomastoid muscle. When injury to the great auricular nerve is recognized during surgery, an immediate, meticulous repair should be performed in an attempt to restore as much sensory function as possible and to prevent the development of a painful neuroma.

Permanent injury of the facial nerve (cranial nerve VII) is the most dreaded fear of surgeons performing facialplasty. The incidence of all intraoperative facial nerve injuries during rhytidectomy is reported in the literature to range between 0.4 (Stark, 1977) and 2.6 per cent. Baker (1983) reviewed the literature and compiled statistics on 1500 patients with an incidence of facial nerve injury of 0.9 per cent. It is mandatory that the surgeon performing rhytidectomy be familiar with the anatomy and common variations of the facial nerve. Fortunately, permanent injury to the facial nerve is rare. Most patients regain full motor function after an injury to a branch of the facial nerve within a few weeks to a year, although in an occasional patient it may take up to 2½ years for function to return to normal (Spira, Gerow, and Hardy, 1967; Rees and Wood-Smith, 1973; Baker and associates, 1977).

Immediate postoperative paresis or paralysis of muscles supplied by the facial nerve is not uncommon. If due to the infiltration of local anesthetic, complete return of function occurs within several hours as the drug is metabolized. A more persistent paresis lasting 24 hours to a few weeks may occur from nerve trauma during blunt dissection, injection of anesthetic solution into the nerve, edema within the nerve sheath, or cautery trauma.

The nerve branch injured most often varies with different reports in the literature. According to Mcgregor and Greenberg (1972), one of the *buccal branches* of the facial nerve is injured most often. Injuries to buccal branches usually occur in the loose areolar tissue anterior to the parotid gland. When injury occurs, it is most often to a small peripheral branch arising after the buccal branch arborization. Loss of muscle function may be subtle because of multiple connections between the nerve branches.

If transection of a facial nerve branch is detected during the surgical procedure, immediate, meticulous microsurgical repair should be performed. Most often a motor nerve injury is not recognized during surgery and the surgeon and patient are placed in the difficult position of waiting for return of function.

Injury to the *marginal mandibular branch* causes paresis or paralysis of the lip depressor muscles and produces an obvious facial distortion with most attempts at facial animation. The marginal mandibular nerve innervates the lip depressor muscles and the upper medial portion of the platysma muscle, which function synchrononously with the depressor labii inferioris and depressor anguli oris. The main body of the platysma muscle is innervated by the cervical branch of the facial nerve. Ellenbogen (1979) reported that transection of the midcervical platysma may sever the motor branches to the remaining proximal platysma, thus producing a temporary "pseudoparalysis" of lip depressor function.

Injury to the *temporal (frontal) branch* of the facial nerve occurs if the dissection is carried too deep to the SMAS. The nerve is vulnerable in front of the temporal hairline, at a position midway between the lateral canthus of the eye and the superior auricular angle, where the nerve crosses over the zygomatic arch (Fig. 43–62). If the nerve has

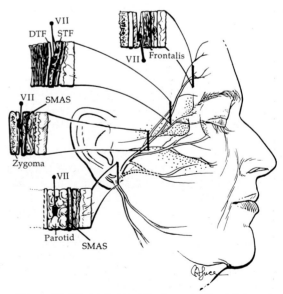

Figure 43–62. Anatomy of the temporal (frontal) branch of the facial nerve. The relationship to the parotid gland, zygomatic arch, superficial temporal fascia (STF), deep temporal fascia (DTF), and frontalis is shown. Note that the nerve is deep to the SMAS, the STF, and the frontalis, which are contiguous structures.

been traumatized but not divided, frontalis muscle function will usually return within six to eight weeks. If even a trace of muscle movement is seen, complete recovery can usually be expected, but in some patients it may take 12 to 24 months. If total paralysis remains after this time, transection of the contralateral frontal nerve may produce forehead-brow symmetry. Without the benefit of frontalis muscle function, there may be sufficient brow ptosis to make a forehead-brow lift necessary. However, not all the facts on frontalis innervation are understood. Miller, Anstee, and Snell (1976) reported a patient with scalp avulsion who regained bilateral frontalis function after the flap was replaced as a free flap with anastomosis of only blood vessels.

Mcgregor and Greenberg (1972) also cautioned against excessively deep dissection over the posterior margin of the sternocleidomastoid muscle, to avoid injury to the accessory nerve (cranial nerve XI). Dissection in this area is not indicated during face lifting.

ALOPECIA

Some degree of hair loss occurs after rhytidectomy in 1 (Cohen and Webster, 1983) to 3 per cent (Leist, Masson, and Erich, 1977) of patients, depending on the report. Most hair loss after facialplasty is due to (1) excess flap tension, (2) superficial dissection destroying the hair follicles, or (3) electrocautery burn of the hair follicles. Patients with thinning hair and those having a tendency to alopecia are prone to greater hair loss. Hair treated with dyes and harsh chemicals tends to break off adjacent to the incisions. Most hair loss is corrected by new growth within four to six months.

The sideburns and temporal hair pattern must be protected in both males and females undergoing primary or secondary face lifts. The temporal extension of the face lift incision should be placed at least 4 to 5 cm behind the anterior temporal hairline to leave an adequate camouflage of the scar. A transverse incision beneath the temporal hairline (sideburn) allows rotation of the flap without elevation of the temporal hairline.

The mastoid portion of the face lift incision must be placed in the hair so as to be hidden and to leave maximal hair on the cervical-mastoid flap. If the incision is placed low, it is easily visible and will significantly affect future hairstyles for the patient.

SCARS

Most scars after facialplasty are relatively inconspicuous. Excess tension and vascular compromise of the skin are the two major causes of obvious scars. Skin flaps must be trimmed and sutured with minimal tension. This is especially true in the preauricular area and around the earlobe, where even moderate tension causes widened scars and distorts the earlobe. Tension along the scar in the hair-bearing areas may produce a widened, hairless scar. Two points of maximal flap tension should be established: (1) at the apex of the postauricular-mastoid incision and (2) in the temporal area just above the ear. All remaining portions of the incision should have minimal tension.

Skin flap vascular compromise with partial- or full-thickness skin loss produces visible scars. This is especially true when there is a slough along the posterior border and below the earlobe, because there is a tendency for scars in this area to become hypertrophic. Small injections of 0.2 to 0.4 mg of triamcinolone help to flatten such scars, but telangiectasias frequently occur in the injected areas.

The postauricular incision is the most frequent site of hypertrophic scars. Several small injections of triamcinolone, as noted above, spaced three to four weeks apart tend to resolve the scars. Hypertrophic scars in the temporal, preauricular, and mastoid areas are uncommon, but they can occur. True keloids are extremely rare. They are most likely to occur in darkly pigmented individuals.

Submental skin incisions should be placed transversely in or near the submental skin crease and should be limited in length so as to remain hidden under the chin. Elliptic skin excision in the submental area tends to produce dog-ears at the lateral poles of the submental scars. Wide undermining, limiting the amount of skin excision, and incision closure from a lateral to a medial direction are factors that help to reduce the occurrence of dog-ears. Vertical scars on the anterior surface of the neck, such as arise from Z-plasties, H-plasties, and W-plasties, rarely give an acceptable appearance and should be avoided except in unusual situations when there is an excessive amount of skin and the patient is willing to accept a highly visible scar in trade for skin removal.

PIGMENTATION

Hyperpigmentation caused by hemosiderin deposits usually occurs at the site of ecchymosis. Patients who bruise easily have a greater tendency to hyperpigmentation. Small, unevacuated hematomas that are noted only after most edema subsides are frequent sites of hyperpigmentation. Hyperpigmentation from hemosiderin deposits usually resolves after six to eight months, but occasionally is permanent.

Patients who have multiple facial telangiectasias frequently have an increase in the number of telangiectasias in the areas of undermined skin. Electrocoagulation with a small needle is the best treatment for larger lesions, but there is a high incidence of recurrence. Small lesions are best covered with make-up.

PAIN

Pain after rhytidectomy is unusual. In the immediate postoperative period, pain is a sign of hematoma formation until it is proved otherwise.

Discomfort and tightness in the submental area, over the neck, and along the mandibular border and postauricular and mastoid areas are not uncommon and may occur with movement of the head and neck for two to four months postoperatively. Anesthesia or hypoesthesia in the cheeks, in the earlobes, and along the course of the great auricular nerve usually occur for several days to several months. Paresthesias over the course of the great auricular nerve suggest its division. A painful neuroma may develop at the unrepaired cut nerve ends. If this occurs, the nerve should be explored, the neuroma resected, and the nerve ends approximated.

FOREHEAD-BROW LIFT

Attempts at esthetic surgery of the forehead and brow were reported by several well-known surgeons in the early part of the twentieth century. Passot (1919) described a temporal lift procedure for lateral brow laxity and in 1930 reported supraciliary brow resec-

tion to improve ptosis. In 1931 Passot described resection of skin posterior to the hairline to improve forehead wrinkles, and subsequently recommended denervation of the frontalis muscle by severing the temporal branch of the facial nerve to further improve results (Passot, 1933). Hunt (1926) described a coronal skin resection. Joseph (1931) reported forehead excisions both anterior to and within the hairline.

All the early forehead lift procedures were performed without interrupting the frontalis muscle, and the results were less than desired. Bames (1957) reported a direct eyebrow lift with corrugator resection, forehead undermining to the hairline, and crosshatching of the frontalis muscle. Regnault (1972) and Gonzalez-Ulloa (1974) described frontalis incisions. Marino (1964, 1971), Griffiths (1974), Skoog, (1974), Hinderer (1975), and Viñas, Caviglia, and Cortinas (1976) recommended partial frontalis and galea excision to (1) decrease the ability of the frontalis to wrinkle the forehead and (2) permit a superior lift of the forehead by increased expansion of the skin and subcutaneous tissue. In a cadaver study, Washio (1976) concluded that transverse frontalis excision and interruption of the fibrous septa between the frontalis and the dermis are necessary in order to permit significant passive elevation of the forehead. Pitanguy (1979) recommended frontalis, corrugator, and procerus crosscutting to decrease muscle function without producing a depression or contour defect.

Complete frontalis resection was suggested by Tessier (1968) and Le Roux and Jones (1974). However, complete loss of forehead animation is not usually a desirable result.

Forehead-Brow Anatomy

The paired frontalis muscles are vertically oriented extensions of the galea aponeurotica that begin at approximately the level of the anterior hairline, extend inferiorly to cover almost the entire forehead, and insert into the dermis of the forehead skin in the supraorbital region. The function of the frontalis is to elevate the eyebrows, an essential component of facial expression. Transverse forehead lines result from repeated frontalis contraction, producing an accordion effect on the forehead skin. The frontalis muscle is innervated by the frontal (temporal) branch of the facial nerve (Fig. 43–62). Loss of frontalis innervation always results in brow ptosis on the affected side.

In opposition to the brow-lifting activity of the frontalis muscles is the pull of the corrugator supercilii, procerus, and orbicularis oculi muscles. Contraction of these muscles pulls the forehead and brow in an inferior direction. The three muscles interdigitate in the medial aspect of the suprabrow and glabellar areas.

The *corrugator supercilii* muscles arise from the periosteum along the superior medial orbital rim, and insert into the dermis of the medial brow. Contraction of the corrugator and procerus muscles pulls the brow medial and downward, producing a scowling or angry appearance. Glabella creases, which can be long and deep depending on the extent of corrugator activity, develop as a result of repeated corrugator contraction. The *procerus* muscles originate from the surface of the upper lateral cartilage and nasal bones, insert into the skin in the glabellar area, and interdigitate with the frontalis, corrugator, and orbicularis oculi muscles. Contraction of the procerus muscle pulls the forehead down, elevates the root of the nose skin, and causes transverse wrinkles at the root of the nose. The orbicularis oculi muscles interdigitate medially with the procerus, corrugator, and frontalis muscles. The sphincter-like contraction of the orbital portion of the orbicularis oculi muscle pulls the brow down, especially the lateral brow where there is absence of a direct lifting effect of the frontalis muscle.

The frontal branch of the facial nerve exits its parotid covering on a line extending from a position 0.5 cm below the tragus of the ear to a point 1.5 cm above the lateral brow (Pitanguy and Ramos, 1966), passing over the zygomatic arch deep to the SMAS. The nerve ascends superficially to the temporalis muscle and deep temporal fascia, remains beneath the SMAS at the lateral brow edge, and enters the frontalis muscle on its deep surface (Fig. 43–62) (Liebman and associates, 1982). In some patients the nerve is visible on the posterior surface of a bicoronal flap.

Indications for Brow Lift

Most often the primary indications for forehead-brow lift are forehead-brow ptosis and lateral upper lid ptosis. However, a forehead-brow lift also helps to correct transverse forehead lines and creases, glabella creases, transverse folds at the root of the nose, upper nasal and medial eyelid fullness due to forehead-brow ptosis, and (to a lesser degree) nasal tip droop. Many patients have upper lid fullness that cannot be corrected by blepharoplasty alone, even with an extended incision.

In some patients correction of transverse forehead lines and/or glabella creases, rather than brow ptosis, may be the main indication for a forehead-brow lift procedure. In such patients, attention is aimed at interrupting muscle activity with minimal brow elevation. The patients in the latter category are usually younger than the usual candidate for a forehead-brow lift.

Patient Evaluation

Some patients requesting facialplasty or blepharoplasty have forehead-brow deformities that are more important in their overall appearance than the deformity for which they are seeking correction.

Patients are examined in repose while standing or sitting and looking straight ahead. Attention is first directed to the upper eyelids and brow position. The contribution of brow ptosis to upper lid fullness is determined by gentle fingertip elevation of the brow and observation of the upper lid. Forehead-brow ptosis is frequently the main component of upper eyelid fullness. Some patients have relatively little excess upper eyelid skin when the brow is manipulated to the anticipated postoperative position, and therefore upper blepharoplasty may provide little or no improvement. If excess upper eyelid skin is present with the brow elevated, upper blepharoplasty will be needed in addition to forehead-brow lift and can be performed at the same time. The brows are observed for position and symmetry. Often one brow is higher than the other, which may be due to (1) asymmetry in orbital anatomy or (2) more often, involuntary unilateral frontalis muscle contraction. If the difference in brow position is mild, the asymmetry can be improved by asymmetric dissection along the orbital rim. Thinning the frontalis in the area of unilateral contraction reduces muscle spasm and excessive brow elevation.

Normal brow position is variable. Congenitally low eyebrows are not uncommon, making forehead-brow lift useful for the younger patient requesting correction of heaviness of the upper lids. In some of these patients, upper blepharoplasty is not indicated. Ellenbogen (1983) delineated the criteria for the ideal eyebrow: (1) the brow begins medially at a vertical line drawn perpendicular through the alar base; (2) the brow terminates laterally at an oblique line drawn through the lateral canthus of the eye and the alar base; (3) the medial and lateral ends lie at approximately the same horizontal level (the medial end has a clubhead configuration that gradually tapers laterally); (4) the apex of the brow lies on the vertical line directly above the lateral limbus of the eye; and (5) the brow arches above the supraorbital rim in women and lies at approximately the level of the rim in men.

The root of the nose is examined for ptosis. Often, skin redundancy causes a heavy, wide appearance of the upper nose and can contribute to fullness and webbing in the upper medial canthus that will not be corrected by upper blepharoplasty. Elevation of the forehead-brow can decrease the width of the nasal root.

The glabellar area is examined for lines and creases, which usually are significantly increased by facial animation. Some patients have an almost permanent frown or scowl due to the corrugator, procerus, and orbicularis oculi muscle contraction. The involuntary habit of contracting these muscles is not easily broken.

The forehead is examined for transverse lines. The length and location of the lines should be noted, as improvement depends on changing the frontalis muscle function directly beneath the lines. The anterior hairline contour is observed along with hair texture, thickness, and style. Any evidence of alopecia should be documented.

Bicoronal Technique

Either a bicoronal or a modified anterior hairline incision can be used for almost all patients undergoing forehead-brow lift. A bicoronal incision is the procedure of choice for patients with a low or normal anterior hairline and normal to thick hair growth (Fig. 43–63). When the hairline is high, a modified anterior hairline incision is used. It follows the frontal hair pattern in the middle portion of the forehead, and turns posteriorly for 7 to 9 cm before curving downward in the temporal area to the junction of the superior helix of the ear with the temporal scalp (Fig. 43–64). If a facialplasty is being performed at the time of the brow lift, the face lift is performed first, and the forehead-brow lift incision joins the temporal extension of the face lift incision.

Before intravenous medication, with the patient in the sitting position, the glabella and transverse forehead lines are marked. Outlining of the bicoronal incision begins in the midline of the scalp. The scalp is evaluated for looseness and anticipated mobility. The midpoint of the incision is marked at a location 7 to 9 cm behind the middle anterior hairline. After scalp resection at least 5 cm of hair-bearing scalp should remain anterior to the incision in the midline, and a greater width in the temporal areas in order to (1)

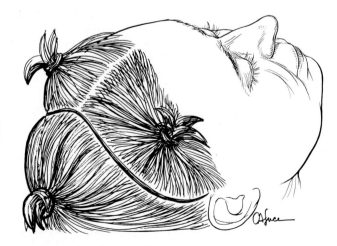

Figure 43–63. Standard incision for forehead-brow lift. The incision must be placed far enough posteriorly so that *after resection* of redundant scalp it will be 5 cm behind the hairline.

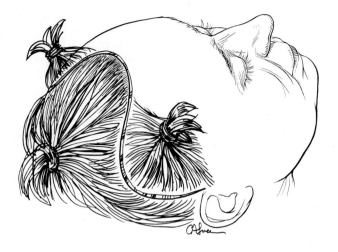

Figure 43–64. Modified or anterior hairline incision for forehead-brow lift. The incision must be made directly at the hairline and not anterior to it.

camouflage the incision and (2) leave an adequate amount of hair for styling. From the midline the incision curves posterolaterally to join the temporal extension of the face lift incision. If a face lift is not being performed, the incision extends to the attachment of the superior pole of the ear in the temporal scalp. The hair is parted along the incision and also down the midline on the anterior side of the incision so as to make a pigtail on the right and left sides, secured with rubber bands (see Fig. 43–63). The posterior scalp hair is made into a ponytail with a rubber band. It is neither necessary nor advantageous to shave or cut the hair.

Local anesthetic solution (0.5 per cent lidocaine with 1:200,000 epinephrine) is infiltrated along the incision line, the entire forehead area, the supraorbital rims, and the dorsum of the nose, regardless of whether general endotracheal anesthesia or intravenous sedation technique is being used. Seven to eight minutes are permitted to elapse in order to achieve the maximal vasoconstrictive effect. During this time plastic lenses are placed in the eyes to protect the corneas from injury when the forehead flap is turned down over the orbital rims. This maneuver is particularly important if an upper blepharoplasty has been performed, because the eyes will be open and especially vulnerable to injury.

The incision is beveled parallel to the hair follicles down to the pericranium in a single movement. Flap dissection is made with a scalpel in the thin areolar plane between the galea and pericranium, and carried down to the supraorbital rims. Blunt dissection or scalp avulsion can easily be performed, but should be avoided because (1) it causes irregular tearing and stripping of the galea and pericranium, which clinically causes an increase in postoperative pain and discomfort; and (2) sensory nerve branches are avulsed, resulting in long-term complaints of scalp anesthesia and paresthesia.

There is a zone of transition between the subgaleal temporal dissection and the subcutaneous dissection in the cheek region (Fig. 43–65). The superficial temporal vessels are always divided and ligated since they lie on the superficial temporal fascia.

As the supraorbital rims are approached, care is taken to identify the supraorbital neurovascular bundles. The anatomy of the supraorbital nerve is variable. There is usually one large nerve and an associated nerve of approximately one-third the size. However, several supraorbital nerves may be present. The supratrochlear nerve lies in the corrugator muscle and is not visualized until the deepest portion of the corrugator muscle has been resected (Figure 43–66).

When the dissection reaches the supraorbital rims and the supraorbital nerves have been identified, blunt dissection releases the flap from the supraorbital rims. The flap is mobilized around the orbital rim to the lateral canthus. The pericranium is incised along the orbital rim and dissected over the edge of the orbital rim, releasing the periorbita on the immediate undersurface of the orbital rim. In the midline the dissection is extended onto the nasal process of the frontal bone. Large, blunt-tipped scissors are passed down the dorsum to the tip of the nose and

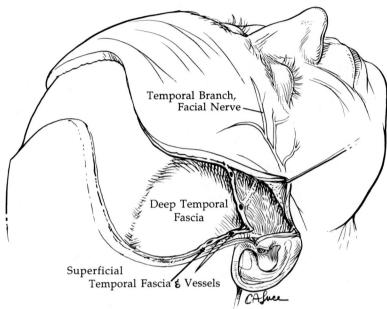

Figure 43–65. The transition point in the temporal scalp between the subgaleal dissection and the subcutaneous dissection of the face lift. The superficial temporal vessels run in the superficial temporal fascia and are divided during this procedure.

Figure 43–66. Supraorbital anatomy. The forehead flap is dissected in a subgaleal (supraperiosteal) plane. The supraorbital neurovascular (NV) bundles are clearly visible as the supraorbital rims are approched. The supratrochlear nerves run within the corrugator muscles and are not visible until the muscle fibers are separated. Scissors are used to identify the supratrochlear branches by spreading in the direction of the corrugator fibers before the muscles are divided.

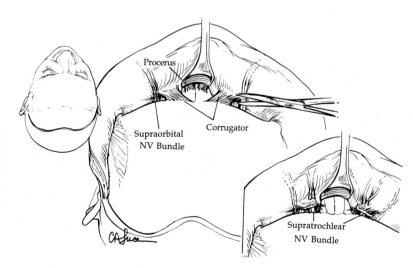

spread to release soft tissue attachments on the upper one-half of the nose.

The corrugator muscles, which are easily identified, are dissected from their periosteal origins and amputated (Fig. 43–66). All corrugator muscle fibers attaching the flap to the skull must be freed if maximal flap mobility is to be obtained. Approximately one-half of the corrugator muscle is left on the forehead flap to prevent a postoperative skin depression. Resection of the medialmost portion of the corrugator muscles actually involves resection of a portion of the procerus and orbicularis oculi muscles, since they interdigitate in this area.

A periosteal elevator is passed down the dorsum of the nose, freeing all remaining muscle attachments to the nasal bones. Complete flap mobility is now established.

Attention is next carried to the glabella creases, which are usually two or three in number (Fig. 43–67). On occasion, there is one large crease. Needles are passed through the flap from outside to inside at the upper and lower limits of the previously marked creases, and the location of the crease on the undersurface of the flap is thereby marked between the upper and lower needles. A sharp scalpel is used to incise through muscle down to subcutaneous tissue on all four sides (right, left, superior, and inferior) of each glabella crease, thus forming an island of soft tissue under each crease that has been isolated from the surrounding muscle. In most patients this technique eliminates or significantly reduces the glabella creases.

Frontalis muscle resection serves three purposes: (1) to reduce frontalis activity, thereby decreasing the depth of the transverse lines; (2) to permit greater flap expansion; and (3) to provide a raw surface for adherence to the pericranium, which helps to stabilize the flap in its elevated position. Care must be taken to resect the galea and frontalis down to the subcutaneous tissue without violating the subcutaneous tissue. Inadvertent subcutaneous excision results in depressions and irregularities on the forehead.

During frontalis resection the sensory nerves must be preserved. The supraorbital nerves, which can be visualized running through the flap, are protected by marking the course of the nerve with ink. The supratrochlear nerves pass through the flap at a slightly more superficial level (relative to the skin) and are more easily seen as the galea and frontalis muscle are resected.

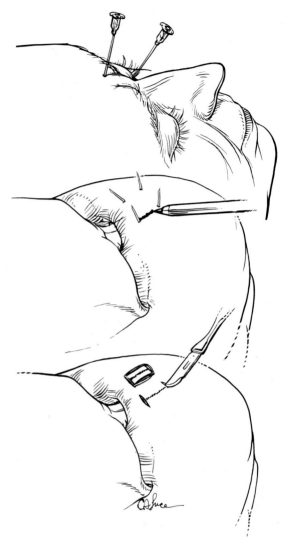

Figure 43–67. Treatment of the glabella creases. Needles are passed from outside to inside the forehead flap to identify the exact area to be treated. Lines are drawn on the galea corresponding precisely to the creases on the skin, and the needles are removed. The frontalis muscle is interrupted in all directions around the crease.

The frontalis is resected as a rectangle of varying size, depending on the nature of the forehead wrinkles to be improved (Fig. 43–68). To correct numerous transverse wrinkles, frontalis resection extends vertically from 1 cm above the medial eyebrow up to the hairline and transversely across the entire forehead, preserving the supraorbital and supratrochlear nerves. For reduction of only a few middle forehead wrinkles, the resection begins 1 cm above the eyebrow and extends superiorly to the hairline and laterally as far as the supraorbital nerves, but does not extend beyond the nerves. When the deformity

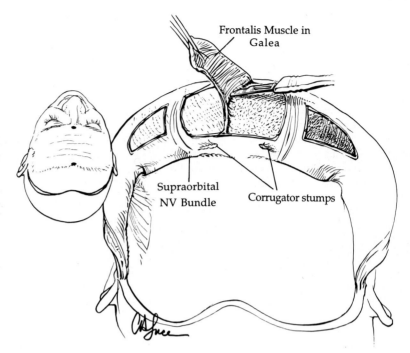

Figure 43–68. Excision of the frontalis muscle. Care is taken to excise only the muscle and no subcutaneous fat. Laterally the resection must begin 3 cm above the brow to preserve sufficient frontalis so as not to interfere with brow function.

is limited to brow ptosis and there are no transverse forehead lines, resection of the galea and only a few frontalis fibers in the central forehead area gives a raw surface for flap adherence to the pericranium. Needles passed through the flap from the outside to the inside help to define the superior, inferior, medial, and lateral extents of the planned frontalis-galea resection.

The forehead-brow flap is redraped in a posterior direction overlapping the cut edge of the posterior scalp flap (Fig. 43–69). Three key fixation points are established: the midline and on the right and left sides of the flap on a line extending vertically from the lateral limbus of the eye. The fixation points are secured with a surgical staple, and all overlapping excess flap is excised. The fixation points are established with slight tension, and the remainder of the flap is trimmed so as to exert minimal tension on the flap closure.

Flap closure in the temporal area from the superior pole of the ear to the top of the temporalis muscle is accomplished using a single layer of surgical staples. Across the top of the head (from temporalis muscle to temporalis muscle), where the flap is almost

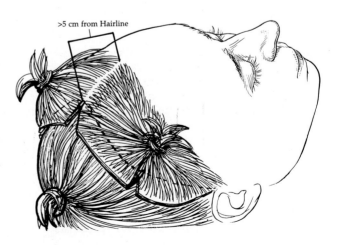

Figure 43–69. Redraping and trimming of the forehead flap. The forehead is suspended from three key points and the remainder of the closure is performed under minimal tension.

twice the thickness of the temporal areas, the galea is closed with a running 4.0 Vicryl suture and the skin is approximated with surgical staples. Drains are not used.

When wound closure is complete, the hair is combed over the incision to cover it, remove any cut hair, and prevent tangles and snarls. A gauze bandage is placed over the incision line and secured in place with a stockinette dressing as described for the face lift.

Mild analgesics are prescribed for postoperative pain. While patients may complain of pressure and discomfort, pain is not a usual complaint. Any complaints of pain must be evaluated for possible hematoma. The eyelids usually do not close completely for the first 12 to 24 hours postoperatively, especially if an upper blepharoplasty has been performed concomitantly. Generous application of ophthalmic lubricating ointment is necessary to prevent desiccation of the corneas. The dressing is removed on the first postoperative day if the forehead-brow lift is performed as an isolated procedure, and on the second postoperative day if it is done in conjunction with a face lift.

Swelling and periorbital ecchymosis are frequently worse on the second or third postoperative day and the patient should be so advised. The hair can be washed on the second postoperative day and daily thereafter. Prophylactic antibiotics are administered only preoperatively. All staples and sutures are removed between the eighth and tenth postoperative day. Selected patients who underwent brow lifting are illustrated in Figures 43–70, 43–71, and 43–72.

Complications

HEMATOMA

Hematoma after a forehead-brow lift is rare, occurring less often than after face lifting. There are two main areas requiring careful hemostasis: (1) the medial periorbital area and root of the nose after muscle resection and (2) the vessels in the cut flap edge. Careful coagulation, combined with stapling of the thin flap in the temporal area and closure of the galea and subcutaneous tissue with a running suture across the top of the scalp, effectively controls bleeding.

Complaints of significant pain suggest a hematoma. A collection of blood under the flap can be easily detected because of the unyielding skull. An unevacuated hematoma can conceivably lead to flap necrosis and alopecia.

ALOPECIA

Significant alopecia is rare. If it occurs, the primary reason is tension on the flap. The blood supply to the forehead flap is abundant and must be significantly decreased by tension to contribute to hair loss. If suture fixation points are utilized, small areas of alopecia frequently occur as the suture penetrates the scalp. Patients who use strong chemicals and dyes for permanents and hair coloring frequently have very brittle hair shafts that break along the incision line, and sometimes throughout the flap anterior to the incision. Patients are advised against using any chemicals except regular shampoo for three weeks before surgery and three weeks postoperatively. Hairs that break off at the scalp surface return at the rate at which the patient normally grows hair. If scars widen from tension on the flap, the hair follicles will die and the scars will be visible.

Patients with thin, fine hair, especially those experiencing daily hair loss with routine brushing and combing, may have more hair loss in the first three to six weeks after surgery. Some patients feel that their hair never returns to its preoperative thickness. Patients experiencing significant hair loss preoperatively may not be satisfactory candidates for forehead-brow lift.

FRONTAL NERVE PARALYSIS

Frontal nerve paralysis is rare. Injury to the frontal branch of the facial nerve can occur during flap dissection at the lateral orbital rim if the dissection is too superficial. In the lateral orbital area the frontal nerve lies on the deep surface of the frontalis muscle and is frequently visualized when the flap is dissected. Resection of the frontalis muscle on the lateral portion of the flap, to correct forehead wrinkles, should be performed at least 3 cm above the lateral orbital rim in order to avoid injury to the temporal nerve. During combined face lifting and forehead-brow lifting the frontal branch must be avoided during the subcutaneous face lift dissection superior to the zygomatic arch. The superficial temporal artery is routinely divided. The transition point from the subcu-

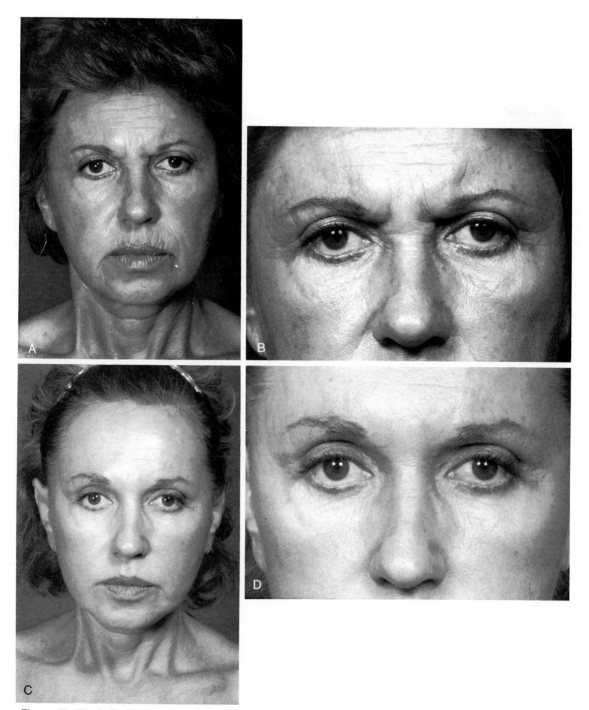

Figure 43–70. *A, B,* Preoperative views of a patient with facial and neck laxity, forehead and brow ptosis, glabella creases, laxity at the root of the nose, corrugator hypertrophy, and transverse forehead lines. *C, D,* Improvement in facial and neck laxity, correction of forehead-brow ptosis, reduction of corrugator bulk, elevation of the laxity of the soft tissue at the root of the nose, and improvement in forehead transverse lines by a combination of facialplasty, coronal forehead-brow lift, and chemical peeling of the upper lip.

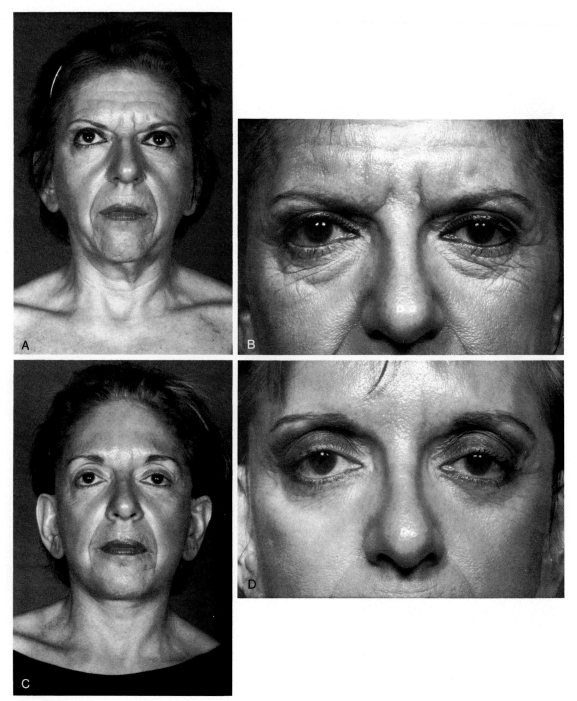

Figure 43–71. *A, B,* Preoperative views of a patient with facial and neck laxity, forehead and brow ptosis, deep glabella creases, and deep transverse forehead creases. *C, D,* Correction of facial and neck laxity, elevation of the forehead and brow, reduction of vertical glabella creases, and reduction of transverse forehead creases by a combination of facialplasty, lower blepharoplasty, and coronal forehead-brow lift.

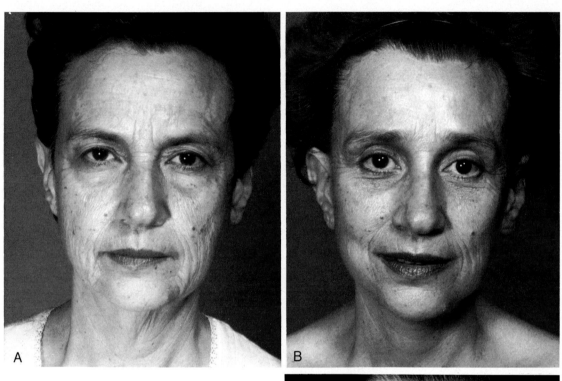

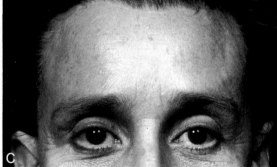

Figure 43–72. *A,* Preoperative view of a patient with facial and neck laxity, blepharochalasis, forehead-brow ptosis, glabella creases, and high forehead. *B, C,* Improvement in facial laxity, correction of blepharochalasis, and elevation of the forehead-brow by a combination of facialplasty, four-lid blepharoplasty, and a modified anterior hairline type of brow lift. Postoperative views show a well-healed, modified anterior hairline incision.

taneous dissection for the face lift to the deeper dissection above is at approximately the level of the lateral canthus of the eye (see Fig. 43–65). Frontalis paralysis or weakness is usually transient. If any movement is present, full return of function can be expected with time, but full muscle recovery may require 10 to 12 months. Frontalis muscle paralysis was discussed in the section on Face lift complications.

SENSORY CHANGES

Sensory innervation to the forehead and anterior scalp is primarily provided by the supraorbital and supratrochlear nerves. The skin incision divides the sensory branches and frequently results in an area of hypoesthesia behind the incision. Sharp dissection in the thin areolar plane between the galea and pericranium minimizes nerve injury, as noted above. The nerve branches within the flap can be visualized and avoided during frontalis muscle resection.

Patients usually complain of hypoesthesia or itching. Reasonably normal sensation usually returns to the forehead and brow area within six weeks to six months. There may be some evidence of permanent hypoesthesia of the scalp posterior to the bicoronal or modified anterior hairline incision.

LAGOPHTHALMOS

Incomplete eyelid closure during the first 24 to 48 hours after surgery is usual. Generous use of ophthalmic ointment helps to prevent drying of the corneas. Patients undergoing simultaneous forehead-brow lift and upper blepharoplasty must be carefully evaluated. Excess lid skin is measured and marked with the forehead lifted to its anticipated postoperative position. Upper blepharoplasty can then be performed as if it is an isolated procedure, followed immediately by the forehead-brow lift. Upper lid edema occurring during forehead-brow lifting makes upper lid skin evaluation inaccurate if this is attempted immediately after the forehead-brow lift.

If the patient has had a previous upper blepharoplasty, careful upper lid evaluation is mandatory. A history of postoperative lagophthalmos and inability to close the lids completely when the brow is manually elevated may be a contraindication to forehead-brow lifting.

Alternative Brow Lift Techniques

In addition to bicoronal or modified coronal incisions, several other approaches to forehead-brow lifting have been advocated.

Passot (1930) and Castañares (1964) described supraciliary excision of skin for direct brow elevation. Lozenge-shaped resections of this kind remove more skin laterally than medially, producing an elevated, arched brow. Although the scar is designed to be hidden by the eyebrow, it is usually visible, occasionally deteriorating with time as the scar contracts. This procedure may have application in elderly patients to correct functional brow ptosis with visual impairment.

Sokol and Sokol (1982) reported a transblepharoplasty technique to suspend a soft tissue eyebrow flap to a superiorly based orbital rim periosteal flap. The long-term results with this procedure are uncertain. Lewis (1983) reported brow elevation by direct suture technique using permanent sutures placed through small incisions within the eyebrow. Again, long-term efficacy is not known. Gurdin and Carlin (1972) described a middle forehead skin excision between two transverse forehead lines with a resultant single transverse line. This approach should probably be reserved for males with deep transverse forehead lines. The resulting scar usually remains red for weeks and is in an obvious location.

Attempts to elevate the brow from a temporal approach, dating from Passot in 1919 to Gleason in 1973, involve extensive undermining in the temporal and lateral canthal area. The minimal brow elevation, the risk of alopecia, and the possibility of frontalis muscle paralysis render the use of this technique undesirable.

REFERENCES

Adamson, J. E., Horton, C. E., and Crawford, H. H.: The surgical correction of the "turkey gobbler" deformity. Plast. Reconstr. Surg., 34:598, 1964.

Anderson, R. L., and Gordy, D. D.: The tarsal strip procedure. Arch. Ophthalmol., 97:2192, 1979.

Aston, S. J.: Platysma muscle in rhytidoplasty. Ann. Plast. Surg., 3:529, 1979.

Aston, S. J.: Platysma cervicofacial rhytidoplasty: correction of obtuse cervicomental angle (videotape). Presented at the Symposium of American Society for Aesthetic Plastic Surgery, 1980.

Aston, S. J.: Male cervicofacial rhytidoplasty. *In* Courtiss, E. (Ed.): Male Aesthetic Surgery. St. Louis, C. V. Mosby Company, 1981.

Aston, S. J.: Lifting cheeks and neck. *In* Lewis, J. R. (Ed.): Atlas of Aesthetic Plastic Surgery. Boston, Little, Brown & Company, 1982.

Aston, S. J.: Problems and complications in platysma-SMAS cervicofacial rhytidectomy. *In* Kaye, B., and Gradinger, G. (Eds.): Symposium on Problems and Complications in Aesthetic Plastic Surgery of the Face. St. Louis, C. V. Mosby Company, 1983.

Aston, S. J., and Pober, J. M.: Basic principles of aesthetic surgery of the face, neck, and brow area. *In* Georgiade, N., Georgiade, G., Riefkohl, R., and Barwick, W. (Eds.): Essentials of Plastic, Maxillofacial, and Reconstructive Surgery. Baltimore, Williams & Wilkins Company, 1987.

Aufricht, G.: Surgery for excess skin of the face and neck. *In* Wallace, E. B. (Ed.): Transactions of the International Society of Plastic Surgeons. Second Congress. Edinburgh, London, E. & S. Livingstone, 1960, pp. 495–502.

Baker, D. C.: Complications of cervicofacial rhytidectomy. Clin. Plast. Surg., *10:*543, 1983.

Baker, D. C., Aston, S. J., Guy, C. L., and Rees, T. D.: The male rhytidectomy. Plast. Reconstr. Surg., *60:*514, 1977.

Baker T. J., and Gordon, H. L.: Complications of rhytidectomy. Plast. Reconstr. Surg., *40:*31, 1967.

Baker, T. J., and Gordon, H. L.: Rhytidectomy in males. Plast. Reconstr. Surg., *44:*219, 1969.

Baker, T. J., Gordon H. L., and Mosienko, P.: Rhytidectomy. Plast. Reconstr. Surg., *59:*24, 1977.

Baker, T. J., Gordon, H. L., and Whitlow, D. R.: Our present technique for rhytidectomy. Plast. Reconstr. Surg., *52:*232, 1973.

Bames, H.: Truth and fallacies of face peeling and face lifting. Med. J. Reconstr., *126:*86, 1927.

Bames, H. O.: Frown disfigurement and ptosis. Plast. Reconstr. Surg., *19:*337, 1957.

Barker, D. F.: Prevention of bleeding following a rhytidectomy. Plast. Reconstr. Surg., *54:*651, 1974.

Barton, Jr., F.: Rhytidectomy. *In* Selected Readings in Plastic Surgery. Vol. 3, No. 2, June, 1985.

Barton, Jr., F.: The aging face/rhytidectomy. *In* Selected Readings in Plastic Surgery, Vol. 4, No. 20, June, 1987.

Beare, R.: Surgical treatment of senile changes in the eyelids. The McIndoe-Beare technique. *In* Smith, B., and Converse, J. M.: Proceedings of the Second International Symposium on Plastic and Reconstructive Surgery of the Eye and Adnexae. St. Louis, C. V. Mosby Company, 1967, pp. 362–366.

Beekhuis, G. J., Klegon, R. B., and Kahn, D. L.: Anesthesia for facial cosmetic surgery: Low dose betamine-diazepam anesthesia. Laryngoscope, *88:*1709, 1978.

Beighton, P., and Bull, J. C.: Plastic surgery in the Ehlers-Danlos syndrome. Plast. Reconstr. Surg., *45:*606, 1970.

Bentley, J. P.: Aging of collagen. J. Invest. Dermatol., *73:*80, 1979.

Berner, R. E., Morain, W. D., and Noe, J. M.: Postoperative hypertension as an etiological factor in hematoma after rhytidectomy. Plast. Reconstr. Surg., *57:*314, 1976.

Bettman, A. G.: Plastic and cosmetic surgery of the face. Northwest. Med., *19:*205, 1920.

Bourguet, J.: La disparipion chirurgicale des rides et plis du visage. Bull. Acad. Méd. (Paris), *82:*183, 1919.

Bourguet, J.: La chirurgie esthétique de la Face. Le Concours Medical, 1921, pp. 1657–1670.

Bourguet, J.: Les hernies graisseuses de l'orbite. Notre traitement chirurgical. Bull. Acad. Méd. (Paris), *92:*1270, 1924.

Bourguet, J.: Chirurgie esthétique de la face: les nez concaves, les rides et les (poches) sous les yeux. Arch. Prov. Chir., *28:*293, 1925.

Bourguet, J.: La chirurgie esthétique de l'oeil et des paupières. Monde Méd., 1929, pp. 725–731.

Butler, R. N., Freedman, A. M., and associates: Psychiatry and psychology of the middle aged. *In* Kaplan, I. H., and Sadock, B. J. (Eds.): Modern Synopsis of Comprehensive Textbook of Psychiatry II. Baltimore, Williams & Wilkins Company, 1975.

Cannon, B., and Pantazelos, H. H.: W-plasty approach to submental lipectomy. *In* Hueston, J. T. (Ed.): Transactions of the Vth International Congress of Plastic and Reconstructive Surgery. Australia, Butterworths, 1971, p. 113.

Cardoso de Castro, C.: The anatomy of the platysma muscle. Plast. Reconstr. Surg., *66:*680, 1980.

Castañares, S.: Blepharoplasty for herniated intraorbital fat. Anatomical basis for a new approach. Plast. Reconstr. Surg., *8:*46, 1951.

Castañares, S.: Forehead wrinkles, glabellar frown, and ptosis of the eyebrows. Plast. Reconstr. Surg., *34:*406, 1964.

Castañares, S.: Facial nerve paralysis coincident with or subsequent to rhytidectomy. Plast. Reconstr. Surg., *54:*637, 1974.

Castañares, S.: Classification of baggy eyelids deformity. Plast. Reconstr. Surg., *59:*629, 1977.

Cohen, S. R., and Webster, R. C.: "How I do it"—head and neck and plastic surgery. A targeted problem and its solution. Primary rhytidectomy—complications of the procedure and anesthetic. Laryngoscope, *93:*654, 1983.

Conley, J.: Face-lift Operation. Springfield, IL, Charles C. Thomas, 1968, p. 105.

Connell, B. F.: Cervical lifts: the value of platysma muscle flaps. Ann. Plast. Surg., *1:*34, 1978a.

Connell, B. F.: Contouring the neck in rhytidectomy by lipectomy and a muscle sling. Plast. Reconstr. Surg., *61:*376, 1978b.

Conway, H.: The surgical face lift—rhytidectomy. Plast. Reconstr. Surg., *45:*124, 1970.

Courtiss, E. H.: Suction lipectomy of the neck. Plast. Reconstr. Surg., *76:*882, 1985.

Craig, S., and Rees, T. D.: The effects of smoking on experimental skin flaps in hamsters. Plast. Reconstr. Surg., *75:*842, 1985.

Cronin, T. D., and Biggs, T. M.: The T-Z-plasty for the male "turkey gobbler" neck. Plast. Reconstr. Surg., *47:*534, 1971.

de Jong R. H.: Local Anesthetics. 2nd Ed. Springfield, IL, Charles C Thomas, 1977.

DeMere, M., Wood, T., and Austin, W.: Eye complications with blepharoplasty or other eyelid surgery. Plast. Reconstr. Surg., *53:*634, 1974.

Dingman, R. O., Grabb, W. C., and Oneal, R. M.: Cutis laxa congenita—generalized elastosis. Plast. Reconstr. Surg., *44:*431, 1969.

Dupuytren, G.: De l'oedéme chronique des tumeurs enkystées des paupières. *In* Leçons Orales de Clinique Chirurgicale. 2nd Ed. Vol. III. Paris, Germer-Bailliere, 1839, pp. 377–378.

Ellenbogen, R.: Pseudo-paralysis of the mandibular branch of the facial nerve after platysmal face-lift operation. Plast. Reconstr. Surg., *63:*364, 1979.

Ellenbogen, R.: Transcoronal eyebrow lift with concomitant upper blepharoplasty. Plast. Reconstr. Surg., 71:490, 1983.

Fenske, N. A., and Lober, C. W.: Structural and functional changes of normal aging skin. J. Am. Acad. Dermatol., 15:571, 1986.

Fleischmajer, R., and Nedwich, A.: Werner's syndrome. Am. J. Med., 54:111, 1973.

Flowers, R. S.: Anchor blepharoplasty. *In* Transactions of the Sixth International Congress of Plastic Surgery. Paris, Masson et Cie, 1976, pp. 471–472.

Freeman, R. G.: Effects of aging on the skin. *In* Helwig, E. B., and Mostofi, F. K. (Eds.): The Skin. Baltimore, Williams & Wilkins Company, 1971.

Fry, H. J. H.: Reversible visual loss after proptosis from retrobulbar hemorrhage. Plast. Reconstr. Surg., 44:480, 1969.

Fuchs, E.: Ueber Blepharochalasis (Erschlattung der Lidhaut). Wien Klin. Wochenschr., 9:109, 1896.

Furnas, D.: Festoons of orbicularis muscle as a cause of baggy eyelids. Plast. Reconstr. Surg., 61:540, 1978.

Gilchrest, B. A.: Age-associated changes in the skin. J. Am. Geriatr. Soc., 30:139, 1982.

Gilchrest, B. A.: Aging. J. Am. Acad. Dermatol., 11:995, 1984.

Gleason, M. C.: Browlifting through a temporal scalp approach. Plast. Reconstr. Surg., 52:141, 1973.

Goin, J., and Goin, M.: Changing the Body: Psychological Effects of Plastic Surgery. Baltimore, Williams & Wilkins Company, 1981.

Goin, M. K., Burgoyne, R. W., Goin, J. M., and Staples, F. R.: A prospective psychological study of 50 female face-lift patients. Plast. Reconstr. Surg., 65:436, 1980.

Gonzalez-Ulloa, M.: Facial wrinkles. Plast. Reconstr. Surg., 29:658, 1962.

Gonzalez-Ulloa, M.: A trend of new operations to improve the results of rhytidectomy. Internat. Micr. J. Aesth. Plast. Surg. (Facial Plasty, 1974-A).

Gonzalez-Ulloa, M.: The history of rhytidectomy. Aesthetic Plast. Surg., 4:1, 1980.

Gonzalez-Ulloa, M., Simonin, F., and Flores, E. S.: The anatomy of the ageing face. *In* Hueston, J. T. (Ed.): Transactions of the Fifth International Congress of Plastic and Reconstructive Surgery. Australia, Butterworths, 1971, p. 1059.

Gonzalez-Ulloa, M., and Stevens, E. F.: Senility of the face. Basic study to understand its causes and effects. Plast. Reconstr. Surg., 36:239, 1965.

Griffiths, C. O.: A new approach to the operative management of forehead, brow, and frown rhytidectomies. Internat. Micr. J. Aesth. Plast. Surg. (Facial Plasty, 1974-B).

Guerrero-Santos, J.: The role of the platysma muscle in rhytidoplasty. Clin. Plast. Surg., 5:29, 1978.

Guerrero-Santos, J.: Surgical correction of the fatty fallen neck. Ann. Plast. Surg., 2:389, 1979.

Guerrero-Santos, J., Espaillat, L., and Morales, F.: Muscular lift in cervical rhytidoplasty. Plast. Reconstr. Surg., 54:127, 1974.

Gurdin, M. D., and Carlin, G. A.: Aging defects in the male: a regional approach to treatment. *In* Master, F. W., and Lewis, J. R. (Eds.): Symposium on Aesthetic Surgery of the Face, Eyelid, and Breast. St. Louis, C. V. Mosby Company, 1972.

Guy, C. L., Converse, J. M., and Morello, D. C.: Esthetic surgery for the aging face. *In* Converse, J. M. (Ed.): Reconstructive Plastic Surgery. Philadelphia, W. B. Saunders Company, 1977, p. 1868.

Hamra, S. T.: The tri-plane face lift dissection. Ann. Plast. Surg., 12:268, 1984.

Hetter, G. P.: Facial lipolysis. *In* Hetter, G. P. (Ed.): Lipolysis: The Theory and Practice of Blunt Suction Lipectomy. Boston, Little, Brown & Company, 1984.

Hinderer, U. T.: Malar implants for improvement of the facial appearance. Plast. Reconstr. Surg., 56:157, 1975.

Holländer, E.: Cosmetic surgery. *In* Joseph, M. (Ed.): Handbuch der Kosmetik. Leipzig, Verlag von Veit, 1912.

Holländer, E.: Plastische (kosmetische) Operation: Dritische Darstellung ihres gegenwärtigen Standes. *In* Klemperer, G., and Klemperer, F. (Eds.): Neue Deutsche Klinik. Berlin, Urban & Schwarzenberg, 1932.

Huang, T. T., Horowitz, B., and Lewis, S. R.: Retrobulbar hemorrhage. Plast. Reconstr. Surg., 59:39, 1977.

Hugo, N. E.: Rhytidectomy with radical lipectomy and platysmal flaps. Plast. Reconstr. Surg., 65:199, 1980.

Hugo, N. E., and Stone, E.: Anatomy for a blepharoplasty. Plast. Reconstr. Surg., 53:381, 1974.

Hunt, H. L.: Plastic Surgery of the Head, Face and Neck. Philadelphia & New York, Lea & Febiger, 1926.

Illouz, Y. G., and Fournier, P.: Illouz's technique: collapsing surgery and body sculpture. Paris, April, 1983.

Jelks, G. W., and McCord, C. D., Jr.: Dry eye syndrome and other tear film abnormalities. Clin. Plast. Surg., 8:803, 1981.

Johnson, J. B., and Hadley, R. C.: The aging face. *In* Converse, J. M. (Ed.): Reconstructive Plastic Surgery. Philadelphia, W. B. Saunders Company, 1964, p. 1329.

Joseph, J.: Hängewangenplastik (Melomioplastik). Dtsch. Med. Wochenschr., 47:287, 1921.

Joseph, J.: Nasenplastik und sonstige Gesichtsplastik. Nebst einen Anhang über Mammaplastik. Leipzig, Curt Kabitsch, 1931, pp. 507–509.

Jost, G., and Levet, Y.: Parotid fascia and face lifting: a critical evaluation of the SMAS concept. Plast. Reconstr. Surg., 74:42, 1984.

Kaufman, T., Eichenlaub, E. H., Levin, M., Hurwitz, D. J., and Klain, M.: Tobacco smoking: impairment of experimental flap survival. Ann. Plast. Surg., 13:468, 1984.

Kaye, B. L.: The extended neck lift: the "bottom line." Plast. Reconstr. Surg., 65:429, 1980.

Kaye, B. L.: The extended face-lift with ancillary procedures. Ann. Plast. Surg., 6:335, 1981.

Kligman, L. H.: Photoaging. Manifestations, prevention and treatment. Dermatol. Clin., 4:517, 1986.

Kolle, F. S.: Plastic and Cosmetic Surgery. New York, Appleton, 1911, pp. 116–117.

Lassus, C.: Ostectomy of superior orbital rim in cosmetic blepharoplasty. Plast. Reconstr. Surg., 63:481, 1979.

Lawrence, W. T., Murphy, R. C., Robson, M. C., and Heggers, J. P.: The detrimental effect of cigarette smoking on flap survival: an experimental study in the rat. Br. J. Plast. Surg., 37:216, 1984.

Leist, F. D., Masson, J. K., and Erich, J. B.: A review of 324 rhytidectomies, emphasizing complications and patient dissatisfaction. Plast. Reconstr. Surg., 59:525, 1977.

Lemmon, M. L.: Superficial fascia rhytidectomy. A restoration of the SMAS with control of the cervicomental angle. Clin. Plast. Surg., 10:449, 1983.

Lemmon, M. L., and Hamra, S. T.: Skoog rhytidectomy: a five-year experience with 577 patients. Plast. Reconstr. Surg., 65:283, 1980.

Le Roux, P., and Jones, S. H.: Total permanent removal

of wrinkles from the forehead. Br. J. Plast. Surg., 27:359, 1974.

Lewis, C. M.: Lipoplasty of the neck. Plast. Reconstr. Surg., 76:248, 1985.

Lewis, J. R., Jr.: A method of direct eyebrow lift. Ann. Plast. Surg., 10:115, 1983.

Lexer, E.: Die gesamte Wiederherstellungschirurgie. Vol. 2. Leipzig, J. A. Barth, 1931, p. 548.

Liebman, E. P., Webster, R. C., Berger, A. S., and DellaVecchia, M.: The frontalis nerve in the temporal brow lift. Arch. Otolaryngol., 108:232, 1982.

Lisman, R. D., Rees, T. D., Baker, D. C., and Smith, B.: Experience with tarsal suspension as a factor in lower lid blepharoplasty. Plast. Reconstr. Surg., 79:897, 1987.

Loeb, R.: Fat pad sliding and fat grafting for leveling lid depressions. Clin. Plast. Surg., 8:757, 1981.

Marino, H.: Treatment of wrinkles of forehead. Prensa Med. Argent., 51:1368, 1964.

Marino, H.: The surgery of facial expression. In Hueston, J. T. (Ed.): Transactions of the Fifth International Congress of Plastic and Reconstructive Surgery. Australia, Butterworths, 1971, p. 1102.

Matsunaga, R. S.: Rhytidectomy employing a two-layered closure: improved results with hidden scars. Otolaryngol. Head Neck Surg., 89:496, 1981.

McDowell, A. J.: Effective practical steps to avoid complications in face lifting. Plast. Reconstr. Surg., 50:563, 1972.

Mcgregor, M. W., and Greenberg, R. L.: Rhytidectomy. In Goldwyn, R. M. (Ed.): The Unfavorable Result in Plastic Surgery. Avoidance and Treatment. Boston, Little, Brown & Company, 1972.

McKinney, P.: Use of tarsal plate resection in blepharoplasty and atonic lower lids. Plast. Reconstr. Surg., 59:649, 1977.

McKinney, P., and Gottlieb, J.: The relationship of the great auricular nerve to the superficial musculoaponeurotic system. Ann. Plast. Surg., 14:310, 1985.

McKinney, P., and Katrana, D. J.: Prevention of injury to the great auricular nerve during rhytidectomy. Plast. Reconstr. Surg., 66:675, 1980.

McKinney, P., and Tresley, G. E.: The "maxi-SMAS": management of the platysma bands in rhytidectomy. Ann. Plast. Surg., 12:260, 1984.

Millard, D. R., Pigott, R. W., and Hedo, A.: Submandibular lipectomy. Plast. Reconstr. Surg., 41:513, 1968.

Miller, C. C.: The excision of bag-like folds of skin from the region about the eyes. Med. Brief, 34:648, 1906.

Miller, C. C.: Semilunar excision of the skin at the outer canthus for the eradication of crow's feet. Am. J. Dermatol., 11:483, 1907a.

Miller, C. C.: The Correction of Featural Imperfections. Chicago, Oak Printing Company, 1907b.

Miller, C. C.: Cosmetic Surgery: The Correction of Featural Imperfections. 2nd Ed. Chicago, Oak Printing Company, 1908, pp. 40–42.

Miller, C. C.: Cosmetic Surgery: The Correction of Featural Imperfections. Philadelphia, F. A. Davis Company, 1925, pp. 30–32.

Miller, G. D., Anstee, E. J., and Snell, J. A.: Successful replantation of an avulsed scalp by microvascular anastomoses. Plast. Reconstr. Surg., 58:133, 1976.

Mitz, V., and Peyronie, M.: The superficial musculoaponeurotic system (SMAS) in the parotid and cheek area. Plast. Reconstr. Surg., 58:80, 1976.

Morel-Fatio, D.: Cosmetic surgery of the face. In Gibson, T. (Ed.): Modern Trends in Plastic Surgery. Washington, Butterworth, 1964, p. 221.

Morgan, B. L.: The aftercare of rhytidectomies with the "no dressing" technique. Plast. Reconstr. Surg., 51:576, 1973.

Noël, A.: La Chirurgie Esthétique. Son Rôle Social. Paris, Masson et Cie, 1926, pp. 62–66.

Noël, A.: La Chirurgie Esthétique. Clermont (Oise), Thiron et Cie, 1928.

Nolan, J., Jenkins, R. A., Kurihara, K., and Schultz, R. C.: The acute effects of cigarette smoke exposure on experimental skin flaps, Plast. Reconstr. Surg., 75:544, 1985.

Owsley, J. Q., Jr.: Platysma-fascial rhytidectomy: a preliminary report. Plast. Reconstr. Surg., 60:843, 1977.

Owsley, J. Q., Jr.: SMAS-platysma face lift. Plast. Reconstr. Surg., 71:573, 1983.

Owsley, J. Q., Jr.: Re.: Vilain: Dallas platysmas (letter). Ann. Plast. Surg., 14:98, 1985.

Panneton, P.: Le blepharochalasis. À propos de 51 cas dans la même famille. Arch. Ophthalmol., 58:725, 1936.

Passot, R.: La chirurgie esthétique des rides du visage. Presse Med., 27:258, 1919.

Passot, R.: Chirurgie Esthétique Pure: Techniques et Resultats. Paris, Gaston Doin et Cie, 1930.

Passot, R.: Chirurgie Esthétique Pure (Techniques et Resultats). Paris, Gaston Doin et Cie, 1931.

Passot, R.: Quelques generalités sur l'operation correctif des rides du visage. Rev. Chir. Plast., 3:23, 1933.

Pennisi, V. R., and Capozzi, A.: The transposition of fat in cervicofacial rhytidectomy. Plast. Reconstr. Surg., 49:423, 1972.

Pensler, J. M., Ward, J. W., and Parry, S. W.: The superficial musculoaponeurotic system in the upper lip: an anatomic study in cadavers. Plast. Reconstr. Surg., 75:488, 1985.

Peterson, R.: Cervical rhytidoplasty—a personal approach. Presented at the Annual Symposium on Aesthetic Plastic Surgery, Guadalajara, Mexico, October, 1974.

Peterson, R.: American Society of Aesthetic Surgery Meeting, Las Vegas, NV, 1982.

Pitanguy, I.: Section of the frontalis-procerus-corrugator aponeurosis in the correction of frontal and glabellar wrinkles. Ann. Plast. Surg., 2:422, 1979.

Pitanguy, I., Cansancao, A., and Daher, J.: Resultados desfavoraveis em cirurgia plastica, hematomas pos ritidectomies. Rev. Bras. de Cir., 61:155, 1971.

Pitanguy, I., Pinto, A. R., Garcia, L. C., and Lessa, S. F.: Ritodoplastia em homens (rhytidoplasty in men). Rev. Bras. Cir., 63:209, 1973.

Pitanguy, I., and Ramos, A. S.: The frontal branch of the facial nerve: the importance of its variations in face lifting. Plast. Reconstr. Surg., 38:352, 1966.

Prockop, D. J., Kivirikko, K. I., Tuderman, L., Guzman, N. A.: The biosynthesis of collagen and its disorders. Part II. N. Engl. J., Med., 301:77, 1979.

Rees, T. D.: Correction of ectropion resulting from blepharoplasty. Plast. Reconstr. Surg., 50:1, 1972.

Rees, T. D.: The "dry eye" complication after a blepharoplasty. Plast. Reconstr. Surg., 56:375, 1975.

Rees, T. D.: Aesthetic Plastic Surgery. Vol. II. Philadelphia, W. B. Saunders Company, 1980, pp. 498–499.

Rees, T. D.: Prevention of ectropion by horizontal shortening of the lower lid during blepharoplasty. Ann. Plast. Surg., 11:17, 1983.

Rees, T. D., and Aston, S. J.: Complications of rhytidectomy. Clin. Plast. Surg., 5:109, 1978.

Rees, T. D., and Dupuis, C.: Baggy eyelids in young adults. Plast. Reconstr. Surg., 43:381, 1969.

Rees, T. D., and Jelks, G. W.: Blepharoplasty and the dry eye syndrome: guidelines for surgery. Plast. Reconstr. Surg., 68:249, 1981.

Rees, T. D., and LaTrenta, G.: The role of the Schirmer's test and orbital morphology in predicting dry eye syndrome after blepharoplasty. Plast. Reconstr. Surg., 82:619, 1988.

Rees, T. D., Lee, Y. C., and Coburn, R. J.: Expanding hematoma after rhytidectomy. Plast. Reconstr. Surg., 51:149, 1973.

Rees, T. D., Liverett, D. M., and Guy, C. L.: The effect of cigarette smoking on skin-flap survival in the face lift patient. Plast. Reconstr. Surg., 73:911, 1984.

Rees, T. D., and Tabbal, N.: Lower blepharoplasty with emphasis on the orbicularis muscle. Clin. Plast. Surg., 8:643, 1981.

Rees, T. D., and Wood-Smith, D.: Cosmetic Facial Surgery. Philadelphia, W. B. Saunders Company, 1973.

Rees, T. D., Wood-Smith, D. and Converse, J. M.: The Ehlers-Danlos syndrome. Plast. Reconstr. Surg., 32:39, 1963.

Regnault, P.: Complete face and forehead lifting with double traction on "crows-feet." Plast. Reconstr. Surg., 49:123, 1972.

Reus, W. F., Robson, M. C., Zachary, L., and Heggers, J. P.: Acute effects of tobacco smoking on the blood flow in the cutaneous micro-circulation. Br. J. Plast. Surg., 37:213, 1984.

Rogers, B. O.: A brief history of cosmetic surgery. Surg. Clin. North Am., 51:265, 1971.

Rogers, B. O.: The development of aesthetic plastic surgery: A history. Aesthetic Plast. Surg., 1:3, 1976.

Rogers, B. O.: A chronologic history of cosmetic surgery. Bull. N.Y. Acad. Med., 47:265, 1977.

Rudolph, R., and Woodward, M.: Ultrastructure of elastosis in facial rhytidectomy skin. Plast. Reconstr. Surg., 67:295, 1981.

Rybka, F. J., and O'Hara, E. T.: Surgical significance of the Ehlers-Danlos syndrome. Am. J. Surg., 113:431, 1967.

Sichel, J.: Aphorismes pratiques sur divers points d'ophthalmologie. Ann. Oculist, 12:185, 1844.

Singer, R.: Improvement of the "young" fatty neck. Plast. Reconstr. Surg., 73:582, 1984.

Skoog, T.: Rhytidectomy—a personal experience and technique. Presented and demonstrated on live television at the Seventh Annual Symposium on Cosmetic Surgery at Cedars of Lebanon Hospital, Miami, FL, February, 1973.

Skoog, T.: Plastic Surgery—New Methods and Refinements. Philadelphia, W. B. Saunders Company, 1974.

Smith, B.: Postsurgical complications of cosmetic blepharoplasty. Trans. Am. Acad. Ophthalmol. Otolaryngol., 73:1162, 1969.

Smith, B., and Lisman, R. D.: Cosmetic correction of eyelid deformities associated with exophthalmos. Clin. Plast. Surg., 8:777, 1981.

Sokol, A. B., and Sokol, T. P.: Transblepharoplasty brow suspension. Plast. Reconstr. Surg., 69:940, 1982.

Spira, M.: Lower blepharoplasty—a clinical study. Plast. Reconstr. Surg., 59:35, 1977.

Spira, M., Gerow, F. J., and Hardy, S. B.: Cervicofacial rhytidectomy. Plast. Reconstr. Surg., 40:551, 1967.

Stark, R. B.: Follow-up clinic: Deliberate hypotension for blepharoplasty and rhytidectomy. Plast. Reconstr. Surg., 49:453, 1972.

Stark, R. B.: A rhytidectomy series. Plast. Reconstr. Surg., 59:373, 1977.

Stasior, O. G.: Blindness associated with cosmetic blepharoplasty. Clin. Plast. Surg., 8:793, 1981.

Straith, R. E., Raju, D., and Hipps, C.: The study of hematomas in 500 consecutive face lifts. Plast. Reconstr. Surg., 59:694, 1977.

Teimourian, B.: Face and neck suction-assisted lipectomy associated with rhytidectomy. Plast. Reconstr. Surg., 72:627, 1983.

Tenzel, R. R.: Treatment of lagophthalmos of the lower lid. Arch. Ophthalmol., 81:366, 1969.

Tessier, P.: Ridectomie frontale—lifting frontale. Gazette Med. France, 75:5565, 1968.

Thompson, D. P., and Ashley, F. L.: Face-lift complications. A study of 922 cases performed in a 6-year period. Plast. Reconstr. Surg., 61:40, 1978.

Tipton, J. B.: Should the subcutaneous tissue be plicated in a face lift? Plast. Reconstr. Surg., 54:1, 1974.

Uitto, J.: Connective tissue biochemistry of the aging dermis. Age-related alterations in collagen and elastin. Dermatol. Clin., 4:433, 1986.

Vinas, J. C., Caviglia, C., and Cortinas, J. L.: Forehead rhytidoplasty and brow lifting. Plast. Reconstr. Surg., 57:445, 1976.

Vinnik, C. A.: An intravenous dissociation technique for outpatient plastic surgery. Tranquility in the office facility. Plast. Reconstr. Surg., 67:799, 1981.

Vistnes, L. M., and Souther, S. G.: The anatomical basis for common cosmetic anterior neck deformities. Ann. Plast. Surg., 2:381, 1979.

Washio, H.: Rhytidoplasty of the forehead—an anatomical approach. In Marchac, D. (Ed.): Transactions of the Sixth International Congress of Plastic and Reconstructive Surgery. Paris, Masson et Cie, 1976, p. 430.

Webster, G. V.: The ischemic face lift. Plast. Reconstr. Surg., 50:560, 1972.

Webster, R. C., Kazda, G., Hamdan, U. S., Fuleihan, N. S., and Smith, R. C.: Cigarette smoking and face lift: conservative versus wide undermining. Plast. Reconstr. Surg., 77:596, 1986.

Webster, R. C., Smith, R. C., Papsidero, M. J., Karolow, W. W., and Smith, K. F.: Comparison of SMAS plication with SMAS imbrication in face lifting. Laryngoscope, 92:901, 1982.

44

Kitaro Ohmori

Esthetic Surgery in the Asian Patient

As in Western countries, the demand for esthetic surgery has increased in Asia and various surgical procedures are being carried out. Most of the procedures employ the same standards as in the West, and the general principles are basically no different from those outlined in other chapters of this text. However, the one unique characteristic of esthetic surgery in the Orient is the popularity of two procedures commonly referred to as the double eyelid operation and augmentation rhinoplasty. These surgical procedures are often viewed as representative of esthetic surgery in Asia. Nevertheless, the procedures performed under these titles can differ widely in intention or indication, depending on the individual surgeon.

HISTORY

The first efforts at esthetic surgery shortly followed the introduction of Western medicine in Asia (Mikamo, 1986), but the history is confusing. Even with a review of the literature, it is impossible to gain a clear perspective of the whole subject. One important reason is the fact that in Asia, even after the organization of professional surgical societies, there were no academic organizations in the field of esthetic surgery and there were no opportunities for professional discussion. Progress in this area tended to be made by the individual practitioner who carried out the procedures. At the same time, one must not forget that the medical community, and society at large, did not necessarily sanction the concept of esthetic surgery.

The fundamental concepts for contemporary esthetic surgical procedures of the eyes and nose were developed by Nishihata (1955) and Uchida (1957). The variations that have followed represent only modifications of their basic principles. However, since Uchida was an ophthalmologist and Nishihata an otorhinolaryngologist, it is apparent that cosmetic surgery of the eyes and nose in Asia has not developed from the mainstream of plastic and reconstructive surgery.

In Japan, the development of plastic and reconstructive surgery lagged behind other surgical disciplines. It first emerged as a branch of dermatology and urology under S. Ohmori and his colleagues during the 1950's, decades after a departmentalized system of medical care had been developed on the German model (Ohmori, 1954).

The Japan Society of Plastic and Reconstructive Surgery was established by surgeons who gathered around Miki and others (Ohmori, 1954). They were keenly aware that plastic surgery needed to be developed by surgeons trained by international authorities in this field. Development of plastic surgery in Asia proceeded rapidly thereafter until it reached its present state. In general, esthetic plastic surgery has developed into an integral aspect of plastic surgery, and today it carries the same commitment to excellence based on surgical principles, clinical experience, and research.

STANDARDS OF BEAUTY

The change in a person's appearance as the result of a surgical procedure designed to make her more attractive might be called "beautification." The basic nature of these operations cannot be separated from such cosmetic concepts as "minor touch-up," "minor changes," and "scarless surgery." In contrast, because esthetic surgery developed as a branch of Western plastic surgery, its vocabulary is basically "scientific." For example, a hump nose is designated as a deformity, as are the changes in the face that take place with aging. The goal of Western esthetic surgery has been the correction of such "deformities."

In the Orient, cosmetic surgery of the eyes and nose is perceived as giving a normal face additional beauty, whereas in Western thinking deformities are corrected to attain a more complete physical self.

It should be noted that the Orient is changing rapidly. This phenomenon is not unrelated to the Westernization of the East through education and the mass media. However, the Orient is also changing on its own. For example, the social understanding of cosmetic surgery has evolved to the point where the old philosophy that nothing should be done no longer prevails. The younger generation is beginning to believe that if there is a way to improve something, there is no reason why one should not take advantage of it. Thus, it is not difficult to predict that esthetic surgery in the Orient will in time change its orientation from beautification to the concept of the correction of deformity.

In the past, various reasons have been proposed to explain why facial cosmetic surgery in the Orient is preoccupied with procedures of the eyes and nose. The Japanese face is fairly round in shape and lacks contour, compared with the Caucasian face. Therefore, the evaluation of beauty was not based on the overall impression of the facial profile, but on esthetic standards that empha-

sized limited regions, such as the eyes and nose. However, this argument is specious. Rhinoplasty is a procedure that fundamentally determines the profile view. In other words, the popularity of augmentation rhinoplasty in the Orient indicates that great importance is placed on the profile in evaluating a face. Orientals also judge facial appearance by the "proportions" of the face, i.e., the beauty of individual features such as the eyes and nose. Therefore, if surgeons in Asia have developed more efficacious procedures for the eyes and nose in general, it can be assumed that these procedures should probably be considered representative of esthetic surgery in the Orient.

While the face is only a single attribute of the human body, it is the one most easily recognized. The beauty of a face is related to factors that vary with trends in fashion and ethnic considerations. Nevertheless, a face that is beautiful beyond a certain level is usually accepted universally, transcending temporal, geographic, and racial factors. In a modern nation with well-developed communications media, a beautiful face is judged not only by the unique ethnic standards peculiar to that nation, but also by criteria for beauty that are common to other nations and races.

In what may be termed a "below average face," many ethnically unique features may be prominent. For example, in Japan the face and cephalometric radiograph illustrated in Figure 44–1 are generally accepted as "attractive" by modern-day Japanese. There is no evidence of bimaxillary protrusion or bimaxillary prognathism. The facial proportion and nasal angles measured for such an "attractive face" seem to be no different from those obtained from a Western "attractive face." However, many Orientals still seem to feel positively about a woman's face which retains juvenile features, referring to it as slim and innocent.

The quantification and analysis of features that determine the beauty of a face constitute an important and necessary subject of research. However, the ability to calculate average values from data derived from "attractive faces," to formulate a model matching these values, and to lead the patient toward such a single goal is not the objective of esthetic surgery. The more extensive the measurements derived from the study of the "attractive face," the more variety one finds

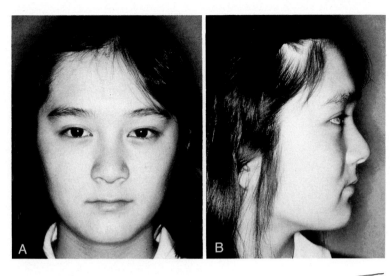

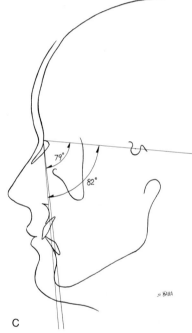

Figure 44–1. An "attractive" Japanese female. *A*, Frontal view. *B*, Profile view. *C*, Cephalometric radiograph. The SN distance is 70, the SNA 82 degrees, and the SNB 79 degrees. There is no evidence of bimaxillary protrusion or prognathism.

C

in the data (Farkas, Kolar, and Munro, 1986). If the average numerical values pertaining to the "attractive face" were correct, esthetic surgery would merely be producing a great number of similar faces. This would mean that the individuality of people would be lost, and that, in itself, would be a fundamental flaw. Moreover, there are quantitative limitations to what can be accomplished with a surgical procedure. More important, if a numerical value were derived from a database that was itself imperfect, or if these values were somehow manipulated for a particular purpose, the numbers not only would be meaningless but could have a harmful effect.

Uchida (1957) developed a "beauty index" for the eyes and nose in Japan, and although he was doubtful of the validity of the proposed numerical values, his index gained a life of its own. The result was that both physicians and patients became possessed of the illusion that esthetic surgery existed merely to satisfy such numerical standards. A reexamination of the various items that formed the basis for these calculations demonstrated that the numbers rested on a somewhat biased foundation. For example, in items that comprised the beauty index of the nose, the craniofacial framework was not evaluated by cephalometric technique. A popular actress of the day

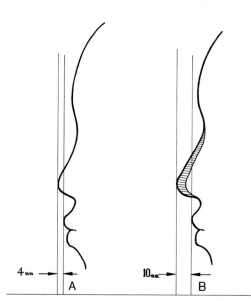
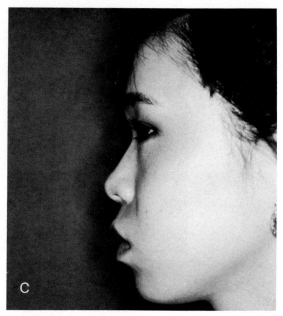

Figure 44–2. The beauty index of Uchida (1957) and the role of nasal augmentation. In an "attractive" Japanese face, the distance between the nasal tip and the medial portion of the upper lip is between 10 and 14 mm. In the below average face, it may be as low as 0 to 4 mm. Therefore, to satisfy the beauty index, it is necessary to augment the nasal tip and dorsum. A, Below average profile. B, Intended change with nasal augmentation. C, Clinical example of a patient with bimaxillary protrusion who had undergone nasal augmentation.

was made the model of the "attractive face." The data for the "below average face" were derived from a patient population thought to have deformities not only in the nose but also in the facial framework. Thus, the numerical values were determined mainly by measurements derived from the surface of the face and from personal impression. Consequently, it was first thought that orthopedic deformities of the face, such as bimaxillary protrusion, were often seen in patients seeking cosmetic surgery of the nose.

In the cases cited by Uchida (1957), the height of the nasal tip is at the same level as that of the medial portion of the upper lip in many patients, certainly a characteristic not found on the "attractive face." Even though Uchida was aware that the fundamental cause of such features lay in the craniofacial skeleton of regions other than that of the nose, the indices were formulated on the premise that this was strictly a nasal problem. Therefore, esthetic surgery in Japan came to rest on a foundation based on a beauty index that confused deformities of the craniofacial framework with problems of the external nose. This approach allowed augmentation procedures to be applied to the nasal dorsum to increase the height differ-

ential between the nasal tip and the medial portion of the upper lip, i.e., to correct maxillary protrusion without surgically correcting the maxilla (Fig. 44–2). This surgical philosophy was probably also related to the prevailing surgical technology of the times, in which surgeons were trained only in nasal augmentation procedures using a prosthesis. Moreover, many surgeons believed it appropriate to respond to the patient's every demand and to increase the height of the nasal dorsum if the patient so desired. This led to the mass production of the so-called *seikeibijin* ("plastic surgery beauty"). Although there is no clear definition of the seikeibijin, the term is widely used within Japanese society. "Seikei" means to organize the shape, and "bijin" means a beauty, in the sense of a beautiful person. Thus, the term would mean a "beauty whose shape has been organized."

A slight maxillary protrusion, common among Japanese, and a concave nasal dorsum were the primary indications for augmentation of the nasal dorsum with a silicone prosthesis. In order to balance the augmented nose and to deemphasize the slight bimaxillary protrusion, the chin was also augmented. Such surgeons then reasoned that to balance all facial features after the above two procedures, the forehead must also be augmented. In addition, a double eyelid operation with excessive defatting was performed on the upper lids. The final result was the creation of a *seikeibijin* (Fig. 44–3). When one looks at

such a face, one immediately detects the unnatural appearance. The female face, which should be small and delicate, has been enlarged by augmentation, and the result is that the feminine characteristics have been

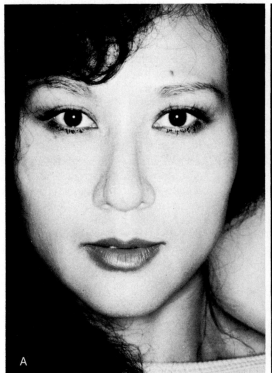

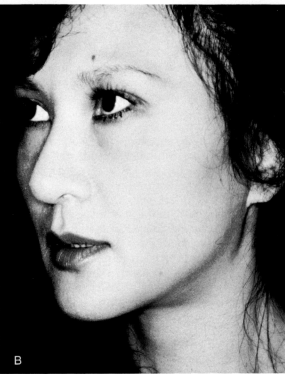

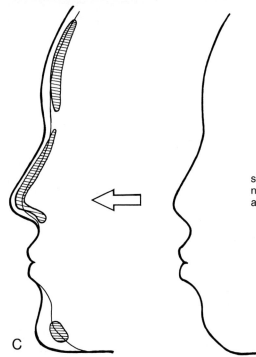

Figure 44–3. *Seikeibijin* is a term used to describe a face whose shape has been created by silicone augmentation of the forehead, nose, and chin. *A,* Frontal view. *B,* Profile view. *C,* Outline of the areas of silicone prosthesis augmentation.

erased. Faces categorized by the term *seikei-bijin* are unfortunately mass produced, despite the fact that the society that uses the term does not necessarily feel positively about either the face or the word.

PATIENT SELECTION

It is well known that patients seeking esthetic surgical treatment can also have psychologic problems. Thus, in examining a patient, one must never forget the caveats of patient selection (see also Chap. 3).

If a patient brings a picture of a movie star but uses it only to supplement his or her own explanation, this behavior alone is not a contraindication to surgery. However, when the patient wishes to change her face to be exactly like that in the picture, or believes that the operation will make her a "beauty," the surgeon should consider the matter carefully before agreeing to perform surgery. There are also times when an Oriental patient brings a photograph of a Caucasian movie star and asks to be changed into an exact replica. No procedure can accomplish this and it would be inappropriate to carry out any surgical procedure to that end. Of course, it is also readily understandable that the requests made by an Oriental patient may differ somewhat depending on whether she is living in the East or the West.

Esthetic eye surgery and profileplasty profoundly change the impression that the face gives postoperatively. Thus, another issue is whether the patient is psychologically prepared to accept such a degree of postoperative change. Once a face has been accepted and recognized by society, one must be aware of the risk of taking away an individual's entire social identity by fundamentally changing that face. Unless a patient is living under exceptional circumstances, this type of radical surgical change should be made before the patient begins to lead an active social life. If the patients are still young, the possibility is greater that they will be able to accept and absorb these changes as a part of the other changes that come with growth and development. In contrast, in the casè of middle-aged or older individuals, such facial changes are accepted with great difficulty by them and their associates. However successful the operation may have been, patients may not be able to return to their usual social life.

SURGERY FOR THE DOUBLE EYELID

Esthetic surgery for the upper eyelids of the Oriental is a combination of a double eyelidplasty, defatting, and correction of the epicanthal fold.

The difference between the blepharoplasty of the West and the double eyelidplasty of the Orient is the objective. In the former, it is to correct the palpebral aging changes. In the latter, the main objective is to create a double eyelid by reconstructing a superior palpebral sulcus. However similar the double eyelid operation may be to the procedure that alters the slant of the palpebral aperture in the West (Ortiz-Monasterio and Rodriguez, 1985), the double eyelid operation is also a procedure designed to change the impression that the eyes create. As noted, operations to change the overall expression of the eyes are relatively infrequent in Western countries.

The oldest report of the creation of a double eyelid was in a patient with a double eyelid on the right eye and a single lid on the left. The correction was achieved by suturing the left upper lid (Mikamo, 1986). The fact that such operations were conducted to obtain symmetry of the eyelids, creating a double lid in one lid, emphasizes that the double eyelid itself was nothing new or strange to the Oriental. In the following years, the technique of the double eyelid operation was developed mainly by ophthalmologists. The basis for the operation was related to the prevalence of trachoma. Before World War II, treatment of the posttrachoma cicatricial entropion was one of the greatest tasks faced by the ophthalmologist. As represented by the Hotz (1981) technique, procedures to correct the entropion were executed widely. Having conducted these operations frequently, surgeons began to realize that when adhesion occurred between the tarsus and the skin of the upper lid, a double eyelid was created. Consequently, they modified the existing procedure into one with cosmetic considerations. The result was the formation of a prototype of what is presently known as the double eyelid operation (Hayashi, 1939; Hotz, 1981).

Anatomic Considerations

A double eyelid is attributed to a fold in the skin of the upper eyelid that is present when the eye is open. The *superior palpebral*

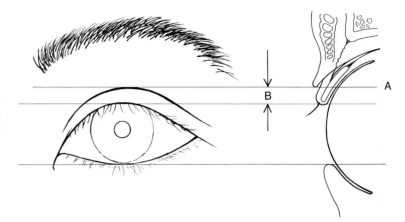

Figure 44–4. Double eyelid line *(A)*. The distance between the line and the lid margin is referred to as the width of the double eyelid *(B)*.

fold appears almost parallel to the lid margin. The line below the fold is called the *double eyelid line,* and the distance between the line and the margin of the lid is called the *width* of the double eyelid (Fig. 44–4).

The anatomic explanation for the presence of the superior palpebral fold was provided by Sayoc (1954), who noted that the expansion of the levator muscle runs through the orbicularis oculi muscle to insert into the dermis (Figs. 44–5, 44–6). However, accord-ing to Ide (1979), it is extremely difficult to identify the muscle branches by light micros-copy; thus, the theory remains somewhat speculative. However, since the double eyelid becomes apparent as the superior palpebral fold is pulled upward by the contraction of the levator muscle, it is logical to imagine that a double eyelid would appear if there were a connection between the levator and skin of the fold.

Westerners generally assume that the up-

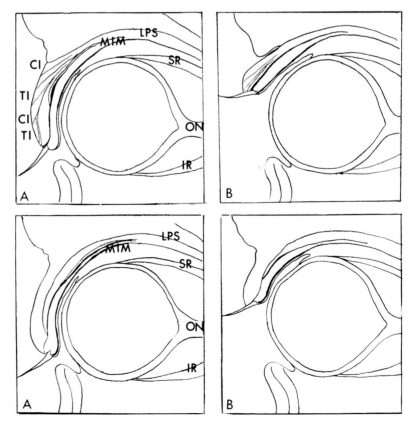

Figure 44–5. Sayoc's concept of anatomic variations between the Caucasian and Oriental eye-lid. *Upper,* sagittal section of a Caucasian eyelid, showing the in-sertion of the levator aponeurosis expansion above the upper edge of the tarsal plate into the dermis of the superior palpebral fold. *Lower,* Sagittal section of an Ori-ental foldless eyelid. Note the lev-ator expansion terminates at the septum orbitale. *A,* Closed posi-tion. *B,* Open position. LPS = levator palpebrae superioris; ON = optic nerve; IR = inferior rectus muscle; SR = superior rectus muscle; TI = tarsal insertion of the aponeurosis of the LPS; CI = cutaneous insertion of the apo-neurosis of the LPS; MIM = Mül-ler's involuntary muscle.

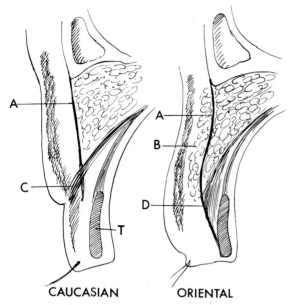

Figure 44–6. Anatomic variations in the Caucasian and Oriental eyelids. *A,* The septum orbitale. *B,* The submuscular fat. *C,* The expansion of the levator palpebrae superioris aponeurosis through the septum orbitale and orbicularis oculi muscle to attach to the skin of the superior palpebral fold in the Caucasian lid. *D,* In the Oriental lid, the levator expansion terminates at the septum orbitale. (After Fernandez.)

CAUCASIAN   ORIENTAL

per eyelid of the Oriental is always a single eyelid. This is a misunderstanding. To date, there have been many anatomic studies, but in summary it can be stated that approxi-

mately 50 per cent or more of the Japanese population possess double eyelids. They are more frequent in females than in males, and the wider ones occur more often in females (Nakagawa and associates, 1974). Thus, among Orientals, it is not unusual for the upper lids to vary between being double and single in the same individual, depending on such variables as fatigue.

In contrast, the epicanthus appears in all races between the third and sixth fetal months, but disappears in Caucasians usually at the time of birth or by adolescence at the latest, unless there is a congenital deformity. While the existence of the epicanthus after maturity in the Caucasian signifies deformity, in the Oriental at least 50 per cent of individuals retain this fold after maturity. Moreover, if slight traces are included, almost all Orientals retain the fold, and thus it may be said that the epicanthal fold is a unique feature of the Oriental face. The anatomic differences between the Caucasian and the Oriental eyelid are summarized in Table 44–1.

Preoperative Considerations

One of the most common reasons why the double eyelid operation is requested is related to make-up techniques for the eyelashes. In

Table 44–1. Anatomic Differences

Caucasian Eyelid	Oriental Eyelid
Well developed	Less developed
Palpebral fold present	No fold present
With deep-seated look	With full upper lid look
Wider and longer palpebral fissure	Narrower and shorter palpebral fissure
Corneal overlap about 3 mm with iris well exposed	Corneal overlap 5 mm or more with iris at 12 o'clock border or partly hidden
Canthal angles obtuse	Canthal angles somewhat acute
Epicanthus rare	Epicanthus very common
Caruncle well exposed	Caruncle partly or wholly hidden
Eyelashes longer and roots well exposed, tilted slightly	Eyelashes shorter and roots usually covered by sagging skin, not tilted
Languorous appearance	No languorous appearance; mysterious look
Past middle age, sagging starts over preseptal portion of orbicularis muscle just above fold line	Sagging starts at edge or just above ciliary line
Insertion of levator to skin present	Insertion of levator to skin absent
Lid fold is formed when levator contracts	No lid fold formed, instead skin rolls in upward
Septum orbitale interrupted by insertion of aponeurosis of levator to skin	Septum orbitale not interrupted as it inserts on aponeurosis of levator muscle
Presence of full upper eyelid rare	Presence of full upper eyelid common
Septum orbitale inserts usually high, about 10–12 mm above superior border of tarsus	Insertion on aponeurosis usually low, just above superior border of tarsus (5–7 mm)
When lids are closed, palpebral fissure appears horizontal, although temporal portion is 1 mm higher than nasal portion	When lids are closed, edge appears slightly slanting in temporal portion, because it is higher by 2–3 mm, giving what is called Oriental slant

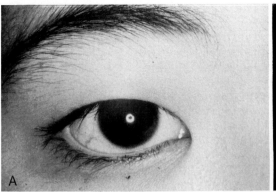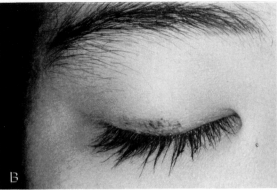

Figure 44–7. *A, B,* Make-up applied to the cilia rubs off on the skin of a single upper eyelid or incomplete double eyelid.

individuals with incomplete double eyelid folds or with single eyelids, the make-up applied to the cilia rubs off on the skin of the upper eyelids when the eye opens (Fig. 44–7).

Before establishing whether the double eyelid or the single eyelid is preferred by the Oriental, an attempt should be made to illustrate the features that are disliked. A less than attractive eye (Fig. 44–8A) has an epicanthal fold that is too prominent, even for the Oriental face, and the eyelid is excessively thick. The superior palpebral fold is unclear, and a portion of skin overhangs the true margin of the lid as a curtain. On the other hand, in what is perceived as an attractive eye (Fig. 44–8B), the epicanthal fold does not directly cross the aperture of the lids (palpebral aperture), and the lid thickness appears minimal. In such an eye, a superior orbitopalpebral sulcus of moderate depth is often found along with one or more obvious superior palpebral sulci above the area between the orbital and palpebral portions of

the orbicularis oculi muscle. When the eye is opened, a natural double eyelid is formed in most cases.

Technique

The so-called double eyelid operation is often explained as one that transforms a single eyelid into a double eyelid. The procedure is executed with the aim of creating a missing palpebral sulcus. The procedures of defatting that may be performed concomitantly with superior palpebral sulcusplasty must be understood as being separate from the double eyelid operation proper.

In the planning of the fold construction, a method of defining the distance in millimeters from the lid margin (limbi palpebrales anteriores) is generally used. The specific distances are usually based on the clinical experience of the individual surgeon. However, it is preferable to establish the exact position of the fold using anatomic defini-

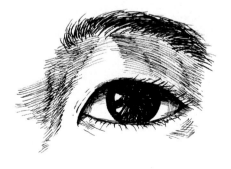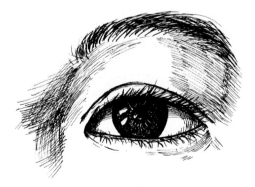

A   B

Figure 44–8. The Japanese esthetics of an "unattractive" *(A)* and "attractive" (B) eye.

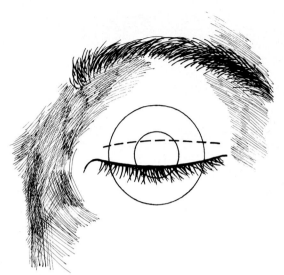

Figure 44–9. Relationship of the line of the superior palpebral sulcus on the upper eyelid and the underlying globe.

tions. The natural palpebral fold of the Oriental face lies at the border between the orbital and palpebral portions of the upper eyelid. At this position, the eyelid begins to lose the roundness or bulge created by the globe at the center of the lid when the eye is closed. An obvious horizontal line is apparent at this location, even for the single eyelid. Consequently, the double eyelid fold should be established as a more or less horizontal line that passes along this location (Fig. 44–9).

The *width of the double eyelid* in the double eyelid procedure must simulate what occurs naturally in the Oriental. The sulcus (suprapalpebral) is covered by the plica (skin) that hangs over the front of it. The degree of coverage may vary: in some the skin covers only slightly, while in others the skin hangs down until it almost reaches the cilia. Since this variation exists naturally, the surgeon must consider not only his own esthetic sense but also the preferences of the patient.

The procedure for establishing the *width of the double eyelid* fold can be summarized as follows. After the position of the fold is determined in the supine position, the patient is asked to sit upright. In this position the patient closes his eyes. With an applicator stick the surgeon presses the fold toward the globe while the patient opens his eyes again slowly. If this maneuver results in a satisfactory width for the double eyelid, it will not be necessary to resect any skin during the operation. However, if the double eyelid lacks adequate width at this point, the stick is gently moved upward until the desired breadth is reached (Fig. 44–10). The tip is pressed in toward the eyeball with slight pressure, and the patient is asked to open his eyes. In doing this, the impression made by the tip of the stick is left above the previously determined fold. The distance between the sulcus and the point of the impression is measured. The plica or skin fold that hangs over the front of the sulcus begins at the

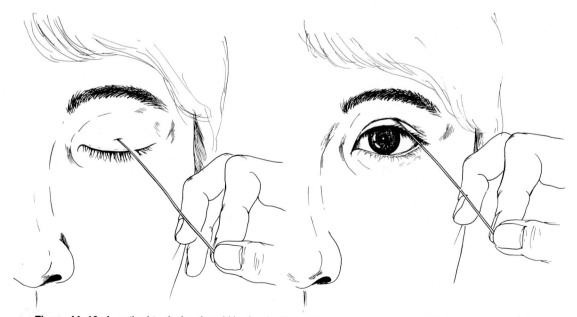

Figure 44–10. A method to design the width of a double eyelid using an applicator stick. See text for details.

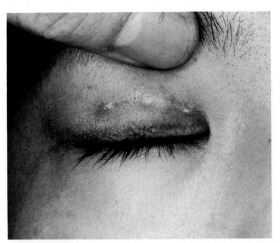

Figure 44–11. Postoperative result of the buried suture (nonincision) method of creating double eyelids. The visible lumps are located where the buried sutures were placed.

sulcus and runs toward the eyebrow, with the double eyelid line as its lowest point. It can be deduced that the amount of skin to be resected is twice this distance. A basic principle of the double eyelid operation involves placing a spindle-shaped incision with the latter value as its greatest width, located immediately above the sulcus (Fig. 44–10).

Creation of the Fold (Palpebral Sulcus). Many procedures have been outlined for the creation of a palpebral sulcus. These procedures can be divided roughly into nonincision and incision methods.

The *nonincision* method is usually separated into the suture method and the buried suture method. The suture method is one in which the fold is fixed by the scar whose appearance follows a tissue reaction to a plain catgut ligature. The buried suture method calls for an anchor suture to be placed between the dermis of the superior palpebral skin and the levator or the tarsus that moves with the levator. Unfortunately, there are several disadvantages to the nonincision method. For example, the suture method is usually applied to eyelids that already possess a tendency toward a double lid, e.g., those that vary between double and single lids. Since the upper lids in such individuals already have many of the elements necessary to form a double eyelid, this operation may be effective if patients are well chosen and the operating surgeon is well versed in the application of this method. In many cases, however, there is a strong possibility that the palpebral sulcus will disappear with the passage of time.

In the buried suture method, absorbable suture material is used. However, in some patients the anchor suture, or cysts originating from the suture, stand out as small lumps when the eyes are closed. This is most common in patients with thin upper eyelids, ironically those who are also the best candidates for this technique (Fig. 44–11). Furthermore, in individuals in whom the width of the double eyelid needs to be adjusted, the only way to do it with the nonincision method is to create an unnatural fold far above the original fold. With so many disadvantages, the technique of choice for double eyelidplasty is the incision method. Many different incision methods have been reported, but the technique of the author will be emphasized.

The Incision Method of Double Eyelidplasty. Accurate preoperative planning is

Figure 44–12. The suture (incision) method of double eyelidplasty. *A,* Cross sectional view. Note that each skin suture must include the expansion of the levator muscle. *B,* The suture line at completion of the procedure.

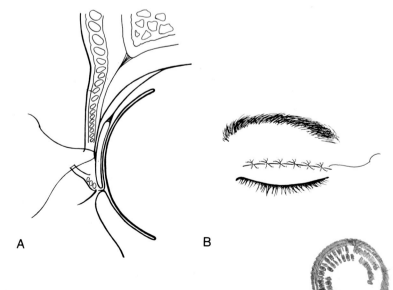

A

B

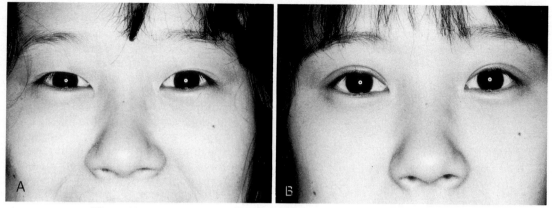

Figure 44–13. Double eyelidplasty. *A,* Preoperative view. *B,* Postoperative view.

crucial for the incision method. In patients in whom skin needs to be excised, the incision is made according to the preoperative measurements (see Fig. 44–10). When excision is unnecessary, the incision is made above the established fold. After the skin is incised, the incision is extended through the muscle layer at the height of the sulcus, and the tarsus is exposed. Following this, the attachment of the expansion of the levator palpebrae superioris to the tarsus via the ciliary bundle is undermined. At this point any deposit of fat above the tarsus is removed. After complete hemostasis, the skin below the incision—the expansion of the levator muscle—and the skin above the incision are joined by fixation sutures. At least six sutures are necessary between the skin and levator expansion. Fol-

lowing this procedure, continuous sutures are used to coapt the skin (Fig. 44–12). A patient who underwent this technique is illustrated in Figure 44–13.

Alternative techniques have been described by Sayoc (1956) (Fig. 44–14) and Fernandez (1960) (Fig. 44–15).

CORRECTIVE PROFILEPLASTY

It is generally accepted that the most common cosmetic nasal procedure in the West is reduction rhinoplasty; in the Orient it is the augmentation rhinoplasty. However, as stated earlier, there is confusion over what constitutes augmentation rhinoplasty. The actual operation termed augmentation rhi-

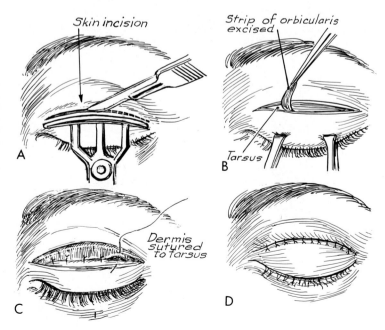

Figure 44–14. Sayoc technique. *A,* Line showing the height and shape of the fold to be constructed. Lid fixation forceps in place, indicating just above it the incision made through the skin, subcutaneous tissue, and orbicularis down to the anterior surface of the tarsal plate. *B,* The narrow strip of orbicularis muscle (1 to 2 mm) excised from the nasal to the temporal poles of the incision. *C,* Suturing of the dermal layer of the lower skin flap to the anterior surface of the exposed tarsus. *D,* Closed incision.

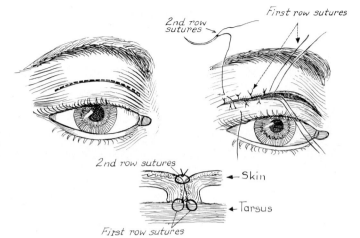

Figure 44–15. Fernandez technique. Operation for the formation of a superior palpebral fold. Skin is incised. A strip of orbicularis muscle and septum orbitale is excised and excess orbital fat is removed. The levator muscle is sutured to the skin at the lower border of the skin incision. Note the two-layer closure.

noplasty will be described first. This will be followed by a discussion that divides the profile into its component parts: the external nose and the facial framework other than the external nose.

Augmentation Rhinoplasty

The present techniques that implant a prosthesis to augment the nose were developed by Nishihata (1955). At one time, augmentation rhinoplasty was attempted by the injection of synthetic material such as silicone fluid. However, there were serious disadvantages to this procedure, including migration of the injected material and the formation of surface irregularities (Fig. 44–16). An operative technique that gave more stable results was sought, and augmentation rhinoplasty that involved the implantation of a block of material evolved as the preferred method.

Surgeons chose to rely on nasal augmentation involving implantation with inorganic material. The main reason was that the Oriental nose is fatty and lacks the full development of the nasal framework, including the alar cartilage. Thus, it responds poorly to correction of the nasal bone and cartilage framework as in the so-called corrective rhinoplasty. Furthermore, the Japanese nose is perceived as lacking in height, making dorsal augmentation of some sort unavoidable. Autogenous bone or cartilage graft has not been selected as the preferred augmentation material for two reasons. First, there is the risk that such material would undergo resorption, and second, patients seeking esthetic surgery

to enhance their appearance would oppose any procedure that left a second (donor site) operative scar.

The original materials used to augment the nasal dorsum were ivory and resin. Subsequently, silicone rubber implants have been demonstrated to be relatively stable on the nasal dorsum, and, when silicone material became readily available, it formed an inseparable element of rhinoplasty in the Orient. Uchida's (1957) beauty index of the nose had inherent problems, but this situation was further distorted by many cosmetic surgeons

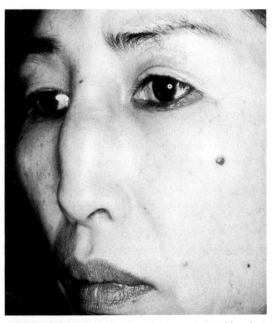

Figure 44–16. Complication of augmentation rhinoplasty by the injection method. An unesthetic hard lump has formed over the nasal dorsum.

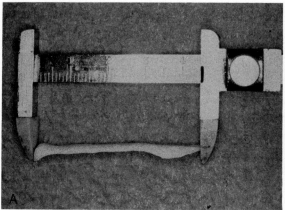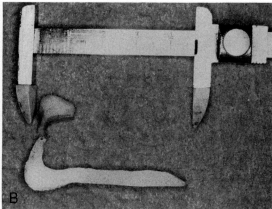

Figure 44–17. The two basic shapes of silicone implants used for augmentation rhinoplasty. *A,* Bar type. *B,* L-shaped type.

who firmly believed that augmentation by a silicone implant was absolutely unavoidable. Thus, the index itself began to be used as one of the justifications for silicone prosthesis augmentation. Subsequently, most of the research on rhinoplasty conducted in the Orient dealt with the characteristics of the implant material, the surgical techniques for creating shapes to fit the nasal framework, and the actual methods of implantation. Furthermore, variously shaped nasal implants began to be used as the surgical solution not only to nasal problems but also to every conceivable issue related to profile correction (Fig. 44–17).

However, there have been objections to the uncontrolled use of the silicone nasal implant. The first arguments were directed against the silicone material itself. Critics stressed that the Oriental patient did not possess any special tolerance to silicone and that the reactions to it were no different from those in Caucasians. Capsule formation has been frequently observed, and at times the implant may become exposed. In addition, long-term studies (Shirakabe, Shirakabe, and Kishimoto, 1985) demonstrated cases in which the implant has migrated, and others in which the implant is not fixed but mobile (Fig. 44–18).

In recent years, doubts have also been expressed about the wisdom of augmentation rhinoplasty itself. First, there is the question of using a rhinoplasty technique to camouflage deformities of the facial framework other than the external nose. An example of this is the substitution of the rhinoplasty procedure for the correction of maxillary protrusion; the result is a nasal tip height that

approaches the same level as the medial portion of the upper lip (see Fig. 44–2). Second, there are objections to the unnatural impression given by a face after augmentation rhinoplasty. This tendency is seen most strikingly in patients in whom the implant has been extended beyond the nasion in order to make the nasal dorsum look longer. Third, the growth and development of the external nose in Orientals in recent years have been more favorable (Iwanaga, 1957). Formerly there were numerous cases of a moderate saddle nose, the most common indication for augmentation rhinoplasty. This is no longer the usual shape of the external nose of the Oriental. Under these circumstances, it is

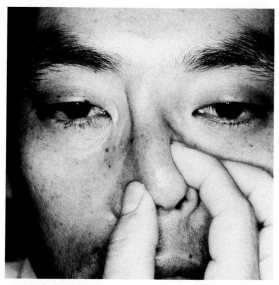

Figure 44–18. A complication of augmentation rhinoplasty using a silicone implant. The implant is movable over the nasal dorsum.

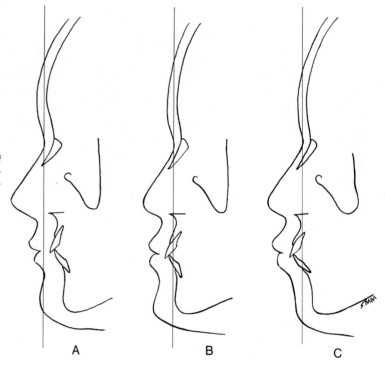

Figure 44–19. Three variations of the Oriental face. *A,* Face with a satisfactory skeleton. *B,* Bimaxillary prognathism. *C,* Bimaxillary protrusion.

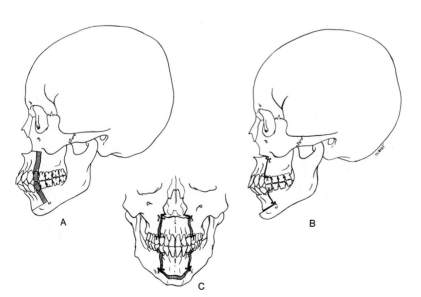

Figure 44–20. Operative technique for the correction of bimaxillary protrusion. *A,* Lines of osteotomy, and tooth extractions. *B, C,* After osteotomy, mobilization of the segments and fixation.

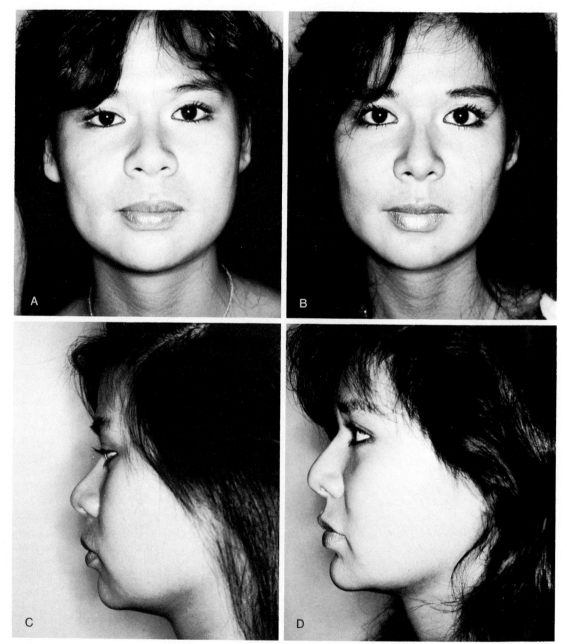

Figure 44–21. Bimaxillary protrusion treated by maxillomandibular dentoalveolar setback osteotomy. *A,* Preoperative frontal view. *B,* Postoperative frontal view. *C,* Preoperative profile. *D,* Postoperative profile.

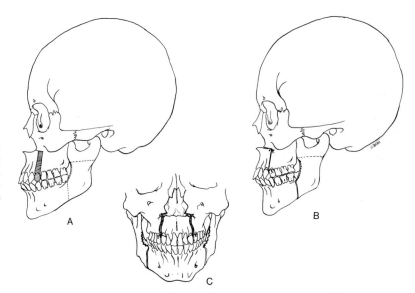

Figure 44–22. Operative technique for the correction of bimaxillary prognathism. *A,* Proposed osteotomies include a maxillary premolar setback and bilateral sagittal split of the mandible (recession). *B, C,* After osteotomy, mobilization of the segments and fixation.

difficult to understand why augmentation techniques still account for almost 100 per cent of all rhinoplasty operations. In fact, in the light of recent statistics based on the morphology of the external nose in Japan, a significant decrease in the frequency of saddle nose may be anticipated.

Furthermore, when one looks closely at patients in whom augmentation rhinoplasty has been performed, it is apparent that many could have been treated quite adequately by reduction rhinoplasty. An example would be the correction of a small dorsal hump by a silicone implant with a smooth outer surface and an undersurface contoured to fit the surface structure of the nasal framework. The use of a silicone implant in such cases should be seriously reconsidered.

The above discussion highlights some of the limitations to augmentation rhinoplasty using silicone prostheses. If the mainstay of profileplasty were to be changed from rhinoplasty to profile orthopedics, how would esthetic surgery for Orientals change?

Orthopedic Profileplasty

In order to facilitate an understanding of what is generally accepted as the "normal range" of facial features for the Oriental profile, the face has been arbitrarily divided into three categories: the desirable face, the bimaxillary protrusion type, and the bimaxillary prognathism type. The respective ceph-

alometric radiographs and features are outlined in Figure 44–19.

In the *bimaxillary protrusion type*, the menton is within the spatial framework that is appropriate for the Oriental face, but the SNA angle is larger than the SNB angle. Both exceed 80 degrees. In *bimaxillary prognathism,* there is a forward projection of the menton; the SNA angle is over 80 degrees, and the SNB angle is equal to or greater than the SNA angle. In both cases, the morphology of the occlusion and the S–N distance fall within the normal range (see Chap. 29 for cephalometric details).

Correction of Bimaxillary Protrusion. Bimaxillary protrusion may be defined as one of the more common forms of the Oriental face. However, it can also be regarded as a deformity necessitating corrective treatment. Since the position of the anterior nasal spine cannot be corrected orthodontically, it is necessary to apply surgical orthopedic measures to the maxilla and the mandible (Ohmori, 1983). The most common procedure is a segmental dentoalveolar osteotomy of the maxilla and mandible (see also Chap. 29) after the extraction of both the upper and lower first premolars (Fig. 44–20). An example of the results of such corrective procedures is shown in Figure 44–21.

Correction of Bimaxillary Prognathism. Like bimaxillary protrusion, bimaxillary prognathism is one of the basic facial features in the Oriental. In these cases, the menton is more forward than in the desirable

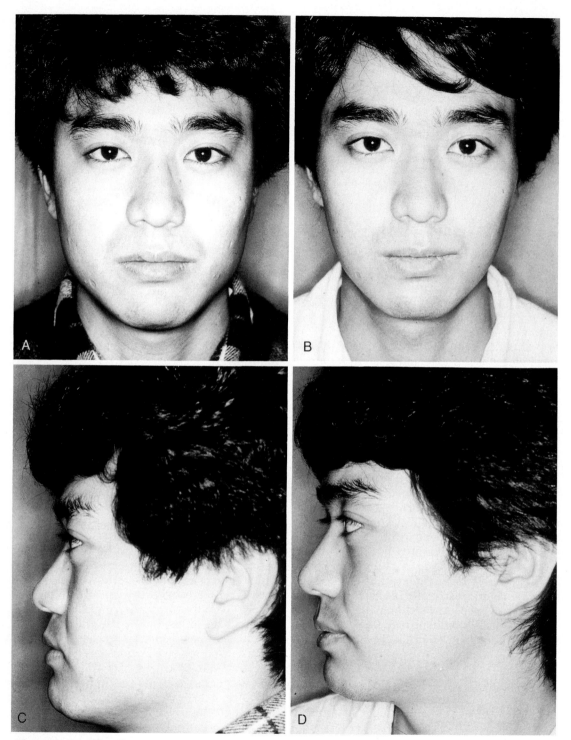

Figure 44–23. Bimaxillary prognathism treated by a segmental setback osteotomy of the maxilla and sagittal split osteotomies (setback) of the rami of the mandible. *A,* Preoperative frontal view. *B,* Postoperative frontal view. *C,* Preoperative profile. *D,* Postoperative profile.

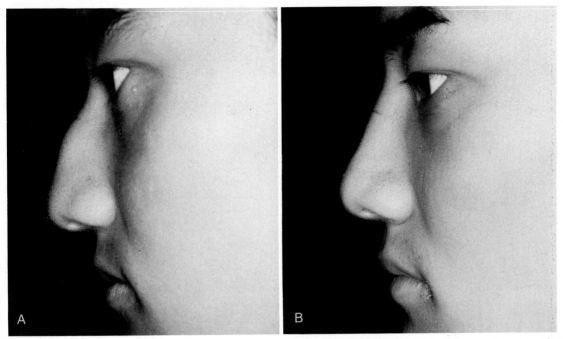

Figure 44–24. Surgical correction of an Oriental hump nose. *A,* Preoperative view. *B,* Postoperative view after modification of the nasal dorsum (hump removal) and osteotomies.

face (see Fig. 44–19), and this may thus be considered a deformity. To correct bimaxillary prognathism, one must choose between a Le Fort I osteotomy and a segmental osteotomy of the maxilla with a setback osteotomy of the mandible (Fig. 44–22). A patient who underwent such a procedure is illustrated in Figure 44–23.

Esthetic Rhinoplasty

There is no clear-cut evidence that the shape of the external nose preferred by Orientals has any unique values or angles that are different from those favored by Caucasians. Neither are there marked differences between East and West in the favored contour

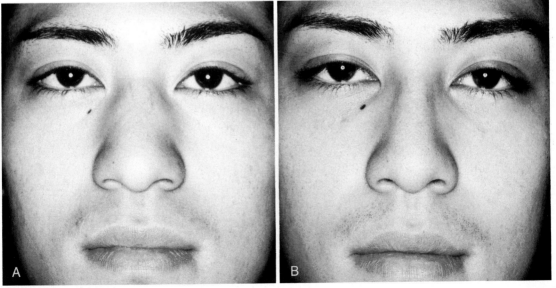

Figure 44–25. Surgical correction of an Oriental wide nose. *A,* Preoperative view. *B,* Postoperative view after lateral osteotomies and nasal bone infractures.

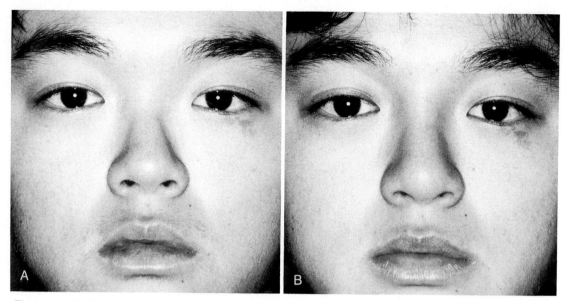

Figure 44–26. Posttraumatic saddle nose deformity corrected by augmentation rhinoplasty. *A,* Preoperative view. *B,* Postoperative view.

of the nasal dorsum. For example, the convex-shaped external nose projects a more masculine impression, and the concave shape gives a more feminine impression in the Orient as well as in the West.

Therefore, every operation to correct the structure of the external nose should be based on the concepts of corrective rhinoplasty: deformities should be handled by augmenting deficiencies and removing excesses. The de-

tails of such rhinoplastic techniques are outlined in Chapters 35, 36, and 37.

The author has found that rhinoplasty utilizing the silicone implant is generally unnecessary for the following reasons:

1. Orthopedic profileplasty should be used for patients with problems involving the craniofacial skeletal framework.

2. A small hump nose or an external nose with a wide base for the pyramid, previously

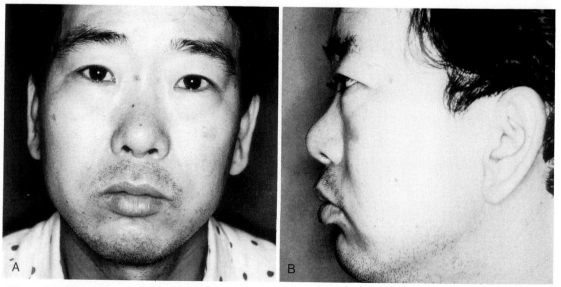

Figure 44–27. *A, B,* An example of an Oriental foreshortened saddle nose. This type of nose is observed less frequently among the Japanese. It is the type best treated by augmentation rhinoplasty. *A,* Frontal view. *B,* Profile.

considered as suitable for silicone implantation, is preferably repaired by classical corrective rhinoplasty techniques, such as nasal bone osteotomy and/or hump removal (Figs. 44–24, 44–25).

3. The trend in recent years is that fewer Oriental patients are requiring augmentation rhinoplasty. The only nasal augmentation procedures performed by the author were two cases of saddle nose, one created by excessive nasal hump reduction, the other resulting from childhood trauma (Fig. 44–26).

There, nevertheless, remain patients with a foreshortened saddle nose (Fig. 44–27). Although it is rare today to find such an external nose among the Japanese, this is the type of nose best managed by augmentation rhinoplasty. As long as such cases exist, there will be a role for augmentation rhinoplasty.

REFERENCES

Farkas, L. G., Kolar, J. C., and Munro, I. R.: Geography of the nose: a morphometric study. Aesth. Plast. Surg., *10*:191, 1986.

Fernandez, L. R.: Double eyelid operation in the Oriental in Hawaii. Plast. Reconstr. Surg., *25*:257, 1960.

Hayashi, K.: A modification of the Hotz method for double eyelid plasty. Jpn. Rev. Clin. Ophthalmol., *34*:369, 1939.

Hotz, F. C.: Surgery of the eyelids. *In* Wingate, R. B. (Ed.): An Atlas of Ophthalmic Surgery. 3rd Ed. Philadelphia, J. B. Lippincott Company, 1981, p. 62.

Ide, C. H.: Congenital anomalies of the eye and its adnexa. Ear Nose Throat J., *58*:463, 1979.

Iwanaga, M.: Anatomical study of the nose in Japan. Kumamoto Igakkai Zasshi, *31*:155, 1957.

Mikamo, K.: A method of palpebral plasty. J. Chugaishinpo, *396*:9, 1986.

Nakagawa, T., Shiga, M., Ohkawa, T., and Takeda, M.: Morphometric and levator function of the Japanese upper eyelid. Clin. Ophthalmol., *28*:689, 1974.

Nishihata, K.: Rhinoplasty. Nihon Jibilinkoka Zensho. Vol. 2. Tokyo, Kanehara & Co., 1955, p. 65.

Ohmori, K.: Atlas of Cranio-maxillofacial Surgery. Tokyo, Kanehara & Co., 1983, p. 118.

Ohmori, S.: Skin Surgery. Tokyo, Kanehara & Co., 1954.

Ortiz-Monasterio, F., and Rodriguez, A.: Lateral canthoplasty to change the eye slant. Plast. Reconstr. Surg., *76*:1, 1985.

Sayoc, B. T.: Plastic construction of the superior palpebral fold. Am. J. Ophthalmol., *38*:556, 1954.

Sayoc, B. T.: Simultaneous construction of the superior palpebral fold in ptosis operation. Am. J. Ophthalmol., *41*:1040, 1956.

Shirakabe, Y., Shirakabe, T., and Kishimoto, T.: The classification of complications after augmentation rhinoplasty. Aesth. Plast. Surg., *9*:185, 1985.

Uchida, J.: Biyougeka no Jissai (Techniques of Plastic Aesthetic Surgery). Tokyo, Kanehara & Co., 1957.

Index

Index

Note: Page numbers in *italics* refer to illustrations; page number followed by *t* refer to tables.

Arm
  amputation of
    prostheses for, 4405, *4406, 4407*
    replantation surgery for, 4376–4377
  congenital anomalies of. *See also* Hand anomalies.
    incidence of, 5225, 5229, 5231, 5229*t*, 5230*t*
    intercalated phocomelia, 5242–5243, 5245, *5243, 5244*
    timetables and, 5223, 5225
    ultrasound examination of, *5234–5235*
    uncertain etiology of, 5236
  cutaneous arteries of, 359, *360*
  embryology of
    experimental studies of, 5217, 5219–5220, *5218, 5219*
    morphologic development in, 5216–5217, 5216*t*, *5217, 5218*
    of muscles, 5220–5221, *5222–5229*
    of nerves, 5221, 5223
    of vascular system, 5220, *5221*
    skeletal development in, 5220
  replantation of, 20
  suction-assisted lipectomy of, complications of, 3977, 3978
  upper, transverse absences of, 5241–5242
Arm flaps
  for nose resurfacing, 2202–2203
  lateral
    anatomy of, 4471, *4472*
    for free flap transfer in upper extremity, 4471–4472, *4472*
    for sensory reconstruction of hand, 4867–4868, *4868*
  medial
    anatomy of, 4470–4471, *4471*
    for free flap transfer in upper extremity, 4469–4471, *4471*
  upper distal, for nasal reconstruction, 1971, *1971–1973*
Armenoid nose, 1853
Arterial ligation
  for lymphedema, 4112
  selection, for control of facial wound hemorrhage, 877
Arterial malformations, of hand, 5324, *5325, 5326, 5327*
Arterial revascularization, for erectile dysfunction, 4219
Arteries. *See also specific arteries.*
  cutaneous
    classification of, 352–353
    regional anatomy of, 355, 358–359, 362–363, 367–368, 371–374, *356, 357, 360, 361, 364–366, 369–371*
    damage to, microscopic signs of, 4367–4368, *4368*
    interconnections of, 346–347, *348–350*
    musculocutaneous, 277, *278, 283,* 283–284
    of lower extremity, 4033–4035, *4034*
Arteriography, for free flap transfer in upper extremity, 4460
Arterioles, microstructure of, 449, *450*
Arteriovenous fistulas
  microsurgical concerns for, 452–453
  of hand, 5502–5503, *5503*
Arteriovenous malformations
  clinical findings in, 3255–3256

Arteriovenous malformations *(Continued)*
  histology of, 3255
  of hand, 5324, 5326, *5325*
  of wrist, 5008, *5008*
  physiology of, 3255
  terminology for, 3254–3255
  treatment of, 3256–3258, *3258*
Arthritis
  correction of systemic abnormalities of, 4698
  incidence of, 4695
  of hand. *See* Hand, arthritis of.
  of temporomandibular joint, 1498–1501, *1500, 1501*
  patient education for, 4697–4698
  treatment problems in, 4695–4696
Arthrodesis
  for degenerative arthritis of hand, 4699, 4700, *4701,* 4701–4702
  historical aspects of, 4686
  of small joints
    complications of, 4677–4678
    fixation techniques for, 4673–4677, *4674–4677*
    general considerations for, *4672,* 4672–4673
    indications for, 4671–4672
  of wrist
    complications of, 4681–4682
    for rheumatoid arthritis, 4715–4716
    general considerations for, 4678
    indications for, 4678
    limited, 4682–4686, *4683–4685*
    operative techniques for, 4678–4681, *4680, 4681*
Arthrography, of temporomandibular joint, 1503–1505, 1504*t, 1505*
Arthrogryposis
  clinical presentation of, 5378–5380, *5378–5379*
  treatment of, 5380–5381
Arthroplasty
  gap, for temporomandibular ankylosis, 1494–1495
  interpositional with alloplastic or biologic materials, for temporomandibular ankylosis, *1495,* 1495–1496
  resection implant
    for degenerative arthritis of hand, 4702
    for rheumatoid arthritis, 4716–4718, *4717, 4720*
Articulation tests, for evaluation of velopharyngeal incompetence, 2912–2913
Artificial synapse theory, 4898, *4899*
Asch forceps, 985, *987*
Asian patients
  beauty standards for, 2416–2420, *2417–2419*
  cleft lip/palate susceptibility and, 2529–2530
  corrective rhinoplasty in, 1879–1880
  esthetic surgery for
    for double eyelids, 2423–2426, *2424–2426*
    for upper double eyelids, 2420–2422, *2421*
    historical perspective of, 2415–2416
    of corrective profileplasty, 2426–2428, *2427, 2428,* 2431
    of orthopedic profileplasty, *2429–2432,* 2431, 2433
    patient selection for, 2420
    preoperative considerations of, 2422–2423, *2423*
    rhinoplasty for, 2433–2435, *2433–2435*
  nose shape of, 1926, *1926*
  nose size of, 1926, *1926*
Aspirin, craniofacial cleft formation and, 2929
Ataxia-telangiectasia, 3227, *3238,* 3239
Atheroma, 3569, 3572

Breast cancer
  breast reconstruction for. *See* Breast reconstruction.
  chemotherapy for, 3900
  incidence of, 3897
  local management of, 3898–3899
  prophylactic mastectomy for, 3922–3924, *3925*
  risk factors for, 3897, 3897*t*
  staging of, 3899, 3899*t*, 3900
  survival from, 3898
Breast feeding, augmentation mammoplasty and, 3892
Breast flaps, for chest wall reconstruction, 3703, *3706*
Breast reconstruction
  after mastectomy, psychosocial aspects of, 126–128
  by tissue expansion, 482–491, *484–487, 489, 490,*
        3906–3908, *3906–3910,* 3911
    advantages of, 482
    bilateral technique for, 485, *485*
    disadvantages of, 482–483
    for congenital breast abnormalities, 488–489, *489,*
        490, 491
    for tuberous breast, 489, 491
    permanent expansion prostheses for, 486–487, *487*
    reconstruction in conjunction with distant flaps,
        487, 487–488
    surgical technique for, 483, *484,* 485
  complications of, 3905–3906, 3916, 3922
  immediate, by tissue expansion, 485–486, *486*
  management of opposite breast in, 3924–3925
  muscle and musculocutaneous flaps for, 387–393,
        389, 390, 392, 393
  nipple-areola reconstruction for, 3926–3927, *3926,*
        3927
  preoperative planning for, 3900–3901, 3913–3914,
        3919–3920
  selection of method for, 3901–3902
  suction-assisted lipectomy for, 3988, *3995*
  timing of, 3901, *3902*
  TRAM flap for, 3916–3920, *3917–3921,* 3922, 3925
  with available tissue, 3902–3906, *3903–3905*
  with gluteus maximus flap, 3922, *3923, 3924*
  with latissimus dorsi flap, 3911–3914, 3916, *3912–*
        3916
Breast reduction
  complications of, 3877, 3879
  dermal pedicles for, 3847, *3848, 3849*
    superior based, 3847, 3849, *3850–3854,* 3853
  development of, 3847
  for massively hypertrophied breasts, 3877, *3881*
  for moderately hypertrophied and ptotic breasts,
        3877, *3879, 3880*
  free nipple graft for, 3854, 3856, *3858, 3859*
  inferior pyramidal dermal flap technique for, 3856,
        3860–3863, 3861
  psychosocial aspects of, 126
  vertical bipedicle dermal flap technique for, 3853–
        3854, *3856, 3857*
  with abdominoplasty, 3953, *3960–3961*
Breastfeeding, problems of, for cleft palate infant, 2731
Brephoplasty, 54
Bronchopleural fistula, chest wall reconstruction and,
        3726, *3727–3730*
Brooke formula, 788, 792*t,* 793
  modified, 792*t,* 793
Brow lift. *See* Forehead-brow lift.
Brow suspension, for eyebrow ptosis, 1759, *1759*
Brucellosis, 5550

Buccal fat pad excision, with facialplasty, 2384
Buccal mucosa, cancer of, 3452, *3453–3455*
Buccal sulcus
  deficiency of, correction of, 2796–2797, *2797*
  restoration of, 3508
    by skin graft inlay technique, *1452, 1453,* 1457
    secondary abnormalities of, from bilateral cleft lip
        repair, 2853, 2855, *2855*
Buccopharyngeal membrane, persistence of, 1998
Buffalo hump deformity, suction-assisted lipectomy for,
        3981, *3983*
Bullet wound, nerve injury from, 678
Burkitt's lymphoma, 3359
Burn contractures
  contraction process and, 167, *167*
  history of treatment for, 787–788
  of axilla, 5471, 5473, *5474, 5475*
  of elbow, 5469, 5471, *5472*
  of hand
    dorsal, 5458, 5460–5461, *5460*
    volar, 5464–5465, *5465*
  of oral commissure, 2229, 2231
  true vs. apparent defect of, *24,* 24–25, *25*
Burn injuries
  causes of, 2153–2154
  deaths from, 2153
  of ear, 2204–2207, *2207–2209,* 2209–2210
  of eyebrows, 2218–2222, *2219–2220*
  of hand
    amputations for, 5467, 5469, *5469–5471*
    complications of, *5415,* 5415–5416
    depth categories for, 5404*t*
    historical aspects of, 5399–5402
    inpatient treatment of, 5405–5414, *5411, 5412,*
        5414–5416
    outpatient treatment of, 5405
    pathology of, 5402–5403
    physical examination of, 5403–5405, *5404*
    reconstruction for. *See* Hand reconstruction, after
        burn injury.
  of male genitalia, *4234,* 4234–4235
  of upper lip, 2183–2184
  scalp alopecia from, 2223–2226, *2227, 2228*
  to face. *See* Facial injuries, from burns.
Burn wound sepsis, *807,* 807–808
Buttock, cutaneous arteries of, 368, 371, *369*
Buttonhole incision, for cancellous chips, 610

Cable grafting, 4769
Calcaneal artery fasciocutaneous flap, lateral, 4085,
        4087
Calcitonin, for reflex sympathetic dystrophy, 4910–
        4911
Calcium channel blockers, in postoperative treatment
        of skin flaps, 316–317
Calcium gluconate injection, for acid burns, 5437–5438
Calculi, salivary, 3290, *3291, 3292,* 3312–3313
Caldwell projection
  for plain films, 884–885, *885*
  of orbit, 1584
Calf flap, posterior, for sensory reconstruction of hand,
        4871, 4871–4872
Caloric needs, of burn patients, 798–799, 799*t*

Cold injuries *(Continued)*
  localized, historical background for, 851–852
    late sequelae of, 857–858
    pathophysiology of, 852–854, 854t
    treatment of, 854–857, *856*
    with systemic hypothermia, 865
  predisposing factors of, 849–851, *850*
Collagen
  components of, 169, *170*
  degradation of, in abnormal scars, 737
  dermal, turnover in skin grafts, 244
  epithelial migration and, 164
  fibers of, structure of in dermis, 208, *208, 209,* 210
  in biologic dressings, for thermal burns, 805
  in Dupuytren's contracture, 5057
  in remodeling process, 4434
  in scar tissue, 169
  in tendon, 529
  injectable, 781–782
    complications of, 783–784
    histopathology of, 782
    indications for, 782–783
    technique for, 783
  metabolism of, 169–171
    factors affecting, 175, 178–179
  production of
    hypoxia and, 735
    in abnormal scars, 736–737
  regenerated, in suture material for alloplastic implants, 719–720
  remodeling of, 172, 175, *172–174, 176, 177*
  synthesis, in tendon graft healing, 531
  tensile strength of skin and, 161–162, *174*
  types of, in abnormal scars, 737
Collagen-GAG membranes, 726, *728,* 729
Colles' fascia, 4190
Colles' fracture, 4635–4637, *4635t, 4636, 4637*
Colloid resuscitation, 793
Coloboma, correction of, in Treacher Collins syndrome, 3116, *3116*
Color transparencies, 37–38
Columella
  anatomy of, 1788, 1797, *1797*
    in cleft lip and palate, 2583
  deformities of, in unilateral cleft lip and palate, 2590
  growth of, relationship to bilateral cleft lip repair, 2856
  hanging, correction of, 1857, *1858*
  lengthening of, 2667, 2673, 2675–2676, *2674, 2675*
    in bilateral cleft lip nasal deformity, 2856–2857, *2857–2867,* 2859, 2863–2864
  reconstruction of, 1985–1987, *1986, 1987*
  retracted, correction of, 1857–1858, *1859–1861,* 1860
  wide base of, correction of, 1860–1861, *1861*
Columella-ala triangle, resection of, *1837,* 1837–1838
Columellar-lobar junction, 1788
Coma, 870
Commissure, reconstruction of, 2025, 2027, *2026*
Compartment syndromes
  anatomic considerations of, 4032–4033, *4033*
  treatment of, 4067–4068
Competence, embryological, 2454
Complement system, 191–192, *192*
Composite flaps
  concept of, for facial reconstruction, 306, *307*
  historical aspects of, 376–377

Composite grafts
  for eyelid reconstruction, 1715, *1717*
  of scalp, for alopecia treatment, 1520–1527, *1521–1523, 1525, 1526*
    round punch types of, 1520–1523, *1521–1523*
    square or hexahedral types of, 1523–1524
    strip scalp types of, 1524, 1526–1527, *1525, 1526*
  of skin and adipose tissue, for nasal reconstruction, 1932
  of skin and cartilage, for nasal reconstruction, 1930–1932, *1931*
Compression arthrodesis, for small joints, 4675–4677, *4676, 4677*
Compression garments, as adjuncts for fat suctioning, 4026, *4027*
Compression syndromes
  anterior interosseous nerve syndrome, 4831–4833, *4832*
  costoclavicular, 4998–4999, *4999*
  of hand, evaluation by wick catheter, 4287, *4287*
  of median nerve, 4823. *See also* Carpal tunnel syndrome.
  of upper extremity
    anatomic structures associated with, 4998, *4998*
    diagnosis of, 4999–5000, 5002–5005, *4999–5004*
  pronator syndrome, 4833–4834, *4834*
Compression therapy, for hemangiomas, 3213
Computed tomography
  in computer-aided surgical planning, 1212, 1214, *1214*
  of facial injuries, 899
  of nasoethmoido-orbital fractures, 1090–1091, *1090, 1091*
  of optic nerve injury, 1118, *1119*
  of orbit, 1584–1586
  of temporomandibular joint, 1505
  of velopharyngeal sphincter, 2914
  of zygoma fractures, 998, *999, 1000*
Computer-aided surgical planning
  three-dimensional, 1209
  with three-dimensional cephalometrics, 1209, *1211,* 1212, 1212t, *1213*
Concha, alteration of, 2116, *2117*
Conchamastoid sutures, for reducing auricular prominence, 2116–2117, *2117*
Conduction test, evaluation of facial nerve function, 2253
Condylar growth, process of, 2505–2506
Condylar region, osteotomies of, 1235, *1236*
Condyle
  dislocations of, 1487–1489, *1487–1489*
  fractures of
    classification of, *1490,* 1496
    closed or conservative management of, 1497, *1497*
    diagnosis of, 1496
    open reduction for, 1497–1498, *1499*
    roentgenography of, 1497
  hyperplasia of
    and unilateral mandibular macrognathia, 1294, *1294, 1295–1296, 1297*
    with osteochondroma, 1490–1494, *1491–1493*
  hypoplasia of, *1291,* 1292, *1293,* 1294. *See* Craniofacial microsomia.
  idiopathic osteonecrosis of, 1502
  movement of, 147–148

HLA. *See* Histocompatibility antigens (HLA).
Hockeystick incision, 1843–1844
Hodgkin's lymphoma, staging classification for, 3185
Holocrine glands. *See* Sebaceous glands.
Holoprosencephaly
  dysmorphic facies associated with, *73*
  embryogenesis of, 2458, 2517, *2517*, 2926, *2926*
  fetal alcohol syndrome, pathogenesis of, 2458–2459,
    2458, 2459
  malformation sequence in, 72, *72t*
  MNP deficiencies and, 2529
  types of, 2935, *2935t*
Homans-Miller procedure, 5028, *5028, 5029*
Horizontal buttresses, 1021
Hormones
  breast development and, 3841–3842, *3842*
  for transsexualism therapy, 4240–4241
Horner's syndrome, 1754
  as nerve block complication, 4307
  development of, after brachial plexus block, 4313–
    4314
Hubbard tank immersion, for treatment of generalized
  cold injury, *863*, 863–864
Human growth hormone (hGH), 798
Human papillomavirus
  malignant transformation of, 3563
  types of, *3561t*
Humby knife, 237, *237*
Hurler syndrome, 84, *88*, 98
Hyaluronidase (Wydase), 5442
Hydralazine, postoperative treatment of skin flaps, 316
Hydrocephalus, in craniosynostosis, 3025
Hydrodistention, for vasospasm, 456
Hydrofluoric acid burns, 5437, *5437, 5438*
  treatment of, 5437–5438
Hydrogel, 722–723, *723, 724*
Hydron, 805
Hydroxyapatite, for alloplastic implants, 715–716, *716*,
  725, *726*
Hydroxyzine, 4315
Hyperabduction maneuver, 5002, *5002*
Hyperalimentation, for thermal burn patients, 798–
  799, *799*, 800t, 800–801
Hyperbaric oxygen, for postoperative skin flap treat-
  ment, 318
Hyperhidrosis, from cold injury, 858
Hyperkalemia, from fluid resuscitation, 793, 795
Hypernasality, functional/hysterical, velopharyngeal
  incompetence and, 2906–2907
Hypernatremia, from fluid resuscitation, 793, 794–795
Hyperostosis, gigantism of, 5365, *5368–5369*
Hyperpigmentation
  after dermabrasion, 780–781
  after facialplasty in male, 2399
  blotchy, after chemical peeling, 770
  chemical peeling for, 758, *760, 761*
  familial, after blepharoplasty, 2349
Hyperplasia
  cellular, 242–243
  facial, *1300*, 1301
Hypersensitivity, delayed, from injectable collagen, 783
Hypertelorism, orbital, post-traumatic, 1088, 1625,
  1628, *1628*
Hyperthyroidism
  orbital pathology in, 1630
  "scleral show" of, 2327, 2328, 2330, *2328*
  spasm of Müller's muscle in, 2327, 2328, *2328*, 2330

Hypertonic solutions
  extravasation injuries from, 5440
  of saline, for fluid resuscitation, 793
Hypertrophic scars
  after chemical peeling, 769, *770, 771*
  biochemical observations of, 735–738
  dermabrasion for, 773–774, *774–776*
  diagnosis of, 738
  formation of
    after dermabrasion, 781
    after thermal burn injury, 810
    causes of, 172, *173*
    in split-thickness donor site, 246–247
  from hand burns, 5458, 5460–5461, *5462*
  inhibition of, by mechanical pressure, 740–741
  microvasculature of, 735
  vs. keloids, 732, *733*, 737–738
Hypertrophy syndromes, with vascular malformations,
  3258–3260, *3260–3263*, 3263–3264
Hypodermis, anatomy of, 224
Hypoglossal nerve
  anatomy of, 3280, *3280*
  injury of, from salivary gland surgery, 3314
Hypoglossal-facial nerve anastomoses, for facial paralysis, 2277–2278, *2278t*, *2278–2282*, 2281, 2283–
  2284
Hyponatremia, from fluid resuscitation, 793, 794, 795
Hypopharynx
  anatomy of, 3416, *3416*
  cancers of, 3460–3462, *3461*
Hypoplasia
  condylar, *1291*, 1292, *1293*, 1294
  mandibular, 1260. *See also* Mandibular hypoplasia.
  variations of, functional disturbances associated
    with, 1262
  maxillary, 1360
  preoperative planning for, 1362, *1362*
Hypospadias
  anatomic description of, 4156, *4156*
  complications of, 4166–4167
  embryology of, 4154–4155
  incidence of, 4155
  one-stage repairs for, 4159–4161, *4160*
    by flip-flap method
      with distal flap chordee, 4162–4163, *4163*
      without chordee, 4161–4162, *4162*
    by meatal advancement glansplasty, 4161, *4161*
    by repair of proximal shaft, using full-thickness
      skin graft, 4163–4164, *4164*
    by vascularized preputial island flap, 4164–4165,
      4165
  postoperative care for, 4165–4166
  preoperative considerations for, 4157
  two-stage repairs of, techniques for, 4157–4159, *4158*,
    4159
Hypothenar muscles, 4271–4272, *4272, 4273*
Hypothenar space infections, 5543
Hypothermia
  acute, 859
  chronic, 859
  subacute, 859
  systemic
    late sequelae of, 864–865
    pathophysiology of, 862
    physiologic responses in, 860t-861t
    predisposing diseases, 858
    treatment of, 862–864, *863*

Hypothermia *(Continued)*
  with frostbite, 865
Hypotonia
  in Down syndrome, 3163
  Robin sequence and, 94
Hypovolemic shock, 4330
  prevention of, after thermal burn injury, 791
Hypoxia
  abnormal scar formation and, 735
  and pathogenesis of cleft lip/palate, 2533
Hypoxia-selectivity hypothesis, of abnormal scar formation, 736–737

Ibuprofen, 317
Iliac bone grafts
  for frontal bone repair and contouring, 1564–1565, *1565*
  for mandibular defect, *1444–1446*
  for secondary rhinoplasty, 1911
  nonvascularized type of, 605
    for children, 610, 612, *609–611*
    technique of, 606, 608, 610, *606–608*
  vascularized, 612
  vs. split rib grafts, for mandibular defects, 1422, *1431*
Iliac crest free flap, 603
Imbibition, serum, 250–252
Imidazole, 317
Immunogenicity, of alloplastic implants, 702
Immunoglobulins, classes of, 191
Immunologic tolerance, 194
Immunology
  defects of, in Down syndrome, 3161–3162
  graft survival and, 193–194
  in abnormal scar formation, 733, 735, 735*t*
  of thermal burn injury, 801–802
Immunosuppressant drugs, 195–196
Immunosuppression
  basal cell carcinoma and, 3617, 3619
  modification of allograft rejection mechanism, 194–196
  orthotopic composite tissue allografts with, 203*t*
  squamous cell carcinoma and, 3629
  transplantation and, 194–196
Immunotherapy, for malignant melanoma, 3651–3652
Implants. *See* Alloplastic implants; *specific implants.*
  exposure of, 505–506
  failure of, 505
  for augmentation mammoplasty, 3884–3885
  for reconstruction of orbital floor fracture, 1075–1077, *1077*
  historical aspects of, 54–55
  osteointegrated, for retention of denture, in reconstructed mandible, 1456
Impotence
  nonsurgical treatment options for, 4219
  pathophysiology of, 4213–4215, *4214, 4215*
  surgical treatment options for, 4219–4220
Imuran (azathioprine), 195
Incisions
  bicoronal, *1592*, 1593
  bicoronal scalp, 1657, 1659
  choice of site for, 44
  conjunctival, 1594, *1595*
  Converse subciliary, *1035*, 1072

Incisions *(Continued)*
  coronal, 1098, 1100–1101, *1099–1101*
  external, for rhinoplasty, 1847
  eyelid
    transconjunctival, 1593–1594, *1594*
    transcutaneous, 1593, *1593, 1594*
  for abdominal wall reconstruction, 3763–3764
  for classical radical neck dissection, *3429*, 3429–3430
  for face lift, 2369–2370, *2370*
  for facialplasty, in male, 2392–2393
  for flexor tendon repair, 4522–4524
  for forehead-brow lift, 2400, *2401*, 2402
  for full abdominoplasty, 3937, 3939, *3942–3945*
  labiobuccal vestibular, 1226, *1226*, 1363
  lateral brow, 1594, *1595*
  local types of
    general considerations for, 4443, *4443*
    midlateral, *4442*, 4442–4443
    on dorsum of hand, 4443
    zigzag, 4441–4442, *4442*
  medial canthal, 1594, *1595*
  midlateral, *4442*, 4442–4443
  mucogingival, 1226, *1226*, 1363
  of lower extremity, 374
  preauricular, 1227
  submandibular, 1225, *1237*
  technique for making, 48
  to expose orbital floor, *1035*, 1072–1073, *1073*
  transcartilaginous nasal tip, 1844, *1845*
  vertical midline nasal, 1097–1098
Incisive foramen/papilla, 2726, *2726*
Inclusion cysts
  of hand, 5485–5486, *5486*
  of nail bed or distal phalanx, *4510*, 4511
Inderal (propranolol), 315, 4910
Indomethacin, 317
Induction, primary embryonic, *2453*, 2454
Inert buried appliances, for mandibular fixation, 3507–3508
Infant(s). *See also* Children.
  feeding problems of
    for cleft palate infant, 2731
    in Robin sequence, 3128
  orthostatic feeding of, 3130–3131
  soft tissue injuries in, 1154–1155
Infection
  after treatment of mandibular fractures, 976
  craniofacial cleft formation and, 2928
  effect on patency of microvascular anastomoses, 454
  from orthognathic surgery, 1404–1405, *1408*
  from radiation injury, 835–836, *836, 837*
  postoperative, 1881. *See under specific surgical procedure.*
    after tissue expansion, 505
    from maxillary tumor surgery, 3332
  potentiation of, by alloplastic implant, 703
Inflammatory lesions, of perionychium, 4512
Inflammatory mediators, 4897
Infraclavicular block, performance of, *4319*, 4320
Infraorbital nerve
  anatomic relations of, 996, *996*
  injury of, 1131
Infraorbital nerve block, 147–148, *147, 148*, 1609–1610, *1610*
  after orbital or nasoethmoido-orbital fractures, 1106–1107

Rasp technique
  for corrective rhinoplasty, 1841–1842, *1841, 1842*
  for resection of bony hump of nose, 1827–1828, *1828, 1829*
Rathke's pouch, 2477–2478, *2477*
Ravitch's technique
  for chondrogladiolar deformity, 3742, 3745, *3746, 3747*
  for chondromanubrial deformity, 3745, *3747, 3748*
  for pectus excavatum deformity, 3733, *3734–3736,* 3737–3738
Raynaud's phenomenon, initiation of, 5013–5014, *5014.* *See also* Vasospastic disorders.
Receptor blockers
  and prostaglandins, for postoperative treatment of skin flaps, 317
  for postoperative treatment of skin flaps, 315–316
Reciprocal clicking, 1481–1482, *1482*
Reconstructive surgery. *See also specific types of reconstruction.*
  planning of, 24–26
  vs. esthetic surgery, 1–2
Rectus abdominis flap
  anatomy of, 390–391, 393, *393*
  for abdominal wall defects, 397
  for abdominal wall reconstruction, 3768
  for chest wall and pulmonary cavity reconstruction, 396–397
  for chest wall reconstruction, 3694, 3696–3697, *3695*
  for genital reconstructive surgery, 4137, *4139–4141*
    advantages of, 4139, 4141
    disadvantages of, 4139
    regional flap comparisons of, 4141, *4142, 4143*
  for groin and perineum reconstructions, 399
  myocutaneous type of, anatomy of, 299–300, *300*
Rectus abdominis muscle, microneurovascular transfer of, 2299
Rectus femoris flap
  applications of, 4039–4040, *4041*
  for abdominal wall defects, 397
  for genital reconstructive surgery, 4149, 4152, *4149–4151*
  for groin and perineum reconstructions, 398–399
  motor innervation of, 4039
  origin and insertion of, 4039
  vascular supply of, 4039
Recurrent laryngeal nerve, anatomy of, 4314
Recurrent laryngeal nerve block, complications of, 4307–4308
Recurrent-pattern syndromes, 82, *83,* 84*t*
Red glass test, 1599
Reduction methods, for zygoma fractures, 1000–1001, *1001*
Reese dermatome, 230, *232–235,* 235–236
Reflex sympathetic dystrophy
  clinical forms of, 4891–4894, *4893, 4895*
  definition of, 4884–4886, 4885*t*
  diagnosis of, 4885–4886, 4886*t*
  diagnostic techniques for, 4903–4904
  differential diagnosis of, 4904–4906, *4906*
  endogenous opioid pain control system in, 4901–4902
  etiology of
    peripheral anatomic basis of, 4898–4903, *4899*
    psychophysiologic basis of, 4902–4903
  historical aspects of, 4886–4887
  incidence of, 4887

Reflex sympathetic dystrophy *(Continued)*
  mechanism of onset for, 4903
  myofascial dysfunction and, 4894–4896
  pain of, 4888–4889
  precipitating causes of, 4888
  prevention of, 4914–4916
  prognosis for, 4887–4888
  psychologic findings in, 4900–4901, 4901*t*
  stages of, physical findings in, 4889–4891, 4890*t,* *4890–4892*
  sympathetic nervous system and, 4897–4898
  treatment of, 4907
    by acupuncture, 4912
    by hand therapy, 4912–4914
    by pharmacologic agents, 4909–4911
    by psychotherapy, 4914
    by surgical control of peripheral nerve irritants, 4912
    by sympathectomy, 4908–4909
    by sympathetic block, 4907–4908
    by transcutaneous electrical nerve stimulation, 4911–4912
  trophic changes in, biologic mechanisms of, 4896–4898
"Registration peptide," 171
Regitine (phentolamine), 5019–5020, 5442
Reichert's cartilage, 2487–2488, 3059
Reinnervation, in muscle transfer, 4973, *4973*
Rejection, of limb allografts, 198–200
Relative afferent pupillary defect (Marcus Gunn pupil), 1583
Religion, plastic surgery and, 117
Relocation, of bone, 2500, 2502
Remodeling, 531
  of mandible, 2502, 2504
  of maxilla, 2508–2509, *2508*
Remodeling growth, 2499
Remodeling process, 4434
Rendu-Osler-Weber syndrome, 3227, 3238–3239, *3238*
Repair. *See also specific types of repair.*
  choice of method of, 46–48
  timing of, 45–46
Replantation
  centers for, 4356–4357
  definition of, 54, 4356, *4356*
  for arm amputations, 4376–4377
  for degloving or ring avulsion, 4374–4375
  of forearm, 4375–4376, *4375, 4376*
  of hand, 4289, 4375–4376, *4375, 4376*
  of lower extremity, 4068–4069
    indications for, 4070–4071
    ischemia time and, 4069
    nature of amputation injury and, 4070
    operative technique for, 4071, 4073
    postoperative management for, 4073
    replacement of lost tissue in, 4070
    salvage technique for, 4071, *4072*
    surgical problems in, 4069
    zone of injury in, 4069–4070
  postoperative care for, 4377
  psychosocial aspects of, 132–134
  secondary procedures for, 4377–4378
  techniques of, *4362*
  with absent venous drainage, 4374
Research, in plastic surgery, 19

Short face deformity, 1384, *1385–1388*, 1386–1387
Shoulder, cutaneous arteries of, 359, *360*
Shoulder cable powered active prostheses, 4394–4395, *4395*
Shoulder flap, for neck resurfacing, 2197, *2198–2199*
Shoulder-hand syndrome, *4893*, 4893–4894
Sialadenitis, 3178
Sialadenoma papilliferum, 3299
Side cross finger flap
  for coverage of fingertip amputations, 4490, *4491–4493*, 4492–4493
  for dorsal digital defects, *4495*, 4496
Silastic epidermis, 805
Silastic wrap, 679
Silicone, for alloplastic implants, 708–709, 708*t*, *710*
Silicone sling, for eyelid paralysis, 2310, *2311*
Silk sutures, for alloplastic implants, 719*t*, 719–720
Silvadene, 802, 803*t*, 803–804
Silver nitrate, 803, 803*t*
Silver sulfadiazine, 802, 803*t*, 803–804
Simianism, 1347, *1348–1351*, 1351
Simonart's band, 2557, 2593, *2593, 2594*
Sjögren's syndrome, 3282
Skeletal distortions, secondary to hemangiomas, 3210
Skeletal hypertrophy, in lymphatic malformations, 3243, *3244*
Skeletal maxillary protrusion, 1333, *1335*
Skeletal muscle
  blood supply to, 550
  fibers of, 546–547, *547*
  grafting of, 547, 551–555, *552, 554*
  injury to, 551
  innervation of, 547–549, *547, 548*
  microneurovascular transfers, 555–556, *556*
  tenotomy and, 547–548
Skeletal osteotomy, 1233, *1237, 1248, 1370*
Skeletal system, complication of, from electrical injuries, 828–829
Skeletal tissues, development of 2487–2488, *2487, 2489, 2491*
Skin
  aging process of, 44–45, 2360–2361
    histology of, 749–751, *750, 751,* 2362, 2362*t*
  anatomy of
    in foot vs. in hand, 5156, 5159, *5156–5159*
    skin grafts and, 221–224, *222*
  biologic functions of, 207–208
  blanching of, 214
  blood supply of, regional patterns of, 286, *287,* 288
  circulation of, 335, *336–344,* 344
  collagen fiber structure in, 208, *208, 209,* 210
  color and texture matching of, 46
  color of
    after cold injury, 858
    as index of flap perfusion, 319*t,* 320
  condition of, after chemical peeling, 770–771
  conductance of, for diagnosis of reflex sympathetic dystrophy, 4903
  crease lines in, 213
  cutaneous receptors in, 4859–4860, *4860*
  depigmentation of, after chemical peeling, 769
  disorders of. *See specific disorders.*
  extensibility of, 215
    cleavage lines and, 218–220, *219*
  functions of, 221
  mechanical studies of, *212*
  microcirculation of, 308–309, *309*

Skin *(Continued)*
  nonliving, storage of, 247
  of scalp, 1516, 1538
  physical properties of, 210
    directional variations in, 215–220, *216–219*
  problems of
    from amputation, 4332
    in rheumatoid arthritis, 4704
  stress-strain curve of, 210, *210*
  stretching or expansion of, 214
  striae formation in, 214
  structural studies of, *211*
  sun-damaged, histology of, 749–751, *750, 751*
  tattoos of, 3608–3610, *3609*
  tension properties of, 213–214
  thickness of, 224
  types of, 45
  venous drainage of, 353, 355, *354, 355*
  viscoelastic properties of, 210, 213, *213*
Skin closure, Steri-tape technique of, 49, *49*
Skin flap, 2348. *See also specific types of flaps.*
  alteration of rheology and, 317
  arterial cutaneous, *292,* 292–295, *293, 294*
  axes of, 374–375, *375*
  classification of
    by blood supply, 277–278, *278*
    by composition, *278,* 278–279
    by method of movement, 276–277, 277*t*
  dimensions of, *375,* 375–376
  drainage of lymphedema through, 4113, *4114*
  expanded, for neck, after burn injury, 2197, 2200
  expansion of, for cheek resurfacing, 2174–2178
  fasciocutaneous types of, 295–299, *296, 297, 298*
  folded, for nasal lining restoration, 1979, *1980*
  for abdominal wall reconstruction, 3765–3766, *3766, 3767*
  for cervical contractures, complete, 2068, *2069–2075,* 2073–2074, 2076
  for cheek reconstruction, 2049–2050, *2050, 2051*
    in zone 2, 2042–2043, *2044–2048,* 2045–2048
  for chest wall reconstruction, 3683, *3685, 3686, 3687,* 3688
  for correction of Cupid's bow, 2648, *2648*
  for lymphedema therapy, 4111
  for nasal reconstruction
    historical perspective on, 1932–1934
    local nasal flaps, 1934–1936, *1935–1940,* 1940
    nasolabial cheek flaps, 1940, *1941–1949,* 1943
  free, for nasal reconstruction, 1971, 1974, *1974*
  hypervascular planes of, 377
  hypovascular planes of, 377
  Limberg flap, modified, for cheek reconstruction, 2038–2040, *2039–2043,* 2042
  local vs. distant, 275, 277
  myocutaneous, *299,* 299–301, *300, 301*
  nasal turn-in, for nasal lining restoration, 1979, *1980*
  pathophysiologic changes in, 309–313, *310, 311, 312, 313*
    anatomic, 310, *310*
    hemodynamic, 311–312, *311, 312*
    metabolic, 312–313, *313*
  perfusion, monitoring of, 318–323, 319*t*
  pharmacologic studies of, 314–318
    increasing tolerance to ischemia and, 317–318
  radial innervated dorsal type, for soft tissue injuries of thumb, 5100, *5102*
  random cutaneous, *288–291,* 288–292